McCRACKEN'S

Removable partial prosthodontics

McCRACKEN'S

Removable partial prosthodontics

DAVIS HENDERSON, B.S., D.D.S., F.A.C.D.

Professor and Chairman, Division of Removable Partial Prosthodontics,
University of Florida College of Dentistry, Gainesville, Florida;
formerly Chairman, Department of Prosthodontics,
University of Kentucky College of Dentistry, Lexington, Kentucky;
Fellow, Academy of Denture Prosthetics; Member, American Prosthodontic Society;
Member, Southeastern Academy of Prosthodontics;
Member, American College of Prosthodontists; Charter Member, Carl O. Boucher
Prosthodontic Conference; Member, International Association for Dental Research;
Diplomate, American Board of Prosthodontics

VICTOR L. STEFFEL, D.D.S., F.A.C.D., F.A.D.P.

Professor Emeritus and former Chairman, Division of Removable Partial Prosthodontics,
The Ohio State University College of Dentistry, Columbus, Ohio;
Past President: The Ohio Dental Association, Academy of Denture Prosthetics,
American Prosthodontic Society; and the Federation of Prosthodontic Organizations;
Executive Director-Treasurer, The American Prosthodontic Society;
Honorary Sponsoring Fellow, Carl O. Boucher Prosthodontic Conference;
Recipient, The Ohio State University Centennial Achievement Award (1970);
Past Supreme Grand Master, Psi Omega Fraternity

FOURTH EDITION

with 585 illustrations

The C. V. Mosby Company   ST. LOUIS   1973

Dedicated to the memory of

Dr. William Lionel McCracken

educator, author, researcher

Preface to fourth edition

In keeping with the noble educational objectives of the late Dr. William L. Mc-Cracken, this book as revised still has the original purpose of supplying the student—undergraduate, graduate, or postgraduate—with a better understanding of fundamental principles and procedures involved in removable partial prosthodontics. Additionally, with a comprehensive presentation of both clinical and dental laboratory aspects of practice, it should furnish dentists and dental technicians with the means of avoiding pitfalls as well as the solution to many problems when they do arise.

In the past, the dental profession has been remiss in recognizing and acknowledging the true treatment value of removable partial restorations. Frequently, dentists have not been comfortable in diagnosis, treatment planning, and surveying, and then designing and constructing such dentures. Possibly the dental schools have been delinquent in developing teaching methodologies that are better than conventional approaches in order to stimulate learning in less time so that a realistic objective can be fulfilled. Where a fixed partial denture is not feasible, a properly constructed removable partial denture can be a very effective vehicle of function over an indefinite period of time—protecting remaining supporting structures from destructive forces. It is our hope, therefore, that with a simplified classification, a common language of nomenclature, and text clarity, much confusion may be eliminated and, by a study of this book, an increase in knowledge may be readily obtained by those interested.

While all in this fourth edition is not new, with the recent active period in research, improved materials, and techniques, many progressive changes have been introduced. In places, refinements of previously advanced methods constitute the modernizing. However, inasmuch as learning is in constant change, a textbook likewise must be kept dynamic. It has very often been stated that, with a dearth of specialists in prosthodontics, if the need for removable partial denture service is to be satisfactorily met, it will of necessity come largely from the general practitioners. In this era, longevity further complicated the service problem.

In assembling the subject matter for this fourth edition, we thoroughly evaluated all the preceding considerations and wish to stress that successful removable partial dentures depend upon the dentist's knowledge and application of all the basic sciences. We contend further that this phase of mouth reconstruction involves application of a greater number of clinical disciplines and skills than any other restorative process. A thoughtful treatment plan involves not only a thorough diagnosis but also a consideration of bone, soft tissues, periodontal ligaments, occlusion of both natural and artificial teeth, crowns, fixed partial dentures, oral surgery, individual restorations, biomaterials, and biomechanics. We have tried to make this new edition as complete as possible in relation to all the above. Obviously, any one single book must be kept too limited in size to encompass every aspect of the subject; for example—behavioral patterns of patients.

In summary, in this fourth edition we have incorporated some practices that have proved relatively successful and rewarding during our years of experience; chapters have been rearranged in an orderly sequence of learning; the study, demonstration, and interpretation of biomechanics (abutment engineering) as relating to denture components, guide planes, and abutments have been freshly covered; terminology has been standardized throughout to hasten (hopefully) the eventuality of unanimity in the usage of terms; sound fundamentals (which do not change) have been meticulously retained, while materials and procedures which require a constant re-evaluation have been updated; new up-to-

date illustrations have entirely replaced unclear and obsolete ones; the bibliography has been revised—obsolescent references having been deleted and contemporary ones added; a comprehensive coverage of the surveying procedure and a chapter for guidance of the dentist in writing work authorizations have been rearranged in a more convenient order of succession; and since such varied aspects of removable partial denture service as relining and repairing, cleft palate, and maxillofacial restorations are merely related to the main theme, we have relocated such subject matter near the end of the text.

Grateful acknowledgment is expressed to Doctors Sharry, Bohannon, Carman, Costich, and White for their continuing contributions to this fourth edition. We are truly appreciative of the constructive criticism and compliments of the reviewers of the third edition. Their counsel and suggestions are embodied in this textbook to the greatest extent possible.

Davis Henderson
Victor L. Steffel

Preface to first edition

Although I welcomed the invitation to author a textbook on the subject of partial denture construction, I realized from the outset that such a book would follow closely in the wake of several excellent textbooks on this subject. I therefore approached the task with a sense of great responsibility. However, I would not have accepted the challenge had I not felt sincerely that I could add something to what had already been written and thus produce a text in this field which is sorely needed and which provides the dental student, the dental practitioner, and the dental laboratory technician with the information necessary to produce a partial denture that is in itself a definitive restorative entity. It is my sincere hope that this textbook will be used not only by teachers of prosthetic dentistry but also by practicing dentists and dental technicians, and that in this book the dentist and dental technician may find a common meeting ground for better solution of the problems associated with the partially edentulous patient.

I am deeply grateful for the opportunities that I have had to combine private practice with teaching and for the knowledge that has evolved from this experience. Although I have attempted to present various philosophies and techniques in order that the reader may select that which to him seems most applicable, it is inevitable that certain preferences will be obvious. These are based upon convictions evolved through experience both in private practice and in the teaching of clinical prosthodontics. It is only logical, then, that I should therefore state my own personal beliefs, which are as follows:

1. I believe that the practice of prosthetic dentistry must forever remain in the hands of the dentist and that he must therefore be totally competent to render this service. In the fabrication of a partial denture restoration, the dentist must be competent to render a comprehensive diagnosis of the partially edentulous mouth and, utilizing all of the mechanical aids necessary, plan every detail of treatment. He must either personally accomplish whatever mouth preparations are necessary or delegate to his colleagues such specialized services as surgical, periodontal, and endodontic treatment. In any case, primary responsibility for adequate mouth preparations remains his alone. He must undertake whatever impression procedures are necessary and must be primarily responsible for the accuracy of any casts of the mouth upon which work is to be fabricated. He must provide the laboratory technician with an adequate prescription in the form of diagrams and written instructions and with a master cast which has been completely surveyed with a specific design outlined upon it. He must be solely responsible for the accuracy and adequacy of any jaw relation records and must specify all materials and, in many instances, the exact

method by which occlusion is to be established on the finished restoration. Finally, he must be competent to judge the excellence of the finished restoration or recognize its inadequacies and must assume the responsibility for demanding a degree of excellence from the technician that will continually raise rather than lower the standards of dental laboratory service.

2. I believe that the dental laboratory technician has a responsibility to his profession to demand a quality of leadership from the dentist which he can respect and follow without question. The responsibility for providing adequate prosthetic dentistry service to the patient must be shared by both dentist and technician, and each has not only a right to expect that the other do his part competently but also an obligation to demand a quality of service from the other that will not jeopardize the finished product. The technician therefore would do dentistry a great service if he would reject inadequate material from the dentist and respectfully suggest whatever improvements are necessary for him to produce an acceptable piece of work. As long as the technician accepts inadequate material from the dentist and the dentist is willing to place an inadequate product in the patient's mouth, the quality of removable prosthetic appliances will continue to be, as it all too frequently is, a far poorer service than the dentist and technician together are capable of rendering.

I believe also that dental laboratories should always be willing to adopt newer techniques and philosophies developed by the dental profession and being taught to dental graduates. Too often the commercial dental laboratory insists upon using stereotyped techniques that suit its production methods and actively attempts to discourage the recent graduate from putting into practice modern methods and techniques that were painstakingly taught to him in dental school by instructors whose knowledge of the subject far exceeds that of the laboratory technician who depreciates it.

3. I believe that any free-end partial denture must have the best possible support from the underlying edentulous ridge and that the design of the abutment retainers must apply a minimum of torque to the adjacent abutment teeth. I believe that some kind of secondary impression is necessary to obtain adequate support for the denture base, both through tissue placement and from the broadest possible coverage compatible with biologic requirements and limitations.

4. I believe in the functional, or dynamic, registration of occlusal relationships rather than in relying upon intraoral adjustment of an established centric occlusion or upon the ability of an instrument to simulate articulatory movements. I believe that the occlusion on a partial denture, be it fixed or removable, should be made to harmonize with the existing adjusted natural occlusion, and that this can best be accomplished by the registration of functional occlusal paths. For this to be done adequately, occlusion on the partial denture must be established upon either the final denture base(s) or upon an accurate substitute for the final base(s). The practice of attempting to submit jaw relation records to the technician prior to the fabrication of the denture framework is therefore, with few exceptions, strongly condemned.

5. I believe that a partial denture, when properly designed, carefully made, and serviced when needed, can be an entirely satisfactory restoration and can serve as a means of preserving remaining oral structures as well as restoring missing dentition. Unless a partial denture is made with adequate abutment support, with optimal base support, and with harmonious and functional occlusion, it should be clear to all concerned that such a denture should be considered only a temporary, treatment, or interim denture rather than a restoration representative of the best that modern prosthetic dentistry has to offer.

W. L. McCracken

Contents

McCRACKEN'S

Removable partial prosthodontics

CHAPTER 1

Terminology

Prosthodontic terminology has been neglected until only recently, resulting in much confusion because of conflicting terms. As a result of the efforts of the Academy of Denture Prosthetics and its Nomenclature Committee, a *Glossary of Prosthodontic Terms* has been made available to the profession.* The efforts of the Nomenclature Committee are continuing in an endeavor to provide an authentic and acceptable glossary of prosthodontic terminology.

The Bureau of Library and Indexing of the American Dental Association has published a *Vocabulary of Dentistry and Oral Science.*† This was the first dental vocabulary to be published since 1936 and was the result of three workshops sponsored by the American Dental Association ("Concepts of Occlusion" in 1952, "Supplementing the Dental Dictionary" in 1953, and "Troublesome Terms" in 1954) and of Denton's efforts toward compiling a comprehensive review of dental nomenclature.

More recently, a glossary of accepted terms in all disciplines of dentistry, *Current Clinical Dental Terminology,** has been published. This glossary is an important step toward efficient spoken and written communication in dentistry.

Many conflicting or indefinite terms in common usage in prosthodontics require definition and clarification. Many of these are used synonymously; others are used incorrectly. Whereas the following is not meant to be a complete glossary of partial denture terminology, some definitions will be given, based upon available reference material.

A *prosthesis* is the replacement of an absent part of the human body by some artificial part such as an eye, a leg, or a denture. *Prosthetics,* then, is the art or science of supplying missing parts of the human body.

When applied to dentistry, the term *prosthetics* becomes *prosthodontics* and denotes the branch of dental art or science that treats specifically with the replacements of missing dental and oral tissues. The term *prosthodontics* is somewhat preferable to the term *prosthetic dentistry*. The latter is defined by the American Dental Association as "the science or art of pro-

---

*This glossary first appeared in the March, 1956, issue of The Journal of Prosthetic Dentistry (published by The C. V. Mosby Company, St. Louis, Mo.). The latest reprint, published in 1968, may be obtained from Dr. W. Les Warburton, Secretary, Educational and Research Foundation of Prosthodontics, 807 Medical Arts Bldg., Salt Lake City, Utah 84111.

†Denton, G. B.: The vocabulary of dentistry and oral science, Chicago, 1958, American Dental Association.

---

*Boucher, C. O., editor: Current clinical dental terminology; a glossary of accepted terms in all disciplines of dentistry, St. Louis, 1963, The C. V. Mosby Co.

viding suitable substitutes for the coronal portions of teeth, or for one or more lost or missing natural teeth and their associated parts, in order that impaired function, appearance, comfort, and health of the patient may be restored." This definition is broad and may be applied to all restorative dentistry.

The replacement of missing teeth in a partially edentulous arch may be accomplished by a fixed, or cemented, prosthesis or by a removable prosthesis. The former may be in two pieces, with a locking joint between, or all in one piece and is not designed to be removed by the patient. This type of restoration is a *fixed partial denture*. On the other hand, a *removable partial denture* is designed so that it can be removed conveniently from the mouth and replaced by the patient.

A *complete denture prosthesis* is entirely supported by the tissues (mucous membrane, connective tissues, and underlying bone) to which it is attached. A *removable partial denture* either may be entirely tooth supported or may derive its support from both the teeth and the tissues of the residual ridge. The denture base of a tooth-borne removable partial denture derives its support from abutment teeth at each end of the edentulous area. The tissue that it covers is not used for support. A tooth-tissue–supported removable partial denture has at least one denture base that extends anteriorly or posteriorly, terminating in a denture base portion that is not tooth supported. Such a base extending posteriorly on a removable partial denture qualifies the restoration as a *distal extension denture*.

Sufficient points of difference exist between the tooth-supported and the tooth-tissue–supported removable restorations to justify a distinction between them. Principles of design and techniques employed in construction may be completely dissimilar. The points of difference are as follows:

1. Manner in which the prosthesis is supported

2. Impression methods required for each
3. Types of direct retainers best suited for each
4. Denture base material best suited for each
5. Need for indirect retention

A distinction between these two types of removable restorations is adequately made by an acceptable classification of removable partial dentures. It seems cumbersome to refer to the tooth-supported removable restoration as a removable bridge to distinguish it from a tooth-tissue–supported removable partial denture.

The term *appliance* is correctly applied only to a device worn by the patient in the course of treatment, such as splints, orthodontic appliances, and space maintainers. A denture, an obturator, a fixed partial denture, or a crown is properly called a *prosthesis*. The terms *prosthesis, restoration,* and *denture* generally will be used synonymously in this book to avoid tiresome repetition of the single word *prosthesis*.

An *interim denture* is a dental prosthesis to be used for a short interval of time for reasons of esthetics, mastication, occlusal support, and convenience or for conditioning of the patient to the acceptance of an artificial substitute for missing natural teeth until more definite prosthetic dental treatment can be provided.

A *transitional denture* is a removable partial denture that serves as a temporary prosthesis to which teeth will be added as more teeth are lost and that will be replaced after postextraction tissue changes have occurred. A transitional denture may become an interim denture when all the teeth have been removed from the dental arch.

A *treatment denture* is a dental prosthesis used for treating or conditioning the tissues that are called upon to support and retain a denture base.

Use of the term *acrylic* as a noun will be avoided. Instead, it will be used only as an adjective, such as *acrylic resin*. The word *plastic* may be used either as an adjective or a noun; in the latter sense it refers to any of various substances that harden and retain their shape after being molded. The term *resin* will be used as a broad term for substances named according to their chemical composition, physical structure, and means for activation or curing, such as *acrylic resin.*

The term *denture base* will be used to designate the part of a denture, either of metal or of a resinous material, that supports the supplied teeth and/or receives support either from the abutment teeth or the residual ridge, or both. The word saddle is considered objectionable terminology when used to designate a denture base.

The tissues underlying the denture base will be mentioned as the *residual ridge* or *edentulous ridge,* referring to the residual alveolar bone with its soft tissue covering. The exact character of this soft tissue covering may vary, and it includes the mucous membrane and the underlying fibrous connective tissue.

Resurfacing of a denture base with new material to make it fit the underlying tissues more accurately will be spoken of as *relining. Rebasing* refers to a process that goes beyond relining and involves the refitting of a denture by the replacement of the denture base with new material without changing the occlusal relations of the teeth.

Perhaps no other terms in prosthodontics have been associated with more controversy than have *centric relation, centric occlusion,* and *centric position.* All confusion could be terminated by acceptance of one definition of centric relation and one definition of centric occlusion and then using these respective positions as references for other horizontal locations of the mandible or other relationships of opposing teeth. The following definitions, which are given in the *Glossary of Prosthodontic Terms,* are selected as meaningful:

"*centric relation:* The most retruded relation of the mandible to the maxillae at a given degree of vertical opening."

"*centric occlusion:* The relation of opposing occlusal surfaces which provides the maximum planned contact and/or intercuspation."

"*centric position:* The position of the mandible in its most retruded relation to the maxillae."

For complete dentures, centric occlusion should be made to coincide with centric relation for that patient. In adjusting natural occlusion, the objective may be to establish harmony between centric relation and centric occlusion. On removable partial dentures, the objective is to make the artificial occlusion coincide and be in harmony with the remaining natural occlusion. Ideally, the natural occlusion first must have been adjusted to maximum contact at centric relation and be free of eccentric interference before establishing a similar occlusion on the partial denture.

In describing the various component parts of the partial denture, conflicting terminology must be recognized and the preferred terms defined. A *retainer* is defined as "any form of attachment applied directly to an abutment tooth used for the fixation of a prosthetic restoration."[*] Thus the attachment may be either intracoronal or extracoronal and may be used as a means of retaining either a removable or a fixed restoration. A solder joint also may be considered to be an attachment. The term *internal attachment* will be used in preference to precision attachment, frictional attachment, and other terms to describe any mechanical retaining device that depends upon frictional resistance between parallel walls of male and female (key and keyway) parts. Precision attachment is discarded because its usage implies that all other types of retainers are less precise in their design and fabrication.

Clasp will be used in conjunction with the words *retainer, arm,* or *assembly* whenever possible. The clasp assembly will con-

---

[*]From Academy of Denture Prosthetics, Nomenclature Committee: Glossary of prosthodontic terms, St. Louis, 1968, The C. V. Mosby Co.

sist of a *retentive clasp arm* and a *reciprocal* or *stabilizing clasp arm,* plus any minor connectors and occlusal rests from which they originate or with which they are associated. *Bar clasp arm* will be used in preference to Roach's name to designate this type of extracoronal retainer and is defined as a clasp arm that originates from the base or framework, traverses soft tissue, and approaches the tooth undercut area from a gingival direction. In contrast, the term *circumferential clasp arm* will be used to designate a clasp arm that originates above the height of contour, traverses a portion of the suprabulge portion of the tooth, and approaches the tooth undercut from an occlusal direction. Both types of clasp arms terminate in a retentive undercut lying gingival to the height of contour, and both provide retention by the resistance of metal to deformation rather than frictional resistance of parallel walls.

A *continuous bar retainer* is a component of the partial denture framework that augments the major connector(s) and lies on the lingual or facial surface of several teeth. It is most frequently used on the middle third of the lingual slope of lower anterior teeth. If connected to the lingual bar major connector with a thin, contoured apron, the major connector is then designated as a *linguoplate.*

Any thin, broad palatal coverage used as a major connector is called a *palatal major connector* or, if of lesser width, a *palatal bar.* A palatal major connector may be further described according to its anteroposterior location on the palatal surface, for example, an anterior palatal major connector or a posterior palatal bar. The term *anatomic replica* will be used to designate cast metal palatal major connectors that duplicate the topography of that portion of the patient's mouth. This is in keeping with a desire to use descriptive terminology whenever possible.

The term *rest* will be used to designate any component of the partial denture that is placed on an abutment tooth, preferably in a seat prepared to receive it, so that it

limits movement of the denture in a gingival direction. When a rest is placed on the occlusal surface of a posterior tooth, it is designated as an *occlusal rest.* If the rest occupies a position on the lingual surface of an anterior tooth, it is referred to as a *lingual rest.* A rest placed on the incisal edge of an anterior abutment tooth is called an *incisal rest.* All these rests function to prevent movement of the denture toward the soft tissues and to assist in providing occlusal support for the prosthesis.

An *abutment* is a tooth used for the support or anchorage of a fixed or removable prosthesis.

The term *height of contour* is defined as the line encircling a tooth at its greatest bulge or diameter with respect to a selected path of placement.

An *undercut,* when referring to an abutment is that portion of a tooth that lies between the height of contour and the gingivae; when referring to other oral structures an undercut means the contour or cross section of a residual ridge or dental arch that would prevent the placement of a denture.

Two or more parallel surfaces of abutment teeth so shaped as to direct a prosthesis during placement and removal are called *guiding planes.* Guiding planes are parallel axially; however, they may or may not be divergent facially.

The terms *canine* (tooth) and *premolar* (tooth) will be used to designate those teeth commonly called cuspid and bicuspid teeth. Denton gives the chief arguments for the use of the word *canine* as "(1) it is the term used in other sciences, and (2) other terms in standard usage can be understood only in relation to *canine* tooth; for example canine eminence, canine fossa, etc." For the use of *premolar* he gives the following arguments: "(1) the term bicuspid is not descriptive of all teeth in that class, and (2) the acceptance of premolar makes uniform the terminology of dentistry and comparative dental anatomy."

In describing an impression and resulting cast of the supporting form of the edentulous ridge, *functional impression* and *functional ridge form* will be used in the absence of a more descriptive terminology. These terms have become accepted as meaning the form of the edentulous ridge when it is supporting a denture base. It is artificially created by the use of an impression material that displaces those tissues that can be readily displaced and that would be incapable of rendering support to the denture base. Firm areas are not displaced due to the flow characteristics of the impression material. Thus the tissues are recorded more nearly in the form that they will assume when supporting a functional load. In contrast, the static form of the edentulous ridge, as often recorded in a soft impression material such as hydrocolloid, rubber-base material, or metallic oxide impression paste, is referred to as the *anatomic ridge form.* This is the surface form of the edentulous ridge when at rest or when not supporting a functional load.

Functional occlusal registration is sufficiently descriptive and is used to designate a dynamic registration of opposing dentition rather than the recording of a static relationship of one jaw to another. While centric position is found somewhere in a functional occlusal registration, eccentric positions are also recorded, and the created occlusion is made to harmonize with all gliding and chewing movements that the patient is capable of making.

The word *cast* may be used as a verb (to cast) or as an adjective (cast framework or cast metal base). It is used most frequently in this text as a noun to designate a positive reproduction of a maxillary or mandibular dental arch made from an impression of that arch. Such an objective is further designated according to the purpose for which it is made, such as *diagnostic cast, master cast,* or *investment cast.* An investment cast also may be referred to as a *refractory cast,* since it is compounded to withstand high temperatures without disintegrating and, incidentally, to perform certain functions relative to the burnout and expansion of the mold. A *refractory invest-*

ment is an investment material that can withstand the high temperatures of casting or soldering. Plaster of Paris or artificial stone also may be considered *investment* if it is used to invest any part of a dental restoration for processing it.

A *wax pattern* is converted to a *casting* by the elimination of the pattern by heat, leaving a mold into which the molten metal is thrown by centrifugal force or other means. *Casting* is therefore used most frequently as a noun, meaning "a metal object shaped by being poured into a mold to harden." It is used primarily to designate the cast metal framework of a partial denture but also may be used to describe a molded denture base, which is also actually cast into a mold.

Cast in dentistry should always imply that it is an accurate reproduction of the tissues being studied or upon which a restoration may be fabricated. Any cast that is admittedly inaccurate is unpardonable and unacceptable in modern dentistry because of the excellence of impression and cast materials available today.

The word *cast* is preferable to the term *model,* which should be used only to designate a reproduction for display or demonstration purposes. A model of a dental arch or any portion thereof may be made of durable and attractive material. It need not be an accurate reproduction but should be a reasonable facsimile of the original. It is frequently made of tooth-tissue–colored acrylic resin.

Mold is also incorrect when applied to a reproduction of a dental arch or a portion thereof. It is used to indicate either the cavity into which a casting is made or the shape of an artificial tooth.

Dental stones are used to make an artificial stone reproduction from an impression, and occasionally they are used as an investment or for mounting purposes. All dental stones are gypsum products. Use of the word *stone* in dentistry should be applied only to those gypsum materials that are used for their hardness, accuracy, and/or abrasion resistance.

Some controversy exists over the use of the terms *x-ray, radiograph,* and *roentgenogram* in dentistry. The American Academy of Oral Roentgenology has indicated its preference for the use of roentgenogram, at the same time admitting that it may leave much to be desired as descriptive terminology. Examination of several recent textbooks on dental subjects finds usage divided between all three terms. However, in deference to the terminology preferred by the American Academy of Oral Roentgenology, the terms *roentgenogram, roentgenographic survey,* and *roentgenographic interpretation* are used herein.

Stability is defined as the quality of a denture to be firm, steady constant, and not subject to change of position when forces are applied. Stability becomes more meaningful when thought of as a denture base to supporting bone relationship.

Retention is spoken of as that quality inherent in the denture that resists the force of gravity, the adhesiveness of foods, and the forces associated with opening the jaws. Retention, considered in terms of complete dentures, should be considered a denture base to soft tissue relationship. In removable partial prosthodontics we speak in terms of direct retention. *Direct retention* is the retention obtained in a removable partial denture by the use of attachments or direct retainers (clasps) that resist their removal from the abutment teeth.

Balanced occlusion is a term that describes the contact of opposing teeth. It is defined as the simultaneous contacting of upper and lower teeth on the right and left in the anterior and posterior occlusal areas in centric or any eccentric position.

Many other terms used in prosthetic dentistry might be defined in this chapter, but such an undertaking is worthy of the efforts of those who have recently directed their thoughts to that end. The Nomenclature Committee of the Academy of Denture Prosthetics is to be commended for their continuing efforts in compiling a current glossary that may be used for guidance in prosthodontic terminology.

Familiarity with accepted prosthodontic terminology should be acquired by the student dentist because once a vocabulary is established it is always difficult to change.

CHAPTER 2

The clasp-retained partial denture

The clasp-type partial denture, utilizing the extracoronal direct retainer, is probably used a hundred times more frequently than is the intracoronal, or internal attachment, partial denture (Fig. 2-1). Although the clasp partial denture has disadvantages, for reasons of economy and time involved, it will probably continue to be used because it is capable of providing physiologically sound treatment for the greatest number of patients needing partial denture restorations in keeping with their ability to pay for such treatment. Some of the possible disadvantages of a clasp partial denture are as follows:

1. Caries may develop beneath clasp components, especially if the abutments are not protected with cast restorations and if the patient fails to keep the prosthesis and the abutments clean.

2. Strain too often is placed on the abutment teeth by improper clasp designs.

3. Clasps are often unesthetic, particularly when placed on visible tooth surfaces.

Despite these disadvantages, the use of removable prostheses may be preferred whenever there are tooth-bounded edentulous spaces of greater magnitude than can be restored safely with fixed prostheses or when cross-arch stabilization and wider distribution of stress loading is desirable. The removable partial denture retained by internal attachments eliminates some of the disadvantages of clasps, but it has other disadvantages, one of which is too great a cost for a large percentage of patients needing partial dentures. *Fixed partial dentures should always be used whenever indicated.*

When the alignment of the abutment teeth is favorable, the clinical crown is of sufficient length, the pulp size is diminished by tooth maturity, and the economic status of the patient permits, an internal attachment prosthesis is unquestionably preferable for esthetic reasons. In most instances, if the internal attachment denture is designed properly, this is its only advantage, since abutment protection and bracing components should be used with both internal and external retainers. However, economics permitting, esthetics alone may justify the use of an internal attachment denture.

We do not believe in the routine use of hinges or other types of stressbreakers for distal extension partial dentures, much less in conjunction with internal attachments. It is not because they are ineffective but because they are more frequently misused and substituted for adequate support for the partial denture base. Particularly in the mandibular arch, in the absence of the cross-arch stabilization inherent in a rigid denture design, a stress-broken distal extension denture frequently subjects the edentulous ridge to excessive trauma from horizontal forces.

Because it must be used in conjunction with some form of stressbreaker, the locking or dovetail type internal attachment is not indicated when one or more distal extension edentulous spaces exist. A rigid de-

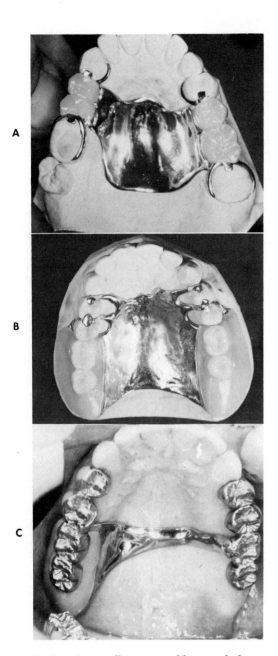

Fig. 2-1. A, Maxillary removable partial denture that is entirely supported by the abutment teeth adjacent to each edentulous area. **B,** Maxillary bilateral distal extension denture supported by both the natural teeth and the residual ridges. **C,** Maxillary unilateral distal extension denture supported by the natural teeth and residual ridge but utilizing internal attachments rather than extracoronal retainers. (**C,** Courtesy Dr. P. K. Thomas.)

sign is preferred, and therefore some type of extracoronal retainer must be used. Of these retainers, the clasp retainer is still the most frequently used, and it seems likely that its use will continue until a more widely acceptable retainer is devised.

FOUR PHASES OF PARTIAL DENTURE SERVICE

Partial denture service logically may be divided into four phases. The first phase is related to *patient education.* Included in the second phase are *treatment planning, design of the partial denture framework,* and *execution of mouth preparations.* The third phase is the *obtaining of adequate support for the distal extension denture base.* The fourth and final phase is the *establishment of harmonious occlusal relationships with the opposing and remaining natural teeth.*

Patient education

The term patient education is described in Current Clinical Dental Terminology as follows: "Effective communication between the dentist and/or his auxiliaries and the patient concerning dentistry and the principles of treatment and prevention. The procedure of increasing the patient's knowledge of the oral cavity and its care to the point where he can understand the reasons for proposed dental services."

Responsibility for the ultimate success of a removable partial denture service is shared by the dentist and the patient. It is folly to assume that a patient will have an understanding of the benefits of a removable partial denture service unless he is so informed. It is also unlikely that he will have the knowledge to avoid misuse of the restoration or be able to provide the required oral care and maintenance procedures to ensure the success of the partial denture unless he is adequately advised.

The finest biologically oriented removable partial denture is often doomed to failure if the patient relaxes proper oral hygiene habits or fails to respond to recall appointments. A partial denture created to fulfill a primary role of *preservation* will assume a much less desirable role with only token cooperation on the part of the patient.

Patient education should begin at the initial contact with the patient and continue throughout his treatment. This educational procedure is especially important when the treatment plan and prognosis are discussed with the patient. The limitations imposed upon the relative success of the partial denture through failure of the patient to accept his responsibility must be explained before definitive treatment is undertaken. A patient will not usually retain all the information presented in the oral educational instructions. For this reason he should be presented with written suggestions to reinforce the oral presentations.

Treatment planning and design

After a complete oral examination, including interpretation of roentgenograms, evaluation of the occlusal relations of the remaining natural teeth, and survey of diagnostic casts, a treatment plan is evolved that is based upon the support available for the partial denture. Distal extension situations in which no posterior abutments remain and in which extension bases must derive their principal support from the underlying residual ridge require an entirely different partial denture design than does one in which total abutment support is available. This is apparent from visual examination, but roentgenographic interpretation and the surveying of abutments must take into consideration the greater torque and tipping leverages of the distal extension partial denture.

Basically, the same principles apply to the unilateral distal extension denture as to the bilateral distal extension denture. On the other hand, entirely different principles of design apply to a prosthesis that is totally tooth supported. Each type must be designed according to the manner of support.

The dental cast *surveyor* is necessary in any dental office in which patients are being treated with removable partial dentures. There is no more reason to justify its omission from a dentist's armamentarium than to ignore the need for roentgenographic equipment or the mouth mirror and explorer or the periodontal probe used for diagnostic purposes.

Several moderately priced surveyors, which will adequately accomplish the diagnostic procedures necessary for designing the partial denture, are on the market. And yet, in many dental offices today, this most important phase of dental diagnosis is delegated to the commercial dental laboratory because of the absence of a single necessary piece of equipment or apathy on the part of the dentist who does include removable partial prosthodontics in his practice. This is a deplorable and degrading situation, which makes no more sense than relying upon the technician to interpret roentgenograms and to render a diagnosis therefrom.

After treatment planning, mouth preparations may be performed with a definite goal in mind. Through the aid of diagnostic casts upon which the tentative design of the partial denture has been outlined and the mouth changes have been indicated in colored pencil, occlusal adjustments, abutment restorations, and abutment modifications can be accomplished providing for adequate support and retention and a harmonious occlusion for the partial denture.

Selected proximal tooth surfaces should be made parallel to provide guiding planes during placement and removal of the prosthesis. Occlusal rest seats that will direct occlusal forces along the long axis of the supporting teeth as nearly as possible should be established so that neither the tooth nor the denture will be displaced under occlusal loading. This dictates that the floor of the rest preparation be made to incline toward the center of the tooth and be spoon shaped, with the marginal ridge lowered to permit sufficient bulk without occlusal interference.

Retentive areas must be identified or

created, which will provide, as far as is feasible, for relatively equal and uniform retention on all abutment teeth, sufficient only to resist reasonable dislodging forces. *Reciprocal tooth surfaces upon which bracing clasp arms may be placed also must be identified or created.*

After mouth preparations are believed completed, an impression should be made in irreversible hydrocolloid and a cast poured in quick-setting stone. This cast can then be surveyed, with the patient still present, to ascertain whether the planned abutment contours have been accomplished or if additional recontouring is necessary. When mouth preparations have been completed, the impression for the master cast should be made and the cast poured immediately. The master cast must then be surveyed so that the design of the denture framework can be drawn upon it.

The final design of the denture framework should be outlined in pencil on the master cast, including the location of clasp arms in relation to the height of contour of the abutment teeth. It must be remembered that the location of clasp arms will be determined by the height of contour of the abutment teeth and that this exists for a given path of placement only; hence, proximal guiding planes and accurate blockout of proximal tooth surfaces are desirable. The position of the cast in relation to the surveyor must be recorded so that the technician may similarly place the cast on his surveyor to parallel the blockout material. This is easily done by scoring the base of the cast on three sides parallel to the path of placement or by tripoding the cast, but this must be done before the cast is removed from the surveyor.

It is necessary that a specific design be planned carefully in advance of mouth preparations and that these mouth preparations be carried out with care, as outlined on the diagnostic cast. Then specific and exact mouth preparations, including abutment restorations, will dictate the final form of the denture framework to be outlined on the master cast. This should be

drawn accurately onto the master cast after surveying so that there will be no doubt in the mind of the technician as to the exact design of the partial denture framework that he is to construct under guidance and supervision of a dentist.

Surveying the master cast, recording the relationship of the cast to the surveyor, and drawing a definite outline on the master cast are still not enough. It is difficult to draw all the details of the denture design upon the master cast. This should be done by labeling a colored pencil drawing upon a chart, which provides the technician with an outline of the partial denture framework and allows for instructions for the technician to follow in fabricating the denture. From this information it is possible for the technician to return a casting *that the dentist can superimpose* upon the outline as drawn on the master cast. From any lesser instructions the technician cannot be criticized for returning a more stereotyped partial denture design.

The dentist should be responsible for the design of the partial denture framework from the beginning to the finish; therefore, he is accountable for providing the technician with all the information needed. It is the responsibility of the technician to follow the written instructions given him by the dentist, but at the same time it is his prerogative to demand that these instructions be so informative that he can follow them without question.

Up to this point the treatment planning and preliminary design of the partial denture, the mouth preparation procedures, and the design of the denture framework have been accomplished by the dentist. Given thorough written instructions and the master cast upon which the dentist has drawn precisely the denture design, the technician then may fabricate the metal framework. The finished framework should be returned to the dentist so that he can evaluate its fit in the mouth and make any necessary occlusal adjustments on the framework.

When laboratory procedures are correctly executed, the framework should fit the master cast as planned. If the framework does not fit the mouth as planned, the dentist then can determine whether or not the error is due to a faulty impression on his part or an inaccurate master cast or a laboratory procedure. In any event adequate support for distal extension denture bases and the need for exact occlusal records make it necessary for the denture framework to be returned to the dentist for further records before completion of the restoration.

Adequate support for distal extension denture bases

The third of the four phases in the construction of a partial denture is adequate support for distal extension bases; therefore it does not apply to tooth-borne removable partial dentures. In the latter, support comes entirely from the abutment teeth through the use of rests.

For the distal extension partial denture, however, a base made to fit the anatomic ridge form does not provide adequate support under occlusal loading. Neither does it provide for maximum border extension nor accurate border detail. Therefore some type of correction impression is necessary. This may be accomplished by several means, all of which satisfy the requirements for support of any distal extension partial denture base.

Foremost is the requirement that certain soft tissues should be recorded or related under some loading so that the base may be made to fit the form of the ridge when under function, thereby providing support and assuring a maintenance of that support for the longest possible time. This requirement makes the distal extension partial denture unique in that the support from the tissues underlying the distal extension base must be made as equal to and compatible with the tooth support as is possible.

A complete denture is entirely tissue supported and the entire denture can move tissueward under function. In contrast, any movement of a partial denture base is inevitably a rotational movement, which may result in a loss of planned occlusal contacts and the application of uncontrolled forces to the abutment teeth. Therefore, every effort must be made to provide the best possible support for the distal extension base to minimize these forces.

No single impression technique can adequately record the anatomic form of the teeth and adjacent structures, and at the same time record the supporting form of the edentulous ridge. Therefore some method must be used that will record these tissues either in their supporting *form* or in a supporting *relationship* to the rest of the denture. This may be accomplished by one of several methods. One method is to reline the finished denture to provide adequate support. Another is to make a combination impression by finger loading a previously made anatomic impression at the time that it is related to the rest of the arch in an overall elastic impression. The latter method does not attempt to record a different surface form of the ridge but, instead, records the relationship of the ridge to the rigid parts of the denture in the same manner that it will be related to the rest of the arch when an occlusal load is applied. This method presumes that there will be some rebound of the tissues when an occlusal load is released.

A third method records the supporting form of the ridge with a secondary impression through the use of a mouth-temperature wax. Although there are minor variations in this technique, the one most commonly used is the making of the wax impression in a resin base attached to the denture framework. Anatomic ridges are cut away and discarded and that portion of the master cast repoured to conform to the new wax impression. This provides a corrected master cast upon which the denture base will be processed.

A fourth method of recording also involves the correction of the edentulous areas of the master cast. Special acrylic resin trays that cover the edentulous areas are attached to the mental framework. The trays are modified with modeling plastic placed on the tissue surface to stabilize the trays during border molding procedures. Then borders are molded in modeling plastic to obtain their correct contour and extension. The modeling plastic inside the tray is relieved in selected areas, and a secondary impression is made with a free-flowing impression material.

The *corrected master cast* impression procedures are usually related to the lower distal extension removable partial denture. The same procedures are applicable to the maxillary arch. However, adequate support for the distal extension maxillary denture base can be obtained by the use of a specially prepared individual acrylic resin impression tray that will record the teeth and basal surfaces in a one-piece impression. Larger support areas are available on the maxillary arch than exist on the lower edentulous ridge. It is important that those tissues in either arch that can better bear additional stress be made to do so. The tissues that are easily displaced cannot adequately support a denture base.

When a distal extension partial denture is to be made with a metal base, the master cast is usually corrected prior to making the denture casting. In this instance a resin tray technique is used, utilizing three or more occlusal stops to position the resin tray in the mouth and then back onto the master cast with the same degree of accuracy as the returning of a cast denture framework to the master cast. Thus, the master cast may be corrected prior to the making of the denture casting.

Establishment of occlusal relations

Whether or not the partial denture is tooth borne or has one or more distal extension bases, the recording of occlusal relationships comprises the final step in the construction of a partial denture. For the tooth-borne partial denture, ridge form is of little significance since it is not called upon to support the prosthesis. For the distal extension base, however, jaw relation records should be made only after obtaining the best possible support for the denture base. This necessitates the making of a base or bases that will provide the same support as the finished denture. Therefore, jaw relations cannot be recorded until after the denture framework has been returned to the dentist and a secondary impression has been made. Then either a new resin base or a corrected base must be used to record jaw relations.

Occlusal records for a removable partial denture may be made by several methods. The one most frequently used is the recording of static relationships with the opposing teeth. This method involves the use of a face-bow to correctly orient the maxillary cast to an adjustable articulator, a centric relation record to mount the lower cast, and protrusive and lateral eccentric records to adjust the articulator.

A second method, which is a graphic one, may be used to record centric jaw relation, but only where the opposing teeth and the remaining natural teeth are or can be made noninterfering. This is because a graphic record is usually made on one plane and does not allow for cuspal inclinations. Therefore, this method is generally used only where a removable partial denture is being made to an opposing complete denture.

A third method is the registration of functional paths. This records the opposing teeth in function and allows the occlusion on the partial denture to be made to conform to the cuspal influence of the remaining natural teeth. Such a wax record is converted to a stone template, and the denture teeth are modified to occlude with the template. When there are natural teeth remaining in contact, they will influence jaw movements by cuspal guidance rather than by condylar guidance as in the completely edentulous mouth. Registration of functional paths permits seating of the denture under a functional relationship with the opposing teeth and in cuspal harmony with the remaining natural teeth.

REASONS FOR FAILURE OF THE CLASP PARTIAL DENTURE

Experience with the clasp type partial denture made by methods herein outlined has proved its merit and justifies its continued use. The occasional objection to the visibility of retentive clasps can be minimized through the use of wrought-wire clasp arms. There are few contraindications for use of the clasp partial denture when properly designed. Practically all objections to this type of denture can be disposed of by pointing to deficiencies in its design and fabrication and to deficiencies related to patient education. These are as follows:

1. Inadequate diagnosis and treatment planning
2. Failure to use the surveyor during diagnosis and treatment planning
3. Inadequate mouth preparations, usually due to insufficient planning of the design of the partial denture
4. Failure to provide the technician with a specific design and the necessary information for executing this design
5. Failure of the technician to follow the design and instructions outlined (This is either due to disagreement as to the wisdom of the dentist's design or to resistance on the part of the dental laboratory to follow other than stereotyped designs, which may be mass produced. Either of these causes can and must be either eliminated or rectified through closer cooperation between the dentist and the technician.)
6. Incorrect use of clasp designs and improper use of cast clasps that have too little flexibility, too broad tooth coverage, and too little consideration for esthetics
7. Failure to provide for adequate tissue support for distal extension denture bases
8. Failure to provide for posterior occlusal forms that are in harmony with the cuspal relationships of the remaining natural teeth
9. Failure on the part of the dentist to carry out necessary patient education procedures
10. Failure on the part of the patient to accept responsibility in his treatment

A removable partial denture that is designed and fabricated so that it avoids the errors and deficiencies listed previously is one that proves the clasp type partial denture can be made functional, esthetically pleasing, and long lasting without damage to the supporting structures. The proof of the merit of this type of restoration lies in the knowledge that (1) it permits treatment for the largest number of patients as the need for this service increases with advances in other phases of dentistry and is made economically possible by the avoidance of elaborate mechanical devices and high laboratory costs; (2) it provides restorations that are comfortable and efficient over a long period of time, with adequate support and maintenance of occlusal contact relations; (3) it provides for healthy abutments, free of caries and periodontal disease; (4) it provides for the continued health of restored, healthy tissues of the basal seats; and (5) it makes possible a partial denture service that is definitive and not merely an interim treatment.

Removable partial dentures thus made contribute to a concept of prosthetic dentistry that has as its goal the preservation of remaining oral structures, the restoration of partially edentulous mouths, and *an ultimate elimination of the need for complete dentures.*

CHAPTER 3

Classification of partially edentulous arches

Several methods of classification of partially edentulous arches have been proposed and are in use today. This has led to much confusion and disagreement concerning which method should be adopted and which method best classifies all possible combinations.

It has been estimated that there are over 65,000 possible combinations of teeth and edentulous spaces in a single arch. It is obvious that no single method of classification can be descriptive of any except the most basic types. Therefore, a basic classification should be sufficient. It is unfortunate that no single method has been universally adopted by the profession. This fact probably has done more to prevent a comprehensive approach to the principles of partial denture design than has any other single factor.

Although classifications are actually descriptive of the partially edentulous arches, the removable partial denture restoring a particular class arch is described as a denture of that class. For example, we speak of a Class III or Class I removable partial denture. Certainly this is acceptable and promotes an economy of words. It is simpler to say "a Class II partial denture" than to say "a partial denture restoring a Class II partially edentulous arch."

The most familiar classifications are those originally proposed by Kennedy, Cummer,

and Bailyn. Still others have been proposed by Beckett, Godfrey, Swenson, Friedman, Wilson, Skinner, Applegate, Avant, and more recently by Miller. It is evident that an attempt should be made to combine the best features of all classifications so that a universal classification can be adopted in the future.

Kennedy's method of classification is probably the most widely accepted classification of partially edentulous arches today. Any method that will satisfy the requirements of a classification is acceptable. In an attempt to simplify the problem and encourage more universal usage of a classification and in the interest of adequate communication and a comprehensive understanding of the principles of removable partial denture design, the Kennedy classification will be used in this textbook. The student is referred to the Selected References section for sources of information relative to other classifications.

REQUIREMENTS OF AN ACCEPTABLE METHOD OF CLASSIFICATION

The classification of a partially edentulous arch should satisfy the following requirements:

1. It should permit immediate visualization of the type of partially edentulous arch being considered.
2. It should permit immediate differenti-

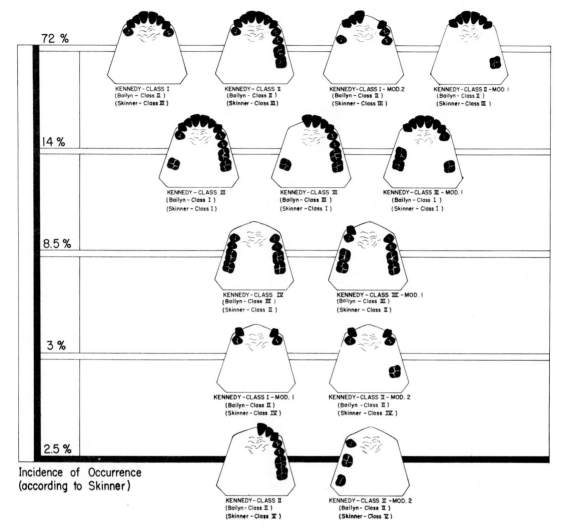

Fig. 3-1. Representative examples of partially edentulous arches classified by the Kennedy, Bailyn, and Skinner methods of classification.

ation between the tooth-borne and the tooth-tissue–supported removable partial denture.

3. It should serve as a guide to the type of design to be used.
4. It should be universally acceptable.

METHOD OF CLASSIFICATION

Kennedy's classification. The Kennedy method of classification was originally proposed by Dr. Edward Kennedy in 1925. Like the Bailyn classification and also the Skinner classification, it attempts to classify the partially edentulous arch in a manner that will suggest, if not govern, the partial denture design for a given situation (Fig. 3-1).

Kennedy divided all partially edentulous arches into four main types. Edentulous areas other than those determining the main types were designated as *modification spaces*. (See Fig. 3-2.)

The Kennedy classification is as follows:

Class I. Bilateral edentulous areas located posterior to the remaining natural teeth

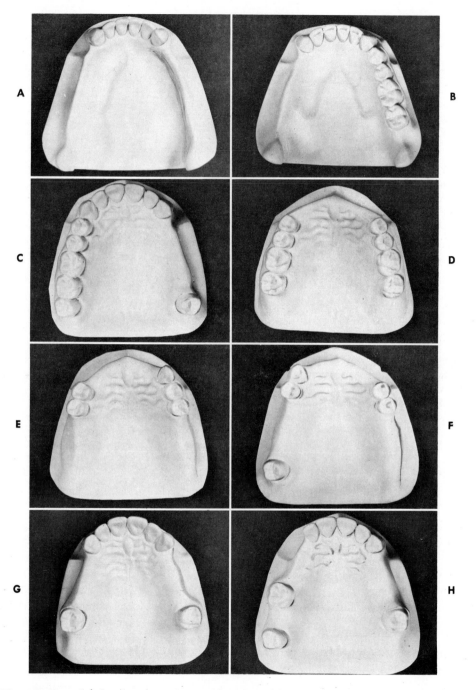

Fig. 3-2. Kennedy classification with examples of modifications. **A,** Class I; **B,** Class II; **C,** Class III; **D,** Class IV; **E,** Class I, modification 1; **F,** Class II, modification 2; **G,** Class III, modification 1; **H,** Class III, modification 2.

Class II. A unilateral edentulous area located posterior to the remaining natural teeth

Class III. A unilateral edentulous area with natural teeth remaining both anterior and posterior to it

Class IV. A single, but bilateral (crossing the midline), edentulous area located anterior to the remaining natural teeth

One of the principal advantages of the Kennedy method is that it permits immediate visualization of the partially edentulous arch. Those schooled in its use and in the principles of partial denture design that are based upon it may immediately compartmentalize their thinking concerning the basic partial denture design that will be used. It permits a logical approach to the problems of design. It makes possible the application of sound principles of partial denture design and is therefore the most logical method of classification.

Applegate's rules for applying the Kennedy classification. The Kennedy classification would be difficult to apply to every situation without certain rules for application. Applegate has provided the following eight rules governing the application of the Kennedy method:

Rule 1. Classification should follow rather than precede any extractions of teeth that might alter the original classification.

Rule 2. If the third molar is missing and not to be replaced, *it is not considered in the classification.*

Rule 3. If a third molar is present and is to be used as an abutment, *it is considered in the classification.*

Rule 4. If a second molar is missing and is not to be replaced, *it is not considered in the classification* (for example, if the opposing second molar is likewise missing and is not to be replaced).

Rule 5. The *most posterior edentulous area* (or areas) always determines the classification.

Rule 6. Edentulous areas other than those determining the classification are referred to as *modifications* and are designated by their number.

Rule 7. The *extent* of the modification is not considered, only the *number* of additional edentulous areas.

Rule 8. There can be no modification areas in Class IV arches. (Another edentulous area lying posterior to the "single bilateral area crossing the midline" would instead determine the classification.)

One suggested change in the order of the Kennedy classification is an attempt to correlate the Class I and Class II partially edentulous arches with the number of edentulous areas involved. Thus Class I would be a unilateral edentulous area posterior to the remaining teeth, and Class II would be a bilateral edentulous area posterior to the remaining teeth.

Whereas it is true that there is some confusion in the mind of the student initially as to why Class I should refer to two edentulous areas and Class II should refer to one, the principles of design make this position logical. Either by design or by accident, presumably the former, Kennedy placed the Class II unilateral distal extension type between the Class I bilateral distal extension type and the Class III tooth-bounded classification. Any change in this order would be illogical for the following reasons. The Class I partial denture is designed as a tooth- *and* tissue-supported denture. Three of the features necessary for the success of such a denture are adequate support for the distal extension bases, flexible direct retention, and some provision for indirect retention. The Class III partial denture is designed as a tooth-borne denture, without need generally, but not always, for indirect retention, without base support from the ridge tissues, and with direct retention, the only function of which is to retain the prosthesis. An entirely different design is therefore common to each class because of the difference in support.

However, the Class II partial denture

must embody features of both, especially when tooth-borne modifications are present. Having a tissue-supported extension base, it must be designed similarly to a Class I denture, but frequently there is a tooth-supported, or Class III, component elsewhere in the arch. Thus the Class II partial denture rightly falls between the Class I and the Class III because it embodies design features common to both. In keeping with the principle that design is based upon the classification, the application of such principles of design is simplified by retaining the original classification of Kennedy.

Another proposed alteration of the Kennedy method is to add the letters A and P to designate modifications. Thus an additional edentulous space is identified specifically as being anterior or posterior. It is doubtful that this change in the original classification adds little, if any, clarification to it. However, if it is used only to supplement the original classification rather than to replace it, there can be little objection to the use of the A and P designations. They cannot be applied to the Class IV arch, however, since Class IV can have no modifications.

CHAPTER 4

Component parts of the removable partial denture: major and minor connectors

COMPONENT PARTS OF THE REMOVABLE PARTIAL DENTURE

A typical removable partial denture will have the following components (Fig. 4-1).

1. Major connector
2. Minor connectors
3. Rests
4. Direct retainers
5. Reciprocal or bracing components
6. Indirect retainers (if the prosthesis has one or more distal extension bases)

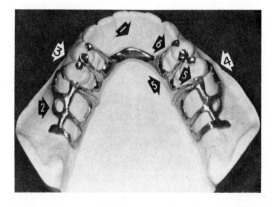

Fig. 4-1. Framework for mandibular removable partial denture with following components: 1, lingual bar major connector, 2, minor connector by which the acrylic resin denture bases will be attached, 3, occlusal rests, 4, direct retainer arm, which is part of the total clasp assembly, 5, reciprocal and bracing components of the clasp assembly, and 6, an indirect retainer consisting of a minor connector and an occlusal rest.

7. One or more bases, each supporting one to several replacement teeth

Major and minor connectors will now be considered separately as to their function, their location, and the acceptable designs, keeping in mind both biologic and mechanical considerations.

Major connector

A major connector is the unit of the partial denture that connects the parts of the prosthesis located on one side of the arch with those on the opposite side. It is that unit of the partial denture to which all other parts are directly or indirectly attached.

The major connector may be compared to the frame of an automobile, and in the construction of a removable partial denture it is just as essential. It might also be compared to the foundation of a building for the same reasons. It must be rigid so that stresses applied to any one portion of the denture may be effectively distributed over the entire supporting area, including abutment teeth and the supporting subjacent tissue areas. Being rigid, the major connector resists torque that would otherwise be transmitted to the abutment teeth as leverage.

It is only through the rigidity of the major connector that all other component parts of the partial denture may be effective. If they are attached to or originate from a flexible major connector, the effectiveness of these components is jeopardized to the detriment of the oral structures and the discomfort of the patient. Many removable partial dentures have failed to serve comfortably and effectively only because the major connector failed to provide rigid support to the rest of the prosthesis. Any removable partial denture design utilizing a nonrigid major connector is doomed to failure, either by causing discomfort to the patient or by subjecting the remaining structures to trauma. Trauma may be manifested by damage to the periodontal support of the abutment teeth, injury to the supporting ridge areas, or impingement of underlying tissues because of flexing of the major connector.

The major connector should be located in a favorable relation to moving tissues and at the same time should avoid impingement of gingival tissues. It also should be located so that areas of bony and tissue prominence are not encountered during placement and removal of the denture. Sufficient relief must be provided beneath a major connector to avoid settling into hard areas such as an inoperable mandibular torus, a palatal torus, or the palatal median suture line. Location and relief must also take into consideration possible impingement of gingival tissues.

Planned relief beneath the major connector, when indicated, avoids the need for later adjustments to provide relief of the prosthesis after tissue damage has occurred. Not only is this time-consuming but also frequently the connector is so weakened by grinding that flexibility and sometimes fracture result. It seems that tissues once impinged by the connector require more relief to avoid recurrence than would have been required originally. To accomplish this, the connector is seriously weakened by adjustment because the original bulk did not provide for the possibility of future reduction.

Margins of major connectors adjacent to gingival tissues should be located far

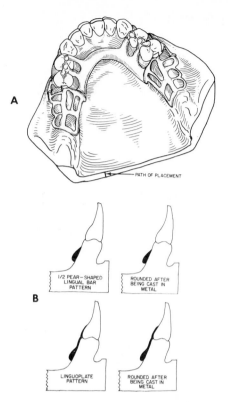

Fig. 4-2. **A,** Lingual bar major connector should be located at least 4 mm. below the gingival margins and more if possible. **B,** The inferior border of both a lingual bar and a linguoplate must be gently rounded after the framework has been cast. Such a configuration is infinitely more kind to the sensitive tissues in the floor of the mouth than is a sharp edge in this area.

enough from those tissues to avoid any possible impingement. The upper border of a lingual bar connector should be located at least 4 mm. below the gingival margin and more if possible (Fig. 4-2). The limiting factor is the height of the moving tissues in the floor of the mouth. Since the connector must have sufficient width and bulk to provide rigidity, a linguoplate must be used in lieu of a lingual bar in many instances.

In the maxillary arch, since there are no moving tissues in the palate as in the floor of the mouth, the borders of the major connector may be placed well away from gingival tissues. Impingement of gingival tissues is not justifiable because adequate sup-

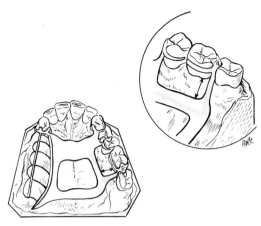

Fig. 4-3. Palatal major connector should be located at least 6 mm. away from gingival margins and parallel to their mean curvature. All adjoining minor connectors should cross gingival tissues abruptly and should join major connectors at nearly a right angle.

port for the connector is most always available elsewhere. Structurally, the tissues covering the palate are well suited for placement of the connector and have adequate deep blood supply. However, when soft tissue covering the median portion of the palate is less displaceable than the tissue covering the residual ridge, varying amounts of relief under the connectors must be provided to avoid impingement of tissue with its resulting sequelae. The gingival tissues, on the other hand, must have an unrestricted superficial blood supply to remain healthy. The borders of the palatal connector should be placed a minimum of 6 mm. away from gingival margins and should be located parallel to their mean curve. Minor connectors that must cross gingival tissues should do so abruptly, joining the major connector at nearly a right angle (Fig. 4-3). In this way the maximum freedom of gingival tissues is assured.

Except for a palatal torus or median suture line, palatal connectors ordinarily require no relief, nor is relief desirable. Intimate contact between the connector and the supporting tissues adds much to the retention and stability of the denture. Except for gingival areas, intimacy of contact

elsewhere in the palate is not of itself detrimental to the health of the tissues, if supported against settling by rests on abutment teeth.

An anterior palatal bar or the anterior border of a palatal plate also should be located as far posteriorly as possible to avoid interference with the tongue in the rugae area. It should be *flat* or *straplike* rather than half-oval and should be located so that its anterior border follows existing valleys between crests of the rugae (Fig. 4-4). The anterior border of such palatal major connectors will therefore be irregular in outline as it follows the valleys between the rugae. The tongue may then pass from one rugae prominence to another without encountering the border of the denture lying between. When a rugae crest must be crossed by the connector border, it should be done abruptly, avoiding the crest as much as possible.

A rule to be used throughout partial denture design is as follows: *Try to avoid adding any part of the denture framework to an already convex surface. Rather, try to utilize existing valleys and embrasures for the location of component parts of the framework. All components should be tapered where they join convex surfaces.*

Mandibular major connectors. The basic form of a mandibular major connector is the *half-pear-shaped lingual bar,* located above moving tissues but as far below the gingival tissues as possible. It is usually made of a reinforced, 6-gauge, half-pear-shaped wax or a similar plastic pattern.

The inferior border of a lingual mandibular major connector must be so located that the tissues in the floor of the mouth will not be impinged as they change elevations during normal activity, that is, swallowing, speech, licking the lips, and so forth. Yet at the same time, it seems logical to locate the inferior border of these connectors as far inferiorly as possible to avoid interference to the resting tongue and trapping of food substances when these are introduced into the mouth. Additionally, the more inferior a lingual bar can be

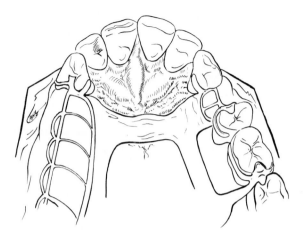

Fig. 4-4. Anterior palatal bar or the anterior margin of a palatal plate should be located as far posteriorly on the rugae as possible, with its anterior border following the natural valley between rugae crests.

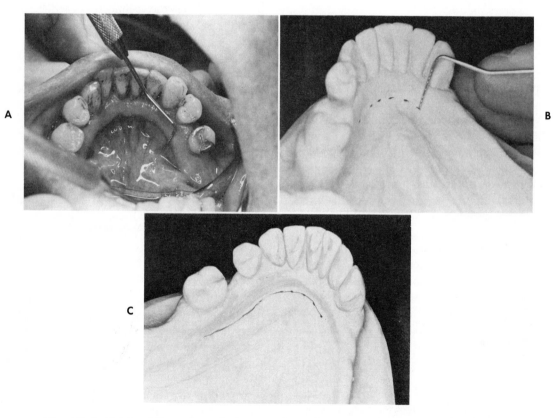

Fig. 4-5. A, Height of floor of mouth (tongue elevated) in relation to lingual gingival sulci measured with a periodontal probe. B, Recorded measurements are transferred to the diagnostic cast and then to the master cast after mouth preparations are completed. C, Line connecting marks is indicative of the location of the inferior border of a major connector. If periodontal surgery is performed, the line on the cast can be related to incisal edges of the teeth and the measurements recorded for subsequent use.

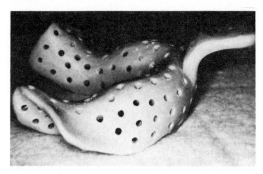

Fig. 4-6. Individualized acrylic resin impression tray. Lingual flanges should be so trimmed that the elevated position of the alveolar lingual sulcus can be accurately recorded in an impression material when the patient touches the vermilion border of the upper lip with the tip of the tongue. Tray was constructed as illustrated in Fig. 14-10.

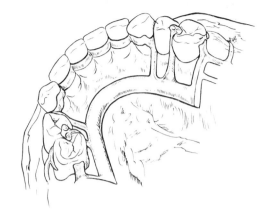

Fig. 4-7. Continuous bar retainer located above the cingula of the anterior teeth may be added for one reason or another, but only when it provides needed stabilization for the teeth or the denture.

located, the farther the superior border of the bar can be placed from the lingual gingival crevices of adjacent teeth, which in itself will avoid impinging the gingival tissue.

There are at least two clinically acceptable methods to determine the relative height of the floor of the mouth to locate the inferior border of a lingual mandibular major connector. The first method is to measure the height of the floor of the mouth with a periodontal probe in relation to the lingual gingival margins of adjacent teeth (Fig. 4-5). During these measurements the tip of the patient's tongue should be just lightly touching the vermilion border of the upper lip. Recording of these measurements permits their transfer to both diagnostic and master casts thus assuring a rather advantageous location of the inferior border of the major connector. The second method is to use an individualized impression tray having its lingual borders about 3 mm. short of the elevated floor of the mouth and then use an impression material that will permit the impression to be accurately molded as the patient licks his lips (Fig. 4-6). The inferior border of the planned major connector can then be located at the height of the lingual sulcus of the cast resulting from such an impression. Of the two methods,

we have found the measuring of the height of the floor of the mouth to be less variable and more clinically acceptable.

Fortunately, there are few situations in which extreme lingual inclination of the remaining lower premolar and incisor teeth prevents the use of a lingual bar connector. By conservative mouth preparations in the form of disking and by blockout, a lingual connector can almost always be used. Lingually inclined teeth may sometimes have to be reshaped by means of crowns. Although the use of a labial major connector may be necessary in rare instances, this should be avoided by resorting to necessary mouth preparations rather than accepting a condition that is otherwise correctable. The same applies to the use of a labial bar when a mandibular torus interferes with the placement of a lingual bar. Unless surgery is definitely contraindicated, interfering mandibular tori should be removed rather than a labial bar connector used.

A continuous bar retainer located above the cingula of the anterior teeth may be added to the lingual bar for one reason or another, but this should never be done without good reason (Fig. 4-7). When a linguoplate is otherwise indicated and the axial alignment of the anterior teeth is such that excessive blockout of interproximal

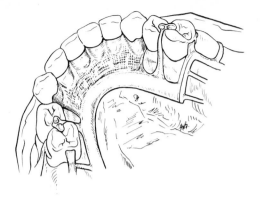

Fig. 4-8. Linguoplate is used when the space between bounding connectors is better filled in than left open. Such an apron does not serve to replace those connectors but, instead, is sometimes added to the fundamental denture design to make the major connector rigid.

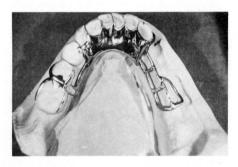

Fig. 4-9. View of a lower Class II design with a contoured linguoplate. The linguoplate is made as thin as possible and follows the contours of the teeth contacted.

undercuts must be made, a continuous bar retainer may be indicated. Additionally, when wide diastemas exist between the lower anterior teeth, a continuous bar retainer may be more esthetically acceptable than a linguoplate.

If the rectangular space bounded by the lingual bar, the continuous bar retainer, and the bounding minor connectors is filled in, a linguoplate results (Figs. 4-8 and 4-9). Again, this should only be done for good reason. The following rule applies: *No component of a partial denture should be added arbitrarily or conventionally. Each component should be added for a good reason and to serve a definite pur-*

pose. The reason for adding a component may be for stabilization against horizontal rotation, retention, support, patient comfort, the preservation of the health of the tissues, esthetics or any one of several other reasons, *but the dentist alone should be responsible for the choice of design used and he should have good reasons, both biologic and mechanical, for doing so.*

A linguoplate should be made as thin as is technically feasible and should be contoured to follow the contours of the teeth and the embrasures. The patient should be made as little aware of added bulk and altered contours in this area as is possible. The upper border should follow the natural curvature of the supracingular surface of the teeth and should not be located above the middle third of the lingual surface except to cover interproximal spaces to the contact points. All gingival crevices and deep embrasures must be blocked out parallel to the path of placement to avoid gingival irritation and any wedging effect between the teeth.

The linguoplate should be something that is added to, not something replacing, the conventional lingual bar. The half-pear shape of a lingual bar should still be present, with the greatest bulk and rigidity at the inferior border. The linguoplate does not in itself serve as an indirect retainer. When indirect retention is required, definite rests must be provided for this purpose. Both the linguoplate and the continuous bar retainer should ideally have a terminal rest at each end regardless of the need for indirect retention. But when indirect retainers are necessary, it is incidental that these rests may serve also as terminal rests for the linguoplate or continuous bar retainer. In such instances, it is the rests and not the linguoplate or continuous bar retainer that function as indirect retainers.

Indications for the use of a linguoplate. The indications for the use of a linguoplate may be listed as follows:

1. *For stabilizing periodontally weakened lower teeth.* Whereas not as effective as fixed splinting and not as effective

as when a labial bar is added, lingual splinting can be of definite value when used in conjunction with definite rests on sound adjacent teeth. A continuous bar retainer may be used to accomplish the same purpose, since it is actually the upper border of a linguoplate without the gingival apron. The continuous bar retainer accomplishes stabilization along with the other advantages of a linguoplate. It is frequently more objectionable to the patient's tongue and is certainly more of a food trap than is the contoured apron.

2. *In the Class I situations in which the residual ridges have undergone excessive vertical resorption.* Flat residual ridges offer little resistance to horizontal rotational tendencies of a denture. The remaining teeth must be depended upon to resist such rotation. A correctly designed linguoplate will utilize remaining teeth to resist horizontal rotations.

3. *When the lingual frenum is high or the space available for a lingual bar is slight.* In either instance, the superior border of a lingual bar would have to be placed objectionably close to gingival tissues. Irritation could be avoided only by generous relief, which would not only be annoying to the tongue but would also create an undesirable food trap. By using a linguoplate, the gingivae may be bridged and the superior border tapered to tooth contact, permitting its inferior border to be placed higher without tongue and gingival irritation and without compromise of rigidity.

4. *When the future replacement of one or more incisor teeth will be facilitated by the addition of retention loops to an existing linguoplate.* Mandibular incisors that are periodontally weak may thus be retained, with the knowledge that future additions to the partial denture are possible.

The same reasons for use of a linguoplate anteriorly apply also to its use elsewhere in the lower arch. If a lingual bar alone is to be used anteriorly, there is no reason for adding an apron elsewhere. However, when auxiliary splinting is used for stabilization

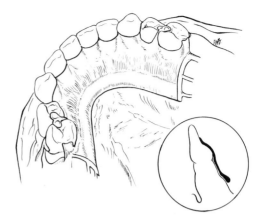

Fig. 4-10. Lingual apron may be extended to include all open spaces lying between the major connector and other component parts of the denture. This should never be done arbitrarily but only when open spaces would be less desirable. The linguoplate is supported anteriorly by lingual rest seats on the canines.

of the remaining teeth and/or for horizontal bracing of the prosthesis, small rectangular spaces sometimes remain. Tissue response to such small spaces is better when bridged with an apron than left open. Generally, this is done to avoid gingival irritation or the entrapment of food debris or to cover generously relieved areas that would be irritating to the tongue (Fig. 4-10).

Maxillary major connectors. Four basic types of maxillary major connectors will be considered: (1) single palatal bar, (2) U-shaped palatal connector, (3) combination anterior and posterior palatal bar-type connectors, and (4) palatal plate-type connectors.

Single palatal bar. This is perhaps the most widely used and yet the least logical of all palatal major connectors (Fig. 4-11). It is difficult to say whether this or the palatal horseshoe is the more objectionable of palatal connectors.

For a single palatal bar to have the necessary rigidity, it must have concentrated bulk. The latter may be avoided only by ignoring the need for rigidity, which is unfortunately too frequently done. For a single palatal bar to be rigid enough to be effec-

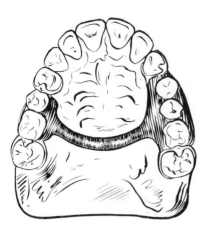

Fig. 4-11. Half-round palatal bar must be bulky to obtain the rigidity required for cross-arch distribution of stress. Its bulk may make it objectionable to the patient's tongue.

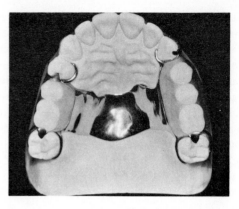

Fig. 4-12. Broad palatal major connector can be made rigid without resorting to bulk since its surface will lie in several planes. Note that the anterior portion of the major connector follows the "valley" of the rugae. The thinness and contour of this single palatal major connector is not uncomfortable to the patient's tongue and it does not interfere with speech.

tive, it must be centrally located between the two halves of the denture. This means that a single palatal bar always must be centrally located with concentrated bulk. Mechanically, this practice may be sound enough, but from the standpoint of patient comfort, it is highly objectionable.

A partial denture made with a single palatal bar is frequently either too flexible or too objectionable to the patients' tongue, or both. The decision to use a single palatal bar should be based on the size of the denture areas being connected and whether or not a single connector located between them would be rigid without objectionable bulk. Bilateral tooth-borne restorations of short spans may be effectively connected with a single, broad palatal connector, particularly when the edentulous areas are located posteriorly (Fig. 4-12). Such a connector can be made rigid, without objectional bulk and interference to the tongue, provided its surface lies in three planes.

For reasons of torque and leverage, a single palatal bar should not be used to connect anterior replacements with distal extension bases. To be rigid enough to resist torque and to provide adequate horizontal and vertical support as well, a single bar would have to be objectionably bulky. When placed anteriorly, this bulk becomes even more objectionable to the patient since it interferes with speech formation.

U-shaped palatal connector. From both the patient's standpoint and a mechanical standpoint, the palatal horseshoe is a poor connector. It should never be used arbitrarily. When a large inoperable palatal torus exists and occasionally when several anterior teeth are to be replaced, the U-shaped palatal connector may have to be used (Fig. 4-13). In most instances, however, other designs will serve more effectively.

To be rigid the U-shaped palatal connector must have bulk where the tongue needs the most freedom, which is in the rugae area. Without sufficient bulk the U-shaped design leads to increased flexibility and movement at the open ends. In distal extension dentures, when posterior tooth support is nonexistent, movement is particularly noticeable and is traumatic to the residual ridge. Many maxillary partial dentures have failed for no other reason except the flexibility of a U-shaped major connector (Fig. 4-14). No matter how well the extension base is supported or how harmonious the occlusion, when horizontal move-

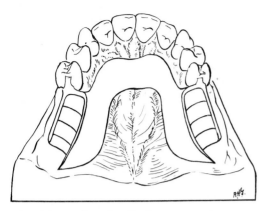

Fig. 4-13. U-shaped palatal connector is a poor major connector that should be used only when a large inoperable palatal torus prevents the use of palatal coverage or a combination anterior-posterior palatal bar-type designed framework.

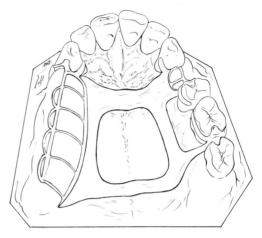

Fig. 4-15. Anterior and posterior palatal bar is the most rigid of palatal major connectors and, when properly designed, is neither objectionable to the patient nor harmful to the adjacent tissues.

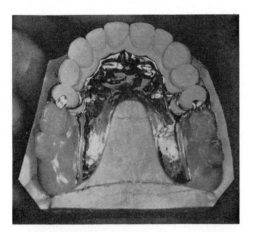

Fig. 4-14. Common partial denture design utilizing an objectionable palatal horseshoe major connector. Such a connector lacks necessary rigidity, places bulk where it is most objectionable to the patient, and impinges gingival tissues lingual to the remaining teeth, resulting in chronic inflammation. This denture failed primarily because of lack of the rigidity in the major connector, provision for indirect rentention, occlusal support, and consideration of gingival health in the location of the anterior border of the major connector.

ment under function is not resisted by a rigid major connector, the residual ridge suffers.

The wider the coverage of a U-shaped major connector, the more it resembles a palatal plate with its several advantages. But when used as a narrow horseshoe, the necessary rigidity is usually lacking. A U-shaped connector may be made rigid by providing multiple tooth support on definite tooth rests. A common error in the design of a U-shaped connector, however, is its proximity to, or actual contact with, gingival tissues. The principle that the borders of major connectors should either be placed on prepared rest seats or be located well away from gingival tissues has been given previously. The majority of U-shaped connectors fail to do either, with resulting gingival irritation and periodontal damage to the tissues adjacent to the remaining teeth.

Combination anterior and posterior palatal bar-type connectors. Structurally, the most rigid of palatal major connectors, the anterior and posterior palatal bar combination, may be used in almost any maxillary partial denture design (Figs. 4-15 to 4-17).

Whenever it is necessary for the palatal connector to make contact with the teeth for reasons of support, definite tooth support must be provided. Anterior tooth support is sometimes necessary, particularly when the denture includes anterior replacements. This is best accomplished by establishing shoulders or ledges on gold restorations using veneer crowns, three-quarter crowns, or pin-ledge restorations. However,

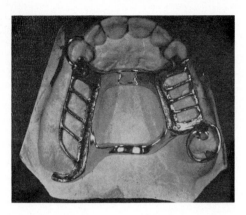

Fig. 4-16. Anterior and posterior palatal bar-type major connectors. The anterior bar is a flat strap located as far posteriorly as possible to avoid rugae coverage and tongue interference. The anterior border of this bar should be located just posterior to a rugae crest or in the valley between two crests. The posterior bar is half-oval (approximately 6-gauge) and is located as far posteriorly as possible yet entirely on the hard palate. It should be located at right angles to the midline rather than on a diagonal, even though its two wings must curve inward as it connects with other components of the denture framework. An 18-gauge wrought-wire retainer arm was used on the right canine because only a mesiolabial undercut existed for retentive purposes.

when the abutment teeth are sound, caries activity is low, and oral hygiene habits are favorable, rest seats in enamel may be used effectively. Multiple rest seats extending over several teeth may be considered to be just as effective as are lesser areas of greater depth. These should be located far enough above the gingival attachment to provide for bridging the gingival crevice with blockout. At the same time they should be low enough on the tooth to avoid unfavorable leverage, and low enough on maxillary incisors and canine teeth to avoid occlusal interference at the cingulum of the tooth. Experience with rest seats placed in sound enamel has been entirely satisfactory, all other factors being favorable.

Connector borders resting on unprepared tooth surfaces can lead only to slippage of the denture along both inclines, or orthodontic movement of the tooth, or both. In any case, settling into gingival tissues is inevitable. When the needed occlusal support ceases to exist, the health of the surrounding tissues is usually impaired. Similarly, interproximal projections resting upon the gingival third of the tooth and upon gingi-

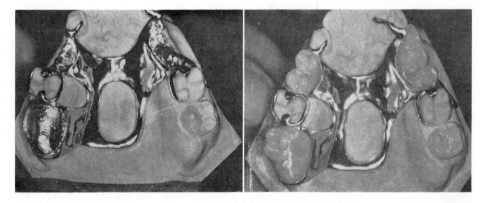

Fig. 4-17. Maxillary Class II, modification 2, partial denture with anterior and posterior palatal bar-type major connectors, before and after artificial teeth have been added. Except for a short distal extension base, this is essentially a tooth-borne restoration. Since a lateral incisor was necessarily used as an abutment on one side, double lingual rests were used on enamel ledges prepared on both the central and lateral incisors. Artificial teeth that would be visible anteriorly are abutted to the ridge to avoid any visible display of the denture base material. Note the posterior location of the half-oval posterior bar crossing the midline at a right angle rather than on a diagonal.

val tissues that are structurally unable to render support can only cause impingement to the detriment of the health of those tissues.

A cardinal rule, then, for the location of the major connector in relation to the remaining teeth and their surrounding gingivae is this: *Either support the connector by definite rests on the teeth contacted, bridging the gingivae with adequate relief, or locate the connector far enough away from the gingivae to avoid any possible restriction of blood supply and entrapment of food debris.* All gingival crossings should be abrupt and at right angles to the major connector, and these should bridge the gingivae with adequate relief.

The major connector must be contoured so that it does not present sharp margins to the tongue and cause irritation or annoyance by its angular form. The superior border of a lingual bar connector should be tapered to the tissues above, with its greatest bulk at the lower border. This results in a contour that is known as a half-pear shape, being flat on the tissue side, tapered superiorly, and having the greatest bulk in the inferior third. Lingual bar patterns, both wax and plastic, are made in this conventional shape. However, the inferior border of the lingual bar should be slightly rounded when the framework is polished. A rounded border will not impinge on the lingual tissue when the denture bases rotate inferiorly under occlusal loads. Frequently, additional bulk is necessary to provide rigidity, particularly when the bar is long or an alloy of lesser rigidity is used. This is accomplished by underlying the ready-made form with a sheet of 24-gauge casting wax rather than altering the original half-pear shape.

Sharp, angular form of any portion of a palatal connector should be avoided, and all borders should be tapered slightly toward the tissues. A posterior palatal bar should be half-oval in shape and located as far posteriorly as possible to avoid interference with the tongue. A posterior bar or the posterior border of any palatal connec-

tor should never be placed on moving tissues and should be located on the hard palate anterior to the line of flexure formed by the junction of the hard and soft palates. The only condition preventing its use is when there is an inoperable maxillary torus extending posteriorly to the soft palate, which prevents the use of a posterior bar. In this situation, a U-shaped major connector must be used.

The strength of this major connector design lies in the fact that the half-oval posterior bar and the flat anterior bar are joined together by longitudinal connectors on either side, forming a square or rectangular frame. Each component braces the other against possible torque and flexure. Flexure is practically nonexistent in such a design.

Ordinarily, both the anterior and posterior connectors should be placed as far posterior as possible to avoid interference with the tongue. The anterior connector may be extended anteriorly to support anterior tooth replacements, or it may be widened to form a thin palatal plate with a posterior brace. In this form a U-shaped connector is made rigid because of the added horizontal brace posteriorly. Frequently, a maxillary torus may thus be encircled by the major connector without sacrificing rigidity.

The combination anterior-posterior connector design may be used with any Kennedy Class of partially edentulous arch. It is used most frequently in Classes II and IV, whereas the single wide palatal bar or strap is more frequently used in Class III situations and the palatal plate or full coverage most frequently in Class I situations for reasons to be explained subsequently.

Both anterior and posterior connectors, and also the anterior and posterior borders of a palatal plate, should cross the midline at a right angle rather than on a diagonal. This is for reasons of symmetry. The tongue, being a bilateral organ, will accept symmetrically placed components far more readily than those placed without regard for bilaterally symmetry. Therefore, any curves in the connector should be placed to one side

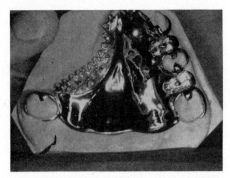

Fig. 4-18. Full palatal coverage with a full lingual apron provides maximum retention and stability in a surgically mutilated mouth. Each remaining tooth is used for support, and all but two incisors for retention to resist the leverage from the edentulous space. This must be considered an entirely tooth-borne restoration despite the length of the edentulous span. Finishing line for acrylic resin is necessarily near the midline of the palate since acrylic resin must be used to restore the normal contour of the palate.

of the midline, so that the connector may pass from one side to the other at right angles to the sagittal plane.

Palatal plate-type connector. For lack of better terminology, the words *palatal plate* are used to designate any thin, broad, contoured palatal coverage used as a maxillary major connector. The older types of thin castings, usually made of 26-gauge wax, were of indefinite thickness. This was due to the wax being thinned during adaptation to the cast and to polishing with abrasive wheels (Fig. 4-18). Newer techniques have resulted in the production of anatomic replica palatal castings that have uniform thickness and strength by reason of their corrugated contours. Thinner castings possessing greater rigidity are possible by this method. Through the use of electrolytic polishing, uniformity of thickness can be maintained and the anatomic contours of the palate faithfully reproduced in the finished denture.

The anatomic replica palatal plate has several advantages over other types of palatal major connectors. Some of these are as follows:

1. It permits the making of a uniformly thin metal plate that reproduces faithfully the anatomic contours of the patient's own palate. Because of its uniform thinness, the fact that it feels familiar to the patient's tongue, and the thermal conductivity of the metal, the palatal plate is accepted more readily by the tongue and underlying tissues than any other type of connector.

2. The corrugation in the anatomic replica adds strength to the casting; a thinner casting with adequate rigidity is thus made possible than could formerly be constructed with adapted sheet wax.

3. Surface irregularities are intentional rather than accidental; therefore, electrolytic polishing is all that is needed. The original uniform thickness of the plastic pattern is thus maintained.

4. Interfacial surface tension between metal and tissues provides the prosthesis with greater retention. Retention must be adequate to resist the pull of sticky foods, the action of moving border tissues against the denture, the forces of gravity, and the more violent forces of coughing and sneezing. These are all resisted to some extent by the retention of the base itself in proportion to the total area of denture contact. The amount of both direct and indirect retention required will depend upon the amount of retention provided by the denture base.

The palatal plate may be used in one of three ways. It may be used as a plate of varying width covering the area between two or more edentulous areas (Figs. 4-19 and 4-20), or it may be used as a full or partial cast palate extending posteriorly to a palatal seal area (Figs. 4-21 and 4-22), or it also may be used in the form of an anterior palatal connector with a provision for extending an acrylic resin denture base posteriorly (Fig. 4-23).

In most Class II and Class III situations the palatal plate will be located anterior to the posterior palatal seal area. Only in extensive Class I situations will it be extended posteriorly to the vibrating line of the soft palate. Little posterior seal is ever necessary with a metal palate because of the accuracy and stability of the cast metal.

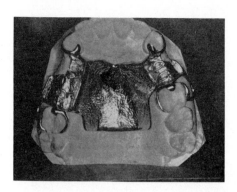

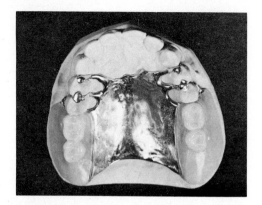

Fig. 4-19. Maxillary Class III partial denture framework with anatomic replica palatal plate major connector. Such a denture is used when bilateral stabilization of abutment teeth is needed. Note the posterior extension of the palatal plate to provide broader coverage and to extend the margin posteriorly where it may be less noticeable to the tongue. Partial metal bases are used with loops and undercut finishing lines for retention, but without visible display of metal anteriorly.

Fig. 4-20. Maxillary Class I partial denture framework with anatomic replica palatal plate. Although retention is increased by using a broad major connector, the need for indirect retainers still exists and they are placed on the mesiocclusal surfaces of the first premolars. Direct retention is furnished by bar-type clasps engaging distobuccal undercuts on the second premolars. A metal extension from the framework contacts prepared guiding planes on the distal surfaces of the second premolars to complete the clasp assembly.

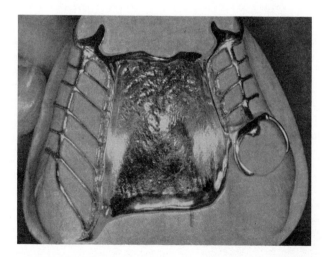

Fig. 4-21. Anatomic replica palatal major connector for a Class II, modification 1, partial denture. The anterior border avoids coverage of the anterior rugae; the posterior border lies well back on the immovable hard palate, crossing the midline at a right angle. Total contact provides excellent auxiliary retention without objectionable bulk. The finishing lines are parallel to the crest of the ridge. All direct retention for this denture is buccal wrought wire. Indirect retention is furnished by the lingual arm (placed in a rest seat) on the canine of the tooth-borne side. A bar-type retainer engaging a distolabial undercut on the patient's right canine would have been preferable for direct retention. However, a tissue undercut cervical to the labial gingival tissue of the canine and the lack of a distolabial undercut required the use of a wrought-wire circumferential retainer arm.

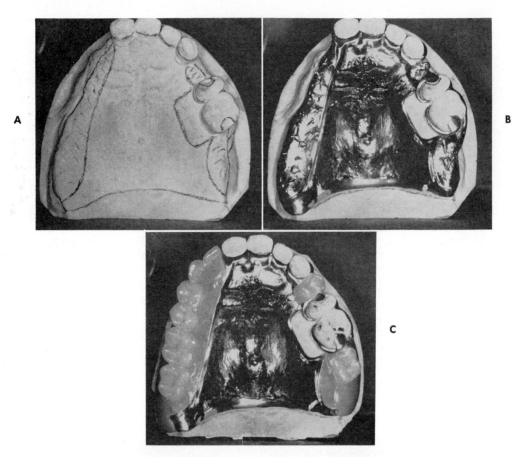

Fig. 4-22. Three views of maxillary Class I, modification 1, partial denture with full palatal major connector extending posteriorly to the vibrating line. Note the apron anteriorly terminating on an enamel ledge prepared on all the anterior teeth. Note the clearance lingual to the premolar and molar abutments. **A,** Design as submitted to the laboratory. **B,** Casting as returned from the laboratory. Note the partial metal base with diagonal spurs and undercut finishing line parallel to the crest of the residual ridge. **C,** Completed restoration. The replaced lateral incisor, canine, and first premolar are abutted to the ridge; but from the second premolar distally a buccal flange of resin is used.

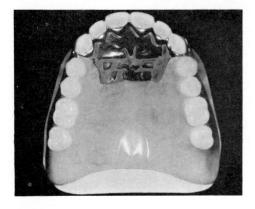

Fig. 4-23. Maxillary major connector (palatal linguoplate) to which the acrylic resin denture base has been attached. The palatal linguoplate is supported by rests occupying lingual rest seats prepared on the canines. This type of major connector will assist in resisting horizontal rotational tendencies of the denture and is particularly applicable when the residual ridges have undergone extreme vertical resorption, when adequate direct retention is difficult to develop, and when terminal abutments have suffered a fair amount of bone loss and splinting is contraindicated.

This is in contrast to the broad posterior palatal seal needed with resin denture bases. The location of the posterior seal, at the junction of the movable and immovable soft palate, is the same for both.

When the last remaining abutment tooth on either side of a Class I arch is the canine or first premolar tooth, full palatal coverage is not only advisable but is also practically mandatory when the residual ridges have undergone excessive vertical resorption. This may be accomplished in one of two ways. One method is to use a casting anteriorly with retention posteriorly for the attachment of a resin denture base, which then extends posteriorly to a palatal seal (Fig. 4-23). The other method is to utilize a full cast palate extending to the posterior palatal seal area (Fig. 4-22). The several advantages of a cast palate over a full resin palate make the full cast palate sufficiently preferable to offset the slight additional cost. However, when the cost and fee must be held to a minimum, the former method may be used satisfactorily. The partial metal palate may also be used when later rebasing is anticipated. In such case the posterior seal can be redone as part of the rebasing procedure.

Whereas the full palatal plate is not a connector that may be used universally, it has become accepted as the most satisfactory palatal connector for many maxillary partial dentures. In all circumstances, the portion contacting the teeth must have positive support from adequate rest seats. The dentist should be familiar with its use and, at the same time, with its limitations, so that it may be used intelligently and to fullest advantage.

In 1953, Dr. Louis Blatterfein described a systematic approach to designing maxillary major connectors. His method involves five basic steps and is certainly applicable to the greatest majority of maxillary removable partial denture situations. With a diagnostic cast in hand and a knowledge of the relative displaceability of the tissues covering the median palatal raphe, the basic steps he recommends are:

Step 1. *Outline of primary bearing areas.* These are the areas that will be covered by the denture base(s) (Fig. 4-24, *A* and *B*).

Step 2. *Outline of nonbearing areas.* The nonbearing areas are the lingual gingival tissues within 5 mm. of the remaining teeth, hard areas of the median palatal raphe (including tori, and palatal tissues posterior to the vibrating line (Fig. 4-24, *C*).

Step 3. *Outline of bar areas.* Steps 1 and 2, when completed, provide an outline or designate areas that are available to place components of major connectors (Fig. 4-24, *C*).

Step 4. *Selection of bar type.* Selection of the type of connecting bar(s) is based on four factors: mouth comfort, rigidity, location of denture bases, and indirect retention. Connecting bars should be of minimum bulk and so positioned that interference to the tongue during speech and mastication is not encountered. Connecting bars must have a maximum of rigidity to distribute stress bilaterally. The double bar type of major connector provides the maximum of rigidity without bulk and total tissue coverage. In many instances the choice of a bar type is limited by the location of the edentulous ridge areas. When edentulous areas are located anteriorly, the use of only a posterior bar is not possible. By the same token, when only posterior edentulous areas are present, the use of only an anterior bar is not a plausible choice. The need for indirect retention influences the outline of the major connector in that provision must be made in its location so that indirect retainers may be attached.

Step 5. *Unification.* After selection of the type bar(s) based on the considerations in Step 4, the denture base areas and connecting bars are joined (Fig. 4-24, *D*).

The indications for the use of full palatal coverage have been previously discussed in this chapter. Although there are many variations in palatal major connectors, a thorough comprehension of all factors influencing their design will lead the dentist to the best design for a particular patient.

The use of a splint bar for denture sup-

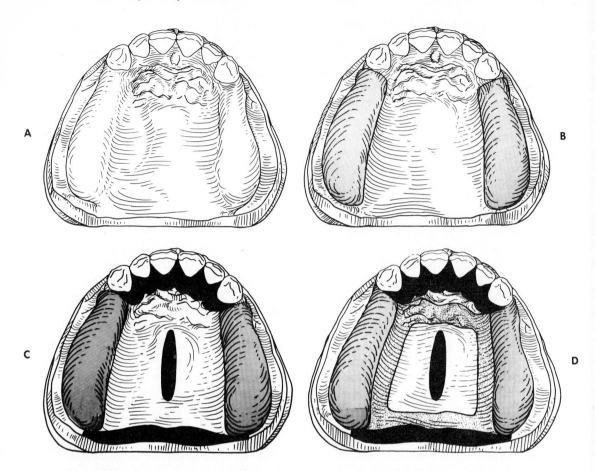

Fig. 4-24. A, Diagnostic cast of partially edentulous maxillary arch. **B,** Denture base areas are outlined. **C,** Nonbearing areas outlined in black, which include lingual soft tissue within 5 to 6 mm. of teeth, an unyielding median palatal raphe area, and the soft palate. The space bounded by the bearing and nonbearing area outlines is available for the placement of a major connector. **D,** Major connector selected will be rigid, noninterfering to the tongue, and cover a minimum of the palate.

port. In Chapter 13 under missing anterior teeth, mention is made of the fact that missing anterior teeth are best replaced with a fixed partial denture rather than with a removable partial denture that replaces posterior teeth elsewhere in the arch. The following is quoted from that chapter: "From a biomechanical standpoint, . . . a removable partial denture should replace only the missing posterior teeth, *after* the remainder of the arch has been made intact by means of fixed restorations."

Occasionally, a situation is found in which, economics aside, it is necessary that several missing anterior teeth be replaced with the removable partial denture rather than by fixed restorations. This may be due to the length of the edentulous span, or to the loss of sufficient residual ridge by resorption, accident, or surgery, or in a situation in which the amount of vertical space prevents the use of a fixed partial denture, or in which esthetic requirements can better be met through the use of teeth added to the denture framework. In such instances it is necessary that the best possible support for the replaced anterior teeth be provided. Ordinarily, this is done through the placement of occlusal and/or lingual rests on the adjacent natural teeth,

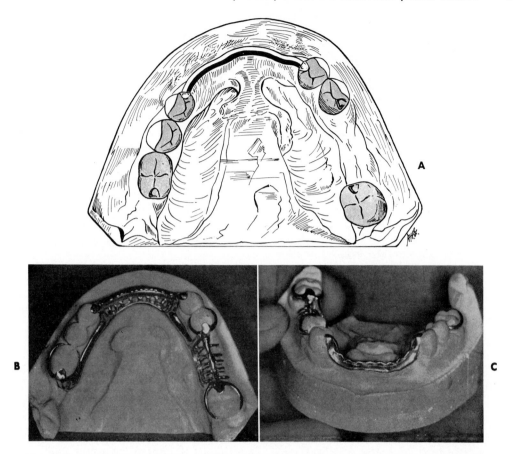

Fig. 4-25. **A,** Splint bar attached to double abutments on either side of the arch. Although this may be made of a hard gold alloy, its rigidity is better assured by making the bar of a chromium-cobalt alloy that fits into recesses prepared in the abutment pieces, attaching it by electric soldering. **B** and **C,** Denture framework designed to fit and be supported by the splint bar.

but when the edentulous span is too large to assure adequate support from the adjacent teeth, another method must be used. This is included in this chapter only because it influences the design of the major connector that must then be used.

An anterior splint bar may be attached to the adjacent abutment teeth in such a manner that a fixed splint results, but with a smooth, contoured bar resting lightly on the gingival tissues to support the removable partial denture. As with any fixed partial denture, the type of abutment retainers and the decision to use multiple abutments will depend upon the length of the span and the

stability of the teeth being used as abutments. Regardless of the type of abutment retainers used, the connecting bar must be cast separately of a rigid alloy or a commercially available bar may be used and attached to the abutments by soldering. Rather than rely upon soldered junctions alone, it is best that recesses be formed in the abutment pieces and that the connecting bar, which rests lightly on the tissues, be cast or made to fit into these recesses; they are then attached by soldering.

Because of the greater rigidity of the chromium-cobalt alloys, the splint bar is preferably cast in one of these materials

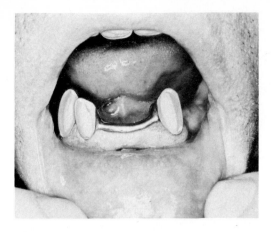

Fig. 4-26. Lower canines and premolar splinted together with a splint bar. The longevity of these teeth is greatly enhanced by splinting. Tissue surfaces are minimally contacted by the rounded form of the lower portion of the bar. The anterior and posterior slopes of the splint bar must be compatible with the path of placement of the denture.

and then attached to the gold abutment pieces by electric soldering. The complete assembly (abutment pieces and connecting bar) is then cemented permanently to the abutment teeth, the same as a fixed partial denture (Fig. 4-25, A). The impression for the partial denture then is made and a master cast obtained that accurately reproduces the contours of the tissue bar. The denture framework is then made to fit this bar by extending the major connector to cover and rest upon the tissue bar. Either retention for the attachment of a resin base or any other acceptable means of attaching the replaced anterior teeth is incorporated into the denture design. (See Fig. 4-25, B and C.)

The resulting partial denture will have the esthetic and other advantages of removable anterior replacements but will have positive support from the underlying splint bar (Fig. 4-26).

Internal clip attachment. The internal clip (or grip) attachment differs from the splint bar in that the internal clip attachment provides both support and retention at the connecting bar.

The connecting bar is made of 11-gauge platinum alloy wire, and the female grip is made of 27-gauge plate metal. Rather than resting on the tissues of the residual ridge as does the splint bar, the wire bar is located slightly above the tissues. Retention is provided by the plate metal grip, which is contoured to fit the bar and is partially embedded by means of retention spurs or loops into the overlying resin denture base.

The internal clip attachment thus provides both support and retention for the anterior modification area and may serve to eliminate both occlusal rests and retentive clasps on the adjacent abutment teeth.

Minor connectors

Arising from the major connector, the minor connector joins the major connector with other parts of the denture. For example, each direct retainer and each occlusal rest are joined to the major connector by a minor connector. In many instances, a minor connector may be identified even though continuous with some other part of the denture. For example, an occlusal rest at one end of a linguoplate is actually the terminus of a minor connector, even though that minor connector is continuous with the linguoplate. Similarly, the portion of a denture base frame that supports the clasp and the occlusal rest is a minor connector, joining the major connector with the clasp proper. Those portions of a denture framework by which the denture bases are attached are minor connectors.

Functions of the minor connectors. In addition to joining denture parts, the minor connector serves two other purposes. These are diametric in function.

One purpose is to *transfer functional stress to the abutment teeth.* Occlusal forces applied to the artificial teeth are transmitted through the base to the underlying ridge tissues, if that base is primarily tissue supported. Occlusal forces applied to the artificial teeth nearer to an abutment are transferred to that tooth through the occlusal rest. Similarly, occlusal forces are transferred to other abutment teeth supporting auxiliary rests and to the abutment teeth supporting a partial denture that is entirely tooth borne. The minor connectors arising from a rigid major connector make possible this transfer of functional stress throughout the dental arch. This, then, is a *prosthesis-to-abutment* function of the minor connector.

Another function of the minor connector is to *transfer the effect of the retainers, rests, and stabilizing components to the rest of the denture.* This is an *abutment-to-prosthesis* function of the minor connector. The effect of occlusal rests on supporting tooth surfaces, the action of retainers, and the effect of reciprocal clasp arms, guiding planes, and other stabilizing components are transferred to the rest of the denture by the minor connectors and then throughout the dental arch. Thus forces applied on one portion of the denture may be resisted by other components placed elsewhere in the arch for that purpose. A bracing or stabilizing component on one side of the arch may be placed to resist horizontal forces originating on the opposite side. This is possible only because of the transferring effect of the minor connector, which supports that stabilizing component, and the rigidity of the major connector.

Form and location of minor connectors. Like the major connector, the minor connector must have sufficient bulk to be rigid; otherwise, the transfer of the stresses and of the effect of other components cannot be effective. At the same time the bulk of the minor connector must be as unobjectionable as possible.

A minor connector contacting the axial surface of an abutment should not be located on a convex surface but, instead, should be located in an embrasure in which it will be the least noticeable to the tongue. It should conform to the interdental embrasure, passing vertically from the major connector to the other components. It should be thickest toward the lingual surface, tapering toward the contact area. The deepest part of the interdental embrasure should have been blocked out to avoid in-

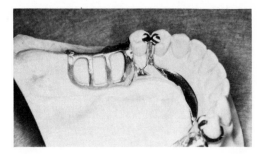

Fig. 4-27. Undercuts in the lingual embrasure between the premolars have been blocked out parallel to the path of placement. The minor connector is V shaped to avoid bulk, the greatest depth of the V being at the junction with the occlusal rests.

terference during placement and removal and to avoid any wedging effect on the teeth contacted.

Generally the minor connector should form a right angle with the major connector so that the gingival crossing may be abrupt and cover as little of the gingival tissues as possible. All gingival crossings should be relieved by blockout of the gingival crevice on the master cast before a refractory cast is made.

When a minor connector contacts tooth surfaces on either side of the embrasure in which it lies, it should be tapered to the teeth so that the tongue may encounter a smooth surface (Fig. 4-27). Sharp angles should be avoided, and spaces should not exist for the trapping of food debris.

It is a minor connector that contacts the guiding plane surfaces of the abutment teeth whether as a connected part of a direct retainer assembly or a separate entity (Fig. 4-28). Here the minor connector must be wide enough to utilize the guiding plane to fullest advantage. When it gives rise to a clasp arm, it should be tapered to the tooth below the origin of the clasp. If no clasp arm originates, such as when a bar clasp arm is originating elsewhere, it should be tapered to a knife edge the full length of its buccal aspect.

When a denture tooth will be placed against a proximal minor connector, its (minor connector) greatest bulk should be

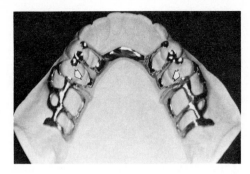

Fig. 4-28. Minor connector (arrows) contacting guiding plane surface is as broad as about two-thirds the distance between the tips of the adjacent buccal and lingual cusps of the abutment tooth. It extends gingivally contacting an area of the abutment from the marginal ridge to two-thirds the length of the enamel crown. Viewed from above it is triangular in shape, the apex of the triangle being buccally located and the base of the triangle lingual. Less interference to the arrangement of the adjacent artificial tooth is encountered with the minor connector so shaped.

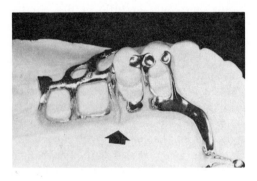

Fig. 4-29. Finishing line (arrow) at the junction of the ladderlike minor connector and major connector blends smoothly into the minor connector contacting the distal guiding plane on the second premolar. Framework is "feathered" toward the tissue anterior to the finishing line to avoid as much bulk in this area as possible—without compromising the strength of the butt-type joint.

located toward the lingual aspect of the abutment tooth. In this manner sufficient bulk is assured with the least interference to the placement of the denture tooth. Ideally, the artificial tooth should contact the abutment tooth with only a thin layer of metal intervening buccally. Lingually, the bulk of the minor connector should lie

in the interdental embrasure the same as between two natural teeth.

The minor connector, then, should be located to pass vertically in an interdental embrasure, whenever possible. Its form should conform to the interdental embrasure, with sufficient bulk to be rigid but tapered to the tooth surface when exposed to the tongue, and it should be designed so that it will not interfere with the placement of an artificial tooth.

As stated previously, those portions of a denture framework by which acrylic resin denture bases are attached are minor connectors. This type of minor connector should be so constructed that it will be completely imbedded within the denture base.

The junctions of these minor connectors with the major connectors should be a strong butt-type joint but without appreciable bulk (Fig. 4-29). Angles formed at the junction of the connectors should not be greater than 90 degrees, thus assuring the most advantageous and strongest connection between the acrylic resin denture base and the major connector.

An open latticework or ladder type of construction is preferable and is conveniently made by using preformed 12-gauge one-half round and 18-gauge round wax strips. The minor connector for the lower distal extension base should extend posteriorly about two thirds the length of the edentulous ridge and have elements on both the lingual and buccal surfaces. Not only will such an arrangement add strength to the denture base but in all probability it will minimize distortion of the cured base from its inherent strains due to processing. The minor connector must be planned with care so that it will not interfere with the arrangement of artificial teeth.

Minor connectors for maxillary distal extension denture bases should extend the entire length of the residual ridge and should also be of a ladderlike and loop construction (Fig. 4-30). The finishing line junction with the major connector should take the from of an angle of less than 90 degrees,

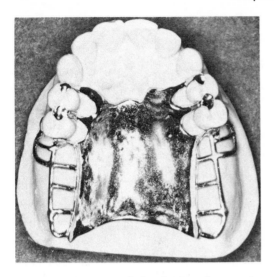

Fig. 4-30. Extension of the finishing line to the area of the hamular notch provides a butt-type joint for attachment of the border portion of the acrylic resin base through the hamular notch.

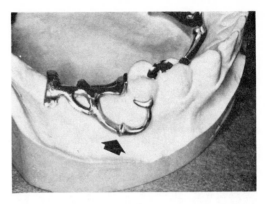

Fig. 4-31. Note that the direct retainer arm tapers from its tip to the finishing line. Without a finishing line (arrow) at the junction of the direct retainer arm and the minor connector for the denture base, the flexing of the direct retainer arm would create minute cracks in the anterior border of the denture base—often contributing to chipping of the border as well as an unhygienic condition from food particle impaction.

therefore being somewhat undercut. Of course the medial extent of the minor connector depends on the lateral extent of the major palatal connector. Too little attention is given this finishing line location in many instances. If the finishing line is located too far medially, the natural contour of the palate will be altered by the thickness of resin supporting the artificial teeth. If, on the other hand, the finishing line is located too far buccally, it will be most difficult to create a natural contour of the acrylic resin on the lingual of the artificial teeth. The location of the finishing line at the junction

of the major and minor connector should be based on restoring the natural palatal shape, taking into consideration the presumed anteroposterior and lateral alignment of the missing natural posterior teeth.

Just as consideration is given the junction of major and minor connectors attaching the denture base, so must equal consideration be given the junction of minor connectors and bar-type direct retainer arms (Fig. 4-31). These junctions are also butt-type joints and when so made possess the same advantages of the butt-type joint previously discussed.

CHAPTER 5

Rests and rest seats

Occlusal support for the partial denture must be provided by some kind of rests placed on the abutment teeth (Fig. 5-1). These always should be located upon tooth surfaces properly prepared to receive them.

Any unit of a partial denture that rests upon a tooth surface to provide vertical support to the denture is called a *rest*. A rest may be placed upon the occlusal surface of a premolar or molar tooth, upon the prepared lingual surface of an anterior tooth that is capable of withstanding the forces applied, or upon an incisal surface. Occlusal support is sometimes obtained upon a tooth surface inclined occlusally or

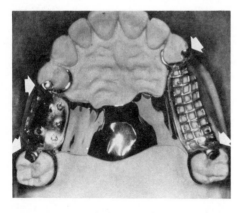

Fig. 5-1. Framework for a tooth-supported removable partial denture. Arrows point to components (rests) located on specifically prepared areas of the abutment teeth. Denture will be supported through three occlusal rests and one incisal rest on the canine.

incisally from its greatest convexity, but any rest so placed upon an unprepared surface is subject to slippage along tooth inclines. This violates one of the basic rules for rest design: *a rest should be designed so that transmitted forces are directed along the long axis of the supporting tooth as nearly as possible*. A second rule is that *a rest must be placed so that it will prevent movement of the restoration in a cervical direction.*

In an all-tooth–borne denture the rests should be capable of transferring *all* the vertical occlusal stresses to the abutment teeth. This is one of the principal functions of a rest, in addition to preventing movement of the partial denture in a cervical direction. A tooth-supported denture may therefore function similar to a fixed partial denture, the rests serving the same purpose as the soldered unions of the pontic with the abutment pieces. For this degree of stability to exist, it is obvious that the rest must be rigid and must receive positive support from the abutment tooth.

In a removable partial denture having one or more distal extension bases, the denture becomes increasingly tissue supported as the distance from the abutment increases. Closer to the abutment, however, the occlusal load is transmitted to the abutment tooth by means of the rest. The load is thereby distributed between the abutment and the supporting residual ridge tissues.

In addition to distributing the occlusal

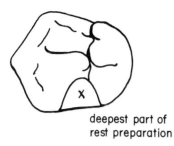

deepest part of
rest preparation

Fig. 5-2. Deepest part of an occlusal rest preparation should be inside the lowered marginal ridge at **X**. The marginal ridge is lowered to accommodate the origin of the occlusal rest with the least occlusal interference without sacrificing bulk.

load the rest serves other purposes. It acts to maintain the occlusal relationship with the opposing teeth by preventing settling of the partial denture. At the same time, settling of the denture against gingival tissues is prevented, thereby avoiding any impingement of the gingival tissues adjacent to the abutment teeth.

By the rest preventing movement of the denture in a cervical direction, the position of the retentive portion of the clasp arm is maintained in its intended relation to the tooth undercut. Although passive when in its terminal position, the retentive portion of the clasp arm should remain in contact with the tooth, ready to resist a vertical dislodging force. Then, when a dislodging force is applied, the clasp arm should immediately become active to resist vertical displacement. If, due to settling of the denture, the clasp arm is standing away from the tooth, some vertical displacement is possible before the retainer can become functional. The rest serves to prevent such settling and thereby helps to maintain the vertical stability of the partial denture. Rests are designated by the surface of the tooth prepared to receive the rest, that is, *occlusal rest, lingual rest, incisal rest*.

Form of the occlusal rest and rest seat. An occlusal rest is located upon the occlusal surface of a molar or premolar tooth that has been prepared to receive it (Fig. 5-2). The outline form of an occlusal rest seat should be a "rounded" triangular shape with the apex nearest the center of the tooth. It should be as long as it is wide and the base of the triangular shape (at the marginal ridge) should be the same dimension as one half the distance between the tips of the adjacent buccal and lingual cusps of the abutment tooth. The marginal ridge of the abutment tooth at the site of the rest seat must be lowered to permit a sufficient bulk of metal for strength and rigidity of the rest and minor connector. This then means that a reduction of the marginal ridge of approximately 1.5 mm. is usually necessary.

The floor of the occlusal rest seat should be inclined slightly toward the center of the tooth and should be concave or *spoon shaped*. Caution should be exercised in preparing a rest seat to avoid creating sharp edges or "line-angles" in the preparation. The angle formed by the occlusal rest and the vertical minor connector from which it originates should be less than a right angle, or less than 90 degrees (Figs. 5-3 and 5-4). Only in this way can the occlusal forces be directed along the long axis of the abutment tooth. An angle greater than 90 degrees fails to transmit occlusal forces along the supporting axis of the abutment tooth. It also permits slippage of the prosthesis away from the abutment and causes orthodontic forces to be applied, which are the resultant of forces applied to an inclined plane (Fig. 5-5).

When an existing occlusal rest preparation on enamel or on an existing cast restoration cannot be modified or deepened because of fear of perforation of the enamel or gold, yet the existing floor is inclined away from the center of the tooth, a secondary occlusal rest must be employed to prevent slippage of the primary rest and orthodontic movement of the abutment tooth. Such a rest should pass over the lowered marginal ridge on the side of the tooth opposite the primary rest and should, if possible, be inclined slightly toward the center of the tooth. However, two opposing occlusal rests on diverging tooth inclines will function to prevent unfavorable forces

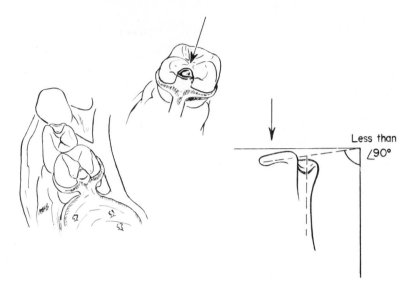

Fig. 5-3. Occlusal rest should be spoon-shaped and inclined slightly toward the center of the tooth on an occlusal surface properly prepared to receive it.

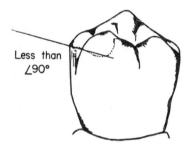

Fig. 5-4. Floor of the occlusal rest should be inclined slightly from the lowered marginal ridge toward the center of the tooth. Any angle less than 90 degrees is acceptable as long as the disking of the proximal surface and the lowering and rounding of the marginal ridge precede the completion of the rest seat itself.

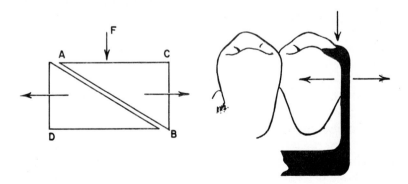

Fig. 5-5. Resultant of a force applied to an inclined plane when the floor of an occlusal rest preparation inclines away from instead of toward the center of the abutment tooth. **F,** Occlusal force applied to abutment tooth. **AB,** Relationship of occlusal rest with abutment tooth when angle is greater than 90 degrees. **ABC,** Partial denture framework. **ABD,** Abutment tooth.

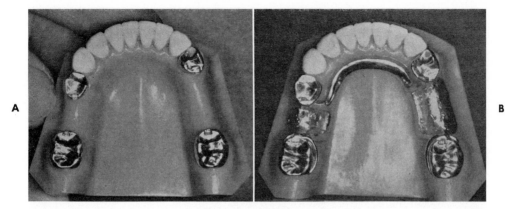

Fig. 5-6. Mandibular internal rest partial denture. **A,** Abutment crowns with internal rests. Both the dovetail design and a gingival well prevent horizontal movement. **B,** Completed partial denture framework with cast lingual retention on all four abutments. A short buccal stabilizing and removal arm is used on the molar abutments.

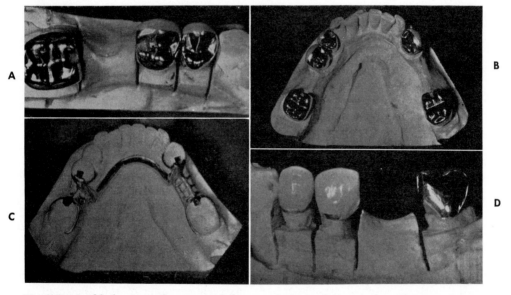

Fig. 5-7. Mandibular internal rest partial denture. **A,** Internal rests in four abutment crowns. **B,** Occlusal view showing proximal guiding planes. **C,** Buccal view showing the machined parallelism of the proximal surface. **D,** Completed gold alloy casting with wrought-wire lingual retention on all four abutments. Use of a buccal stabilizing arm is optional.

if all related connectors are sufficiently rigid.

In any partly tissue-supported partial denture the relation of the occlusal rest to the abutment should be that of a shallow ball-and-socket joint, so shaped to prevent a possible transfer of horizontal stresses to the abutment tooth. The occlusal rest should provide only occlusal support. Stabilization against horizontal movement of the prosthesis must be provided by other components of the partial denture rather than by any locking effect of the occlusal rest, which might cause the application of leverages to the abutment tooth.

Internal occlusal rests. A partial denture

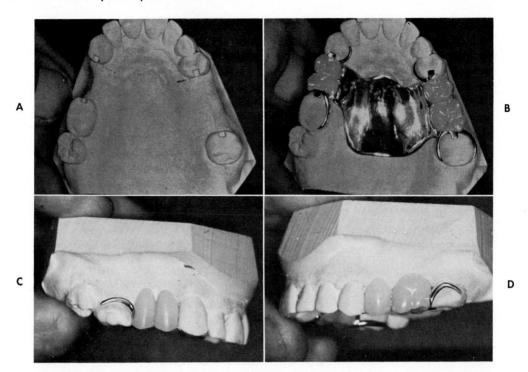

Fig. 5-8. Maxillary internal rest partial denture. **A,** Internal rests in four abutment crowns. **B,** Completed partial denture with lingual retentive clasp arms on canine and premolar abutments. **C** and **D,** Buccal views of the completed restoration showing abutted resin teeth (upon which gold occlusal surfaces will be fabricated) and absence of visible clasp arms on the premolar abutments. (Modified from McCracken's partial denture construction, ed. 3, St. Louis, 1969, The C. V. Mosby Co.)

that is totally tooth-supported by means of cast retainers on all abutment teeth may utilize internal occlusal rests for both occlusal support and horizontal stabilization (Figs. 5-6 to 5-8).

An internal occlusal rest is not in any way a retainer and therefore should not be confused with an internal attachment. The term *precision* is applied to both, *but any element of a partial denture should possess the accuracy and exactness synonymous with precision.*

Occlusal support is derived from the floor of the rest and an additional occlusal bevel if such is provided. Horizontal stabilization is derived from the near-vertical walls. The form of the rest should be parallel to the path of placement, tapered slightly occlusally, and slightly dovetailed to prevent dislodgement proximally. The original Neurohr rest is thus modified to

provide support and stabilization for the partial denture (Fig. 6-39, *A*).

The principal advantages of the internal rest are that it facilitates the elimination of a visible clasp arm buccally and permits the location of the rest seat in a more favorable position in relation to the "tipping" axis (horizontal) of the abutment. Retention is provided by a lingual clasp arm, either cast or of wrought wire, lying in a natural or prepared infrabulge area on the abutment tooth.

Technical obstacles to the use of internal rests are gradually being overcome. Such a rest usually cannot satisfactorily be carved in wax or machined in gold. Ready-made plastic rest patterns are generally too bulky. Assembly of a ready-made rest similar to an internal attachment necessitates soldering operations and added cost. The best solution seems to be the use of a

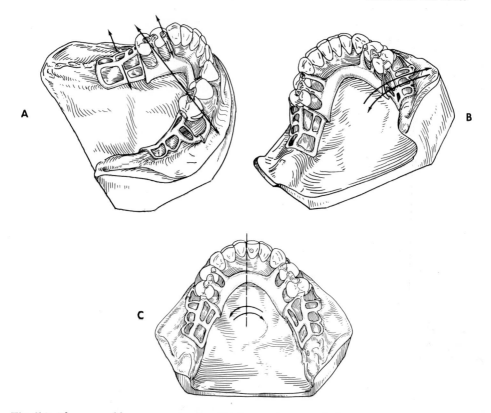

Fig. 5-9. Three possible movements of a distal extension partial denture. **A,** Rotation around the fulcrum line passing through the two principal occlusal rests when the denture base moves toward the supporting residual ridges. **B,** Rotation around a longitudinal axis formed by the crest of the residual ridge. **C,** Rotation around a perpendicular axis located near the center of the arch.

machined mandrel made of chrome-cobalt alloy,* which can be waxed into the crown or inlay pattern, invested, and cast to. The mandrel is easily tapped out leaving the internal rest formed in the abutment casting. Further developments of this technique promise more widespread use of the internal occlusal rest but only for tooth-supported partial dentures unless some form of stressbreaker is used between the abutment tooth and the distal extension denture base.

Possible movements of the partial denture. At least three possible movements of a distal extension partial denture exist. One is rotation about an axis formed by the two principal occlusal rests (Fig. 5-9, *A*).

---

*Ticon PRP mandrel and surveyor fixture, Ticonium Division, CMP Industries, Inc., Albany, N. Y.

This axis, known as the *fulcrum line,* is the center of rotation as the distal extension base moves *toward* the supporting tissues when an occlusal load is applied. The fulcrum line shifts to anteriorly placed rests as the base moves *away* from the supporting tissues as an occlusal load is released and vertical dislodging forces become effective. These dislodging forces are the vertical pull of food between opposing tooth surfaces, the effect of moving border tissues, and the forces of gravity against a maxillary denture. Presuming that the direct retainers are functional and that the occlusal rests remain seated, rotation rather than total displacement occurs. This movement is resisted in one direction by the tissues of the residual ridge, in proportion to the supporting quality of those tissues, the accuracy of the fit of the denture base, and the total amount of occlusal load applied. It is resisted in the opposite direction by the action of occlusal rests serving as *indirect retainers*.

A second movement is rotation about a longitudinal axis as the distal extension base moves in a rotary direction about the residual ridge (Fig. 5-9, *B*). This movement is resisted primarily by the rigidity of the major connector and its ability to resist torque. If the major connector is not rigid or if a stressbreaker exists between the distal extension base and the major connector, this rotation about a longitudinal axis either applies undue stress to the sides of the supporting ridge or causes horizontal shifting of the denture base.

A third movement is rotation about an imaginary perpendicular axis located near the center of the dental arch (Fig. 5-9, *C*). This movement occurs under function as diagonal and horizontal occlusal stresses are brought to bear upon the partial denture. It is resisted by stabilizing or bracing components, such as reciprocal clasp arms and minor connectors that are in contact with vertical tooth surfaces. Such stabilizing components are essential to any partial denture design regardless of the manner of support and the type of direct retention employed. Bracing components on one side of the arch act to stabilize the partial denture against horizontal forces being applied from the opposite side. It is obvious that rigid connectors must be employed to make this effect possible.

Horizontal forces always will exist to some degree because of lateral stresses occurring during mastication and bruxism. The magnitude of lateral stress may be minimized by fabricating an occlusion that is in harmony with the opposing dentition and free of lateral interference during excursive jaw movements. The amount of horizontal shift occurring in the partial denture will therefore depend upon the magnitude of lateral stresses applied and the effectiveness of the stabilizing components.

In a tooth-borne partial denture, movement of the base *toward* the edentulous ridge is prevented by the rests on the abutment teeth. Movement *away* from the edentulous ridge is prevented by the action of direct retainers on the abutments, situated at each end of each edentulous space. Therefore, the first of the three possible movements is nonexistent in the tooth-borne denture. The second possible movement, which is about a longitudinal axis, is prevented by the rigid components of the direct retainers on the abutment teeth as well as by the ability of the major connector to resist torque. This movement is much less in the tooth-borne denture, because of the presence of posterior abutments. The third possible movement occurs in any partial denture; therefore, bracing components against horizontal movement must be incorporated into any partial denture design.

The functions of the occlusal rest are not directly involved in either of the latter two movements. Instead, the occlusal rest should provide occlusal support only. All movements of the partial denture other than in a gingival direction should be resisted by other components. For the occlusal rest to enter into a bracing function would result in a direct transfer of torque to the abutment tooth. Since three movements are possible in a distal extension partial denture, an occlusal rest for such a partial denture should not have steep vertical walls or locking dovetails, which could possibly cause horizontal and torque stresses to be applied intracoronally to the abutment tooth.

In the tooth-borne denture the only movements of any significance are horizontal, and these may be resisted by the stabilizing effect of bracing components placed on the several abutments. Therefore, in the tooth-borne denture the use of intracoronal rests is permissible. In such usage the rests provide not only occlusal support but also horizontal stabilization.

Stress distribution in a tooth-supported partial denture is, or should be, such that each abutment tooth is assisted by others in the dental arch, and possible movements of the partial denture under function are held within acceptable physiologic limitations. It is therefore possible and acceptable to utilize an intracoronal type of occlusal rest if desired in any tooth-supported situation. In such case, vertical walls of an internal occlusal rest may be utilized to transfer horizontal forces to the abutment teeth and, by so doing, stabilize the partial denture against horizontal movement. An internal occlusal rest can thus be substituted for an external stabilizing clasp arm and, by utilizing a retentive clasp arm on the lingual surface of an abutment tooth, eliminate altogether the necessity for a visible clasp arm buccally or labially. This will be discussed further in Chapter 6.

The use of intracoronal rests and intracoronal direct retainers is optional with the tooth-borne denture. However, with the distal extension denture, the ball-and-socket type of rest or the nonlocking internal rest are preferable and should be used whenever possible.

Location of rests. Rests may be placed upon sound enamel, cast restorations, or silver amalgam alloy restorations. The use of a silver amalgam alloy restoration as support for an occlusal rest is the least desirable because of its tendency to flow under pressure and also because of the comparative weakness of a marginal ridge made of this alloy.

Rests placed on sound enamel are not conducive to caries in a mouth with a low caries index, provided good oral hygiene is maintained. Proximal tooth surfaces are much more vulnerable to caries attack than are the occlusal surfaces supporting an occlusal rest. The decision to use abutment coverage is usually based upon proximal and cervical vulnerability of the tooth rather than upon the vulnerability of an occlusal rest area. When pre-carious fissures are found in the occlusal rest areas in teeth that are otherwise sound, they may be removed and restored, preferably with

gold foil, without resorting to more extensive abutment protection.

Whereas it cannot be denied that the best protection from caries for an abutment tooth is full coverage, it must be presumed that such crowns will be contoured properly to provide support and retention for the partial denture and that full coverage restorations will provide subgingival protection to the tooth. Little is accomplished by the placement of full crowns if the more vulnerable cervical areas of an abutment tooth are not fully protected.

In making the decision whether or not to use unprotected enamel surfaces for rests, future vulnerability must be considered, for it is not easy to fabricate full crowns later to accommodate rests and clasp arms. In many instances sound enamel may be used safely for the support of occlusal rests. In such situations the patient should be advised that future caries susceptibility is not predictable and that much will depend upon his oral hygiene and possible future changes in his caries susceptibility. Although the decision to use unprotected abutments logically should be left up to the dentist, economic factors may influence the final decision. The patient should be made aware of the risks involved and of his responsibility for maintaining good oral hygiene and for returning periodically for observation.

Rest preparations in sound enamel. In most instances, disking of proximal tooth surfaces is necessary to provide proximal guiding planes and to eliminate undesirable undercuts when rigid parts of the denture casting must pass during placement and removal. The preparation of occlusal rest seats *always must follow proximal disking*, never precede it. Only after the disking is completed may the location of the occlusal rest seat in relation to the marginal ridge be determined. When disking follows the preparation of the occlusal rest seat, the inevitable consequence is that the marginal ridge is too low and too sharp, with the center of the floor of the rest too close to the marginal ridge. Therefore it is often not possible to correct the rest preparation without making it too deep, and then irreparable damage has been done to the tooth.

Occlusal rests in sound enamel should be prepared with diamond points of approximately the size of Nos. 6 and 8 round burs. The larger of the two diamonds is used first to lower the marginal ridge and to establish the outline form of the occlusal rest. The resulting occlusal rest seat is then complete except that the floor is not deepened sufficiently to be inclined slightly toward the center of the tooth. The smaller diamond point is then used to deepen the floor of the occlusal rest to a gradual incline toward the center of the tooth, at the same time forming the desired spoon shape inside the lowered marginal ridge. Smoothing the enamel rods by the planing action of a round bur of suitable size revolving at moderate speed, followed by the use of an abrasive rubber point, is usually the only polishing needed.

When a small enamel defect is encountered in the preparation of an occlusal rest seat, it is usually best to ignore it until the rest reparation has been completed, and then prepare the remaining defect with small burs to receive a small gold foil restoration. This then may be finished flush with the floor of the rest preparation previously established.

Occlusal rest preparations in existing restorations are treated the same as those in sound enamel. Any proximal disking must be done first, for if the occlusal rest seat is placed first and then the proximal surface is disked, the outline form of the occlusal rest seat is sometimes irreparably altered.

There is always a possibility that an existing restoration may be perforated in the process of preparing an ideal occlusal rest seat. While some compromise is permissible, the effectiveness of the occlusal rest seat should not be jeopardized for fear of perforating an existing inlay or crown. The rest seat may be widened to compensate for its shallowness, but the floor of the rest seat should still be inclined slightly toward the

center of the tooth. When this is not possible, a secondary occlusal rest should be used on the opposite side of the tooth to prevent slipping of the primary rest.

When perforation does occur, it may be filled with gold foil, but occasionally the making of a new restoration is unavoidable. In such a situation the original crown or inlay preparation should be modified to accommodate the occlusal rest, which is then placed in the wax pattern to avoid risking again the perforation of the completed restoration.

Occlusal rest seats in new restorations always should be placed in the wax pattern. The location of the occlusal rest should be known at the time that the tooth is prepared for a crown or an inlay, so that sufficient clearance may be provided in the preparation for the rest. The final step in the preparation of the tooth should be to make sure that such clearance exists, and, if not, to make a depression to accommodate the depth of the rest.

Occlusal rest seats in wax patterns are best made with round steel burs of suitable sizes. A perfectly rounded rest seat is thus possible, whereas carving with an instrument frequently results in an angular or irregular rest preparation. Although a round steel bur in a straight handpiece becomes partially clogged with wax during the first few revolutions, it may be used with light pressure to form the rest seat. The larger of two sizes is used first to create the outline form and to lower the marginal ridge. A slightly smaller bur is then used to deepen the floor of the rest seat, moving it around sufficiently to make one smooth concavity. After casting, an occlusal rest seat thus formed in a wax pattern needs only to be cleaned and burnished with a small finishing bur. Further polishing is usually unnecessary.

Occlusal rest seats in crowns and inlays are generally made somewhat larger and deeper than are those in enamel. Those made in abutment crowns supporting tooth-borne dentures may be made slightly deeper than those in abutments supporting a distal extension base, thus approaching the effectiveness of boxlike internal rests.

Internal rest seats also should be created first in wax, either with suitable burs in a handpiece holder or by waxing around a lubricated mandrel held in the surveyor. In either situation, the rest preparation must be finished on the casting with burs in a handpiece holder or with a precision drill press. Plastic and metal shoes that fit over a mandrel are also available for this purpose, thus assuring a smooth casting and eliminating the need for finishing the inside of the internal rest with burs. Sufficient clearance must have been provided in the preparation of the abutment to accommodate the depth of the internal rest.

Lingual rests on canines and incisor teeth. Whereas the preferred site for an external rest is the occlusal surface of a molar or premolar, an anterior tooth may be the only abutment available for occlusal support of the denture. Also, an anterior tooth occasionally must be used to support an indirect retainer or an auxiliary rest. A canine is much preferred over an incisor for this purpose. When a canine is not present, multiple rests spread over several incisor teeth are preferable to the use of a single incisor. Root form, root length, inclination of the tooth, and ratio of the length of the clinical crown to the alveolar support must be considered in determining the site and form of rests placed on incisors.

A lingual rest is preferable to an incisal rest because it is placed nearer the center of rotation of the abutment and therefore will have less tendency to tip the tooth. In addition, lingual rests are more esthetically acceptable than are incisal rests.

If an anterior tooth is sound and the lingual slope is gradual rather than perpendicular, a lingual rest may be placed in an enamel seat at or just incisally to the cingulum (Fig. 5-10). This type of lingual rest is usually confined to maxillary canines having a gradual lingual incline and a prominent cingulum. In some instances such a rest also may be placed on maxillary central incisors. The lingual slope of the mandibular canine is usually too steep for an adequate lingual rest seat to be placed in the enamel, and some other provision for rest support must be made.

The preparation of an anterior tooth to receive a lingual rest may be accomplished in one of two ways. These are as follows:

1. The proximal marginal ridge is lowered, and the deepest part of the rest seat is made toward the center of the tooth. The surface of the tooth can be reduced and shaped with various diamond stones. A predetermined path of placement for the denture must be kept in mind in preparing the rest seat. The lingual rest seat must not be prepared as though it were going to be approached from a direction perpendicular to the lingual slope. The floor of the rest seat should be toward the cingulum rather than the axial wall (Fig. 5-11). Care must be taken not to create an enamel undercut, which would interfere with placement of the denture.

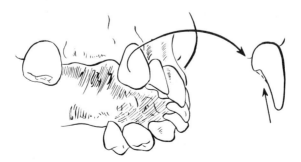

Fig. 5-10. Lingual rest seat placed in the enamel just incisally to the cingulum. Its preparation requires the slight reduction of a portion of the cingulum.

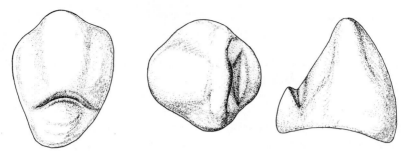

Fig. 5-11. Three views of a lingual rest seat prepared in the enamel of a maxillary canine. The rest seat, from the lingual aspect, assumes the form of a broad inverted V, maintaining the natural contour often seen in a maxillary canine cingulum. Looking at the preparation from an incisal view, it will be noted that the rest seat preparation is broadest at the most lingual aspect of the canine. As the preparation approaches the proximal surfaces of the tooth, it is less broad than at any other areas. A proximal view demonstrates the correct taper of the floor of the rest seat. It also should be noted that the borders of the rest seat are slightly rounded to avoid line angles in its preparation.

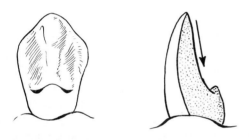

Fig. 5-12. The rest seat preparation can be exaggerated for better support when it is prepared in a metallic restoration.

2. The most satisfactory lingual rest, from the standpoint of support, is one placed on a prepared rest seat in a cast restoration (Fig. 5-12). This is done most effectively by planning and executing a rest seat in the wax pattern rather than attempting to cut a rest in a cast restoration in the mouth. The contour of the denture casting may then restore the lingual form of the tooth.

By accentuating the cingulum in the wax pattern, the floor of the rest seat may be made to incline toward the center of the tooth. A saddlelike shape, which provides a positive rest seat located favorably in relation to the long axis of the tooth, is thus formed. The framework of the denture is made to fill out the continuity of the lingual surface so that the tongue contacts a smooth surface without the patient being conscious of bulk or irregularities.

The lingual rest may be placed on the lingual surface of a cast veneer crown, a three-quarter crown, or some type of inlay (Fig. 5-13). The latter displays less metal than the three-quarter crown, especially on the mandibular canine where the lingual rest placed on a cast restoration is frequently used. The three-quarter crown may be used if the labial surface of the tooth is sound and retentive contours are satisfactory. However, if the labial surface presents inadequate or excessive contours for placement of a retentive clasp arm, or if gingival decalcification or caries is present, a veneered full crown should be used.

Incisal rests and rest seats. Incisal rests are usually placed at the incisal angles of anterior teeth and on prepared rest seats. Although this is the least desirable placement of rest types for reasons previously mentioned, it may be used successfully for selected patients when the abutment is sound and when a cast restoration is not otherwise indicated. Therefore, incisal rests generally are placed on enamel (Fig. 5-14). Incisal rests are used predominantly as auxiliary rests or as indirect retainers.

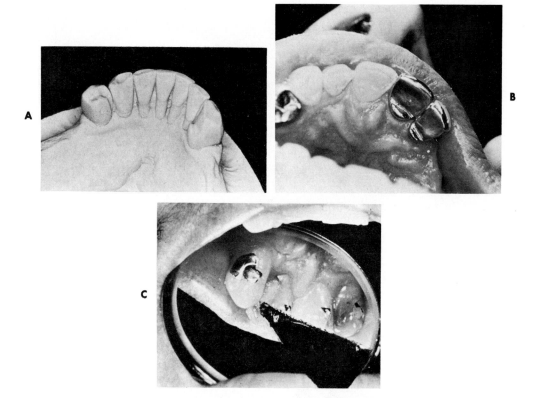

Fig. 5-13. **A,** Master cast from which a removable partial denture framework will be constructed. The properly contoured lingual rest seat was placed in a veneer crown for the canine abutment. **B,** Positive vertical support for the prosthesis is furnished by the rest seats prepared in the splinted three-quarter crowns on the lateral and central incisor. These rest seats are optimally placed as near the center of rotation of the abutment teeth as possible. **C,** Lingual rest seat placed in this pin-retained inlay is cup-shaped and is confined within the inlay itself.

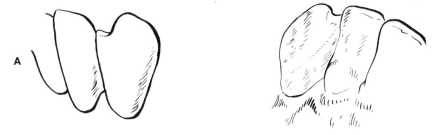

Continued.

Fig. 5-14. **A** and **B,** Incisal rest seat placed in the mesial incisal edge of a lower canine. Note that the contact point is not involved in the preparation of the rest seat to support a linguo-plate (as seen in **C**). **D,** The distal incisal rest on the canine furnished excellent vertical support for the tooth-borne removable partial denture and is not too objectionable esthetically.

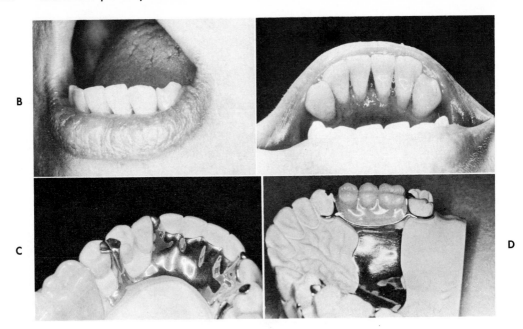

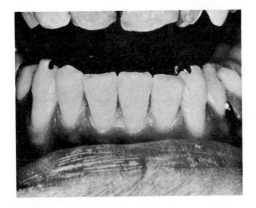

Fig. 5-14, cont'd. For legend see page 51.

Fig. 5-15. Incisal rests are utilized on this removable partial denture and are more acceptable esthetically than three-quarter crowns in which lingual rest seats may be placed.

Although the incisal rest may be used on a canine abutment in either arch, it is more applicable to the mandibular canine. This type of rest provides definite support with relatively little loss of tooth structure and little display of metal. Esthetically, it is preferable to the three-quarter crown (Fig. 5-15). The same criteria apply in deciding whether to use unprotected enamel for an

occlusal rest on a molar or premolar. An incisal rest is more likely to lead to some orthodontic movement of the tooth because of unfavorable leverage factors than is the lingual rest.

An incisal rest seat is prepared in the form of a notch at an incisal angle, with the deepest portion of the preparation toward the center of the tooth (Fig. 5-16). The notch should be beveled both labially and lingually, and the lingual enamel should be partly shaped to accommodate the rest arm. This arm is actually a minor connector, terminating at the incisal rest, and therefore must be rigid.

It is, of course, essential that both the master cast and the casting be accurate if the rest is to seat properly. The incisal rest should be overcontoured slightly to allow for labial and incisal finishing to the adjoining enamel in much the same manner as a three-quarter crown or inlay margin is finished to enamel. In this way minimal display of metal is possible without jeopardizing the effectiveness of the rest.

Care in selecting the type of rest seat to

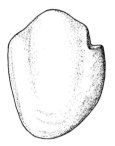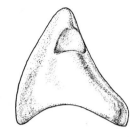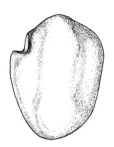

Fig. 5-16. Three views of an incisal rest seat preparation on a mandibular canine. The labial view demonstrates the inclination of the floor of the rest seat so that forces will be directed along the long axis of the tooth as nearly as possible. Note that the floor of the rest seat has been extended slightly onto the labial aspect of the tooth. As seen from a proximal view, the proximal edge of the rest seat is rounded rather than being straight. The lingual view shows that all borders of the rest seat are rounded to avoid sharp line angles. It is especially important to avoid a line angle at the junction of the axial wall of the preparation and the floor of the rest seat. The rest that occupies such a preparation should be able to move slightly in a lateral direction to avoid torquing the abutment tooth.

be used, in preparing it, and in fabricating the framework casting does much to assure the success of any type of rest. The topog-raphy of any rest should be such that it restores the topography of the tooth existing before the rest seat was prepared.

CHAPTER 6

Direct retainers

A removable partial denture must have *support,* derived from the abutment teeth through the use of rests and from the residual ridge through well-fitting bases. It must be *stabilized against horizontal movement* through the use of rigid bracing components such as reciprocal clasp arms and the contact of minor connectors with vertical tooth surfaces. It must be *stabilized against rotational movement and resulting torque* through the use of rigid connectors, indirect retainers, and other bracing components. In addition, the removable partial denture must have sufficient *retention* to resist reasonable dislodging forces.

Retention for the removable partial denture is accomplished mechanically by placing retaining elements on the abutment teeth and by the intimate relationship of denture bases and major connectors with the underlying tissues. The latter is similar to the retention of complete dentures and is proportionate to the accuracy of the impression registration, the accuracy of the fit of the denture bases, and the total area of contact involved.

Retention of denture bases has been described as the result of the following forces: (1) adhesion, which is the attraction of the saliva to the denture and to the tissues; (2) cohesion, which is the attraction of the molecules of the saliva for each other; (3) atmospheric pressure, which is dependent upon a border seal and results in a partial vacuum beneath the denture base when a dislodging force is applied; (4) the plastic molding of the tissues around the polished surfaces of the denture; and (5) the effect of gravity upon the mandibular denture. Boucher, writing on the subject of complete denture impressions, describes these forces as follows:

Adhesion and cohesion are effective when there is perfect apposition of the impression surface of the denture to the mucous membrane surfaces. These forces lose their effectiveness if there is any horizontal displacement of the dentures that breaks the continuity of this contact. Atmospheric pressure is effective primarily as a rescue force when extreme dislodging forces are applied to the denture. It depends on a perfect border seal to keep the pressure applied on only one side of the denture. The presence of air on the impression surface would neutralize the pressure of the air against the polished surface. Since each of these forces is directly proportional to the area covered by the dentures, the dentures should be extended to the limits of the oral cavity.

The plastic molding of the soft tissues around the polished surfaces of dentures helps to perfect the border seal. Also, it forms a mechanical lock at certain locations on the dentures, provided these surfaces are prepared for it. This lock is developed automatically and without effort by the patient if the impression is made with an understanding of the anatomic possibilities.[*]

---

[*]Paraphrased from Boucher, C. O.: Complete denture impressions based upon the anatomy of the mouth, J. Am. Dent. Assoc. 31:1174-1181, 1944.

Although few partial dentures are made without some mechanical retention, retention from the denture bases may contribute significantly to the overall retention of the partial denture and therefore must not be discounted as a retentive force. *Denture bases should be designed and fabricated so that they will contribute as much retention to the partial denture as possible.*

Mechanical retention of removable partial dentures is accomplished by means of direct retainers of one type or another. A direct retainer is any unit of a removable dental prosthesis that engages an abutment tooth in such a manner as to resist *displacement* of the prosthesis away from basal seat tissues. This may be accomplished by frictional means, by engaging a depression in the abutment tooth, or by engaging a tooth undercut lying cervically to the height of contour.

TYPES OF DIRECT RETAINERS

There are two basic types of direct retainers. One is the *intracoronal* retainer, which engages vertical walls built into the crown of the abutment tooth to create frictional resistance to removal. The other type is the *extracoronal* retainer, which engages an external surface of the abutment tooth in an area cervical to the greatest convexity or in a depression created for that purpose. Rather than creating frictional resistance to removal, a flexible arm is forced to deform, or a spring device is compressed, thereby generating resistance to removal. The most common extracoronal attachment is the *retentive clasp arm.*

The intracoronal retainer is usually spoken of as an *internal attachment*, or a *precision attachment*. The principle of the internal attachment was first formulated by Dr. Herman E. S. Chayes in 1906 and the attachment manufactured commercially carries his name. Although it may be fabricated by the dental technician as a cast dovetail fitting into a counterpart receptacle in the abutment crown, the alloys used in manufactured attachments and the precision with which they are constructed make the ready-made attachment much

preferable to any that can be fabricated in the dental laboratory. Much credit is due the manufacturers of precious metals used in dentistry for their continued improvements in the design of internal attachments and to the development of precise techniques for their use.

Some of the better-known internal attachments are the Ney-Chayes attachment, the Stern-Goldsmith attachment, the Brown attachment, the Baker attachment, and the Williams attachment. Descriptive literature and technique manuals are available from the manufacturers.

Internal attachments   INTRACORONAL

The internal attachment has two major advantages over the extracoronal attachment, which is the elimination of a visible retentive component and vertical support through a rest seat located more favorably in relation to the horizontal axis of the abutment tooth. For this reason the internal attachment may be preferable in selected situations. It provides some horizontal stabilization similar to that of an internal rest, but some additional bracing extracoronally is usually desirable. It has been claimed that stimulation to the underlying tissues is greater when internal attachments are used because of intermittent vertical massage. This is probably no more than is possible with extracoronal retainers of similar construction.

Some of the disadvantages of internal attachments are that (1) they require prepared abutments and castings, (2) they require somewhat complicated clinical and laboratory procedures, (3) they eventually wear, with resulting loss of frictional resistance to denture removal, (4) they are difficult to repair and replace, (5) they are effective in proportion to their length and are therefore least effective on short teeth, and (6) they are difficult to place completely within the circumference of an abutment tooth.

Since the internal attachment must be built within the coronal limits of the tooth, a large pulp may be jeopardized by the depth of the receptacle. Since it depends upon frictional resistance for retention, crown length must be sufficient to provide adequate frictional surfaces. The cost of an internal attachment prosthesis is necessarily higher than is a restoration of similar construction utilizing extracoronal retainers, even when the latter utilizes abutment castings. Limitations to the use of internal attachments are (1) size of pulp, which is usually related to age of the patient, (2) length of the clinical crown, which may prevent use on short or abraded teeth, and (3) greater cost to the patient.

Since the principle of the internal attachment does not permit horizontal movement, all horizontal, tipping, and rotational movements of the prosthesis are transmitted directly to the abutment tooth. *The internal attachment therefore may not be used in conjunction with tissue-supported distal extension denture bases unless some form of stressbreaker is used between the movable base and the rigid attachment.* Whereas stressbreakers may be used, they do have some disadvantages, which will be discussed later, and their use adds further to the cost of the partial denture. It is doubtful that the possible advantages of the stress-broken, internal-attachment denture are available to but a small percentage of the population needing a removable partial denture service.

Extracoronal direct retainers

While the extracoronal or clasp direct retainer is used many times more frequently than the internal attachment, it is also all too frequently misused. It is hoped that a better understanding of the principles of clasp design will lead to more intelligent use of this retainer in the future.

Clasp retention is based upon the resistance of metal to deformation. For a clasp to be retentive, it must be placed in an undercut area of the tooth where it is forced to deform when a vertical dislodging force is applied. It is this resistance to deformation that generates retention. Such resistance is proportionate to the flexibility of the clasp arm.

It should be clearly understood that a retentive undercut exists only in relation to a given path of placement and removal, for if the path of escapement of the retentive clasp is parallel to the path of removal of the prosthesis, no retentive undercut exists.

A positive path of placement and removal is made possible by the contact of rigid parts of the denture framework with parallel tooth surfaces that act as guiding planes. It is also made possible, to some extent, by simultaneous tooth contact on either side of the dental arch as the prosthesis is placed and removed. If some degree of parallelism does not exist during placement and removal, trauma to the teeth and supporting structures, as well as strain on the denture parts, is inevitable. This ultimately results in damage either to the teeth and their periodontal support, or to the denture itself, or both. Therefore, without guiding planes, clasp retention will either be detrimental or nonexistent. If clasp retention is only frictional, due to an *active* relationship of the clasp to the teeth, orthodontic movement and/or damage to periodontal tissues will result. *Instead, a clasp should bear a passive relationship to the teeth except when a dislodging force is applied.*

To be retentive, a tooth must have a height of contour cervical to which the surface converges. Although any single tooth, when surveyed, will have a height of contour or an area of greatest convexity, areas of cervical convergence may not exist when that tooth is viewed in relation to a given path of placement. Also, certain areas of cervical convergence may not be available for the placement of retentive clasps because of their proximity to gingival tissues.

This is best illustrated by mounting a spherical object such as an egg on the adjustable table of a dental surveyor (Fig. 6-1, *A*). The egg now represents the cast of a dental arch or, more correctly, one tooth of a dental arch. The egg is first placed perpendicular to the base of the

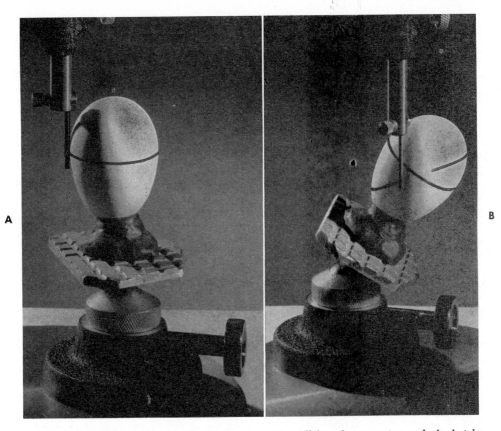

Fig. 6-1. **A,** When an egg is placed with its long axis parallel to the surveying tool, the height of contour is found at its greatest circumference. Similarly, the height of contour may be identified on a single tooth when its long axis is placed parallel to the surveying tool. Rigid parts of the partial denture framework may be located in the suprabulge areas above the height of contour, whereas only the flexible portions of clasp retainers may be placed in the infrabulge areas below. Those infrabulge surfaces that will be crossed by rigid parts of a partial denture framework must be eliminated either during mouth preparations or by block-out. **B,** If the same egg is tilted in relation to the vertical arm of the surveyor, areas formerly infrabulge are now found to be suprabulge and will accommodate nonretentive denture components. At the same time, however, areas formerly suprabulge or only slightly infrabulge are found to be so severely undercut that the design and location of clasp retainers must be changed. Unfortunately, no single tooth in a partially edentulous arch may govern the relation of the cast to the surveyor and thus the path of placement of the partial denture. A compromise position must be found which, following mouth preparations, will satisfy all four factors: (1) no interference to placement, (2) effective location of retentive components, (3) most esthetic placement of all component parts, and (4) existence of guiding planes that will assure a definite path of placement and removal. (Courtesy J. M. Ney Co., Hartford, Conn.)

surveyor and surveyed to determine the height of convexity. The vertical arm of the surveyor represents the path of placement that a denture would take and, conversely, its path of removal.

With a carbon marker, a circumferential line is drawn on the egg at its greatest circumference. This line, which Kennedy called the height of contour, is its greatest

convexity. Cummer spoke of it as the guideline, since it is used as a guide in the placement of retentive and nonretentive clasps. To this, DeVan added the terms suprabulge, denoting the surfaces sloping superiorly, and infrabulge, denoting the surfaces sloping inferiorly. Prothero proposed that the height of convexity of a tooth be considered as the common base of two cones, the apex of one cone being somewhere above the occlusal surface and the apex of the other being somewhere below the cervical circumference of the tooth.

Any areas cervical to the height of contour may be utilized for the placement of retentive clasp arms, whereas areas occlusal to the height of contour may be utilized for the placement of nonretentive reciprocating, or stabilizing components. Obviously, only flexible components may be placed gingivally to the height of contour because if rigid elements were to be so placed, the under cut areas would be areas of interference to placement and removal rather than areas of retention.

With the original guidelines on the egg, the egg is now tilted from the perpendicular to an angular relation with the base of the surveyor (Fig. 6-1, *B*). Its relation to the vertical arm of the surveyor has now been changed, just as a change in the position of a dental cast would bring about a different relationship with the surveyor. The vertical arm of the surveyor still represents the path of placement, but its relation to the egg is totally different.

Again, the carbon marker is used to delineate the greatest convexity or the height of contour. It will be seen that areas that were formerly infrabulge are now suprabulge, and vice versa. A retentive clasp arm placed below the height of contour in the original position may now be either excessively retentive or totally nonretentive, whereas a nonretentive reciprocal arm located above the height of contour in the first position now may be located in an area of undercut.

The location and degree of a tooth undercut available for retention is therefore relative to the path of placement and removal of the partial denture; at the same time, nonretentive areas upon which rigid components of the clasp may be placed exist for a given path of placement only.

When the theory of clasp retention is applied to the abutment teeth in a dental arch, each tooth may be considered as an entity as far as the design of retentive and reciprocating components is concerned. This is possible because its relationship to the rest of the arch and to the design of the rest of the prosthesis has been considered previously in selecting the most suitable path of placement. Once the relation of the cast to the surveyor has been established, the height of contour on each abutment tooth becomes fixed, and the clasp design for each may be considered separately.

When the surveyor blade contacts a tooth on the cast at its greatest convexity, a triangle is formed. The apex of the triangle is at the point of contact of the surveyor blade with the tooth, and the base is the area of the cast representing the gingival tissues (Fig. 10-19). The apical angle is called the angle of cervical convergence (Fig. 6-2). This angle may be measured as described in Chapter 10, or it may be estimated by observing the triangle of light visible between the tooth and the surveyor blade. For this reason, a wide surveyor blade rather than a small cylindrical tool is used so that the triangle of light may be more easily seen.

The following factors determine the amount of retention that a clasp is capable of generating:

1. Size of the angle of cervical convergence
2. How far into the angle of cervical convergence the clasp terminal is placed
3. Flexibility of the clasp arm, which is the product of:
   a. Its length, measured from its point of origin to its terminal end
   b. Its relative diameter, regardless of its cross-sectional form
   c. Its cross-sectional form or shape, that is, whether it is round, half-round, or some other form
   d. The material of which the clasp is made, that is, whether it is made of a cast gold alloy, cast chrome alloy, wrought gold alloy, or wrought chrome alloy (each alloy

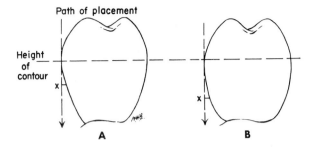

Fig. 6-2. Angle of cervical convergence on two teeth presenting dissimilar contours. The greater angle of cervical convergence on tooth **A** necessitates the placement of a clasp terminus nearer the height of contour than when a lesser angle exists, as in **B**. It is apparent that uniform clasp retention depends upon the degree of tooth undercut rather than on the distance below the height of contour at which the clasp terminus is placed.

has its own characteristics in both cast or wrought form)

Relative uniformity of retention. The size of the angle of convergence will determine how far into that angle a given clasp arm will be placed. Disregarding, for the time being, variations in clasp flexibility, relative uniformity of retention will depend upon the location of the clasp terminal—not in relation to the height of contour but in relation to the angle of cervical convergence.

The retention on all principal abutments (of which there will be two in Class I and Class II situations and three or more in Class III situations) should be as nearly equal as possible. Whereas esthetic placement of clasp arms is desirable, it may not be possible to place all clasp arms in the same occlusocervical relationship because of variations in tooth contours. The only exceptions are when retentive surfaces may be made similar by altering tooth contours or when two cast restorations are made with similar contours.

Instead, the retentive clasp arms must be located so that they lie in the same approximate degree of undercut on each abutment tooth. In Fig. 6-2 this is at point *X* on both teeth, *A* and *B*, despite the variation in the distance below the height of contour. Should both clasp arms be placed equidistantly below the height of contour, the higher location on tooth *B* would have too little retention, whereas the lower location on tooth *A* would be too retentive.

The measurement of the degree of undercut by mechanical means is therefore most important. Although experience with undercut gauges is most important, the student should graduate with a thorough comprehension of *all* the factors influencing clasp retention and be able to apply them intelligently.

Flexibility of the clasp arm. The following factors influence the flexibility of a clasp arm.

LENGTH. The longer the clasp arm the more flexible it will be, all other factors being equal. The length of a circumferential clasp arm is *measured from the point at which a uniform taper begins.* The retentive circumferential clasp arm should be tapered uniformly from its point of origin. The length of this uniform taper is the full length of the clasp arm (Fig. 6-3).

The length of a bar clasp arm also is measured from the point at which a uniform taper begins. Generally, the taper of a bar clasp arm should begin at its point of origin from a metal base or at the point at which it emerges from a resin base (Fig. 6-4). While a bar clasp arm will usually be longer than a circumferential clasp arm, its flexibility will be less because its half-round form lies in several planes, which prevents its flexibility from being proportionate to its total length. Table 6-1 gives an approximate depth of undercut that may be used for the cast gold retentive clasp arms of the circumferential and bar-type clasps. Based

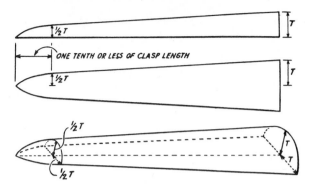

Fig. 6-3. Clasp arm should be tapered uniformly from its point of attachment at the clasp body to its tip. The dimensions at the tip are about half those at the point of attachment. A clasp arm so tapered is approximately twice as flexible as one without any taper. In the illustration, **T** is clasp thickness. (Courtesy J. F. Jelenko & Co., Inc., New York, N. Y.)

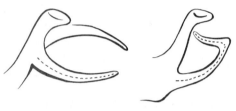

Fig. 6-4. Length of a clasp arm is measured along the center portion of the arm until it either joins the clasp body (circumferential) or until it becomes a part of the denture base or is embedded in the base (bar-type clasp).

Table 6-1. Permissible flexibilities of circumferential and bar-type clasp arms*

Circumferential		Bar-type	
Length (inches)	Flexibility (inches)	Length (inches)	Flexibility (inches)
to 0.3	0.01	to 0.7	0.01
0.3 to 0.6	0.02	0.7 to 0.9	0.02
0.6 to 0.8	0.03	0.9 to 1.0	0.03

*Based on the approximate dimensions of Jelenko "pre-formed" plastic patterns, J. F. Jelenko & Co., Inc., New York, N.Y.

on a proportional limit of 60,000 psi and on the assumption that the clasp arm is properly tapered, the clasp arm should be able to flex repeatedly within the limits stated without strain hardening or rupturing.

DIAMETER OF THE CLASP ARM. The greater the average diameter of a clasp arm, the less flexible it will be, all other factors being equal. If its taper is absolutely uniform, the average diameter will be at a point midway between its origin and its terminal end. If its taper is not uniform, a point of flexure and therefore a point of weakness will exist that will then be the determining factor in its flexibility regardless of the average diameter of its entire length.

CROSS-SECTIONAL FORM OF THE CLASP ARM. Flexibility may exist in any form, but it is limited to only one direction in the case of the half-round form. The only universally flexible form is the round form, which is practically impossible to obtain by casting and polishing.

Since all cast clasps are essentially half round in form, they may flex away from the tooth, but edgewise flexing (and edgewise adjustment) is limited. For this reason, cast retentive clasp arms are more acceptable in tooth-borne partial dentures in which they are called upon to flex only during placement and removal of the prosthesis. A retentive clasp arm on an abutment adjacent to a distal extension base must not only flex during placement and removal but also must be capable of flexing during functional movement of the distal extension base. It must have either universal flexibility to avoid transmission of tipping stresses to the abutment tooth or be capable of disengaging the undercut when vertical forces directed against the denture are toward the residual ridge. A round clasp form is the only circumferential clasp form that may be safely used to engage a tooth undercut on the side of an abutment tooth *away* from the distal extension base. *The location of the undercut is perhaps the most important single factor in selecting a clasp for use with distal extension partial dentures.*

MATERIAL USED FOR CLASP ARM. Whereas all cast alloys used in partial denture construction possess flexibility, their flexibility is proportionate to their bulk. If this were not true, other components of the partial denture could not have the necessary rigidity. The only disadvantage of cast gold partial dentures is that their bulk must be increased to obtain needed rigidity at the expense of added weight. It cannot be denied that greater rigidity with less bulk is possible through the use of chrome alloys.

Although cast gold alloys may have greater resiliency than do cast chrome alloys, the fact remains that the structural nature of the cast clasp does not approach the flexibility and adjustability of the wrought-wire clasp. Having been formed by being drawn into a wire, the wrought-wire clasp arm has toughness exceeding that of a cast clasp arm. It may therefore be used in smaller diameters to provide greater flexibility without fatigue and ultimate fracture.

Advantages and disadvantages of any given clasp design. In selecting a particular clasp arm for a given situation, its advantages must be weighed against its disadvantages. The dentist should not expect the technician to make the decision as to which clasp design is to be used. *The choice of clasp design must be both biologically and mechanically sound, based upon the diagnosis and treatment plan previously established.*

The advantages of any particular clasp design should lie in an affirmative answer to most or all of the following questions:

1. Is it flexible enough for the purpose for which it is being used? (On an abutment adjacent to a distal extension base will tipping and torque be avoided?)
2. Does the clasp arm cover a minimum of tooth surface?
3. Will the clasp arm be as inconspicuous as possible?
4. Will tooth dimension not be increased, which would relatively increase the width of the occlusal table?
5. Is the clasp design applicable to malposed or rotated abutment teeth?
6. Can it be used despite the presence of tissue undercuts?
7. Can the clasp terminal be adjusted to increase or decrease retention?
8. Will adequate stabilization be provided to prevent horizontal and rotational movements?
9. Will rigidity be provided where it is needed?
10. Is the clasp arm likely to become distorted or broken? If so, can it be replaced?

The disadvantages of any given clasp design are generally the opposite of the advantages listed above. These are as follows:

1. The retentive arm is too rigid for an abutment adjacent to a distal extension base.
2. Too much tooth surface is covered, resulting in the trapping of food debris and possible caries attack.
3. There will be an objectionable display of metal, resulting in poor esthetics.
4. Tooth dimension will be increased, resulting in an increased functional load on the abutment.
5. Tooth undercuts on malposed teeth cannot be approached without encountering other disadvantages.
6. Tissue undercuts will have to be blocked out excessively, resulting in poor esthetics, annoyance to cheek and tongue, and the trapping of debris.

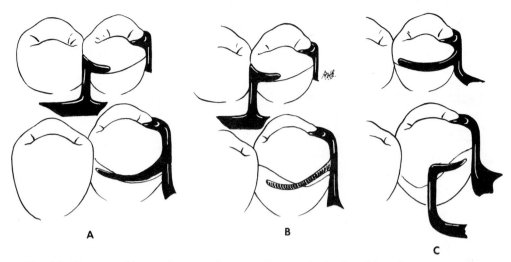

Fig. 6-5. Class assembly may be a combination of circumferential and bar clasp arms in one of several possible combinations. **A,** Cast circumferential retentive clasp arm with a nonretentive bar clasp arm on the opposite side for reciprocation. **B,** Wrought-wire circumferential retentive clasp arm with a nonretentive bar clasp arm on the opposite side for reciprocation. **C,** Retentive bar clasp arm with a nonretentive cast circumferential clasp arm on the opposite side for reciprocation.

7. Edgewise adjustment to increase or decrease retention is impossible.
8. Orthodontic movement of the abutment tooth is possible because of inadequate stabilization.
9. Horizontal stabilization of the partial denture is inadequate because of insufficient rigidity of stabilizing components.
10. The clasp arm may be easily distorted by careless handling.
11. If broken, the clasp arm may be difficult to replace.

With this background the various types of clasps will be considered. The choice of a clasp is like the choice of a tool to be used in a given situation. Knowing what types are available and being familiar with their various advantages and disadvantages, a clasp design may be selected that best meets the needs of the individual situation.

Although there are some rather complex designs for clasp arms, they may all be classified as falling into one of two categories. One is the *circumferential clasp arm*, which approaches the retentive undercut from an occlusal direction. The

other is the *bar clasp arm*, which approaches the retentive undercut from a cervical direction.

Circumferential clasp designs include the C-type clasp, the embrasure clasp, the ring clasp, the back-action clasp, and the combination clasp.

Bar clasp designs include the infrabulge clasp, all bar clasp designs, such as the T, Y, L, C, I, U, E, and S clasp arms, and the mesiodistal clasps.

Clasp assembly may be a combination of circumferential and bar clasp arms in one of several possible combinations, some of which are (1) a cast circumferential retentive clasp arm with a nonretentive bar clasp on the opposite side for reciprocation (Fig. 6-5, *A*), (2) a wrought-wire circumferential retentive clasp arm with a nonretentive bar clasp arm on the opposite side for reciprocation (Fig. 6-5, *B*), and (3) a retentive bar clasp arm with a nonretentive cast circumferential clasp arm on the opposite side for reciprocation (Fig. 6-5, *C*).

No confusion should exist between the choice of clasp arm and the purpose for which it is used. Either type of cast clasp arm may be made tapered and retentive or

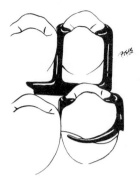

Fig. 6-6. Auxiliary occlusal rest may be used rather than a reciprocal clasp arm without violating any priciple of clasp design. Its greatest disadvantages are that a second rest seat must be prepared and an enclosed tissue space results. An auxiliary occlusal rest is also sometimes used to prevent slippage when the principal occlusal rest cannot be inclined toward the center of the tooth.

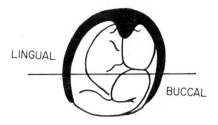

Fig. 6-7. The line drawn through the illustration represents more than 180° of the greatest circumference of the abutment from the occlusal rest. Unless portions of the lingual reciprocal arm and the retentive buccal arm are extended beyond the line, the clasp would not accomplish its intended purpose. If the respective arms of the retainer were not extended beyond the line, the abutment could move away from the retainer or the removable partial denture could move away from the abutment.

rigid and nonretentive, depending upon whether it is used for retention or reciprocation. A clasp assembly should consist of (1) one or more minor connectors from which the clasp arms originate, (2) a principal rest, (3) a retentive clasp arm engaging a tooth undercut with a retentive terminal, (4) a nonretentive clasp arm on the opposite side of the tooth for reciprocation and stabilization against horizontal movement of the prosthesis. Rigidity of this clasp arm is essential to its purpose. An auxiliary occlusal rest may be used rather than a reciprocal clasp arm if it is located to accomplish the same purpose (Fig. 6-6). The addition of a lingual apron to a cast reciprocal clasp arm neither alters its primary purpose nor the need for proper location to accomplish that purpose.

Basic principles of clasp design. Any clasp assembly must satisfy the basic principle of clasp design, which is that *more than 180 degrees of the greatest circumference of the crown of the tooth must be included, passing from diverging axial surfaces to converging axial surfaces* (Fig. 6-7). This may be in the form of continuous contact when circumferential clasp arms are used or broken contact when bar clasp arms are used. At least three areas of tooth contact must be embracing more than one

half the tooth circumference. These are the occlusal rest area, the retentive terminal area, and the reciprocal terminal area.

Other principles to be considered in the design of a clasp are as follows:

1. The occlusal rest must be designed so that movement of the clasp arms cervically is prevented.

2. Each retentive terminal should be opposed by a reciprocal arm or element capable of resisting any orthodontic pressures exerted by the retentive arm. Reciprocal elements must be rigidly connected bilaterally if reciprocation to the retentive elements is to be realized (Fig. 6-8).

3. Unless guiding planes will positively control the path of removal, retentive clasps should be bilaterally opposed, that is, buccal retention on one side of the arch should be opposed by buccal retention on the other side, or lingual on one side opposed by lingual on the other. In Class II situations, the third abutment may have either buccal or lingual retention. In Class III situations retention may be either bilaterally or diametrically opposed.

4. The path of escapement of each retentive clasp terminal must be other than parallel to the path of removal of the prosthesis.

5. Amount of retention always should

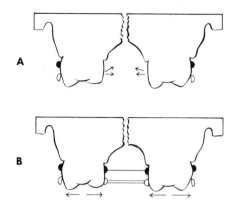

Fig. 6-8. **A,** Flexing action of the retentive clasp arm initiates medially directed pressure on the abutment teeth as its retentive tip springs over the height of contour. **B,** Reciprocation to medially directed pressure is counteracted either by lingually placed clasp arms contacting the abutments simultaneously with the buccal arms and engaging the same degree of undercut or by reciprocal elements of the framework contacting lingual guiding planes when the buccal arms begin to flex.

be the minimum necessary to resist reasonable dislodging forces.

6. Clasp retainers on abutment teeth adjacent to distal extension bases should be designed so that they will avoid direct transmission of tipping and rotational forces to the abutment. In effect they must act as stressbreakers, either by their design or by their construction. This is accomplished by proper placement of the retentive terminal or by the use of a more flexible clasp arm.

7. *Ideally, reciprocal elements of the clasp assembly should be located at the junction of the gingival and middle thirds of the crowns of abutment teeth. The terminal end of the retentive arm is optimally placed in the middle of the gingival third of the crown.* These locations will permit the abutment teeth to better resist horizontal and torquing forces than they could if the retentive and reciprocal elements were located nearer the occlusal or incisal surfaces. As a simile, remember that a fencepost is more easily loosened by applying horizontal forces near its top than

applying the same forces nearer ground level.

The reciprocal clasp arm has two, sometimes three, functions. First, the reciprocal clasp arm should provide reciprocation against the action of the retentive arm. This is particularly important if the retentive arm is accidentally distorted toward the tooth where it would become an active orthodontic force. The retentive clasp arm should be passive until a dislodging force is applied.

During placement and removal, reciprocation is most needed as the retentive arm flexes over the height of contour. Unfortunately, the reciprocal clasp arm does not usually come into contact with the tooth until the denture is fully seated and the retentive clasp arm has again become passive. A momentary tipping force is thus applied to the abutment during each placement and removal. This may not be a damaging force, since it is transient, so long as the force does not exceed the normal elasticity of the periodontal attachments. True reciprocation during placement and removal is possible only through the use of crown surfaces made parallel to the path of placement. The use of a ledge on a cast restoration permits the paralleling of the surfaces to be contacted by the reciprocal arm in such a manner that true reciprocation is made possible. This will be discussed in Chapter 13.

Second, the reciprocal clasp arm should be located so that the denture is stabilized against horizontal movement. This is possible only through the use of rigid clasp arms, rigid minor connectors, and a rigid major connector. Horizontal forces applied on one side of the dental arch are resisted by the stabilizing components on the opposite side. These are not only the reciprocal clasp arms but also all rigid components contacting vertical tooth surfaces. Obviously, the greater the number of such components, within reason, the greater will be the distribution of horizontal stresses.

Third, the reciprocal clasp arm may act to a minor degree as an indirect retainer.

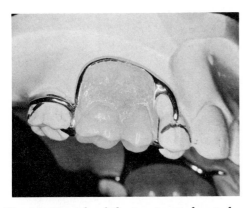

Fig. 6-9. Example of the two types of cast clasps in use. The molar abutment is engaged by a circumferential clasp originating above (or occlusal to) the height of contour, whereas the premolar abutment is engaged by a bar clasp originating from the base below (or gingival to) the height of contour. However, only the terminal tip of this clasp is placed in a measured undercut.

This is only true when it rests on a suprabulge surface of an abutment tooth lying anterior to the fulcrum line. Lifting of a distal extension base away from the tissues is thus resisted by a rigid arm, which is not easily displaced cervically. The effectiveness of such an indirect retainer is limited by its proximity to the fulcrum line, which gives it a relatively poor leverage advantage, and by the fact that slippage along tooth inclines is always possible. The latter may be prevented by the use of a ledge on a cast restoration, but enamel surfaces are not ordinarily so prepared.

Circumferential clasp arms. Although a thorough knowledge of the principles of clasp design should lead to a logical application of those principles, it is better that some of the more common clasp designs be considered individually. The circumferential clasp will be considered first as an all-cast clasp.

The cast circumferential clasp is usually the most logical clasp to use with all tooth-supported partial dentures because of its retentive and bracing ability. Only when the retentive undercut may be approached better with a bar clasp arm or when esthetics will be enhanced should the latter

be used (Fig. 6-9). The circumferential clasp arm does have the following disadvantages:

1. More tooth surface is covered than with a bar clasp arm because of its occlusal direction of approach.

2. On some tooth surfaces, particularly the buccal surface of mandibular teeth and the lingual surfaces of maxillary teeth, its occlusal approach may increase the width of the occlusal surface of the tooth.

3. In the mandibular arch more metal may be displayed than with a bar clasp arm.

4. As with all cast clasps, its half-round form prevents edgewise adjustment to increase or decrease retention. Adjustments in the retention afforded by a clasp arm should be made by moving a clasp terminal cervically into the angle of cervical convergence or occlusally into a lesser area of undercut. Tightening a clasp against the tooth or loosening it away from the tooth increases or decreases frictional resistance rather than adjusting the retentive potential of the clasp. *True adjustment is, therefore, impossible with most cast clasps.*

Despite its disadvantages, the cast circumferential clasp arm may be used effectively, and many of these disadvantages may be minimized by proper design. Adequate mouth preparations will permit its point of origin to be placed far enough below the occlusal surface to avoid poor esthetics and increased tooth dimension (Fig. 6-10). Although some of the other disadvantages listed imply that the bar-type clasp may be preferable, the circumferential-type clasp is actually superior to a bar clasp arm that is improperly used or poorly designed. Experience has shown that the possible advantages of the bar clasp arm are too often negated by faulty application and design, whereas the circumferential clasp arm is less easily misused.

The basic form of the circumferential-type clasp is a buccal and lingual arm originating from a common body (Fig. 6-11). This clasp is used improperly when two retentive clasp arms originate from the body

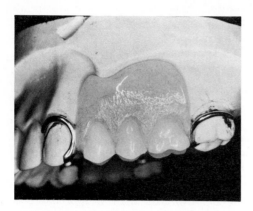

Fig. 6-10. Cast circumferential retentive clasp arms properly designed. They originate on or occlusally to the height of contour, which they then cross in their terminal third, and engage retentive undercuts progressively as their taper decreases and their flexibility increases.

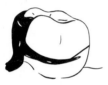

Fig. 6-11. Cast circumferential retentive clasp arm.

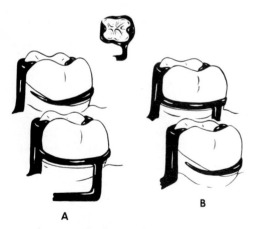

Fig. 6-12. Ring clasp encircling nearly all the tooth from its point of origin. **A,** The clasp originates on the mesiobuccal surface and encircles the tooth to engage a mesiolingual undercut. **B,** The clasp originates on the mesiolingual surface and encircles the tooth to engage a mesiobuccal undercut. In either case a supporting strut is used on the nonretentive side. (Drawn both as a direct view of the near side of the tooth and as a mirror view of the opposite side.)

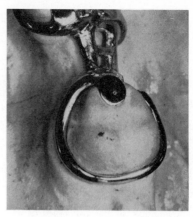

Fig. 6-13. Improperly designed ring clasp lacking necessary support. Such a clasp lacks any reciprocating or stabilizing action, since the entire circumference of the clasp is free to open and close. Instead, a supporting strut should always be added on the nonretentive side of the abutment tooth, which then becomes, in effect, a minor connector from which a tapered and flexible retentive clasp arm originates.

and occlusal rest areas and approach bilateral retentive areas on the side of the tooth away from the point of origin. The correct form of this clasp has only one retentive clasp arm, opposed by a nonretentive reciprocal arm on the opposite side. A common error is to use this clasp improperly by making both clasp terminals retentive. This is not only unnecessary but also disregards the need for reciprocation and bilateral stabilization.

The circumferential-type clasp may be used in several other forms. One is the *ring clasp*, which encircles nearly all of a tooth from its point of origin (Fig. 6-12). It is used when a proximal undercut cannot be approached by other means. For example, when a mesiolingual undercut on a lower molar abutment cannot be approached directly because of its proximity to the occlusal rest area, yet cannot be approached with a bar clasp arm because of lingual inclination of the tooth, the ring clasp encircling the tooth allows the undercut to be approached from the distal aspect of the tooth.

The ring clasp should never be used as an unsupported ring (Fig. 6-13) because

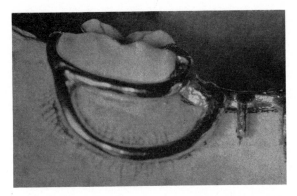

Fig. 6-14. Buccal strut supporting a mesially originating ring clasp. The flexible retentive arms begin at the distal occlusal rest and engage a mesiolingual undercut. Despite its resemblance to a bar-type clasp, this is a circumferential clasp by reason of its point of origin, the strut being actually an auxiliary minor connector.

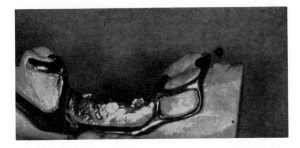

Fig. 6-15. Ring clasp engaging a mesiobuccal undercut on a mesially inclined lower right molar requires a supporting bar on the lingual surface to limit flexure to only the retentive portion of the clasp.

if it is free to open and close as a ring, it cannot provide either reciprocation or bracing. Instead, the ring clasp should always be used with a supporting strut on the nonretentive side, with or without an auxillary occlusal rest on the opposite marginal ridge. The advantage of an auxiliary rest is that further movement of a mesially inclined tooth is prevented by the presence of a distal rest. In any event, the supporting strut should be regarded as being a minor connector from which the flexible retentive arm originates. Reciprocation then comes from the rigid portion of the clasp lying between the supporting strut and the principal occlusal rest. (See Figs 6-14 and 6-15.)

The ring clasp should be used on protected abutments whenever possible because it covers such a large area of tooth surface. Esthetics usually need not be considered on such a posteriorly located tooth.

A ring clasp may be used in reverse on an abutment located anterior to a tooth-bound edentulous space (Fig. 6-16). Whereas potentially an effective clasp, this clasp covers an excessive amount of tooth surface and is esthetically objectionable. The only justification for its use is when a distobuccal or distolingual undercut cannot be approached directly from the occlusal rest area, yet tissue undercuts prevent its approach from a gingical direction with a bar clasp arm.

The *back-action* and *reverse back-action* clasps are modifications of the ring clasp, with all of its disadvantages and no apparent advantages (Fig. 6-17). *It is difficult to ever justify their use.* The undercut can usually be approached just as well with a conventional circumferential clasp, with

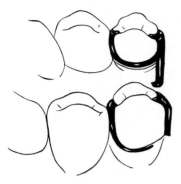

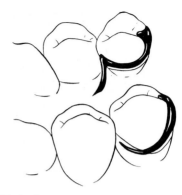

Fig. 6-16. Ring clasp may be used in reverse on an abutment located anterior to a tooth-bound edentulous space.

Fig. 6-17. Back-action circumferential clasp used on a premolar abutment anterior to an edentulous space.

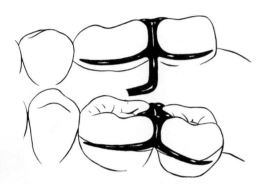

Fig. 6-18. Embrasure clasp is used where no edentulous space exists. Although in this drawing both retentive clasp arms are located on the buccal surface, and the nonretentive arms on the lingual surface, retention and reciprocation can be reversed on both teeth or on either tooth.

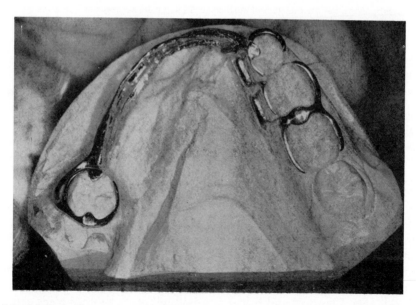

Fig. 6-19. Multiple clasping in a surgically mutilated mouth. On the right are an embrasure clasp, a bar clasp arm, and a conventional circumferential clasp engaging lingual undercuts on three abutment teeth. On the left is a well-designed ring clasp engaging a lingual undercut, with supporting strut on the buccal surface and auxiliary occlusal rest to prevent mesial tipping. Note the rigid design of the major connector.

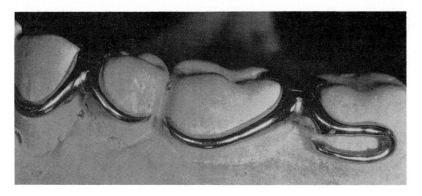

Fig. 6-20. Embrasure and hairpin circumferential retentive clasp arms. The terminus of each engages a suitable retentive undercut. Use of hairpin-type clasp on the second molar is made necessary by the fact that the only available undercut lies directly below the point of origin of the clasp arm.

less tooth coverage and less display of metal. With the C-type clasp, the proximal tooth surface can be used properly as a guiding plane, as it should be, and the occlusal rest can have the rigid support it requires. An occlusal rest always should be attached to some rigid minor connector and should never be supported by a clasp arm alone. If the occlusal rest is part of a flexible assembly, it cannot function adequately as an occlusal rest. *Unfortunately, the back-action clasp is still being used, despite the fact that it is biologically and mechanically unsound.*

In the construction of an unmodified Class II or Class III partial denture, there are no edentulous spaces on the opposite side of the arch to aid in clasping. Mechanically, this is a disadvantage. However, when the teeth are sound and retentive areas are available or when multiple restorations are justified, clasping is accomplished by means of an *embrasure clasp* (Figs. 6-18 and 6-19).

Sufficient space must be provided between the abutment teeth in their occlusal third to make room for the common body of the embrasure clasp (Fig. 6-20), yet the contact area should not be eliminated entirely. Since vulnerable areas of the teeth are involved, abutment protection with inlays or crowns is indicated in almost every instance. The decision to use unprotected

abutments must be made at the time of oral examination and should be based on the age of the patient, caries index, and oral hygiene, as well as on whether or not existing tooth contours are favorable.

The embrasure clasp always should be used with double occlusal rests, even when definite proximal shoulders can be established (Fig. 6-21). This is to avoid interproximal wedging by the prothesis, which could cause separation of the abutment teeth and result in food impaction and clasp displacement. In addition to providing support, occlusal rests also serve to shunt food away from contact areas. For this reason, occlusal rests should always be used whenever food impaction is possible.

Embrasure clasps should have two retentive clasp arms and two reciprocal clasp arms, either bilaterally or diagonally opposed. An auxillary occlusal rest or a bar clasp arm can be substituted for a circumferential reciprocal arm as long as definite reciprocation and bracing result. A lingually placed retentive bar clasp arm may be substituted, if a rigid circumferential clasp arm is placed on the buccal surface for reciprocation.

Other modifications of the cast circumferential clasp are the multiple clasp, the half-and-half clasp, and the reverse action clasp. The *multiple clasp* is simply two opposing C-type clasps joined at the terminal

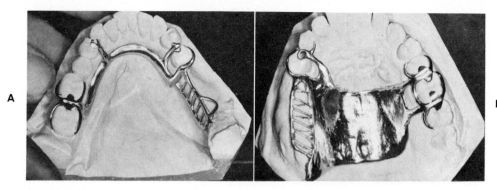

Fig. 6-21. Two examples of the use of embrasure clasps for Class II partially edentulous arches. **A,** Mandibular Class II. Embrasure clasps on two left molar abutments, buccal wrought-wire retention on the right second premolar, and indirect retainer on the left first premolar and canine. **B,** Maxillary Class II. Embrasure clasps on left premolar and first molar with additional occlusal rest and lingual stabilizing arm on the second molar. Buccal wrought-wire retention on the right premolar. The palatal connector avoids the palatal rugae and unnecessary contact with gingival tissues. Posteriorly the connector crosses the midline symmetrically just anterior to the posterior limit of immobile palatal tissues. (Modified from McCracken's partial denture construction, ed. 3, St. Louis, 1969, The C. V. Mosby Co.)

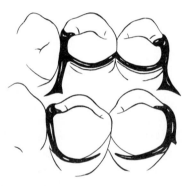

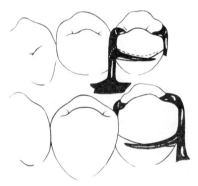

Fig. 6-22. Multiple clasp is actually two opposing "C-type" clasps joined at the terminal end of the two reciprocal arms.

Fig. 6-23. Half-and-half clasp consists of one circumferential retentive arm arising from the distal and a second circumferential arm arising from the mesial on the opposite side, with or without a secondary occlusal rest. The dotted line illustrates a nonretentive reciprocal clasp arm used without a secondary occlusal rest.

end of the two reciprocal arms (Fig. 6-22). It is used when additional retention is needed, usually on tooth-borne partial dentures. It may be used for multiple clasping in instances in which the partial denture replaces an entire half of the dental arch. It may be used rather than an embrasure clasp when the only available retentive areas are adjacent to each other. Its disadvantage is that two embrasure approaches are necessary rather than a single common embrassure for both clasps.

The *half-and-half clasp* consists of a circumferential retentive arm arising from one

direction and a reciprocal arm arising from another (Fig. 6-23). Since the second arm must arise from a second minor connector, this arm is actually a bar clasp used with or without an auxiliary occlusal rest. Reciprocation arising from a second minor connector can usually be accomplished with a short bar or with an auxiliary occlusal rest, thereby avoiding so much tooth coverage. Thus it is apparent that there is little justi-

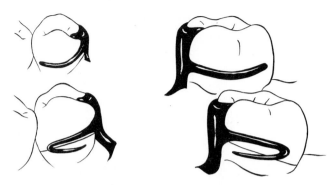

Fig. 6-24. Reverse-action or hairpin clasp arm may be used when a proximal undercut lies below the point of origin of the clasp. It can be used on any posterior abutment, but it may be esthetically objectionable and covers considerable tooth surface.

fication for the use of the half-and-half clasp in bilateral dentures. Its design was originally intended to provide dual retention, a principle that should be applied only to unilateral denture design.

The *reverse action* or *hairpin clasp arm* is designed to permit engaging a proximal undercut from an occlusal approach (Fig. 6-24). Other methods of accomplishing the same result are with a ring clasp originating on the opposite side of the tooth or with a bar clasp arm originating from a gingival direction. However, when a proximal undercut must be used on a posterior abutment and when tissue undercuts or high tissue attachments prevent the use of a bar clasp arm, the reverse action clasp may be used successfully. Although the ring clasp would be preferable, lingual undercuts may prevent the placement of a supporting strut without tongue interference. In this limited situation the hairpin clasp arm serves adequately, despite its several disadvantages. The clasp covers considerable tooth surface and may trap debris; its occlusal origin may increase the functional load on the tooth, and its flexibility is limited. Esthetics usually need not be considered when the clasp is used on a posterior abutment, but the hairpin clasp arm does have the additional disadvantage of displaying too much metal for use on an anterior abutment.

Properly designed, the reverse action clasp should make a hairpin turn to engage an undercut below the point of origin (Fig. 6-24). The upper arm of this clasp should be considered a minor connector giving rise to the tapered lower arm. Therefore only the lower arm should be flexible, with the retentive portion beginning beyond the turn only the lower arm should flex over the height of contour to engage a retentive undercut. The clasp should be designed and fabricated with this in mind.

These are the various types of cast circumferential clasps. As mentioned previously, they may be used in combination with bar clasp arms as long as differentiation is made by their location and bulk between retention and reciprocation. Circumferential and bar clasp arms may be made either flexible (retentive) or rigid (reciprocal) in any combination as long as each retentive clasp arm is opposed by a rigid reciprocal arm.

The use of many of the less desirable clasp forms can be avoided by changing the crown forms of the abutments with full restorations. In fabricating abutment coverage, tooth contours should be established that will permit the use of the most desirable clasp forms rather than reproduce a form that makes necessary the use of less desirable clasp designs.

Bar clasp arms. The term *bar clasp arm* is generally preferred over the less descriptive term *Roach clasp arm*. Reduced to its simplest terms, the bar clasp arm arises from the denture framework or a metal base and approaches the retentive undercut from a gingival direction (Fig. 6-9).

The bar clasp arm has been classified by the shape of the retentive terminal. Thus it has been identified as a T, modified T, Y, C, I, U, E, R, or S clasp arm. All have the same characteristics in common: they originate from the framework or base and approach the undercut from a gingival direction. The form the terminal takes is of little significance as long as it is mechanically and functionally effective, covers as little tooth surface as possible, and displays as little metal as possible.

The T and Y clasp arms are the most frequently misused. It is unlikely that the full area of a T or Y terminal is ever necessary for adequate clasp retention. Whereas the larger area of contact would provide greater frictional resistance, this is not true clasp retention and only that portion engaging an undercut area should be considered retentive. Usually, only one terminal of such a clasp arm is placed in an undercut area. The remainder of the clasp arm is therefore superfluous unless it is needed as part of the clasp assembly to encircle the abutment tooth more than 180 degrees of its greatest circumference, passing from diverging axial surfaces to converging axial surfaces. If the bar clasp arm is made to be flexible

for retentive purposes, it is highly improbable that any suprabulge portion of the clasp will provide stabilization and bracing, since it is also part of the flexible arm. Therefore the suprabulge portion of a T or Y clasp arm may be dispensed with in many instances and the clasp terminal placed in

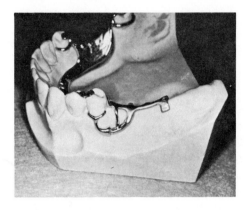

Fig. 6-26. Bar clasp arm on a distal abutment must be made light enough to be flexible and may be used only when it can engage a proximal undercut adjacent to the extension base. The mesial T portion of the clasp arm had to be placed to encompass the abutment by more than 180 degrees. It is placed on the height of contour. Note the finishing line where the clasp and denture base will join.

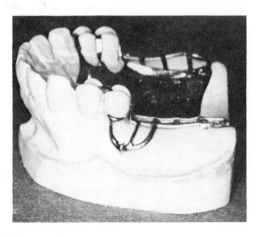

Fig. 6-27. Bar clasp arm on a maxillary terminal abutment. Note the uniform taper from the point where it will emerge from a resin base, and the fact that it engages the tooth undercut on the *side adjacent* to the distal extension base. A butt-type joint for a finishing line between the direct retainer and the acrylic resin base is provided.

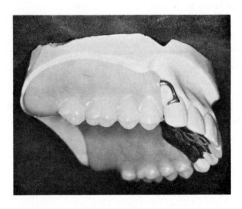

Fig. 6-25. Bar clasp arm properly used on a terminal abutment. A mesial extension or T is neither advantageous nor desirable in this situation since the abutment tooth was encompassed more than 180 degrees.

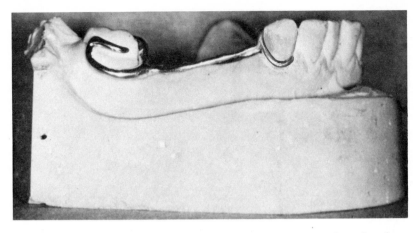

Fig. 6-28. Bar clasp arm on a lower molar abutment engaging a mesiobuccal undercut. Note the proper utilization of parallel proximal guiding planes. (Modified from McCracken's partial denture construction, ed. 3, St. Louis, 1969, The C. V. Mosby Co.)

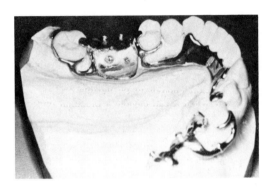

Fig. 6-29. Bar clasps used for both retention and reciprocation. Bar-type retainer on right second premolar engages a distobuccal undercut. The bar-type configuration on the lingual of the molar is utilized for reciprocation and bracing.

a retentive undercut. It matters little whether the arm takes the form of a modified T, the curve of a C, of the more direct approach of an I.

The L clasp is simply an I clasp with a longer arm and the U merely a double I. In the S clasp the arm is given an S turn, supposedly to make it more flexible; actually, its only purpose should be to avoid a tissue undercut. The terminal of the bar clasp should be designed to be biologically and mechanically sound rather than to conform to any alphabetical connotation.

With only one exception, the bar clasp arm should be used only with tooth-borne partial dentures or tooth-borne modification areas. This exception is when an undercut that logically can be approached with a bar clasp arm lies on the side of an abutment tooth adjacent to a distal extension base (Figs. 6-25 to 6-29). If a tissue undercut prevents such use of a bar clasp arm, a mesially originating ring clasp, a cast, or a wrought-wire reverse action clasp may be used.

A bar clasp arm should never be used on a terminal abutment if the undercut lies on the side of the tooth away from the extension base. The bar clasp arm is not a particularly flexible clasp arm because of the effect of its half-round form and its several planes of origin. Although the cast circumferential clasp arm can be made more flexible than can the bar clasp arm, the combination clasp is much preferred for use on all terminal abutments when torque and tipping are possible because of engaging an undercut away from the distal extension base. Occasionally, however, a situation exists in which a bar clasp arm may be used to advantage without jeopardizing a terminal abutment. In this instance alone, a bar clasp arm swinging distally into the undercut is a logical choice, since movement of the abutment, as the distal extension base moves tissueward, is avoided by the distal location of the clasp terminal.

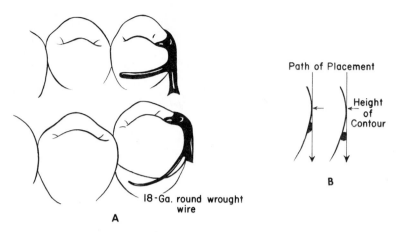

Fig. 6-30. A, Combination clasp consists of a cast reciprocal clasp and a wrought-wire retentive clasp arm. The latter is either cast to or soldered to the cast framework. **B,** In addition to the advantages of flexibility, adjustability, and appearance, the wrought-wire retentive arm makes only a line contact with the abutment tooth, rather than the broader contact of the cast clasp.

The specific indications for using a bar clasp arm are (1) when a small degree of undercut exists in the cervical third of the abutment tooth, which may be approached from a gingival direction, and (2) with a single exception, on abutment teeth when they support tooth-borne partial dentures or tooth-borne modification areas. Thus use of the bar clasp arm is contraindicated when a deep cervical undercut exists or when a severe tissue undercut exists, either of which must be bridged by excessive blockout. When severe tooth and tissue undercuts exist, which must be blocked out, the presence of a bar clasp arm usually results in annoyance to tongue and cheek and in the trapping of food debris.

The combination clasp. The combination clasp consists of a wrought-wire retentive clasp arm and a cast reciprocal clasp arm (Fig. 6-30). Although the latter may be in the form of a bar clasp arm, it is usually a circumferential arm. The retentive arm is almost always circumferential, but it also may be used in the manner of a bar, originating gingivally from the denture base.

The advantages of the combination clasp lie in the *flexibility,* the *adjustibility,* and the *appearance* of the wrought-wire retentive arm. It is used when maximum flexibility is desirable, such as on an abutment

tooth adjacent to a distal extension base or on a particularly weak abutment. It may be used for its adjustability when precise retentive requirements are unpredictable and later adjustment to increase or decrease retention may be necessary. A third justification for its use is its esthetic advantage over cast clasps. Being wrought in structure, it may be used in smaller diameters than a cast clasp with less danger of fracture. Being round in form, light is refracted in such a manner that the display of metal is less noticeable than with the broader surfaces of a cast clasp.

The most common use of the combination clasp is on an abutment tooth adjacent to a distal extension base. When a distal undercut exists that may be approached with a properly designed bar clasp arm or with a ring clasp (despite its several disadvantages), a cast clasp can be located so that it will not cause abutment tipping as the distal extension base moves tissueward. When the undercut is on the side of the abutment away from the extension base, the wrought-wire retentive arm offers greater flexibility than does the cast clasp arm and therefore better dissipates functional stresses. For this reason the combination clasp is preferred (Fig. 6-31).

The combination clasp has two disad-

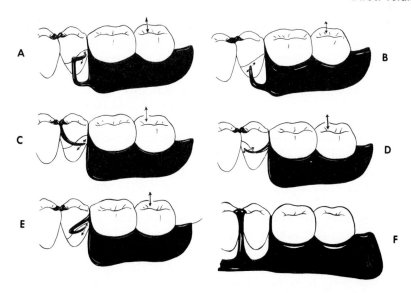

Fig. 6-31. Five types of extracoronal direct retainer assemblies that may be used on an abutment adjacent to a distal extension base. The arrows indicate the general direction of movement of the retentive tips of the retainer arms when the denture base rotates toward and away from the edentulous ridge. **A,** A distobuccal undercut engaged by a one-half T-type bar clasp. The portion of the clasp arm on and above the height of contour will afford some bracing against horizontal rotation of the denture base. **B,** An I bar placed in an undercut at the middle (anteroposteriorly) of the buccal surface. This retainer contacts the tooth only at its tip. Note that the guiding plane on the distal of the abutment is contacted by metal of the denture framework and that a mesial rest is utilized. **C,** An interproximal ring-type clasp engaging a distobuccal undercut. A bar-type retainer cannot be used because of the tissue undercuts inferior to the buccal surface of the abutment. **D,** An 18-gauge wrought-wire circumferential retainer arm engaging a mesiobuccal undercut. A wrought-wire arm, instead of a cast arm, must be used in this situation because of the ability of the wrought wire to flex omnidirectionally. A cast half-round retainer arm would not flex edgewise, resulting in excessive stress to the tooth when rotation of the denture base occurs. **E,** Hairpin-type clasp may be used when the undercut lies cervical to the origin of the retainer arm. Both the hairpin and interproximal ring types of clasps may be used to engage a distobuccal undercut on the terminal abutment of a distal extension denture. However, a distobuccal undercut on the terminal abutment should be engaged by a bar-type clasp in the absence of a gross buccal tissue undercut cervical to the terminal abutment. The hairpin and interproximal ring clasps are the least desirable of the clasping situations illustrated here. **F,** Lingual view shows the use of double occlusal rests, connected to the lingual bar by a minor connector in the illustrated designs. This design eliminates the need for a lingual clasp arm, places the fulcrum line anteriorly to better utilize the residual ridge for support, and provides bracing against horizontal rotation of the denture base.

vantages: (1) the extra steps in fabrication, particularly when high-fusing chrome alloys are used, and (2) the fact that it is easily distorted by careless handling on the part of the patient. The disadvantages of the wrought-wire clasp are offset by its advantages, which are (1) its flexibility, (2) its adjustability, (3) its esthetic advantage over other retentive circumferential clasp arms, and (4) the fact that a minimum of tooth surface is covered because of its line

contact with the tooth rather than the surface contact of a cast clasp arm.

The disadvantages listed previously should not prevent its use regardless of the type of alloy being used for the cast framework. Technical problems are minimized by selecting the best wrought wire for this purpose and then either casting to it or soldering it to the cast framework. Eighteen-gauge round Ticonium wrought wire has proved to be an excellent material. It is tough, yet flexible enough, and not expensive. Gold alloys and Ticonium may be cast to it, and it may be soldered to the higher-fusing chrome alloys. The technique for adapting wrought-wire clasp arms will be given in Chapter 17.

The patient may be taught to avoid distortion of the wrought wire by explaining that the fingernail should always be applied to its point of origin, where it is held rigid by the casting rather than at the flexible terminal end. Frequently, lingual retention may be used rather than buccal retention, especially on a mandibular abutment, so that the wrought-wire arm is never touched by the patient during removal of the denture. Instead, removal may be accomplished by lifting against the cast reciprocal arm located on the buccal side of the tooth. However, this negates the esthetic advantage of the wrought-wire clasp arm, and esthetics may be given preference when the choice must be made between buccal and lingual retention. Frequently, however, retention must be used where it is found and the clasp designed accordingly.

Lingual retention in conjunction with internal rests. The internal rest has been covered in Chapter 5. It has been emphasized that the internal rest is not utilized as a retainer but that its near-vertical walls provide for reciprocation against a lingually placed retentive clasp arm. For this rea-son visible clasp arms may be eliminated, thus meeting one of the principal objections to the extracoronal retainer.

Such a retentive clasp arm, terminating in an existing or prepared infrabulge area on the abutment tooth, may be of any acceptable design. It is usually a circumferential arm arising from the body of the denture framework at the rest area. It should be wrought, for the advantages of adjustability and flexibility make the wrought clasp arm preferable. It may be made of either platinum-gold-palladium or of chrome-cobalt alloy and may be cast-to with gold or chrome-cobalt alloy or be assembled by soldering to one of the higher-fusing chrome-cobalt alloys. In any event, future adjustment or repair is facilitated.

The use of lingual extracoronal retention avoids much of the cost of the internal attachment yet disposes of a visible clasp arm when esthetics must be considered. Frequently its use with a tooth-supported partial denture is employed only on the anterior abutments, and the posterior abutments, when esthetics is not a consideration, are clasped in the conventional manner. (See Figs. 5-6 to 5-8.)

Other types of clasps. Several other types of clasps will be considered briefly. One is the *mesiodistal clasp*. It is sometimes used on isolated abutments when some retention is desired. It should never be used when a

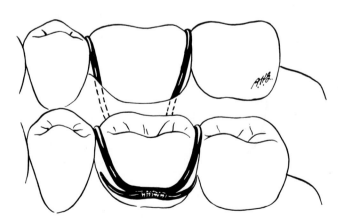

Fig. 6-32. Crib-type clasp used in removable orthodontic appliances and interim partial dentures.

distal extension base is involved, because tipping of the abutment would be inevitable.

In most instances the tooth must be prepared to receive this type of clasp. Its flexibility lies in its ability to open and close as it engages bilateral proximal undercuts. It must be kept thin and flexible. To be effective the tips of the clasp must engage part of the labial or buccal surface, but they should be made wide and flat interproximally to display as little metal as possible. Since adjoining tooth replacements would prevent the intended action of the clasp, the mesiodistal clasp may be used only when interproximal spaces that are not to be filled by other parts of the denture exist.

The *crib clasp* is a wrought-wire clasp frequently used in removable orthodontic appliances (Fig. 6-32). Retention from the crib clasp is not obtained from the crib alone but rather from the retentive terminals attached to it by soldering.

The *infrabulge clasp* is a bar clasp arm arising from the border of the base, either as an extension of a cast base or attached to the border of a resin base (Fig. 6-33). It is made more flexible than the usual bar clasp arm by separating that portion of the cast base that gives rise to the clasp arm from the clasp arm itself, either by making a saw cut or by casting against a separating

shim of matrix metal, which is later removed with acid. It may be made more flexible through the use of wrought wire, which is either attached to a metal base by soldering or embedded in the border of a resin base.

Some of the advantages attributed to the infrabulge clasp are (1) its interproximal location, which may be used to esthetic advantage; (2) increased retention without tipping action on the abutment, and (3) less chance of accidental distortion due to its proximity to the denture border. The infrabulge clasp is not a hygienic clasp design because of the narrow separation that tends to trap debris and is therefore not readily cleaned by tongue and saliva. The wearer should be meticulous in his care of a denture so made, not only for reasons of oral hygiene but also to prevent cariogenic debris from being held against tooth surfaces.

Dr. Vincent J. Oddo, Jr., developed the *"movable-arm" clasp* (Fig. 6-34). Support in the form of occlusal rests and bracing in the form of other elements are used in conjunction with the movable-arm clasp.

The retentive portions of the clasp are placed in undercut regions of the abutment tooth after the denture is seated in the mouth. This of course will eliminate the spring tension exhibited by conventional extracoronal direct retainers when the partial denture is seated and removed.

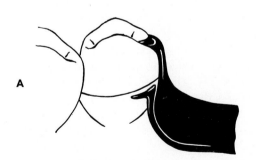
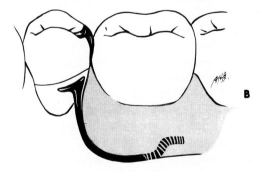

Fig. 6-33. Infrabulge clasp designed by Dr. M. M. DeVan. In **A** the clasp arm arises from the border of a metal base and is separated from it with a saw cut or by having been cast against a separating shim, which is later removed. A wrought-wire retentive arm may be soldered to the metal base to serve the same purpose. In **B** the clasp arm is attached to the border of a resin base. This is usually a wrought-wire clasp arm partially embedded in the resin base at the border.

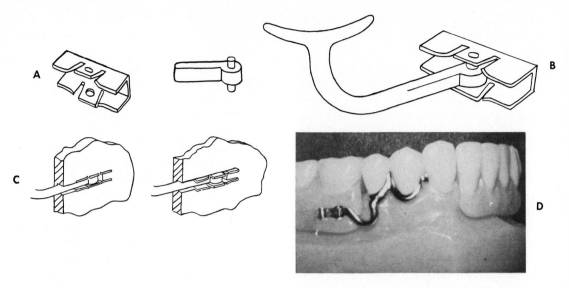

Fig. 6-34. **A,** Components for fabricating the movable-arm clasp is available in kit form. Metal spring-lock box (left) and rigid plastic burnout pattern used to fabricate the cast retentive arm. **B,** Cast retentive arm of direct retainer assembled in spring-lock box (open position). **C,** Assembled unit is located in waxed denture base prior to processing in acrylic resin (right figure). Movable-arm clasp assembly in acrylic resin base (left figure). Projecting portions of spring-lock box are finished flush with resin base. Spring tension on movable-arm can be varied by adjusting the upper and lower edges of the spring-lock box. **D,** Interproximal movable-arm clasp in the closed position. (Redrawn from Oddo, Vincent, J., Jr.: The movable-arm clasp for complete passivity to partial denture construction, J. Am. Dent. Assoc. **74:**1008-1015, April, 1967. **D,** Courtesy Dr. Vincent J. Oddo, Jr.)

Advantages of the movable-arm partial denture as stated by Dr. Oddo include:

(1) Each clasp is treated separately and, as a result, a common path of placement of a number of clasps on one partial denture is no longer a concern.

(2) Clasp tension, loosening, flexibility, and breakage are not considered since passivity eliminates stress and flexibility.

(3) Since the retentive arm can be placed anywhere in the undercut region, esthetics is improved.

The movable-arm principles seem sound and continued clinical evaluation of the movable-arm denture is most worthy. However, the occurrence of inherent problems with movable portions of partial dentures in construction, cost, service, adjustment, and occasional replacement must also be weighed as well as their advantages.

Clasping teeth in sequence. Many removable partial dentures can be designed to great advantage by clasping teeth in sequence, provided these teeth have a proximal contact with each other. Frequently, when all molars are missing in the lower arch, the rest areas may be shifted to the mesial part of the first premolars to avoid the acute tipping angle of the denture base when an occlusal rest is placed on the distocclusal surface of the terminal abutment (Fig. 6-35). The mesial portion of the clasp engages the mesiobuccal surface of the first premolar with a short arm for reciprocation only. As the clasp assembly crosses the occlusal surface, it provides the occlusal rest (placed in a prepared rest seat) and continues along the lingual surface of both premolars at the height of contour. When the clasp reaches its distal surface of the second premolar, it springs into position below the distal marginal ridge of the

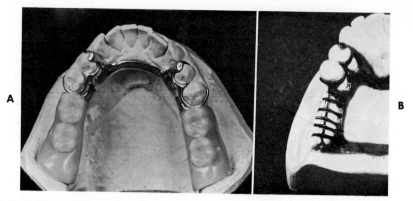

Fig. 6-35. A, Premolars are clasped in sequence. Note that the premolars, as a unit on either side, are engaged by the clasp assembly by over 180 degrees of their collective, greatest circumference. **B,** The same design can be used to esthetic and functional advantage in the maxillary arch that has corresponding edentulous regions and when the premolars are in a marked buccal version. An unsightly display of metal on the buccal surfaces of the premolars is also avoided. (From Steffel, V. L.: J. Prosthet. Dent. **12:**524-535, 1962.)

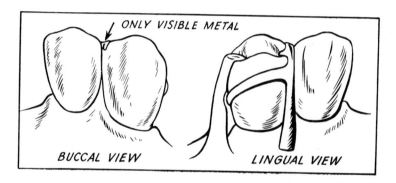

Fig. 6-36. Saddle-Lock principle of hidden clasp retention. This effectively conceals retentive clasps but may do so at the expense of proximal guiding planes and unprotected tooth surfaces. These objections can be overcome by providing parallel guiding surfaces on protective crown or inlay restorations occlusal to the area used for retentive purposes. The vertical minor connector supporting the occlusal rest is separated from the retentive clasp arm by applying a protective coating over the clasp pattern and then waxing the vertical minor connector over it. It should also be noted that the bracing element of the clasp assembly is located disadvantageously, being placed in the occlusal one-third portion of the abutment tooth. (Courtesy Saddle-Lock, Inc., Brooklyn, N. Y.)

tooth and its end engages the distobuccal undercut. Minor connectors join the assembly to the lingual bar at the occlusal rest and between the premolars.

Mesiodistal clasping of posterior abutment teeth. Several dental laboratory companies have stressed the esthetic advantages of mesiodistal clasping (Figs. 6-36 and 6-37). *Whereas esthetics is desirable, it should not be given precedence over biologic considerations.* Such mesiodistal clasp-

ing utilizes the same areas on abutment teeth that are the most vulnerable to caries attack and also those surfaces that ordinarily should be utilized for guiding planes.

When enamel surfaces are sound and other factors are favorable, when the use of guiding planes is not jeopardized, and when adequate reciprocation is provided, proximal undercuts may be used to obtain better esthetic placement of clasp retainers. Such clasps should be designed to include

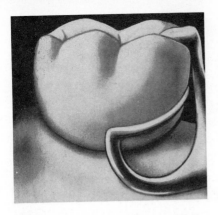

Fig. 6-37. Utilization of a proximal undercut provides excellent and esthetically acceptable retention but prevents effective use of a proximal guiding plane and may jeopardize a surface vulnerable to caries attack unless the crown is protected with a cast restoration. (Courtesy Saddle-Lock, Inc., Brooklyn, N. Y.)

more than half of the greatest tooth circumference, which is difficult to accomplish without some display of metal.

Mesiodistal clasping is most effective when used in conjunction with cast restorations and internal rests. Internal rests eliminate the need for the clasp to include more than 180 degrees of the tooth, since the boxlike rest seat provides adequate stabilization of the abutment tooth. On cast restorations, proximal undercuts may be created without fear of jeopardizing areas that would be vulnerable on the natural tooth. On cast restorations also, guiding planes need not be ignored, even when a proximal undercut is utilized for retention.

In some modern clasp designs the occlusal rest is separated from the clasp retainer to allow flexing into interproximal areas. While accomplishing its intended purpose of better esthetics, this design ignores the need for guiding planes and results in an unhygienic clasp because of the trapping of debris. Such clasps are mechanically sound but biologically objectionable. Moreover, the technician frequently leaves the clasp terminal embedded in resin, rendering it totally inactive as a retentive clasp arm.

The choice of clasp designs should be based upon biologic as well as mechanical principles. The dentist responsible for the treatment being rendered the patient must be able to justify the clasp design used for each abutment tooth in keeping with these principles.

Hart-Dunn attachment for unilateral distal extension partial dentures.[*] Objections to the use of embrasure clasp retainers on the nonedentulous side of a Class II partially edentulous arch can be met with the use of the Hart-Dunn attachment partial denture. Retention is by an embrasure hook consisting of 18- or 19-gauge round wrought wires placed just beneath the contact areas in the mesial and distal areas of the selected abutment tooth, slightly curved to allow easy placement from the lingual direction and protection of the interdental papillae. Stabilization is provided by occlusal rests mesially and distally, which also serve to prevent the wires from settling into the interdental papillae (Fig. 6-38).

Mann has emphasized that, because the Hart-Dunn attachment is placed in a horizontal direction just prior to seating the clasp on the opposite or denture base side, conventional surveying of the abutment teeth cannot be used. This is to say that guiding planes to placement and removal are not used. Instead, a divider is used for surveying the cast. Mann is quoted directly, as follows:

One point of the divider is placed on the center of rotation for the attachment (at a point midway between the embrasure hook and the occlusal rests), and the other end of the divider is swept over the buccal and lingual surfaces of the abutment tooth on the opposite side and over the lingual denture base area on the study [diagnostic] cast. Either a precision [internal] attachment or a circumferential clasp can be used on the denture base side to lock the partial denture in position. However, *these retainers must be on the arc scribed by the divider* in order that the at-

---

[*]Dunn, A. L.: A safe temporary partial denture, J. Am. Dent. Assoc. **23:**96-99, 1936.

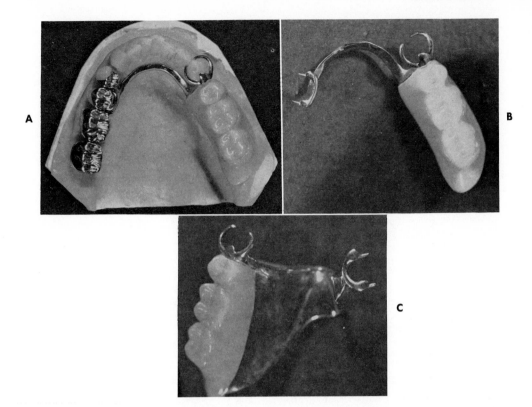

Fig. 6-38. Hart-Dunn attachment for distal extension partial dentures. **A,** Mandibular Class II distal extension partial denture retained by circumferential clasping on the terminal abutment on the edentulous side and embrasure wires on either side of the left second premolar. **B,** The partial denture off of the cast, showing the occlusal rests and embrasure wires. **C,** Maxillary Clasp II partial denture of similar design with split palatal bar stressbreaker leading from the clasp retainer on the edentulous side abutment. The use of a cast circumferential direct retainer on the terminal abutment of the edentulous side in these illustrations is questioned as being sound.

tachment can first be seated horizontally, then the clasp or attachment on the denture base side is seated occlusogingivally. If the abutment on the denture base side is inclined toward the buccal, it presents an undercut problem. This can be solved best by constructing a cast crown to eliminate the undercut. . . .*

Either an internal attachment or a conventional clasp on the denture base side may be used. On the opposite side, the hook may be fitted into the pontic casting of a fixed partial denture rather than embrasure hooks. A prefabricated hook suggested and designed by Dr. George Hollen-

back for this purpose is commercially available.*

Other types of retainers

Numerous other types of retainers for partial dentures have been devised that cannot be classified as being primarily of the intracoronal or extracoronal type. Neither can they be classified as relying primarily on frictional resistance or placement of an element in an undercut to prevent displacement of the denture. However, all these utilize some type of locking device, located either intracoronally or extracoro-

---

*From Mann, A. W.: The lower distal extension partial denture using the Hart-Dunn Attachment, J. Prosthet. Dent. 8:282-288, 1958.

*Williams hook attachment, Williams Gold Refining Co., Buffalo, N. Y.

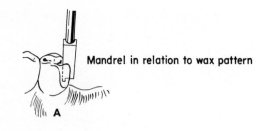

Mandrel in relation to wax pattern

A

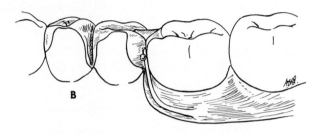

B

Fig. 6-39. Neurohr spring-lock attachment. **A,** The tapered mandrel used in the surveyor to form the vertical rest. **B,** The spring wire lock soldered to the denture base, engaging a depression in the abutment tooth casting.

nally, for providing retention without visible clasp retention. Although the motivation behind the development of other types of retainers has usually been a desire to eliminate visible clasp retainers, the desire to minimize torque and tipping stresses on the abutment teeth has also been given consideration.

All of the few retainers that will be discussed herein have merit, and much credit is due those who have developed specific devices and techniques for the retaining of partial dentures. Unfortunately, not all can be included without devoting considerable space to the history and development of partial denture retaining devices. Also, the use of patented retaining devices and other techniques falls in the same limited category as the internal attachment prosthesis and is, for economic and technical reasons, available to only a small percentage of those patients needing partial denture service.

Neurohr spring-lock attachment. One of the earlier attempts at eliminating partial denture clasps and at the same time providing adequate extracoronal retention was the spring wire lock system of attachment de-

vised by Dr. F. G. Neurohr and patented in 1930 (Fig. 6-39). The Neurohr method employs tapered vertical rests retained within the contours of the abutment tooth. A single buccal clasp arm engages an undercut in the abutment casting and retains the partial denture in place. Occlusal stress is transmitted to the abutment tooth in a near vertical direction. However, some distal tipping force may be applied to the abutment when this attachment is used with a distal extension denture unless adequate support of the denture base by the residual ridge is maintained.

Sherer spring-lock attachment. The Sherer spring-lock attachment also uses a tapered vertical rest but utilizes a dovetail seat to prevent displacement (Fig. 6-40). This attachment was developed by Dr. J. W. Sherer in 1938. An L-shaped flat spring arm is soldered close to the keyed rest where it engages an undercut in the abutment casting. The authors question the use of any locking-type internal attachment for distal extension partial dentures.

Clark attachment. The Clark method of attachment, developed by Dr. E. B. Clark in 1938, makes use of the Neurohr-Williams

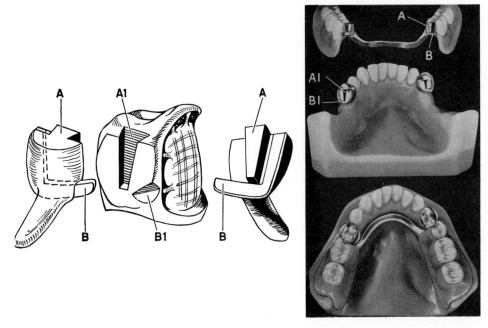

Fig. 6-40. Sherer spring-lock attachment. The tapered male, **A**, attached to the partial denture, slides into the counterpart female at **A1**, which is part of the abutment casting. When these are firmly in place, they are held by the spring lock, **B**, attached to the male, which engages a seat, **B1**, ground into the gold faceplate of the abutment casting. (Courtesy J. F. Jelenko & Co., Inc., New York, N. Y.)

rest shoe, which provides a thin-gauge platinum box for the tapered Neurohr-type rest. The rest shoes are placed in the several abutment castings with the aid of a mandrel held in the surveyor related to the master cast according to a predetermined path of placement. This differs little from the original Neurohr technique and the technique for placing other types of internal attachments. Rather than use a spring lock for retention, however, a lingual clasp arm on the denture casting is used to engage an undercut that has been created in the abutment casting on the side of the tooth away from the tapered rest (Fig. 6-41). Thus occlusal support, stability, and retention are provided without the use of a visible clasp arm. Tipping of the abutment tooth is probable when this attachment, with its cast retentive lingual arm, is used in conjunction with a distal extension denture, thus imposing somewhat the same limitations to the use of this attachment as to some other combinations utilizing in-

ternal attachments. All these are most applicable to tooth-borne restorations and should be used with distal extension dentures only with some type of stress-breaking action in the design of the denture itself or when multiple splinted abutment crowns are used, or when the lingual arm or other retentive element can be made of wrought wire and is long enough to be flexible.

Rybeck[*] has presented the technique for the use of the Clark attachment in detail. In personal correspondence he has further emphasized the stress-breaking action of this design by pointing out that the sidewalls of the attachment are perpendicular to the fulcrum line and thus permit the partial denture to rotate without placing a distal stress on the abutment tooth. He has also emphasized that the design of the clasp arm should be such that only minimal

---

[*]Rybeck, S. A.: Simplicity in a distal extension partial denture, J. Prosthet. Dent. 4:87-92, 1954.

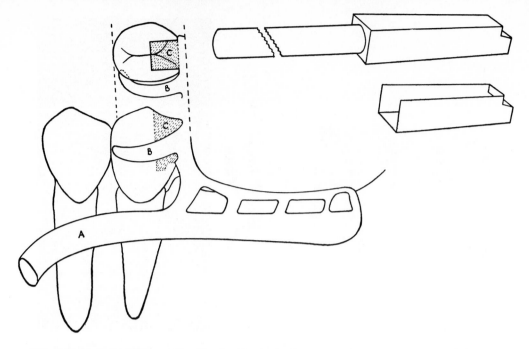

Fig. 6-41. Neurohr-Williams shoe No. 2 with step and corresponding mandrel and a unilateral view of the skeleton of a lower bilateral distal extension partial denture using the Neurohr shoe as a precision rest. **A,** Lingual bar; **B,** lingual clasp arm; **C,** male portion of the attachment, which is cast as part of the skeleton (framework). (Courtesy Williams Gold Refining Co., Inc., Buffalo, N. Y.)

pressure is applied to the abutment tooth at any time.

• • •

Dr. Franklin Smith makes use of the Neurohr-Williams shoe in a manner similar to the Neurohr spring-lock attachment (Fig. 6-42). A single, short retentive clasp arm of 20-gauge wrought wire engages a small distobuccal, horizontal groove in the abutment casting. The lateral walls of the rest shoe are parallel and as such offer some resistance to horizontal rotational tendencies of the denture. Additionally, this attachment permits some vertical rotation of the denture bases toward the residual ridges. It will also resist rotary displacement of the denture bases away from the residual ridges.

Dr. Smith lists the following indications, advantages, contraindications, and disadvantages for his use of the Neurohr-Williams rest shoe. The indications and advantages claimed are:

1. Stress-breaking action in respect to distal rotation
2. Lowered leverage point of applied force
3. Multiple options of retentive area placement
4. Internal reciprocal action and indirect retention
5. Esthetic
6. Stable, simple (in form)
7. Amenable to tilted teeth where "draw" is a problem with conventional approaches
8. Amenable to anterior abutments

The contraindications and disadvantages are as follows:

1. Anticipation of possible tooth (abutment) migration in an anterior direction
2. Cannot be used where poor retentive qualities of an abutment casting is anticipated (for example, short or tapered crowns)

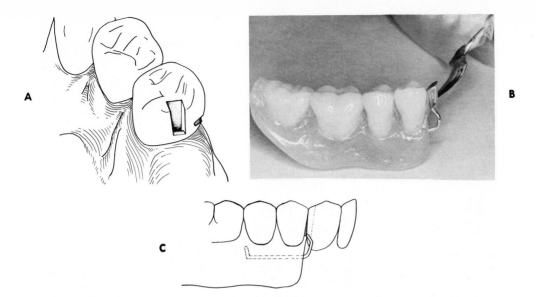

Fig. 6-42. **A,** Premolar abutment crown containing the preformed rest seat. Groove one-half the depth of a #557 bur is prepared at the height of the gingival seat of the female portion. **B,** Retentive arm is fabricated from 20-gauge wrought wire. **C,** Scheme drawing of an assembled unit. Retentive arm is passive until a dislodging force is applied to the denture. (**B,** Courtesy Dr. Franklin Smith.)

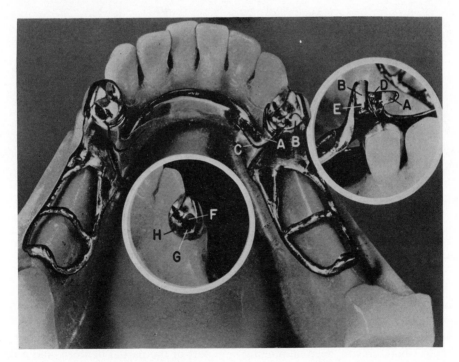

Fig. 6-43. Bilateral dowel rest attachments used on a Class I (bilateral distal extension) cast gold partial denture skeleton. **A,** Stabilizing bar; **B,** lug rest, which fits into notch **F** of the abutment; **C,** slit made with a gold saw to provide spring for the stabilizing bar; **D,** boss, which fits into round recess **H** of the abutment; **E,** dowel, which fits into well **G** of the abutment; **F,** notch into which the lug rest fits; **G,** well into which dowel fits; **H,** round recess into which the boss fits. (From Thompson, M. J.: Solution for specific problems in replacing missing teeth with partial dentures, Illinois State Dental Society's Seminar Manual, 1957.)

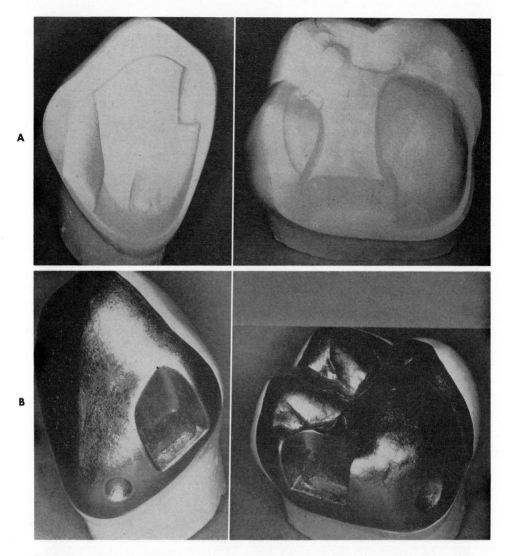

Fig. 6-44. **A,** Preparations for canine and molar abutment teeth upon which dowel rest attachments will be constructed. **B,** Dowel rest attachments constructed on canine and molar abutment teeth. Note the tapered nonlocking rest seat and dimple recessed in the lingual surface, which will be engaged by a corresponding boss on the retentive arm of the denture framework. (From Harris, F. N.: J. Prosthet. Dent. **5:**43-48, 1955.)

3. Any problem of inadequate crown length to retain the casting or house the intracoronal receptable (for example, short crown, deep impinging vertical overlap, large pulps)
4. Time, cost, and complexity of total procedure

Dowel rest attachment. Dr. Morris J. Thompson and others have developed a modification of the Clark attachment,

which is called the *dowel rest attachment* (Figs. 6-43 to 6-46). A boxlike rest seat is machined in the abutment casting for support of the partial denture, and a dimple is provided on the lingual surface of the abutment casting for retention. This dimple is engaged by a boss on a lingual arm on the denture framework, thereby affording retention without the use of a visible clasp arm. The lingual arm is an extension of

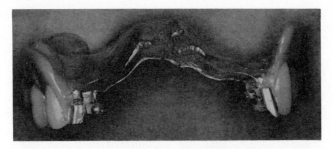

Fig. 6-45. Maxillary partial denture framework with nonlocking rest and lingual retentive arm originating from the palatal major connector but separated from it with a fine saw cut. Note the boss on the spring arm, which engages a corresponding dimple in the abutment restoration. (From Harris, F. N.: J. Prosthet. Dent. **5:**43-48, 1955.)

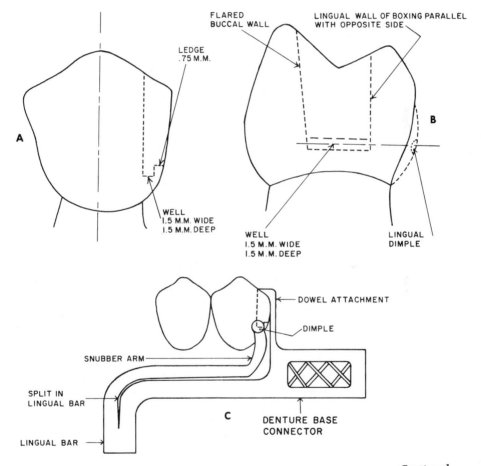

Continued.

Fig. 6-46. A, Schematic drawing of dowel rest preparation in a lower premolar full crown (buccal view). **B,** Schematic drawing of proximal view of dowel rest preparation and lingual dimple in a lower left premolar full crown. **C,** Schematic drawing of a lingual view of the dowel rest attachment. The spring arm terminating in a boss that engages a dimple in the abutment crown is separated from the major connector by a saw cut, or a split lingual bar is cast around a metal shim, which is later eliminated with acid. **D,** Removable partial denture framework incorporating the construction specifications illustrated in **A, B,** and **C.** (**A, B,** and **C,** Courtesy Dr. R. C. Van Dam; **D,** Courtesy Dr. L. E. Knowles.)

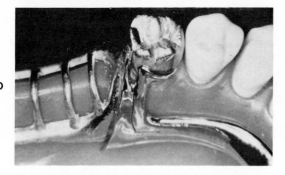

D

Fig. 6-46, cont'd. For legend see page 87.

the major connector, separated from it by a saw cut in the completed casting.

This attachment is most applicable to maxillary partial dentures, when the saw cut may be made in the palatal major connector. A stainless steel shim may be used rather than a saw cut to provide the necessary separation, which is then removed from the casting with acid. Flexibility of the retentive arm will be in proportion to its length as determined by the distance the separation is carried into the major connector.

The advantages that are given for this attachment are (1) no contact of the prosthesis with tooth structure; (2) stress-breaking effect, due to the flexibility of the lingual arm engaging the dimple on the abutment casting; (3) hygienic contours, and (4) no visible clasp arms. One of the most obvious disadvantages of this type of attachment is the lack of other than minimal stabilization against horizontal movement of the partial denture. Abutment torque is avoided by making the rest seat free of any locking effect; but by so doing, since the only external arm is a flexible one, stabilization against horizontal movement may be minimal. Thus, as with many stressbreaker designs, the edentulous ridge is called upon to resist horizontal movement of the prosthesis only slightly aided by two opposing parallel walls and not by any rigid components located on the abutment teeth. The addition of anteriorly placed indirect retainers, one on each lingual side

of the arch, seemingly would add much to the dowel rest denture.

A dowel rest attachment may be used in conjunction with a fixed partial denture (Fig. 6-47). It would not be a complicated procedure provided the fixed restoration was fabricated in conjunction with the re-removable restoration. However, it is doubted that adequate preparation of the rest seat could be accomplished intraorally on an existing pontic. The attachment may also be utilized in the pontic involving only the lingual and lingual occlusal of the pontic.

Coil spring attachment. Lenchner, Handlers, and Weissman have developed a spring retaining device for partial dentures, available as the *TACH E-Z coil spring attachment*. This is a prefabricated device consisting of a metal cylinder that contains a coil spring, a T-shaped cylindrical bar, and an adjustable screw collar. An opening exists in one end of the cylinder through which a portion of the bar protrudes under the action of the spring. This action is limited by the screw collar that is set in the opening of the cylinder through which the bar protrudes. (See Figs. 6-48 and 6-49.)

The attachment is either soldered or welded to the metal partial denture framework. It is set in such a position so that the tip of the bar protrudes and fits into a receptacle (dimple) prepared in the abutment casting. When used with unrestored abutments, the tip of the bar engages the natural undercut of the tooth and requires no receptacle. However, in either case it is necessary to have an opposing occlusal rest in the opposite proximo-occlusal position from the attachment. The receptacle in the abutment casting is located and formed after the denture framework is completed rather than being established previously as with the dowel rest attachment of Thompson.

The advantages claimed for this device are as follows:

1. The device maintains its relation to the abutment during function.
2. No part of the device extends onto

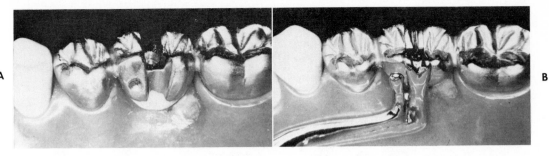

Fig. 6-47. **A,** Dowel rest preparation in the pontic of a fixed partial denture. Preparation provides for a "snubber" arm on the buccal surface of the pontic to facilitate removal of the denture by the patient. **B,** Denture is in its resting position. Note that the occlusal surface of the pontic has been restored by the framework. (Courtesy Dr. L. E. Knowles.)

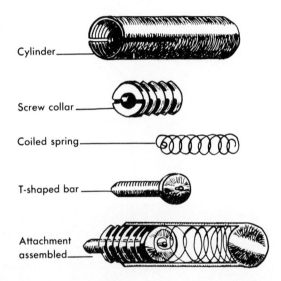

Cylinder

Screw collar

Coiled spring

T-shaped bar

Attachment assembled

Fig. 6-48. Detailed diagram of the modified coil spring attachment. (From Lenchner, N. H., Handlers, M., and Weissman, B.: J. Prosthet. Dent. **8:**973-980, 1958.)

the labial or buccal surfaces of the abutment teeth.

3. No special preparation of the abutment is necessary (although crown restorations are preferable); the use of prepared abutments and castings is optional.

4. It is unnecessary to overbuild abutment castings.

5. It can be used with short abutments.

6. Reduction of contact area reduces the susceptibility to caries (on unprotected abutments).

7. Adjustments are rarely, if ever, necessary.

8. All parts are readily adjustable, removable, and replaceable.

9. Cleanliness is easily maintained by the patient. The exposed portion is readily accessible to brushing.

10. Placement and removal of the denture is easy.

11. It is impossible for the patient to distort the denture during placement and removal.

12. Adequate stabilization against horizontal movement is provided by a lingual stabilizing arm.

The disadvantages of the coil spring attachment are as follows:

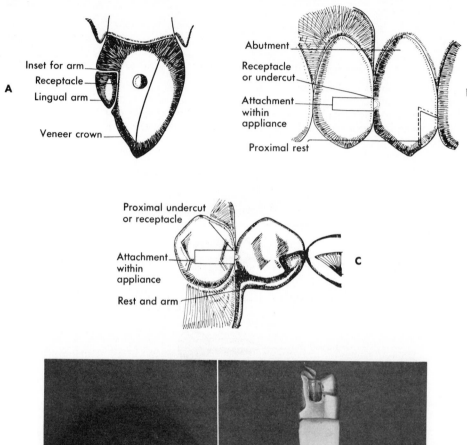

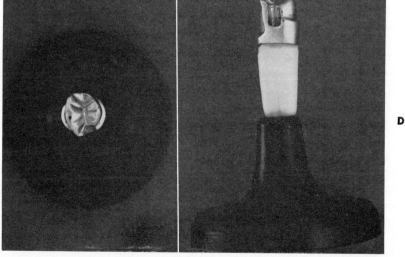

Fig. 6-49. A, Veneer crown designed for use with the coil spring attachment. **B,** The bar of the retaining device, which is attached to the framework, protrudes and engages a receptacle prepared in an abutment tooth casting; or it may engage in a natural tooth undercut. **C,** A diagram of the device in the denture base. Note the relationship with the lingual stabilizing arm and the occlusal rest. **D,** An abutment casting, showing the relation of the rest seat and the inset for the lingual stabilizing arm. (From Lenchner, N. H., Handlers, M., and Weissman, B.: J. Prosthet. Dent. 8:973-980, 1958.)

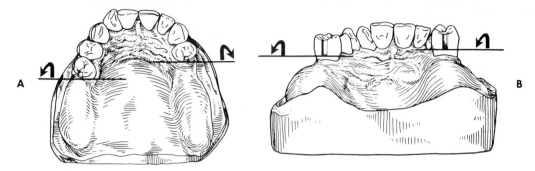

Fig. 6-50. **A,** Axes of rotation, although parallel, are not common since one axis is located anterior to the other axis. **B,** When one nonlocking internal attachment is elevated farther from the residual ridge than its cross-arch counterpart, the axes of rotation do not fall on a common line thus some torquing of abutments should be anticipated. However, in many instances the effect produced by this situation will not exceed the physiologic tolerance of the supporting structures of the abutments—all other torquing factors being equal.

1. The total cost will exceed that of a clasp-retained partial denture.
2. Proximal occlusal rests and guiding planes are not used with this device. However, proximal guiding planes are much more essential to clasp retention, and the presence of an internal rest on the opposite side of the tooth from the retainer, plus paralleled lingual surfaces above a lingual shoulder, should provide all the the stabilization and reciprocation needed.
3. The movable bar may eventually accumulate debris and clog. However, the device may be adjusted or disassembled for cleaning if necessary.

The laboratory technique for the use of the coil spring attachment is provided by the manufacturer. This attachment merits further consideration, and with some modifications it may prove to be a satisfactory type of retainer for removable partial dentures, since it avoids a display of metal yet provides retention against reasonable dislodging forces.

Internal attachments of the locking or dovetail type unquestionably have many advantages over the clasp-type denture for tooth-borne situations. It is, however, questioned that locking type of internal attachments for distal extension removable partial dentures are indicated, with or without stressbreakers or with or without splinted abutments, because of inherent, excessive leverages most often associated with these attachments.

The non-locking type of internal attachments, when used in conjunction with sound prosthodontic principles, can be advantageously used in many instances in Class I and II partially edentulous situations. However, unless the cross-arch axis of rotation is common to the bilaterally placed attachments, torque may be placed on the abutments (Fig. 6-50).

CHAPTER 7

Indirect retainers

Movement of the base of an entirely tooth-borne partial denture *toward* the edentulous ridge is prevented by rests placed on the abutment teeth located at each end of each edentulous space. Presuming that the denture framework is rigid and the rests are properly placed, occlusal forces are transmitted directly to the abutment teeth through the rests placed on those teeth. Movement of the base *away* from the edentulous ridge is prevented by the activation of the otherwise passive direct retainers on the same abutment teeth. Horizontal movement of the partial denture and longitudinal rotational movement of the denture base are prevented by stabilizing components on the same abutment teeth plus any auxiliary abutments contacted for stabilization. Rotation of the tooth-borne partial denture is therefore relatively nonexistent.

In contrast, all Class I and Class II partial dentures, having one or more distal extension bases, are not totally tooth supported; neither are they completely retained by bounding abutments. Any Class III or Class IV partial denture that does not have adequate abutment support falls into the same category. These latter may derive some support from the edentulous ridge and therefore may have a composite support from both teeth and ridge tissues.

Movement of a distal extension base *toward* the ridge tissues will be proportionate to the quality of those tissues, the accu-racy of the denture base, and the total functional load applied. Movement of a distal extension base *away* from the ridge tissues will occur either as a rotational movement about an axis or as displacement of the entire denture. The forces that tend to displace any denture are also the forces that cause rotation of a distal extension partial denture.

Denture rotation about an axis. Presuming that direct retainers are functioning to to prevent total displacement, rotational movement will occur about some axis as the distal extension base or bases either move toward or away from the underlying tissues. This axis is an imaginary line passing through teeth with *direct retainers,* around which line the denture rotates slightly when subjected to various stresses predominantly directed toward residual ridges. It is called the *fulcrum line*. More than one fulcrum line may be present for the same removable partial denture (Fig. 7-1). When the base(s) of an extension denture move away from the basal seat, the fulcrum line will pass through the most anteriorly located supporting elements of the denture framework. In the absence of indirect retainers or components that function as indirect retainers, the fulcrum line will pass through the most posterior and bilaterally located tips of retainer arms engaging an undercut.

For the sake of clarity in discussing the location and functions of indirect retainers,

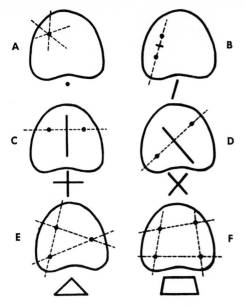

areas and in line with the partial denture. This design derives its stability against tipping from only the short leverages supplied by the clasp arms with no cross-arch assistance. **C,** The imaginary + represents the two clasp, diametrically opposed, distal extension partial denture situation. The fulcrum line forms the cross bar, and the unseating leverage (afforded by the extension bases), combined with the controlling leverage (the indirect retention anterior to the fulcrum line), completes the upright. A partial denture designed to counteract unseating leverages in accordance with this imaginary figure would be stable. **D,** The imaginary × with two diagonally opposed clasps providing the guide for the fulcrum line. The leverage below this line from the single base extension, added to the length of the indirect leverage anterior to the line, completes the geometric figure that represents a stable denture design. **E,** The triangular design results from the use of three clasps, with the abutments being selected as far apart as feasible to include the largest area within the triangle and to provide the longest controlling leverages against tipping strains. Usually, this is a stable design. **F,** The quadrangular figure is representative of a four-clasp restoration. Its area is large enough to circumscribe most unseating stresses so that they would fall within the quadrangle and tend to seat the restoration instead of dislodging it. (From Steffel, V. L.: J. Prosthet. Dent. **12:**524-535, 1962.)

Fig. 7-1. A, Broken lines on the diagram represent imaginary fulcrum lines passing through rest or support areas. The dot represents a single clasp restoration. Any number of fulcrum lines could pass through the one supporting point. Such a restoration could not have stability by means of cross-arch leverage. **B,** A two-clasp unilateral partial denture situation is represented by a straight line, the fulcrum line passing through the rest

---

the term fulcrum line should be considered the axis about which the denture will rotate when the bases move toward the residual ridge.

The fulcrum line is identified on a Class I partial denture as passing through the rest areas of the most posterior abutment on either side of the arch (Fig. 7-2, *A* and *B*). On a Class II partial denture the fulcrum line is always diagonal, passing through the occlusal rest area of the abutment on the distal extension side and the occlusal rest area of the most distal abutment on the other side (Fig. 7-2, *C*). If a modification area is present on that side, the additional abutment lying between the two principal abutments may be used for support of the indirect retainer, if it is far enough removed from the fulcrum line (Fig. 7-2, *D*). In a Class IV partial denture the fulcrum line passes through the two abutments adjacent to the single

edentulous space (Fig. 7-2, *E* and *F*). In a tooth- and-tissue-supported Class III partial denture, the fulcrum line is determined by considering the weaker abutment as nonexistent and that end of the base as being a distal extension (Fig. 7-2, *G* and *H*).

Movement of the denture base away from the tissues and about the fulcrum line is prevented by units of the partial denture framework that are located on definite rest seats on the opposite side of the fulcrum line from the distal extension base and the activation of the retentive element of the direct retainer assembly. These anteriorly located components should be placed as far as possible from the distal extension base affording the best possible leverage advantage against lifting of the distal extension base. Such units are called *indirect retainers.*

An indirect retainer consists of one or

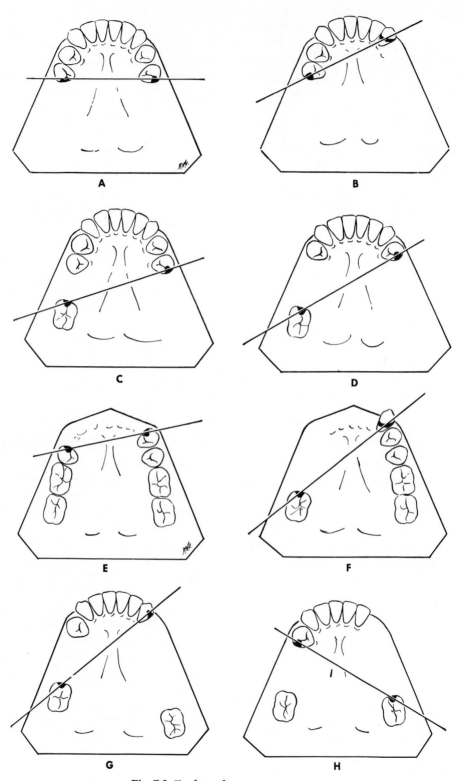

Fig. 7-2. For legend see opposite page.

more rests and their supporting minor connectors. While it is customary to identify the entire assembly as the indirect retainer, it should be remembered that it is the rest that is actually the indirect retainer, united to the major connector by a minor connector. This is to avoid interpreting any contact with tooth inclines as being part of the indirect retainer. *An indirect retainer should be placed as far from the distal extension base as possible in a prepared rest seat on a tooth capable of supporting its function.*

Whereas the most effective location of an indirect retainer is frequently in the vicinity of an incisor tooth, that tooth may not be strong enough to support an indirect retainer and may have steep inclines that cannot be favorably altered to support a rest. In such case, the nearest canine tooth or the mesial occlusal surface of the first premolar may be the best location, despite the fact that it is not as far removed from the fulcrum line. Whenever possible, two indirect retainers closer to the fulcrum line are then used to compensate for the compromise in distance.

Factors influencing effectiveness of an indirect retainer. The factors influencing the effectiveness of an indirect retainer are as follows:

1. Effectiveness of the direct retainers. Unless the principal occlusal rests are held in their seats by the action of the direct retainers, rotation about the fulcrum line will not occur and therefore an indirect retainer cannot act to prevent lifting of the distal extension base away from the tissues.

2. Distance from the fulcrum line. Three areas must be considered:
   a. Length of the distal extension base
   b. Location of the fulcrum line
   c. How far beyond the fulcrum line the indirect retainer is placed

3. Rigidity of the connectors supporting the indirect retainer. All connectors must be rigid if the indirect retainer is to function as intended.

4. Effectiveness of the supporting tooth surface. The indirect retainer must be placed on a definite rest seat on which slippage or tooth movement will not occur. Tooth inclines and weak teeth should never be used for the support of indirect retainers.

Auxiliary functions of an indirect retainer. In addition to preventing movement of a distal extension base away from the tissues, an indirect retainer may serve the following auxiliary functions:

1. It tends to reduce anteroposterior tilting leverages on the principal abutments. This is particularly important when an isolated tooth is being used as an abutment, a situation that should be avoided whenever possible. Ordinarily, proximal contact with the adjacent tooth prevents such tilting of

Fig. 7-2. Fulcrum line found in various types of partially edentulous arches around which the denture will probably rotate when the bases are subjected to forces directed toward the residual ridge. **A** and **B,** In a Class I arch the fulcrum line passes through the occlusal rest areas of the most posterior abutments. **C,** In a Class II arch the fulcrum line is diagonal, passing through the occlusal rest areas of the abutment on the distal extension side and the most posterior abutment on the opposite side. **D,** If an abutment tooth anterior to a modification space lies far enough removed from the fulcrum line, it may be used effectively for the support of an indirect retainer. **E,** and **F,** In a class IV arch the fulcrum line passes through the two abutments adjacent to the single edentulous space. **G,** In a Class III arch with a posterior tooth on one side, which possibly will eventually be lost, the fulcrum line is considered the same as though the posterior tooth were not present. Thus its loss at some future date will not necessitate altering the design of the partial denture. **H,** In a Class III arch with nonsupporting anterior teeth, the adjacent edentulous area is considered to be a tissue-supported end, with a diagonal fulcrum line passing through the two principal abutments as in a Class II arch.

an abutment as the base lifts away from the tissues.

2. Contact of its minor connector with vertical tooth surfaces aids in stabilization against horizontal movement of the denture. Such tooth surfaces, when made parallel to the path of placement, may also act as auxiliary guiding planes.

3. Anterior teeth supporting indirect retainers are splinted against lingual movement.

4. It may act as an auxiliary rest to support a portion of the major connector. For example, a lingual bar may be supported against settling into the tissues by the indirect retainer acting as an auxiliary rest. One must be able to differentiate between an auxiliary rest placed for support for a major connector, one placed for indirect retention, and one serving a dual purpose. Some auxiliary rests are added solely to provide rest support to a segment of the denture and should not be confused with indirect retention.

Forms of indirect retainers. The indirect retainer may take any one of several forms. All are effective in proportion to their *support* and the *distance from the fulcrum line that they are placed.*

Auxiliary occlusal rest. The most frequently used indirect retainer is an auxiliary occlusal rest located on an occlusal surface as far away from the distal extension base as possible. In a mandibular Class I arch this is usually on the mesial marginal ridge of the first premolar on each side (Fig. 7-3). The longest perpendicular to the fulcrum line would be in the vicinity of the central incisors, which are too weak and have lingual surfaces that are too perpendicular to support a rest. Bilateral rests on the first premolars are quite effective, even though located closer to the axis of rotation.

The same principle applies to any maxillary Class I partial denture when indirect retainers are used. Bilateral rests on the mesial marginal ridge of the first premolars are almost always used in preference to rests on incisor teeth (Fig. 7-4). Not only

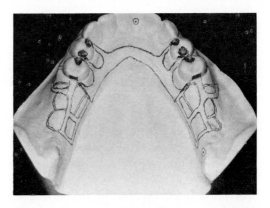

Fig. 7-3. Planning the location for indirect retainers for a Class I partial denture. The greatest distance from the axis of rotation (fulcrum line) would fall on the incisor teeth, which are ill-suited to provide adequate support without tooth movement and/or slippage of the retainer. Dual occlusal rests on prepared rest reats at the mesial marginal ridge of the first premolars provide effective indirect retention with optimal tooth support.

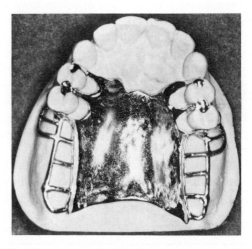

Fig. 7-4. An example of indirect retention used in conjunction with a palatal plate. A secondary function of the auxiliary occlusal rest assemblies is to prevent settling of the anterior portion of the palatal plate and provide stabilization against horizontal rotation.

are they effective without jeopardizing the weaker single-rooted teeth but also interference to the tongue is far less when the minor connector can be placed in the embrasure between canine and premolar rather than anterior to the canine teeth.

Indirect retainers for Class II partial den-

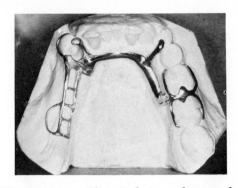

Fig. 7-5. Lower Class II design utilizing embrasure clasping on the nonedentulous side. The indirect retainer on the distal marginal ridge of the rotated first premolar is favorably located in relation to the fulcrum line. Note the use of a wrought-wire retentive clasp arm on the buccal surface of the left first premolar. A bar-type retainer could not be used because of the presence of a gross tissue undercut (buccal) below the first premolar and the absence of a usable undercut on its distobuccal surface. (Modified from McCracken's partial denture construction, ed. 3, St. Louis, 1969, The C. V. Mosby Co.)

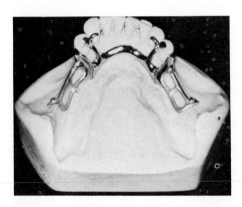

Fig. 7-6. Mandibular Class I design utilizing canine extensions from occlusal rests as indirect retainers. Canine extensions must be placed in prepared rest seats so that resistance will be directed as nearly as possible along the long axes of the canine abutments.

tures are usually placed on the mesial marginal ridge of the first premolar tooth on the opposite side of the arch from the distal extension base (Fig. 7-5). Bilateral rests are seldom indicated except when an auxiliary occlusal rest is needed for support of the major connector or when the prognosis of the distal abutment is poor and

provision must be made for later conversion to a Class I partial denture should that tooth be lost.

Canine extensions from occlusal rests. Occasionally, a finger extension from a premolar rest is placed on the prepared lingual slope of the adjacent canine tooth (Fig. 7-6). Such an extension is used to effect indirect retention by increasing the distance of a resisting element from the fulcrum line. This is particularly applicable when a first premolar must serve as a primary abutment. The distance anterior to the fulcrum line is only the distance between the mesial occlusal rest and the anterior terminal of the finger extension. In this instance, although the extension rests on a prepared surface, it is used in conjunction with a terminal rest on the mesial marginal ridge of the premolar tooth. Tipping leverage on the canine tooth is predominately avoided. *Even when not used as indirect retainers, canine extensions, continuous bar retainers, and linguoplates should never be used without terminal rests because of the resultant forces effective when they are placed on inclined planes alone.*

Canine rests. When the mesial marginal ridge of the first premolar is too close to the fulcrum line or when the teeth are lapped so that the fulcrum line is not accessible, a rest on the adjacent canine tooth may be used. Such a rest may be made more effective by placing the minor connector in the embrasure anterior to the canine, either curving back onto a prepared lingual rest seat or extending to a mesioincisal rest. The same types of canine rests as those previously outlined may be used, which are the lingual or incisal rests. (See Chapter 5.)

Continuous bar retainers and linguoplates. Technically, continuous bar retainers and linguoplates are not indirect retainers, since they rest on unprepared lingual inclines of anterior teeth. The indirect retainers are actually the terminal rests at either end, in the form of auxiliary occlusal rests or canine rests.

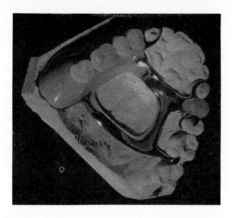

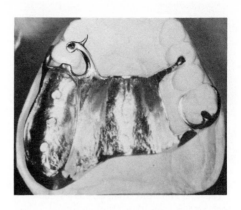

Fig. 7-7. Class II, modification 1, partial denture. The fulcrum line, when the denture base is displaced toward the tissues, runs from the mesioincisal rest on the right canine to the distal rest on the first molar. When the denture base rotates away from the residual ridge the fulcrum line runs from the right canine to the left second premolar since there is no direct retainer on the molar. The only effective indirect retention therefore is on the mesioincisal rest on the left canine. The auxiliary occlusal rest on the molar adds horizontal stabilization and prevents settling of the posterior palatal bar but cannot act as an indirect retainer because it lies posterior to the axis of rotation.

Fig. 7-8. Class II partial denture design with indirect retainer located favorably in relation to the fulcrum line. An additional function of the auxiliary occlusal rest is to prevent tissueward movement of that portion of the palatal plate. Note the use of a bar clasp on the right premolar abutment. This design utilizes a full metal base with nailhead retention and an undercut finishing line all around. (Modified from McCracken's partial denture construction, ed. 3, St. Louis, 1969, The C. V. Mosby Co.)

In Class I and Class II partial dentures a continuous bar retainer or linguoplate may extend the effectiveness of the indirect retainer if used with a terminal rest at each end. In tooth-borne partial dentures they are placed for other reasons but always with terminal rests. (See Chapter 4.)

In Class I and Class II partial dentures especially, a continuous bar retainer or the superior border of the linguoplate should never be placed above the middle third of the teeth so that orthodontic movement during the rotation of a distal extension denture is avoided. This is not so important when the six anterior teeth are in nearly a straight line, but when the arch is narrow and tapering, a continuous bar retainer or linguoplate on anterior teeth extends well beyond the terminal rests, and orthodontic movement of those teeth is more likely. Whereas these are intended primarily to stabilize weak anterior teeth, they may have the opposite effect if not used with discretion.

Modification areas. Occasionally, the occlusal rest on a secondary abutment in a Class II partial denture may be used also as an indirect retainer. This will depend upon how far from the fulcrum line the secondary abutment is located.

The primary abutments in a Class II, modification 1, partial denture are the abutment adjacent to the distal extension base and the most distal abutment on the tooth-borne side. The fulcrum line is a diagonal axis between the principal occlusal rest areas of these two abutments, disregarding any auxiliary occlusal rests that may be present on the same teeth. (See Fig. 7-7.)

The anterior abutment on the tooth-borne side is a secondary abutment, serving to support and retain one end of the tooth-borne segment, as well as adding horizontal stabilization to the denture. If the modification space were not present, as in an unmodified Class II arch, auxiliary occlusal rests and bracing components would still be essential to the design of the denture (Fig. 7-8). But the presence of a modification space conveniently provides an abutment tooth for both retention and support.

If the occlusal rest on the secondary abutment lies far enough from the fulcrum line, it may serve adequately as an indirect retainer. Its dual function, then, is both tooth support for one end of the modification area and support for an indirect retainer. The most typical example is a distal occlusal rest on a first premolar, when second premolar and first molar are missing and the second molar serves as one of the primary abutments. The longest perpendicular to the fulcrum line falls in the vicinity of the first premolar, making the location of the indirect retainer nearly ideal.

On the other hand, if only one tooth, such as a first molar, is missing on the modification side, the occlusal rest on the second premolar abutment is too close to the fulcrum line to be effective. In such case, an auxiliary occlusal rest on the mesial marginal ridge of the first premolar is needed, both for indirect retention and for for support for an otherwise unsupported major connector.

Support for a modification area extending anteriorly to a canine abutment is obtained by any one of the accepted canine rest forms, as previously outlined. In this situation, the canine tooth provides nearly ideal indirect retention, and support for the major connector as well.

Rugae support. Some authorities consider coverage of the rugae area of the maxillary arch as a means of indirect retention, since the rugae area is firm and usually well situated to provide indirect retention for a Class I denture. While it is true that broad coverage over the rugae area can conceivably provide such support, the facts remain that tissue support is less effective than positive tooth support and that rugae coverage is undesirable if it can be avoided.

The use of rugae support for indirect retention is usually part of a palatal horseshoe design. Since posterior retention is usually inadequate in this situation, the requirements for indirect retention are probably greater than can be satisfied by tissue support alone.

Direct-indirect retention. In the mandibular arch, retention from the distal extension base alone is usually inadequate to prevent lifting of the base away from the tissues. In the maxillary arch, where only anterior teeth remain, full palatal coverage is usually necessary. In fact, with any Class I partial denture extending distally from the premolar teeth, except when a maxillary torus prevents its use, palatal coverage may be used to advantage. While full coverage may be in the form of a resin base, the added retention and lesser bulk of the cast metal palate makes the latter preferable. (See Chapter 4.) However, in the absence of full palatal coverage, an indirect retainer should be used with other designs of major palatal connectors for the Class I removable partial denture.

Reaction of tissues to metallic coverage. The reaction of tissues to metallic coverage has been the subject of some controversy between periodontists and prosthodontists. Particular areas over which the controversy is concerned are gingival crossings and broad areas of metal contact with tissues.

From the prosthodontic viewpoint, if oral tissues may not be safely covered with the framework of removable partial dentures, then all parts of the partial denture resting on or crossing soft tissues jeopardize the health of those tissues. If this is true, it is because of several reasons, none of which is the fact of coverage alone.

First of these is *pressure due to lack of support*. If relief over gingival crossings and other areas of contact with tissues, which are incapable of supporting the prosthesis, is inadequate, then impingement of those tissues is inevitable. Impingement will likewise occur if the denture settles due to loss of tooth support. This may be due to failure of the rest areas as a result of improper design, caries involvement, or the flow of amalgam alloy restorations, or to intrusion of abutment teeth under occlusal loading.

It is the responsibility of the prosthodontist to provide and maintain adequate relief and adequate occlusal support.

Settling of the denture also may result in pressure elsewhere in the arch, such as beneath major connectors. Again, the cause of settling must be prevented or corrected if it becomes manifest. Fisher has shown that pressure alone may cause a nonspecific effect on tissues, which has been mistaken for allergic response or the effect of coverage. Pressure then must be avoided whenever oral tissues must be covered or crossed by elements of the partial denture.

The second reason is *uncleanliness*. It is known that tissues respond unfavorably to an accumulation of food debris and to bacterial enzymes. Coverage of oral tissues with dentures that are not kept clean results in irritation of those tissues, not because they are covered but because of the accumulation of irritating factors. This has lead to a misinterpretation of the effect of tissue coverage by prosthetic restorations.

A third explanation of unfavorable tissue response to coverage is the *amount of time the denture is worn*. It is apparent that mucous membrane reverts to connective tissue if isolated from the oral environment for a long enough period of time. Evidence of this is the appearance of tissue, once mucous membrane, beneath the pontics of fixed partial dentures. A raw, denuded surface is visible upon removal of the fixed restoration. The same thing can occur beneath removable prosthetic restorations if they are allowed to remain against the tissues long enough.

Some patients become so accustomed to wearing a removable restoration that they neglect to remove it often enough to give the tissues any respite from constant contact. This is frequently true when anterior teeth are replaced by the partial denture and the individual will not allow the restoration to be out of the mouth at any time except in the privacy of the bathroom during toothbrushing.

The fact remains that living tissue should not be covered all the time or changes in those tissues will occur. *Partial dentures should not be worn upon retiring at night, so that the tissues may rest and be returned to a normal environment at least several hours in the twenty-four hours.* Clinical experience with the use of linguoplates and palatal plates has shown conclusively that when factors of pressure, cleanliness, and time are controlled, tissue coverage is not in itself detrimental to the health of oral tissues.

CHAPTER 8

Denture bases and stressbreakers (stress equalizers)

DENTURE BASES

The denture base supports the supplied teeth and effects the transfer of occlusal stresses to the supporting oral structures.

Although its primary purpose is related to masticatory function, the denture base also may add to the cosmetic effect of the replacement, particularly when modern techniques for tinting and the reproducing of natural-looking contours are used. Most of the modern techniques for creating naturalness in complete denture bases are applicable equally well to partial denture bases.

Still another function of the denture base is the stimulation, by massage, of the underlying tissues of the residual ridge. Some vertical movement occurs with any denture base, even those supported entirely by abutment teeth, because of the physiologic movement of those teeth under function. It is clearly evident that oral tissues placed under functional stress within their physiologic tolerance maintain their form and tone better than do similar tissues suffering from disuse. The term *disuse atrophy* is applicable to both periodontal tissues and the tissues of a residual ridge.

Functions of the tooth-supported partial denture base. Denture bases differ in functional purpose and may differ in the material of which they are made. In a tooth-borne prosthesis, the denture base is primarily a span between two abutments supporting artificial occlusal surfaces. Thus occlusal forces are transferred directly to the abutment teeth through rests. Also the denture base and the supplied teeth serve to prevent horizontal migration of the teeth in the partially edentulous arch and vertical migration of teeth in the opposing arch.

When only posterior teeth are being replaced, esthetics is usually a secondary consideration. On the other hand, when anterior teeth are replaced, esthetics may be of primary importance. Except for esthetic considerations, the tooth-borne partial denture base is essentially a framework supporting occlusal surfaces. Theoretically, occlusal surfaces alone would accomplish masticatory efficiency and maintain the relative position of the natural teeth. However, they would lack desirable esthetics, create undesirable food traps, and deprive the tissues of the stimulation by massage that they would receive from an accurate denture base. The reasons, then, for providing more than only the necessary support for occlusal surfaces in a tooth-borne denture are (1) esthetics, (2) cleanliness, and (3) stimulation of the underlying tissues.

Functions of the distal extension partial denture base. In a distal extension partial denture, the denture bases other than those in tooth-supported modifications must contribute to the support of the denture. Close to the terminal abutment, only a framework supporting occlusal surfaces is necessary. However, farther from the abutment, the support from the underlying ridge tissues becomes increasingly important. Maximum support from the residual ridge may be obtained only by using broad, accurate denture bases, which spread the occlusal load equitably over the entire area that is available for such support. The space that is available for a denture base is controlled by the structures surrounding the space and their movement during function. Maximum support for the denture base therefore can be accomplished only by utilizing a knowledge of the limiting anatomic structures, knowledge of the histologic nature of the basal seat areas, accuracy of the impression, and accuracy of the denture base. A principle as old as the snowshoe is that broad coverage furnishes the best support with the least load per unit area. Therefore, support should be the primary consideration in selecting, designing, and fabricating a distal extension partial denture base. Of secondary importance, but to be considered nevertheless, are esthetics, stimulation of the underlying tissues, and oral cleanliness.

In addition to their difference in functional purpose, denture bases vary in material of construction. This is related to their function because of the need for future rebasing in one instance and usually not in another.

Since the tooth-supported base has an abutment tooth at each end upon which a rest has been placed, future relining or rebasing may not be necessary to reestablish support. Relining is necessary only when tissue changes have occurred beneath the tooth-borne base to the point that poor esthetics and the accumulation of debris result. For these reasons alone, tooth-borne bases that are made soon after extractions should be constructed of a material that permits later relining. Such materials are the denture resins, the most common of which are copolymer and methyl methacrylate resins. Other materials such as styrene

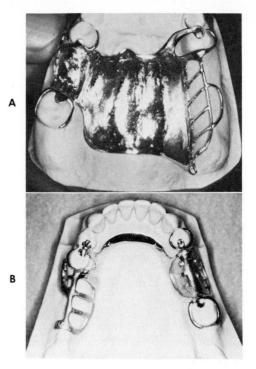

Fig. 8-1. Class II, modification 1, designs utilizing a full metal base on the modification side and retention for a resin base on the opposite side. **A,** Note the design of the undercut finishing line on the distal extension side, parallel to the crest of the edentulous ridge for this maxillary framework. **B,** A mandibular framework with adequate provision for attaching the denture base on the edentulous side. The junction of the major and minor connectors is a strong butt-type joint. (A, Modified from McCracken's partial denture construction, ed. 3, St. Louis, 1969, The C. V. Mosby Co.)

and vinyl-acrylic resins also may be satisfactorily added to for relining.

Resin bases are attached to the partial denture framework by means of a retentive framework designed so that a space exists between it and the underlying tissues of the residual ridge (Fig. 8-1). A blockout of at least 22-gauge thickness over the master cast is used to create a raised platform on the investment cast upon which the pattern for the retentive frame is formed. Thus, after casting, the portion of the retentive framework to which the resin base will be attached will stand away from the tissue surface sufficiently to permit a flow of resin base material beneath the surface.

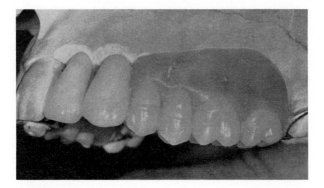

Fig. 8-2. Replaced lateral incisor and canine are abutted to the residual ridge for better esthetics. Occasionally the first premolar is treated similarly, depending on how visible this tooth is. Retentive framework for the resin base must be designed so that interference with the proper placement and arrangement of the artificial teeth will not be encountered.

The retentive framework should be embedded in the base material with sufficient thickness of resin to allow for relieving, if this becomes necessary during denture adjustment over tender areas or during rebasing procedures. Thickness is also necessary to avoid weakness and subsequent fracture of the resin base material surrounding the metal framework.

The use of plastic mesh patterns in forming the retentive framework is generally less satisfactory than is a more open framework. Less weakening of the resin by the embedded framework results from the use of the more open form. Pieces of 12- or 14-gauge half-round wax and 18-gauge round wax are therefore used to form a ladderlike framework rather than the finer latticework of the mesh pattern. The precise design of the retentive framework is not so important as its effective rigidity and strength when embedded in the resin base—free of interference to future adjustment and to arrangement of artificial teeth and open enough to avoid weakening any portion of the attached resin (Fig. 8-2).

The ideal denture base. The requirements for an ideal denture base are as follows:

1. Accuracy of adaptation to the tissues, with low volume change
2. Dense, nonirritating surface that is capable of receiving and maintaining a good finish.

3. Thermal conductivity
4. Low specific gravity; lightness in the mouth
5. Sufficient strength; resistance to fracture or distortion
6. Self-cleansing factor, or easily kept clean
7. Esthetic acceptability
8. Potential for future relining
9. Low initial cost

Obviously such an ideal denture base material does not exist; nor is it likely to be developed in the near future. However, any denture base—whether of resin or metal and regardless of the method of fabrication—should come as close to this ideal as possible.

Advantages of metal bases. Except for those edentulous ridges with recent extractions, metal is preferred to resin for tooth-supported bases because of the several advantages of the metal base. Its principal disadvantage is that it can be rebased only with difficulty, if at all. Nevertheless, the stimulation that it gives to the underlying tissues is so beneficial that it probably prevents some alveolar atrophy that would otherwise occur under a resin base and thereby prolongs the health of the tissues that it contacts. Some of the advantages of a metal base are as follows:

1. *Thermal conductivity.* Temperature changes are transmitted through the metal base to the underlying tissues, thereby help-

ing to maintain the health of those tissues. Freedom of interchange of temperature between the tissues covered and the surrounding external influences (temperature of liquid and solid foods and inspired air) contributes much to the patient's acceptance of a denture and avoids the feeling of the presence of a foreign body. Denture resins, on the other hand, all have insulating properties that prevent interchange of temperature between the inside and the outside of the denture base.

2. *Accuracy and permanence of form.* Cast metal bases, whether of gold or chrome alloys, not only may be cast more accurately than denture resins but also maintain their accuracy of form without change in the mouth. Internal strains that may be released later to cause distortion are not present. Although some resins and some processing techniques are superior to others in accuracy and permanence of form, modern cast alloys are generally superior in this respect. Evidence of this fact is that an additional posterior palatal seal may be eliminated entirely when a cast palate is used, as compared with the need for a definite attempt in this regard when the palate is made of resin. Distortion of a resin base is manifest in the maxillary denture by a distortion away from the palate in the midline and toward the tuberosities on the buccal flanges. The greater the curvature of the tissues, the greater is this distortion. Similar distortions occur in a mandibular denture but are less easily detected. Accurate metal castings are not subject to distortion by the release of internal stains as are most denture resins.

Because of its accuracy, the metal base provides an intimacy of contact, which contributes considerably to the retention of a denture prosthesis. Sometimes called *interfacial surface tension*, direct retention from a cast denture base is significant in proportion to the area involved. This has been previously mentioned as an important factor in both direct and direct-indirect retention of maxillary restorations. Such intimacy of contact is not possible with resin bases.

Permanence of form of the cast base is also assured due to its resistance to abrasion from denture cleaning agents. Cleanliness of the denture base should be stressed; yet constant brushing of the tissue side of a resin denture base, if effective, inevitably causes some loss of accuracy by abrasion. Intimacy of contact, which was never as great with a resin base as with a metal base, is therefore jeopardized further by cleaning habits. The metal bases, particularly the harder chrome alloys, withstand repeated cleaning without significant changes in surface accuracy.

3. *Cleanliness.* Cleanliness is listed apart from resistance to abrasion because the inherent cleanliness of the cast base contributes to the health of the tissues regardless of the patient's cleaning habits. Resin bases tend to accumulate mucinous deposits containing food particles, as well as calcareous deposits. Unfavorable tissue reaction to decomposing food particles and bacterial enzymes and to mechanical irritation from calculus results if the denture is not kept mechanically clean. Whereas calculus, which must be removed periodically, does precipitate on a cast metal base, other deposits do not accumulate as they do on a resin base. For this reason, a metal base is naturally cleaner than is a resin base.

4. *Weight and bulk.* Metal alloys may be cast much thinner than resin and still have adequate strength and rigidity. Still less weight and bulk are possible when the denture bases are made of chrome alloys. Cast gold must be given slightly more bulk to provide the same amount of rigidity but may still be made with less thickness than resin materials.

There are times, however, when both weight and thickness may be used to advantage in denture bases. In the mandibular arch, weight of the denture may be an asset in regard to retention, and for this reason a cast gold base may be preferred. On the other hand, extreme loss of residual alveolar bone may make it necessary to add fullness to the denture base to restore normal facial contours and to fill out the buccal vestibule with a denture contour that will prevent food from being lost in the cheek and from working beneath the denture. In such situations, a resin base may be preferred to the thinner metal base.

In the maxillary arch a resin base may be preferred to the thinner metal base to provide fullness when needed, such as in buccal flanges or to fill a maxillary buccal vestibule. Resin may also be preferred over the thinner metal base for esthetic reasons. In these several instances the thinness of the metal base may be of no advantage, but in areas where the tongue and cheek need maximum room, thinness may be desirable.

Denture contours for functional tongue and cheek contact can best be accomplished with resin. Whereas metal bases are usually made thin to minimize bulk and weight, resin bases may be contoured to provide ideal polished surfaces that contribute to the retention of the denture, restore facial contours, and avoid the accumulation of food at denture borders. Lingual surfaces usually are made concave, except in the distal palatal area. Buccal surfaces are made convex at gingival margins, over root prominences, and at the border to fill the area recorded in the impression. Between the border and the gingival contours, the base is made concave to aid in retention and to facilitate the food bolus being returned to the occlusal table during mastication. Such contours prevent food from being lost in the cheek and from working under the denture. This cannot usually be accomplished with metal bases.

However, the advantages of a metal base need not necessarily be sacrificed for the sake of esthetics or desirable denture contours when the use of such a base is otherwise indicated. Denture bases may be designed to provide almost total metallic coverage, yet with resin borders to avoid a display of metal and to add buccal fullness when needed. The advantages of thermal conductivity are not necessarily lost by covering a portion of the metal base so long as other parts of the denture are exposed to effect temperature changes through conduction.

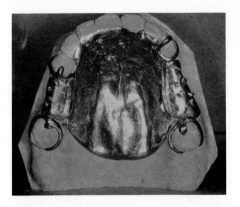

Fig. 8-3. Partial metal bases used with a full palatal plate and "pressed-on" anterior teeth. Attachment of denture with resin is accomplished by diagonal spurs and lingual undercut finishing line. The visible buccal flange will be of resin, yet without sacrificing most of the advantages of a metal base. Support anteriorly is by a mesioincisal rest on a canine and by a lingual rest seat prepared on all remaining anterior teeth.

Attaching artificial teeth to metal bases. Artificial teeth may be added to denture bases by several means. Some of these are as follows:

1. *Porcelain or resin artificial teeth attached to a metal base with resin.* Retention of the resin to the metal base may be accomplished by nailhead retention, retention loops, or diagonal spurs placed at random. Nailheads should be placed so that they will not interfere with the placement of the teeth on the metal base. (See Fig. 8-3.)

Any junction of resin with metal should be at an undercut finishing line or associated with some retentive undercut. Since only a mechanical attachment exists between metal and resin, every attempt should be made to avoid separation and seepage, which results in discoloration and uncleanliness. Denture odors are frequently caused by accretions at the junction of resin with metal when only mechanical union exist. Separation occurring between resin and metal leads eventually to some loosening of the resin base.

2. *Porcelain or resin tube teeth and facings cemented directly to metal bases* (Figs. 8-4 and 9-5). Some disadvantages of this

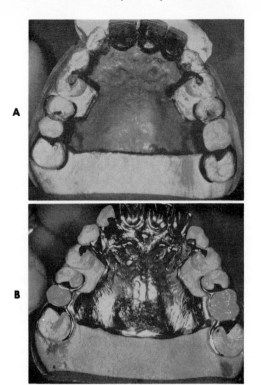

Fig. 8-4. Class III, modification 2, partial denture with palatal plate supporting tubed teeth posteriorly and Steele's facings anteriorly. The design is actually an anatomic replica palatal plate extended anteriorly to support anterior replacements. The entire palatal plate is as thin as mechanically feasible and of uniform thickness, made possible by using an anatomic replica major connector. Esthetics dictated the spacing between the incisor teeth, which could not easily have been accomplished with a fixed partial denture. Note also the clearance lingual to the premolar abutments. **A,** The wax and plastic pattern for this casting, with a plaster index for positioning anterior Steele's facings. The backings are plastic waxed to the anatomic replica palatal pattern. **B,** The completed casting.

type of attachment are the difficulties in obtaining satisfactory occlusion, lack of adequate contours for functional tongue and cheek contact, and unesthetic display of metal at gingival margins. The latter is avoided when the tooth is butted directly to the ridge, but then the retention for the tooth frequently becomes inadequate.

A modification of this method is the attachment of ready-made resin teeth to the metal base with acrylic resin of the same shade. This is called *pressing on* a resin tooth and is not the same as using resin for cementation. It is particularly applicable to anterior replacements, since it is desirable to know in advance of making the casting that the shade and contours of the selected tooth will be acceptable. (See Fig. 8-3.) After making a labial index of the position of the teeth, the lingual portion of the tooth then is cut away to make room for retention on the casting. Subsequently, the tooth is attached to the denture with acrylic resin of the same shade. Being done under pressure, the acrylic resin attachment is comparable to the manufactured tooth in hardness and strength.

Tube or side-groove teeth must be selected in advance of waxing the denture framework. Yet, for best occlusal relationships, jaw relation records always should be made with the denture casting in the mouth. This problem may be solved by selecting tube teeth for width but with occlusal surfaces slightly higher than will be necessary. The teeth are ground to fit the ridge with sufficient clearance beneath for a thin metal base and beveled to accommodate a boxing of metal. If a plastic tube tooth is used, the diatoric hole should be made slightly larger than provided. The casting is completed and tried in, occlusal relationships are recorded, and then the teeth are ground in to harmonious occlusion with the opposing dentition. As will be discussed in Chapter 16, artificial posterior teeth on partial dentures should never be used unaltered but rather should be considered material from which occlusal forms may be created to function harmoniously with the remaining natural occlusion.

3. *Resin teeth processed directly to metal bases.* Modern cross-linked copolymers enable the dentist or technician to process acrylic resin teeth that have satisfactory hardness and abrasion resistance for many situations. Thus occlusion may be created without resorting to the modification of ready-made artificial teeth (Fig.

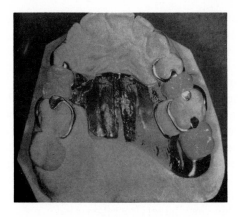

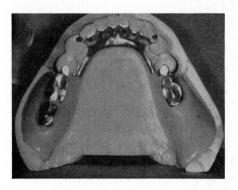

Fig. 8-6. Functional occlusal surfaces cast with inlay-type gold and attached to the denture teeth.

Fig. 8-5. Direct attachment of resin teeth to metal bases. These are waxed to fit the space and opposing occlusion and processed to retention previously provided on the metal framework. Occlusal surfaces of acrylic resin posterior teeth should be duplicated in cast inlay gold.

8-5). Recesses in the denture pattern are either carved by hand or created around manufactured teeth that are used only to form the recess in the pattern. Occlusal relations may be established either in the mouth on the denture framework or by the use of an articulator, and then the teeth are carved and processed in acrylic resin of the proper shade to fit the opposing occlusal record. Better attachment to the metal base than by cementation is thus possible. In addition, unusually long, short, wide, or narrow teeth may be created when necessary to fill spaces not easily filled by the limited selection of ready-made teeth.

Occlusion on resin teeth may be reestablished to compensate for wear or settling by reprocessing new acrylic occlusal surfaces at a later date when this becomes necessary. Distinction always should be made between the need for relining to reestablish occlusion (on a distal extension partial denture) or the need for rebuilding occlusal surfaces on an otherwise satisfactory base (on either a tooth-supported or a tooth-and-tissue supported partial denture).

Reestablishment of occlusion also may be accomplished by placing gold inlays on existing resin teeth. Although this may be done also on porcelain teeth, it is difficult

to cut inlay recesses in porcelain teeth unless air abrasive methods are used. Therefore, if later additions to occlusal surfaces are anticipated, plastic teeth should be used, thereby facilitating the addition of new resin or cast gold surfaces (Fig. 8-6). A simple technique to fabricate cast gold occlusal surfaces and attach them to resin teeth is illustrated in Chapter 17.

4. *Metal teeth.* Occasionally, a second molar tooth may be replaced as part of the partial denture casting. This is usually done when space is too limited for the attachment of an artificial tooth and yet the addition of a second molar is desirable to prevent migration of an opposing second molar. Since the occlusal surface must be waxed prior to casting, perfect occlusion is not possible. Since metal, particularly a chrome alloy, is abrasion resistant, the area of occlusal contact should be held to a minimum to avoid damage to the periodontium of the opposing tooth and the associated discomfort to the patient. Whereas occlusal adjustment on gold occlusal surfaces is readily accomplished, metal teeth made of chrome alloys are difficult to adjust and are objectionably hard for use as occlusal surfaces. Therefore they should be used only to fill a space and to prevent tooth migration and no more.

Need for relining. The distal extension base differs from the tooth-borne base in several respects, one of which is that it must be made of a material that can be relined or rebased when it becomes necessary to reestablish tissue support for the distal extension base. Therefore, resin denture base materials that can be relined are generally used.

Although satisfactory techniques for making distal extension partial denture bases of cast metal are available (see Chapter 15), the fact that metal bases are difficult if not impossible to reline limits their use to stable ridges that will change little over a long period of time.

Changes in ridge form over a period of time may not be visible. Manifestations of change may be seen, however. One of these is a *loss of occlusion* between the distal extension denture base and the opposing dentition, increasing as the distance from the abutment increases. This is proved by having the patient close on strips of 28-gauge green casting wax, or any similar wax, tapping in *centric occlusion* only. Indentations in a wax strip of known thickness are quantitative, whereas marks made with articulating ribbon are only qualitative. In other words, indentations in the wax may be interpreted as being light, medium, or heavy, whereas it is difficult if not impossible to interpret a mark made with articulating ribbon as being light or heavy. In fact, the heaviest occlusal contact may perforate paper articulating ribbon and make a lesser mark than areas of lighter contact. Therefore the use of any articulating ribbon is of limited value in checking occlusion intraorally. In making occlusal adjustments articulating ribbon should be used only to indicate *where* to relieve after the *need for relief* has been established by using wax strips of known thickness. Twenty-eight-gauge green or blue casting wax is usually used for this purpose, although the thinner 30-gauge or the thicker 26-gauge wax may also be used for better evaluation of the clearance between areas not in contact.

Loss of support for a distal extension base will result in a loss of occlusal contact between the denture teeth and the opposing dentition and a return to heavy occlusal contact between the remaining natural teeth. Usually, this is an indication that relining is needed to reestablish the original occlusion by reestablishing supporting contact with the residual ridge. It must be remembered, however, that occlusion on a distal extension base is sometimes maintained at the expense of migration of the opposing natural teeth. In such case, checking the occlusion alone will not show that settling of the extension base has occurred because changes in the supporting ridge may have also taken place.

A second manifestation of change also must be observable to justify relining. This second manifestation of change in the supporting ridge is evidence of rotation about the fulcrum line with the indirect retainers lifting from their seats as the distal extension base is pressed against the ridge tissues. Originally, if the distal extension base was made to fit the supporting form of the residual ridge (see Chapter 15), rotation about the fulcrum line is not visible. At the time the denture is initially placed, no teeter-totter should exist when alternating finger pressure is applied to the indirect retainer and the distal end of a distal extension base or bases. After changes in the ridge form, which causes some loss of support, rotation occurs about the fulcrum axis when alternating finger pressure is applied. This is evidence of changes in the supporting ridge that must be compensated for by relining or rebasing.

If occlusal contact has been lost and rotation about the fulcrum line is evident, then relining is indicated. On the other hand, if occlusal contact has been lost without any evidence of denture rotation, and if stability of the denture base is otherwise satisfactory, then reestablishing the occlusion is the remedy rather than relining. For the latter the original denture base may be used in much the same manner as the original trial base was used to record occlusal relations. Teeth may then be reoccluded to an opposing cast or to an occlusal template, using new teeth or cast gold occlusal surfaces. In any event, new occlusion may be established on the existing bases. Relining in this instance would be the wrong solution to the problem.

More often, however, loss of occlusion is accompanied by settling of the denture base to the extent that rotation about the fulcrum line is manifest. Since relining is the only remedy short of making completely new bases, use of a resin base originally facilitates later relining. For this reason, resin bases are generally preferred for distal extension partial dentures.

The question remains as to when, if ever, metal bases with their several advantages may be used for distal extension partial dentures. It is debatable as to what type of ridge will be the most likely to remain stable under functional loading without apparent change. Certainly the age and general health of the patient will influence the ability of a residual ridge to support function. Minimal and harmonious occlusion and the accuracy with which the base fits the underlying tissues will influence the amount of trauma that will occur under function. Undoubtedly, the absence of trauma plays a big part in the ability of the ridge to maintain its original form.

The best risk for the use of metal distal extension bases is a ridge that has supported a previous partial denture without having become narrowed or flat or consisting primarily of easily displaceable tissues. When such changes have occurred under a previous denture, further change may be anticipated because of the possibility that the oral tissues in question are not capable of supporting a denture base without retrogressive change. Despite every advantage in their favor, apparently there are some such individuals whose ridges respond unfavorably to being called upon to support any denture base.

In other instances, such as when a new partial denture is to be made because of the loss of additional teeth, the ridges may still be firm and healthy. Having previously supported a denture base and having sustained occlusion, bony trabeculae will have become arranged to best support vertical

and horizontal loading, cortical bone will have been formed, and tissue will have become favorable for continued support of a denture base.

Admittedly, there are relatively few instances in which the need for future relining of a distal extension base need not be considered and metal bases may be used. There are, however, many instances that may be considered borderline. In these, metal bases may be used with full understanding on the part of the patient that a new or rebuilt denture may become necessary in the future if unforeseen tissue changes occur. A technique is given in Chapter 15, which permits replacing metal distal extension bases without having to remake the entire denture. This method should be seriously considered any time a distal extension partial denture is to be made with a metal base or bases.

For reasons previously outlined, the possibility that tissues will remain healthier beneath a metal base than they will beneath a resin base may justify its wider use for distal extension partial dentures. Through careful treatment planning, better patient education of the problems involved in making a distal extension denture, and greater care in the fabrication of the denture bases, metal may be used to advantage in some situations in which resin bases are ordinarily used.

STRESSBREAKERS (STRESS EQUALIZERS)

The previous chapters on component parts of a partial denture have presumed absolute rigidity of all parts of the partial denture framework except the direct retainer. All vertical and horizontal stresses applied to the supplied teeth are thus distributed throughout the supporting portions of the dental arch. Broad distribution of stress is accomplished through the rigidity of the major and minor connectors. The effect of the stabilizing components is also made possible by the rigidity of the connectors.

In a distal extension restoration, strain on

the abutment teeth is minimized through the use of functional basing, broad coverage, harmonious occlusion, and flexible direct retainers. Retentive clasp arms may be cast only if they engage undercuts on the abutment teeth in such a manner that tissueward movement of the extension base cannot transmit leverage to the abutment. Otherwise wrought-wire retentive clasp arms should be used because of their greater flexibility. Because of its flexibility, the wrought-wire clasp arm may be said to act as a stressbreaker between the denture base and the abutment tooth.

A concept of stress-breaking exists, however, which insists upon separating the action of the retaining elements from the movement of the distal extension base. Thus, when the term stressbreaker is used, it is generally applied to a device that allows some movement between the denture base or its supporting framework and the direct retainers, whether they are intracoronal or extracoronal in design.

A stressbreaker is also sometimes referred to as a *stress equalizer*. The term *articulated prosthesis* is also frequently applied to a broken-stress partial denture.

More than thirty years ago Kennedy wrote as follows:

Since the advent of the cast clasp and the removable bridge, a great number of men have advocated the use of "stress breakers" between their saddles and the clasps. These have been shown to be absolutely essential by dentists who had used cast clasps for partial dentures. They found that in a short time the teeth to which such clasps were attached loosened, and that this was due mainly to the rigidity of the clasp.

A well-designed round wire clasp is, in itself, a stress breaker, and allows sufficient saddle movement to prevent excessive strain upon the abutment teeth. . . .

In my hands, stress breakers used on partial dentures have permitted so much movement of the saddles, that they produce excessive soreness, and, after many trials, especially after patients have worn them for some time, I found that a greater number of abutment teeth were loosened than where we used the double bar,

. . . the "continuous clasp" [what is now known as the secondary lingual bar or Kennedy bar]. It is only where we have too few teeth in the mouth that it is necessary to use some form of specially designed stress breaker between the clasps and saddles.

. . . Clasps should not be made so rigid that they hold the denture in place. We must depend on the inherent stability of the saddles to prevent strain on the teeth. . . . If there are only one or two teeth present, we would not expect these teeth to do the work of fourteen, without excessive strain being placed upon them, and it is in such conditions that some form of stress breaker becomes useful.*

Several partial denture textbooks have little to say about stressbreakers, as though to avoid a controversial subject. That the subject is controversial is evidenced by the rigid adherence to their use with apparent success by some, whereas properly designed rigid restorations are routinely used by others without harm to abutments. It is only the improperly designed or ineffectively fabricated rigid restoration that has proved to be harmful to abutment teeth. There is little question that some form of mechanical stressbreaker is preferable to a poorly designed and ineffectively fabricated rigid restoration.

It is interesting and significant to note that the development and promotion of stressbreaker designs in this country has been largely through the efforts of the commercial dental laboratory. In most instances this has been due to the failure of the dentist to furnish the laboratory with a master cast that provides for adequate denture base support. If the dentist is not inclined to employ carefully contoured abutment retainers that permit the use of proper clasp designs, and is not willing to take the steps necessary to provide maximum support for tissue-supported denture bases, then he probably should utilize one of the stressbreaker designs offered by the commercial dental laboratory.

---

*From Kennedy, E.: Partial denture construction, Brooklyn, 1942, Denture Items of Interest Publishing Co., Inc.

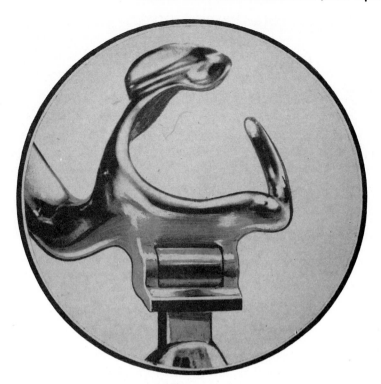

Fig. 8-7. D-E hinge-type stressbreaker utilizing a vertical stop to limit movement of the denture base away from the tissues. Properly applied, this type of stressbreaker permits the effective use of one or more indirect retainers located anterior to the fulcrum line. The trunnion design of the stressbreaker also prevents lateral movement, thus assuring a degree of bilateral stability comparable to that of a one-piece framework. (Courtesy Austenal, Inc., Chicago, Ill.)

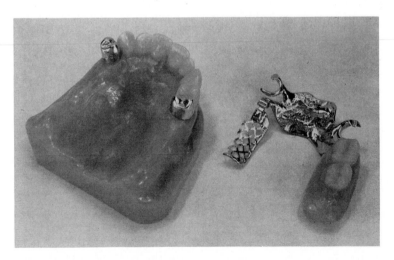

Fig. 8-8. D-E hinge-type stressbreaker before and after the resin denture base has been added. Hinge action is limited to tissueward movement only by the presence of a stop bar. (Courtesy Austenal, Inc., Chicago, Ill.)

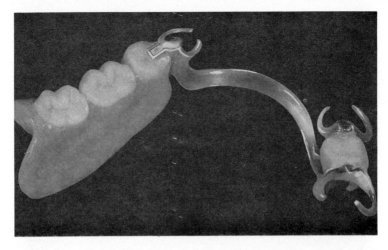

Fig. 8-9. Kennedy Class II, modification 1, partial denture utilizing a hinge stressbreaker of Baca design. Hinge and vertical movements are permitted by the fact that the action is protected by a metal sleeve rather than being embedded in the resin base material. (Courtesy Ticonium Division of CMP Industries, Inc., Albany, N. Y.)

Types of stressbreakers. Stressbreakers may be divided into two groups. In the first group are those having a movable joint between the direct retainer and the denture base (Figs. 8-7 to 8-9). Into this group fall the hinges, sleeves and cylinders, and ball-and-socket devices (some of which are spring-loaded). Being placed between the direct retainer and the denture base, they may permit both vertical movement and hinge action of the distal extension base. This serves to prevent some direct transmission of tipping forces to the abutment teeth as the base moves tissueward under function.

Examples of this group are the various hinges, the Swiss-made Dalbo attachment, the Crismani attachment, the C & M 637 attachment, and the ASC 52 attachment. Most of these attachments are prefabricated, but the laboratory may utilize dual-casting techniques for fabricating the attachment. Because of the rapid wear likely to occur with gold, such attachments are usually made of a harder alloy and therefore are usually machine-made.

The student is referred to three excellent textbooks that describe in detail the use of stressbreakers and articulated partial denture designs: (1) *Precision Attach-ments in Dentistry* by H. W. Preiskel, (2) *Precision Work for Partial Dentures* by Alfred A. Steiger and Raoul H. Boitel of Zurich, and (3) *Protesis Parcial Removible* by Adalberto D. Rebossio of Buenos Aires. The latter is available in Spanish only.

The articulated partial denture designs include those designs having a flexible connection between the direct retainer and the denture base. These include the use of wrought-wire connectors, divided major connectors, and other flexible devices for permitting movement of the distal extension base (Figs. 8-10 and 8-11). Included also in this group are those utilizing a movable joint between two major connectors. These are generally fabricated by the laboratory with a dual-casting technique. The earliest of such connectors were double lingual bars of wrought metal, one supporting the clasps and other components and the other supporting and connecting the distal extension bases. The two bars were usually but not always united at the midline by binding with fine wire and soldering.

The latter principle is still widely used in the form of split major connectors. Instead of using wrought metal, a single cast connector is made flexible by separating a

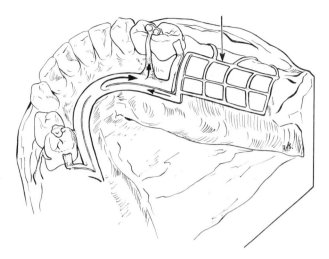

Fig. 8-10. Stress-breaking effect of a split bar major connector. Vertical and diagonal forces applied to the tissue-supported base must pass anteriorly along the lower bar and then back along the more rigid upper bar to reach the abutment tooth. Thus tipping forces that would otherwise be transmitted directly to the abutment tooth are dissipated by the flexibility of the lower bar and the distance traveled.

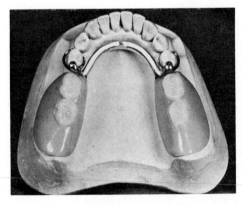

Fig. 8-11. Early type of stress equalizer. The direct retainers (clasps) are connected by a 16-gauge, round, wrought wire. An inferiorly placed cast major connector connects the denture bases. The heavy wrought wire and the cast major connector are joined with solder at the midline only. A need for indirect retention still exists even though a stress equalizer is utilized.

portion of its length. This may be done by making a saw cut part way through a gold casting with a jeweler's saw or by casting to a thin shim; which is then removed leaving a separation. Although mica and other materials have been used for this purpose, stainless steel is usually used (0.02 Tru-

chrome band material), which is then removed by acid. The nature of chrome-cobalt alloys permits the making of one casting first and then waxing and casting the second part to the first without union. This facilitates the making of split bars and movable joints with fine precision and nearly imperceptible junction lines. In any event, the resulting flexibility of the major connector acts to prevent some direct transmission of forces to the abutment tooth.

Double major connectors must be coupled in some manner so that the two parts of the restoration cannot come apart in the mouth, yet will permit freedom of movement of the denture base. Many ingenious connections have been devised, such as a ball-and-socket device developed by Dr. Charles S. Ballard. This is a Vitallium acetabulum that is waxed into the denture in such a manner that a socket, which works freely yet prevents separation, is cast around it. (See Figs. 8-12 and 8-13.)

The principal advantages claimed for partial dentures made with the Ballard stress equalizer attachment are as follows:

1. Occlusal pressures are distributed equally to the edentulous ridges and the supporting abutments.

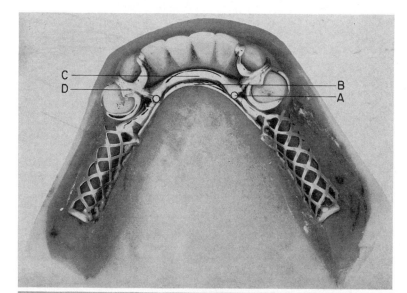

Fig. 8-12

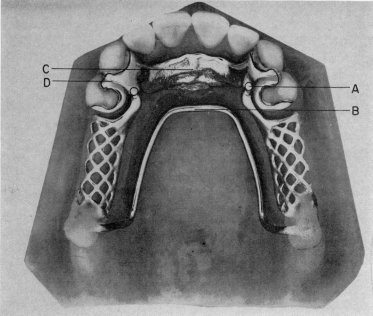

Fig. 8-13

Fig. 8-12. Conventionally clasped lower partial denture framework with lingual bar connecting the rests and clasps. Circles indicate position of Ballard stress equalizer attachment (ball-and-socket joint). **A,** Location of the Ballard stress equalizers; **B,** 14-gauge round (wrought-wire) stabilizing bar; **C,** rigid major connector; **D,** casting, which supports the anterior part by means of clasp attachments. (Courtesy Dr. Charles S. Ballard.)

Fig. 8-13. Upper partial denture framework with palatal bar connecting the rests and clasps, both of which are set into routed portions of the crowns. Circles indicate position of the Ballard stress equalizer attachments. **A,** Location of the Ballard stress equalizers; **B,** 14-gauge round (wrought-wire) stabilizing bar; **C,** rigid major connector; **D,** casting, which supports the anterior part by means of clasp attachments. (Courtesy Dr. Charles S. Ballard.)

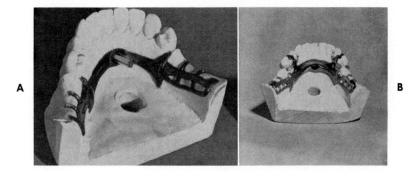

Fig. 8-14. Ticonium hidden-lock partial denture. **A,** The lower half of the framework consisting of the lower half of the lingual bar and the denture base retainer is cast first with a bi-bevel circle formed in the wax pattern by waxing around a lightly oiled mandrel, which is removed to provide a perfect circle within the wax. This half is cast as illustrated. **B,** On a second investment cast, the original bar is replaced and the remainder of the framework is waxed to it. This portion consists of the clasps, indirect retainers, and the remainder of the bar. The hidden-lock and split bar are made possible because of the thin oxide shell that forms during the second casting, leaving an almost imperceptible junction line between the two sections. Hinge movement occurs at the circle in the midline. (Courtesy Ticonium Co., Albany, N. Y.)

2. Individual movement of denture bases is permitted, both perpendicular and lateral, or a combination of both.

3. Torque is eliminated through the action of the universal joints connecting the denture bases and the body of casting.

The equalizer principle may be applied to both upper and lower arches in many different combinations of remaining teeth. It may be used with the conventional lingual bar design or in combination with the continuous bar retainer.

Ideally, the Ballard stress equalizer attachment should be placed on a line between the principal abutments, but it may be placed distogingivally to the posterior abutments. Unlike the hinge, which presumably permits vertical movement only, the denture bases may move laterally also, controlled and stabilized by the presence of a 14-gauge wrought-wire functioning as a "second" bar.

Another design utilizing a dual-casting technique is the Ticonium hidden-lock design (Fig. 8-14). This is a two-piece casting. The top half, which is the major connector supporting the direct retainers and other rigid components, is cast first, and the bottom half, which is the connector between the denture bases, is cast to the first.

The latter is completely independent of the first except that it is locked in by a circle-type retention, prepared in the wax pattern.

The hidden-lock is created by mechanical means, and the split between the two connectors is made possible by the thin oxide shell that forms during the making of the two sections. What appears to be a conventional lingual bar or linguoplate actually is two bars connected by a movable joint at the midline.

Other framework designs utilizing a dual-casting technique are known as the "floating clasp" and "floating saddle" dentures (Fig. 8-15). Such designs have as their objective the distribution of stress to both the residual ridges and abutment teeth within the physiologic tolerance of these supporting structures.

Still other devices permit disassembly of the denture by the patient for cleaning. All mechanical devices that are free to move in the mouth collect debris and become unclean; therefore, disassembly is a desirable feature whether done daily by the patient or periodically by the dentist (some hinged devices have small screws that may be removed for cleaning or adjusting the action of the device).

In addition to the trapping of debris,

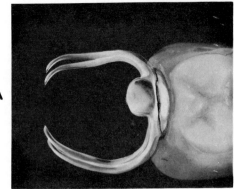

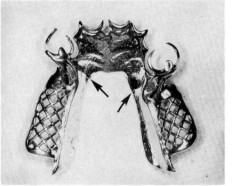

A

B

Fig. 8-15. A, Double-exposed photograph demonstrating the magnitude of vertical movement with a "floating clasp." Some lateral movement of the clasp could also be demonstrated. **B,** Denture base attached to this framework will move independent of the framework both vertically and laterally to a slight degree. The line of junction between the minor connector and framework may be seen (arrows). Such a restoration is commercially described as a "floating saddle" denture. (Courtesy Nobilium Products, Inc., Chicago, Ill.)

some split connectors used as stressbreakers have been known to pinch the underlying soft tissues or the tongue as they open and close under function. Further, such flexible connectors, especially those made of cast alloys, became fatigued through repeated flexing, resulting in permanent distortion of the denture framework and possible ultimate failure through fracture.

Regardless of their design, all stressbreakers effectively dissipate vertical stresses, which is the purpose for which they are used. At the same time their flexibility or mechanical movement eliminates the horizontal stability at the distal extension base that is inherent in a rigid partial denture design. The effectiveness of minor connectors, stabilizing components, occlusal rests, and indirect retainers is either lost or dissipated by the action of the stressbreakers. As a result, consideration of the abutments is at the expense of the tissues of the residual ridge. This is evidenced by the fact that the stress-broken denture will often require relief on the tissue side of the buccal flange. Since horizontal stresses cannot be resisted by rigid stabilizing components elsewhere in the arch, the residual ridge is forced to bear those horizontal forces alone. This and the added cost are the most

obvious disadvantages to the use of stressbreakers in distal extension partial denture designs.

Advantages of stressbreakers. Some of the claimed advantages of the stress-breaking principle may be listed as follows:

1. Since the horizontal forces acting on the abutment teeth are minimized, the alveolar support of these teeth is preserved.

2. By careful choice of the type of flexible connector, it is possible to obtain a balance of stress between the abutment teeth and the residual ridge.

3. Intermittent pressure of the denture bases massages the mucosa, thus providing physiologic stimulation, which prevents bone resorption and eliminates the need for relining.

4. If relining is needed but not done, the abutment teeth are not damaged as quickly.

5. Splinting of weak teeth by the denture is made possible despite the movement of a distal extension base.

Disadvantages of stressbreakers. Some of the disadvantages of the stress-breaking principle are as follows:

1. The broken-stress denture is usually more difficult to construct and therefore more costly.

2. Vertical and horizontal forces are concentrated on the residual ridge, result-

ing in increased ridges resorption. Many stressbreaker designs are not well stabilized against horizontal forces. Proponents of broken-stress dentures claim that this is avoided by the intermittent massage, which stimulates and promotes better health of the residual ridge.

3. If relining is not done when needed, excessive resorption of the residual ridge may result. This is offset to some extent by the fact that such a denture base is no longer in occlusion and therefore resorption may not be progressive.

4. The effectiveness of indirect retainers is reduced or eliminated altogether.

5. The more complicated the prosthesis, the less it may be tolerated by the patient. Spaces between components are sometimes opened up in function, thus trapping food and, occasionally, the tissues of the mouth.

6. Flexible connectors may be bent and distorted by careless handling. Even a slightly distorted connector may induce more stress on the abutment rather than less.

7. Repair and maintenance of any stressbreaker is difficult, costly, and frequently required.

Advantages of a rigid design. Some of the advantages of the rigid partial denture design may be listed as follows:

1. Mechanically, the framework is easier and less costly to make.

2. Equitable distribution of stress between abutments and the residual ridge(s) is possible with a rigid design.

3. The need for relining the rigid prosthesis is less frequent since the residual ridge does not have to carry the functional load unaided.

4. Indirect retainers and other rigid components may act to prevent rotational movement of the denture and will provide horizontal stabilization that is not possible when stressbreakers are used.

5. By reducing the number of flexible or movable parts, there is less danger of distortion by careless handling on the part of the patient.

6. Moving parts being absent, the prosthesis is more easily kept clean.

Disadvantages of a rigid design. Some of the possible disadvantages of the rigid denture design are as follows:

1. Objectionable torque will be applied to the abutment teeth if abutment retainers are not passive and correctly designed.

2. Rigid continuous clasping may be hazardous when stressbreakers are not used.

3. Locking-type (dovetail) intracoronal retainers may not be used at all without stressbreakers on distal extension dentures, because they are locked within the abutment and tipping forces would be transmitted directly to the abutment tooth. Even when used in conjunction with multiple splinting of abutments, coupled with a minimum of occlusion on the distal extension denture base, locking-type retainers are still risky.

4. The use of wrought-wire retentive clasp arms as stressbreakers presents some technical difficulties, particularly when high-fusing chrome alloys are used. Wrought wire may be crystallized by improper application of heat during casting or soldering operations, resulting in early fracture. It also may be easily distorted by careless handling, leading to excessive or insufficient retention, or ultimate fracture due to repeated adjustment.

5. If relining is not done when needed, the abutment tooth may be loosened and suffer permanent periodontal damage because of the repeated application of torque and tipping stresses.

CHAPTER 9

Principles of removable partial denture design

FACTORS INFLUENCING THE DESIGN OF THE REMOVABLE PARTIAL DENTURE

As a direct result of examination and diagnosis, the design of the removable partial denture must originate on the diagnostic cast so that all mouth preparations may be planned and performed with a specific design in mind. This will be influenced by many factors, some of which are listed below:

1. Which arch is to be restored and if both, their relationship to one another.

2. Type of major connector indicated based on existing and/or correctable situations.

3. Whether or not the denture will be entirely tooth borne. If one or more distal extension bases are involved, the following must be considered:
   a. Need for indirect retention
   b. Clasp designs that will best minimize the forces applied to the abutment teeth during function
   c. Need for later rebasing, which will influence the type of base material used
   d. Secondary impression method to be used

4. Materials to be used, both for the framework and for the bases.

5. Type of replacement teeth to be used. This may be influenced by the opposing dentition.

6. Need for abutment restorations, which may influence the type of clasp arms to be used and their specific design.

7. Patient's past experience with a removable partial denture and the reasons for making a new denture. If, for example, a lingual bar has been objectionable, was it due to its design, fit, or the patient's inability to accept it? Frequently, this alone justifies the use of a contoured linguoplate rather than a lingual bar. If an anterior palatal bar has proved objectionable, was it due to its bulk, its location, or its flexibility, or to tissue irritation? A design using a thin palatal major connector located more posteriorly may be preferable to an ante-

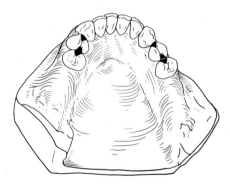

Fig. 9-1. Kennedy Class I partially edentulous arch. The major support for the denture bases must come from the residual ridges, tooth support from occlusal rests being effective only at the anterior portion of each base.

rior bar or palatal horseshoe design located anteriorly.

8. Periodontal condition of the remaining teeth, the amount of abutment support remaining, and the need for splinting. This may be accomplished either by means of fixed restorations or by the design of the denture framework.

9. Method to be used for replacing single teeth or missing anterior teeth. The decision to use fixed restorations for these spaces rather than replacing them with the removable partial denture must be made at the time of treatment planning. Such a decision will necessarily influence the design of the denture framework.

DIFFERENTIATION BETWEEN TWO MAIN TYPES

It is clear that two distinctly different types of removable partial dentures exist. Certain points of difference are present between the Class I and Class II types of partial dentures on the one hand and the Class III type of partial denture on the other. The first consideration is the *manner in which each is supported*. The Class I type and the distal extension side of the Class II type derive their support to a great extent from the tissues underlying the base and only to a limited degree from the abutment teeth (Fig. 9-1), whereas the Class III type derives all its support from the abutment teeth at each end of the edentulous space (Fig. 9-2).

Second, for reasons directly related to the manner of support, the *method of impression registration* required for each type will vary.

Third, the *need for some kind of indirect retention* exists in the distal extension type of partial denture, whereas in the tooth-borne, Class III type there may be no extension base that can lift away from the supporting tissues because of the action of sticky foods and movements of the tissues of the mouth against borders of the denture. This is because each end of each denture base is secured by a direct retainer on an abutment tooth unless anterior teeth

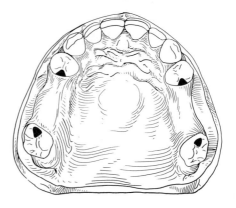

Fig. 9-2. Kennedy Class III, modification 1, partially edentulous arch, which provides total tooth support for the prosthesis. A removable partial denture made for this arch is totally supported by properly prepared occlusal rest seats on the four abutment teeth.

are replaced by the denture. Therefore, the tooth-borne partial denture does not rotate about a fulcrum as does the distal extension partial denture.

Fourth, the manner in which the distal extension type of partial denture is supported often necessitates the *use of a base material that can be relined* to compensate for tissue changes. Acrylic resin is generally used as a base material for distal extension bases. The Class III partial denture, on the other hand, being entirely tooth supported, does not require rebasing except when it is advisable to eliminate an unhygienic, unesthetic, or uncomfortable condition resulting from loss of tissue contact. Metal bases, therefore, are more frequently used in tooth-borne restorations, since rebasing is not as likely to be necessary with them.

Differences in support. The distal extension partial denture, since it derives its major support from the elastic, fibrous connective tissue covering of the residual ridge, is dependent upon the quality of that support for its stability under functional loading. Some areas of this residual ridge are firm, with limited displaceability, whereas other areas are displaceable, depending upon the thickness and structural character of the tissues overlying the residual alveolar bone. The movement of the base under function determines the occlusal efficiency of the partial denture and also the degree to which the abutment teeth are subjected to torque and tipping stresses.

Impression registration. An impression registration for the construction of a partial denture must fulfill the following two requirements:

1. The anatomic form and the relationship of the remaining teeth in the dental arch, as well as the surrounding soft tissues, must be recorded accurately so that the denture will not exert pressure on those structures beyond their physiologic limits and its retentive and stabilizing components may be properly placed. Some impression material that can be removed from undercut areas without permanent distortion must be used to fulfill this requirement. The elastic impression materials such as reversible hydrocolloid agar or irreversible hydrocolloid alginate, mercaptan rubber base (Thiokol), and silicone impression materials are therefore used for this purpose.

2. The supporting form of the soft tissues underlying the distal extension base of the partial denture should be recorded so that firm areas are used as primary stress-bearing areas and readily displaceable tissues are not overloaded. Only in this way can maximum support of the partial denture base be obtained. An impression material that is capable of displacing tissue sufficiently to register the supporting form of the ridge will fulfill this second requirement. One of the fluid mouth-temperature waxes, such as Kerr's Korecta wax No. 4, or any of the readily flowing materials, such as rubber base, zinc oxide–eugenol impression paste, or silicone impression material, provided an individual, corrected tray is used may be employed for registering the supporting form.

No single impression material can satisfactorily fulfill both of the previously mentioned requirements. The compromise by recording just the anatomic form of both

teeth and supporting tissues can result only in inadequate support for the distal extension base of the partial denture.

Differences in clasp design. A fifth point of difference between the two main types of partial dentures lies in their *requirements for direct retention.*

Direct retainers may be classified as being either intracoronal or extracoronal in type. The clasp-type partial denture, utilizing the extracoronal direct retainer, is probably used a hundred times more frequently than is the intracoronal, or internal attachment, partial denture. This is not necessarily an indication of increasing preference for the clasp denture, nor is it a reflection upon the excellence of the internal attachment denture. The fact remains, however, that although the internal attachment was devised more than forty-five years ago, for economic and other reasons the clasp denture is the more widely used. The clasp denture permits the rendering of a physiologically sound partial denture service to the greatest number of patients in keeping with the ability of the majority of patients to pay for such service.

The tooth-borne partial denture, being totally supported by abutment teeth, is retained and stabilized by a clasp at each end of each edentulous space. The only requirement of such clasps is that they flex sufficiently during placement and removal of the denture to pass over the height of contour of the teeth in approaching or escaping from an undercut area. *While in its terminal position on the tooth, a retentive clasp should be passive and should not be called upon to flex except when engaging the undercut area of the tooth for resisting a vertical dislodging force.*

Cast retentive arms are generally used for this purpose. These may be either of the circumferential type, arising from the body of the clasp and approaching the undercut from an occlusal direction, or of the bar type, arising from the base of the denture and approaching the undercut area from a gingival direction. A modification of the latter type is the infrabulge clasp. Each of these two types of cast clasps has its advantages and disadvantages.

The direct retainer adjacent to a distal extension base must perform still another function in addition to that of resisting vertical displacement. Because of the lack of tooth support distally, the denture base will move tissueward under function proportionate to the quality of the supporting tissues, the accuracy of the impression registration, the accuracy of the denture base, and the total occlusal load applied. Because of this tissueward movement, those elements of the circumferential clasp that lie in a mesial undercut area must be able to flex sufficiently to dissipate stresses, which otherwise would be transmitted directly to the abutment tooth as leverage. On the other hand, a bar-type retainer placed to take advanage of a distal undercut moves farther into the undercut and does not overly stress the abutment tooth.

The cast circumferential clasp cannot effectively act to dissipate this stress for two reasons. First, the material itself can have only a limited flexibility, or else other parts of the casting, which must be rigid, such as lingual and palatal bars, would also tend to be flexible. The material employed being the same, the only variable factors are the bulk and diameter used in each component part. Second, and probably more important, the cast circumferential clasp is, of necessity, made half-round in shape. Since edgewise flexing is negligible, the clasp can flex in only one direction and therefore cannot effectively dissipate, by flexing, the torque stresses placed upon it. For this reason some torque is inevitably transmitted to the abutment tooth, which is magnified by the length of the lever arm.

Immediately there comes to mind the stressbreakers, which are often incorporated into the partial denture design for this reason. There are those who strongly believe that a stressbreaker is the best means of preventing leverage from being transmitted to the abutment teeth. It is just as strongly believed by others that a wrought-wire or bar-type retentive arm more effectively accomplishes this purpose with greater simplicity and ease of application. It cannot be denied that a retentive clasp arm made of wrought wire can flex more readily in all directions than can the cast half-round clasp arm and thereby more effectively dissipate those stresses that would otherwise be transmitted to the abutment tooth. The advantages and disadvantages of stressbreakers have been considered in detail in Chapter 8.

Only the retentive arm of the circumferential clasp, however, should be made of wrought metal. Reciprocation and stabilization against lateral movement must be obtained through the use of rigid cast elements that make up the remainder of the clasp. This is called a combination clasp, being a combination of both cast and wrought materials incorporated into one direct retainer. It is frequently used on the terminal abutment for the distal extension partial denture and is indicated where a mesiobuccal but no distobuccal undercut exists or can be made, or where a gross tissue undercut, cervical and buccal to the abutment tooth, exists. It must always be remembered that the factor of length contributes to the flexibiliy of clasp arms. A short wrought-wire arm can be a destructive element because of its reduced ability to flex compared with a longer wrought-wire arm. However in addition to its greater flexibility compared to the cast circumferential clasp, the combination clasp has further advantages of adjustablity, minimal tooth contact, and better esthetics, which justifies its occasional use in tooth-borne designs also.

ESSENTIALS OF PARTIAL DENTURE DESIGN

The design of the partial denture framework should be carefully planned and outlined on an accurate diagnostic cast. After the making of necessary mouth changes to provide for rests, optimal location of framework components, and guiding planes, the master cast is made and carefully surveyed to determine the location of undercut areas that are either to be blocked out or utilized for retention. The design should provide for occlusal rests and rigid reciprocal arms on all abutment teeth to assure vertical and horizontal stability of the partial denture.

The design must include provision for adequate indirect retention that will function to counteract any lifting of the distal extension base away from the tissues. The indirect retainers should be placed in relation to a line drawn through the occlusal rests of the two principal abutments, which is the axis of rotation, or the *fulcrum line*. The indirect retainer may be in the form of an auxiliary occlusal rest, a continuous bar retainer in combination with terminal rests, a linguoplate with terminal rests, or an incisal rest on an anterior tooth. The indirect retainer should be placed as far as possible from this fulcrum line and should not terminate on a tooth incline, such as the lingual surface of an anterior tooth.

Some retentive elements for the attachment of the impression waxes and later the resin bases must be provided for to complete the partial denture framework.

The Class III removable partial denture (Figs. 9-3 to 9-8). The Kennedy Class III removable partial denture, being entirely tooth supported, may be made entirely to fit the anatomic form of the teeth and surrounding structures. It does not require an impression of the functional form of the ridge tissues nor does it require indirect retention. Cast clasps of either the circumferential or the bar type may be used, or the combination clasp may be used if preferred. Unless a need for later rebasing is anticipated, as in the case of recently extracted teeth, the denture base may be made of metal, as it has several advantages.

The Class III partial denture can frequently be utilized as a valuable aid to periodontal treatment because of its stabilizing influence on the remaining teeth (Fig. 9-7).

The Class I, bilateral, distal extension partial denture. The Class I, bilateral, dis-

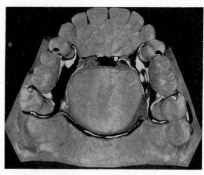

Fig. 9-3. Removable partial denture in a maxillary Class III arch. The design consists of anterior and posterior palatal bar major connectors, resin-supported artificial teeth, and bar clasp arms throughout. (From McCracken, W. L.: J. Prosthet. Dent. 8:71-84, 1958.)

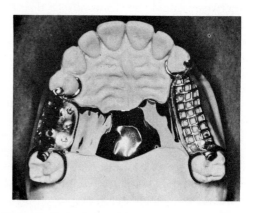

Fig. 9-4. Removable partial denture framework in a maxillary Class III arch. The design consists of a single palatal major connector, bar and circumferential clasp arms and means to attach resin-supported artificial teeth.

tal extension partial denture is just about as unlike the Class III type as any two dental restorations could be. Since it derives its principal support from the tissues underlying its base, a Class I partial denture made to anatomic ridge form cannot have uniform and adequate support. Yet, unfortunately, many Class I mandibular partial dentures are being made from a single hydrocolloid impression. In such situations, both the abutment teeth and the residual ridges suffer because the occlusal load placed upon the remaining teeth is inevita-

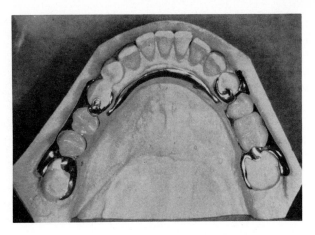

Fig. 9-5. Removable partial denture in a mandibular Class III arch. The design consists of a lingual bar major connector, metal bases and tube teeth, and bar clasp arms. Note the mesially inclined left third molar with onlay-type reciprocal clasp arm. (From McCracken, W. L.: J. Prosthet. Dent. 8:71-84, 1958.)

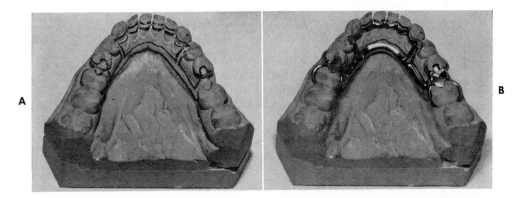

Fig. 9-6. A, Carefully designed tooth-borne denture framework outlined on the master cast, in this particular instance to support anterior teeth in the mouth of a musician being traumatized by constant trumpet playing. Note the positive lingual rest seats on the canines. B, Cast framework as returned from the laboratory, following precisely the design prescribed by the dentist.

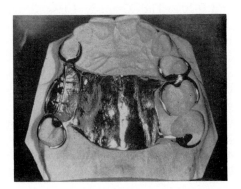

Fig. 9-7. Maxillary Class III partial denture framework designed for maximum periodontal support. The posterior occlusal rest and clasp arm on the nonedentulous side are added for stabilization and to prevent settling of the major connector at that point. A partial metal base is used to avoid any display of base metal anteriorly.

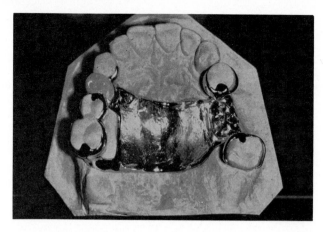

Fig. 9-8. Maxillary Class III, modification 1, denture designed as a periodontal splint. Full crowns on the patient's right premolar and molar are splinted together with continuous lingual ledges. The patient's left premolar is a full crown with lingual ledge. The left molar abutment is unrestored but altered somewhat by recontouring. All gold guiding plane surfaces, lingual and proximal, were machined **parallel to the path** of placement. Unilateral fixed partial dentures would not **provide the bilateral stabilization need**ed for this patient.

bly made greater by the lack of adequate posterior support.

Many dentists, recognizing the need for some type of impression registration that will record the supporting form of the residual ridge, attempt to record this form with a metallic oxide, rubber base, or silicone impression material. Such materials actually only record the anatomic form of the ridge, except when special design of the impression trays permits placement of tissues overlying primary stress-bearing areas. Others prefer to place a base that was made to fit the anatomic form of the ridge under some pressure at the time that it is related to the remaining teeth, thus obtaining functional support. Any impression record will be influenced by the consistency of the impression material and the amount of hydraulic pressure exerted by its confinement within the impression tray. Still others, believing that a properly compounded mouth-temperature wax will displace only those tissues that are incapable of providing support to the denture base, use a wax secondary impression to record the supporting, or functional, form of the edentulous ridge.

The Class II partial denture (Figs. 9-9

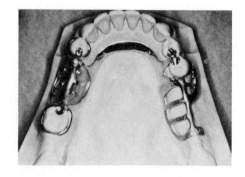

Fig. 9-9. Mandibular Class II, modification 1, partial denture framework for a resin distal extension base and a cast base on the tooth-borne modification space. A bar-type retainer engaging a distobuccal undercut on the right second premolar is used.

and 9-10). The Kennedy Class II partial denture actually may be a combination of both tissue-borne and tooth-borne restorations. The distal extension base must have adequate tissue support, whereas tooth-borne bases elsewhere in the arch may be made to fit the anatomic form of the underlying ridge. Indirect retention must be provided for, but occasionally the anterior abutment on the tooth-borne side will serve to satisfy this requirement. If addition in-

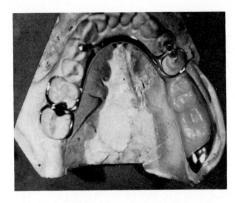

Fig. 9-10. Mandibular Class II partial denture with metal distal extension base. Acrylic resin attachment of the denture teeth to the metal base is with suitable mechanical retention (nailheads, loops, or spurs plus an undercut finishing line). Embrasure clasps are used on the nonedentulous side, with an indirect retainer located favorably in relation to the fulcrum line. Because of a tissue undercut cervical to the buccal surface of the right second premolar and the lack of a distobuccal undercut, a wrought-wire (tapered) retainer arm was used.

direct retention is needed, provisions must be made for it.

Cast clasps are generally used on the tooth-borne side, whereas some clasp design must be used on the abutment tooth adjacent to the distal extension, which will prevent the application of torque to that tooth. *A thorough understanding of the advantages and disadvantages of various clasp designs is necessary in determining the type of direct retainer that is to be used for each abutment tooth.*

The steps in the completion of the Class II partial denture follow closely those of the Class I partial denture, except that the distal extension base is usually made of a resin material, whereas the base for any tooth-borne areas is frequently made of metal. This is permissible because the residual ridge beneath tooth-borne bases is not called upon to provide support for the denture and later rebasing is not as likely to be necessary.

COMPONENT PARTS OF THE PARTIAL DENTURE

All partial dentures have two things in common: (1) they must be supported by

oral tissues and (2) they must be retained against reasonable dislodging forces.

In the Class III partial denture, three components are necessary: the connectors, the retainers, and the bracing or stabilizing components.

The partial denture that does not have the advantage of tooth support at each end of each edentulous space still must have support, but in this instance, the support comes from both the teeth and the underlying ridge tissues rather than from the teeth alone. This is a composite support, and the prosthesis must be fabricated so that the resilient support provided by the edentulous ridge is coordinated with the more stable support offered by the abutment teeth. The three essentials—connectors, retainers, and stabilizing components—must be even more carefully designed and executed because of the movement of tissue-supported denture base areas. In addition, provision must be made for three other essentials, as follows:

1. The best possible support must be obtained from the resilient ridge tissues. This is accomplished by the impression technique more than by the partial denture design, although the amount of area covered by the partial denture is a contributing factor in such support.

2. The method of direct retention must take into account the inevitable tissueward movement of the distal extension base(s) under the stresses of mastication and occlusion. Either some kind of stressbreaker must be used or direct retainers must be designed so that some flexing or stressbreaking under occlusal loading will occur to prevent the direct transmission instead of leverage to the abutment teeth.

3. The partial denture having one or more distal extension denture bases must be designed so that movement of the unsupported and unretained end away from the tissues will be prevented or minimized. This is often referred to as indirect retention and is best described in relation to an axis of rotation through the rest areas of the principal abutments. However, reten-

tion from the partial denture base itself frequently can be made to prevent this movement of the denture base away from the tissues and, in such instances, may be discussed as direct-indirect retention.

The support of the partial denture by the abutment teeth is dependent upon the alveolar support of those teeth, the rigidity of the partial denture framework, and the design of the occlusal rests. Through clinical and roentgenographic interpretation, the dentist may evaluate the abutment teeth and decide whether or not they will provide adequate support. In some instances, the splinting of two or more teeth is advisable, either by fixed partial dentures or by soldering two or more individual restorations together. In other instances, a tooth may be deemed too weak to be used as an abutment, and extraction is indicated in favor of obtaining better support from an adjacent tooth.

Having decided upon the abutments, the dentist is responsible for the preparation of the abutment teeth, for the design of cast restorations, and for the form of the occlusal rest seats. These may be prepared either in sound tooth enamel or in the cast restorations. The technician cannot be blamed for inadequate occlusal rest support. On the other hand, the technician is solely to blame if he extends the casting beyond or fails to include the total prepared area. If a definite occlusal rest seat, with the floor of the seat, inclined toward the center of the tooth, is faithfully recorded in the master cast and delineated in the penciled design, no excuse can be made for poor occlusal rest form on the partial denture if the dentist has sufficiently reduced the marginal ridge area of the rest seat to avoid interference from opposing teeth.

Major connectors. A major connector should be properly located in relation to gingival and moving tissues and should be of such design as to be rigid. Rigidity in a major connector is necessary to provide proper distribution of forces to and from the supporting components.

A lingual bar connector should be tapered superiorly with a half-pear shape in cross section and should be relieved sufficiently but not excessively over the underlying tissues when such relief is indicated. The addition of a continuous bar retainer or a lingual apron does not alter the basic design of the lingual bar. These are added solely for support, bracing, rigidity, and protection of the anterior teeth and specifically are neither connectors nor indirect retainers. The finished inferior border of either a lingual bar or a linguoplate should be gently rounded to avoid irritation to subadjacent tissues when the restoration moves even slightly in function.

The use of a linguoplate is indicated when the lower anterior teeth are weakened by periodontal disease. It is also indicated in Class I partially edentulous arches wherein the need for additional resistance to horizontal rotation of the denture is occasioned by excessively resorbed residual ridges. Still another indication is in those situations in which the floor of the mouth so closely approximates the lingual gingiva of anterior teeth that an adequate lingual bar cannot be positioned without impinging the gingival tissues.

Experience with the linguoplate has shown that with adequate oral hygiene the underlying tissues remain healthy and there are no harmful effects to the tissues from the metallic coverage per se. However, adequate relief must be provided whenever a metal component crosses the gingival margins and the adjacent gingivae. Excessive relief should be avoided because tissues tend to fill a void, resulting in the overgrowth of abnormal tissue. The amount of relief used, therefore, should be only the minimum necessary to avoid gingival impingement.

It does not seem that there are any advantages to be found in the use of the continuous bar retainer that are not enhanced by the use of a linguoplate. In rare instances, when a linguoplate would show through multiple interproximal embrasures, the continuous bar retainer may be preferred for esthetic reasons only. In other instances, when a single diastema exists, a linguoplate may be cut out in this area to avoid display of metal, without sacrificing its use when otherwise indicated.

Rigidity of a palatal major connector is just as important and its location and design just as critical as is rigidity of a lingual bar. A horseshoe-shaped palatal connector is rarely justified except to avoid an inoperable palatal torus. Neither can the routine use of a narrow, single palatal bar be justified. The anterior and posterior palatal bar is mechanically and biologically sound if it is located so that it does not impinge upon tissues. The broad, anatomic palatal major connector is frequently preferred because of its rigidity, better acceptance by the patient, and greater stability without tissue damage. In addition, this type of connector may provide direct-indirect retention that sometimes may, but rarely, eliminate the need for separate indirect retainers.

Direct retainers for tooth-borne partial dentures. Retainers for tooth-borne partial dentures have only two functions, and these are to retain the prosthesis against reasonable dislodging forces without damage to the abutment teeth and to aid in resisting any tendency of the denture to be displaced in a horizontal plane. There can be no movement of the prosthesis tissueward because each terminus is supported by a rest. There can be no movement away from the tissues, and therefore no rotation about a fulcrum, because each terminus is secured by a direct retainer.

Any type of direct retainer is acceptable as long as the abutment tooth is not jeopardized by its presence. Intracoronal (frictional) retainers are ideal for tooth-borne restorations and offer esthetic advantages not to be had with extracoronal (clasp) retainers. Nevertheless, the circumferential and bar-type clasp retainers are mechanically effective and are more economically constructed than are intracoronal retainers. Therefore they are more universally used.

Vulnerable areas on the abutment teeth must be protected by restorations with ei-

ther type of retainer. The clasp retainer must not impinge upon gingival tissues. The clasp must not exert excessive torque upon the abutment tooth during placement and removal. It must be located the least distance into the tooth undercut for adequate retention, and it must be designed with a minimum of bulk and tooth contact.

The bar clasp arm should be used only when the area for retention lies close to the gingival margin of the tooth and little tissue blockout is necessary. If the clasp must be placed high occlusally, or if an objectional space would exist beneath the bar clasp arm because of blockout of tissue undercuts, the bar clasp arm should not be used.

Direct retainers for distal extension partial dentures. Retainers for distal extension partial dentures, while retaining the prosthesis, must also be able to flex or disengage when the denture base moves tissueward under function. Thus the retainer may act as a stress breaker. Mechanical stressbreakers accomplish the same thing, but they do so at the expense of horizontal stabilization. When some kind of mechanical stressbreaker is used, the denture flange must be able to act to prevent horizontal movement. Clasp designs that allow for flexing of the retentive clasp arm may be designed to accomplish the same purpose as that of mechanical stressbreakers, without sacrificing horizontal stabilization and generally with less complicated techniques.

In evaluating the ability of a clasp arm to act as a stressbreaker, one must realize that flexing in one plane is not enough. Rather, the clasp must be freely flexible in any direction, as dictated by the stresses applied. Bulky, half-round clasp arms cannot do this and neither can a bar clasp engaging an undercut on the side of the tooth away from the denture base. Round clasp forms offer advantages of greater and more universal flexibility, less tooth contact, and better esthetics. *Either the combination circumferential clasp with its wrought-wire retentive arm or the carefully located and properly designed bar clasp should be used on all abutment teeth adjacent to extension denture bases.*

Stabilizing components. Stabilizing or bracing components of the partial denture framework are those rigid components that assist in stabilizing the denture against horizontal movement. The purpose of all stabilizing components should be to distribute stresses equally to all supporting teeth without overworking any one tooth.

All minor connectors that contact vertical tooth surfaces (and all reciprocal clasp arms) act as stabilizing components. It is necessary that minor connectors have sufficient bulk to be rigid and yet that they present as little bulk to the tongue as is possible. This means that they should be confined to interdental embrasures whenever possible. When minor connectors are located on vertical tooth surfaces, it is best that these surfaces be parallel to the path of placement. When cast restorations are used, these surfaces of the wax patterns should be made parallel on the surveyor prior to casting.

Reciprocal clasp arms also must be rigid, and they must be placed above the height of contour of the abutment teeth when they will be nonretentive. By their rigidity these clasp arms reciprocate the opposing retentive clasp and they also prevent horizontal movement of the prosthesis under functional stresses. For a reciprocal clasp arm to be placed favorably, some reduction of the tooth surfaces involved is frequently necessary to increase the suprabulge area.

When crown restorations are used, a lingual reciprocal clasp arm may be inset into the tooth contour by providing a ledge on the crown upon which the clasp arm may rest. This permits the use of a wider clasp arm and restores a more nearly normal tooth contour, at the same time maintaining its strength and rigidity.

Guiding planes. The term "guiding planes" is defined as two or more parallel, vertical surfaces of abutment teeth, so shaped as to direct a prosthesis during placement and removal. Upon ascertaining

the most favorable path of placement, vertical surfaces of abutment teeth (retentive and bracing teeth) are found or prepared parallel to the path of placement, and therefore become parallel to each other. Guiding planes may be contacted by various components of the restoration, that is, the body of an extracoronal direct retainer, the stabilizing arm of a direct retainer, the minor connector portion of an indirect retainer, or by a minor connector specifically designed to contact the guiding plane surface.

The functions of guiding plane surfaces are to: (1) provide for one path of placement and removal of the restoration; (2) ensure the planned and intended action of bracing and retentive components; (3) eliminate detrimental strain to abutment teeth and framework components in placing and removing the restoration; (4) eliminate gross food traps between abutment teeth and denture bases; (5) provide retentive characteristics against dislodgement of the restoration when the dislodging force is directed other than parallel to the path of removal; and (6) provide bracing characteristics against horizontal rotation of the denture.

Guiding plane surfaces should be found or created so that they are as nearly parallel to the long axes of abutment teeth as possible. Establishing guiding planes on several abutment teeth (preferably more than two teeth), located at widely separated positions in the dental arch, provides for a more effective use of these surfaces. The effectiveness of guiding plane surfaces is also enhanced if these surfaces lie in more than one common axial surface of the abutment teeth (Fig. 9-11).

As a rule of thumb, proximal guiding plane surfaces should be about two thirds as wide as the distance between the tips of adjacent buccal and lingual cusps and should extend vertically about two thirds the length of the "enamel crown" portion of the tooth from the marginal ridge cervically. In preparing guiding plane surfaces care must be exercised to avoid creating

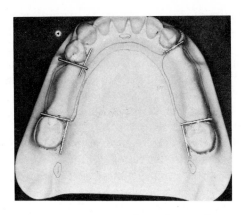

Fig. 9-11. Prospective guiding plane surfaces are indicated by the wires placed on the abutment teeth. All of these surfaces, when utilized, can be made vertically parallel to each other. However, by including guiding plane surfaces, which are divergent cross-arch, resistance to horizontal rotation of the denture is enhanced.

buccal or lingual line angles. Assuming that the bracing or retentive arm of a direct retainer may originate in the guiding plane region, a line angle preparation would weaken either or both components of the clasp assembly. Another precaution that should be observed is to avoid preparing guiding plane surfaces on *both* proximal surfaces of a terminal abutment on the same side supporting a distal extension denture base. A terminal abutment so prepared would be subjected to a "monkey wrench" leverage effect, which could only result in exceeding the physiologic tolerance of the supporting tissues of the abutment.

Ridge support. Support for the tooth-borne denture or the tooth-borne modification space comes entirely from the abutment teeth by means of rests. Support for the distal extension denture base comes primarily from the soft tissues overlying the residual alveolar bone. In the latter, rest support is effective only at the abutment end of the denture base.

The effectiveness of tissue support is dependent upon four things: (1) the quality of the residual ridge, (2) the total occlusal load applied, (3) the accuracy of the denture bases, and (4) the accuracy and type of impression registration.

The quality of the ridge cannot be influenced, except to modify it or improve it by surgical intervention. Such modification is frequently advisable but even less frequently done.

The total occlusal load applied to the residual ridge may be influenced by reducing the occlusal area. This is done by the use of fewer, narrower, and more effectively shaped denture teeth.

The accuracy of the denture base is influenced by our choice of materials and by the exactness of the processing techniques. Inaccurate and warped denture bases influence adversely the support of the partial denture. Materials and techniques that will minimize the possibility of processing errors and assure the greatest dimensional stability should be selected.

The accuracy of the impression technique is entirely in the hands of the dentist. Maximum tissue coverage for support and the use of primary stress-bearing areas should be the primary objectives in any partial denture impression technique. The manner in which this is accomplished should be based upon a biologic comprehension of what happens beneath a distal extension denture base when an occlusal load is applied.

The distal extension partial denture is unique in that its support is derived from both abutment teeth that are comparatively unyielding and from soft tissues that may be comparatively yielding under occlusal forces. Resilient tissues, being unable to provide support for the denture base comparable to that offered by the abutment teeth, are displaced by the occlusal load. Only the projections of the underlying residual bone remain to be traumatized by occlusal forces. This problem of support is further complicated by the fact that the patient has natural teeth remaining upon which he may exert far greater force than he would were he completely edentulous. This fact is clearly evident from the damage often occurring to an edentulous ridge when it is opposed by a few remaining anterior teeth in the other arch and especially when the opposing occlusion of anterior teeth has been arranged so that contact exists in both centric and eccentric positions.

Ridge tissues recorded in their resting or nonfunctioning form are incapable of providing the composite support needed for a denture that derives its support from both hard and soft tissue. It is necessary that three factors be taken into consideration in the acceptance of an impression technique for distal extension partial dentures: (1) the material should record the tissues covering the primary stress-bearing areas in their supporting form, (2) tissues within the basal seat area other than primary stress-bearing areas must be recorded in their anatomic form, and (3) the total area covered by the impression should be as great as possible, to distribute the load over as large an area as can be tolerated by the border tissues. This is an application of the principle of the snowshoe.

Anyone who has had the opportunity of comparing two master casts for the same partially edentulous arch, one cast having the distal extension area recorded in its anatomic or resting, form and the other cast having the distal extension area recorded in its functional form, has been impressed by the differences in the two. A denture base processed to the functional form is generally less irregular, and it has greater area coverage than does a denture base processed to the anatomic, or resting, form. Moreover, and of far greater significance, a denture base made to anatomic form exhibits less stability under rotating forces than does a denture base processed to functional form and thus fails to maintain its occlusal relation with the opposing teeth. By having the patient close onto strips of soft wax, it is evident that occlusion is maintained at a point of equilibrium over a long period of time when the denture base has been made to the functional form. In contrast, evidence exists that there has been a rapid settling of the denture base when it has been made to the anatomic form, with an early return of the occlusion to natural tooth contact only. Such a denture not only fails to distribute the occlusal load equitably but it also allows rotational movement, which is damaging to the abutment teeth and their investing structures.

Indirect retainers. An indirect retainer must be placed as far anteriorly from the fulcrum line as adequate tooth support permits if it is to function to restrict movement of a distal extension base away from the tissues. It must be placed on a rest seat prepared in an abutment tooth that is capable of withstanding the stresses placed upon it. An indirect retainer cannot function effectively on an inclined tooth surface, nor can a single weak incisor tooth be used for this purpose. Either a canine or a premolar tooth should be used for the support of an indirect retainer, and the rest seat must be prepared with as much care as is given any other rest seat. An incisal rest or a lingual rest may be used on an anterior tooth, provided a definite seat can be obtained either in sound enamel or on a cast restoration.

A second purpose that indirect retainers serve in partial denture design is that of support for major connectors. A long lingual bar or an anterior palatal major connector is thereby prevented from settling into the tissues. Even in the absence of a need for indirect retention, provision for such auxiliary support is sometimes indicated.

Contrary to common usage, a continuous bar retainer or a linguoplate does not in itself act as an indirect retainer. Since these are located on inclined tooth surfaces, they serve more as an orthodontic appliance than as support for the partial denture. When a linguoplate or a continuous bar retainer is used, terminal rests should always be provided at either end to stabilize the denture and to prevent orthodontic movement of the teeth contacted. Such terminal rests may function also as the indirect retainers, but these would function equally well in that capacity without the continuous bar retainer or linguoplate.

CHAPTER 10

Surveying

A dental surveyor has been defined as an instrument used to determine the relative parallelism of two or more surfaces of the teeth or other parts of the cast of a dental arch.

Any one of the several moderately priced surveyors on the market will adequately accomplish the procedures necessary in the design and construction of a partial denture. In addition, these surveyors may be used to parallel internal rests and intracoronal retainers. With handpiece holder added, they also may be used to machine internal rests and to parallel guiding plane surfaces of abutment restorations.

DESCRIPTION OF A DENTAL SURVEYOR

Perhaps the most widely used surveyors are the Ney (Fig. 10-1) and the Jelenko (Fig. 10-2) surveyors. Both of these are precision-made instruments but differ principally in that the Jelenko arm swivels whereas the Ney arm is fixed. The technique for surveying and trimming blockout is therefore somewhat different. Other surveyors also differ in this respect, and the dentist may prefer one over another for this reason.

The principal parts of the Ney surveyor are as follows:

1. Platform upon which the base is moved
2. Vertical arm that supports the superstructure
3. Horizontal arm from which the surveying tool suspends
4. Table to which the cast is attached
5. Base upon which the table swivels
6. Paralleling tool or guideline marker (This tool contacts the convex surface to be studied in a tangential manner. The relative parallelism of one surface to another may thus be determined. By substituting a carbon marker, the height of contour then may be delineated on the surfaces of the abutment teeth and also areas of interference requiring reduction on blockout.)
7. Mandrel for holding special tools (Fig. 10-3)

The principal parts of the Jelenko surveyor are essentially the same as those for the Ney surveyor except that by loosening the nut at the top of the vertical arm, the horizontal arm may be made to swivel. The objective of this feature, originally designed by Dr. Noble Wills, is to permit freedom of movement of the arm in a horizontal plane rather than to depend entirely upon the horizontal movement of the cast. To some, this is confusing because two horizontal movements must thus be coordinated. For those who prefer to move the cast only in a horizontal relationship to a fixed vertical arm, the nut may be tightened and the horizontal arm used in a fixed position. The jointed horizontal arm of the Williams surveyor (Fig. 10-4) differs from

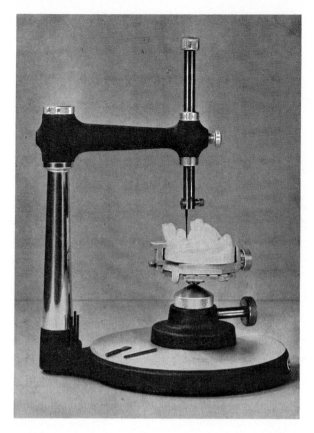

Fig. 10-1. Ney surveyor is a widely used surveyor because of its simplicity and durability. Dental students should be required to own such a surveyor. By becoming familiar with and dependent upon its use, they are more likely to continue using the surveyor in practice as a necessary piece of equipment toward more adequate diagnosis, effective treatment planning, and the performance of many other aspects of prosthodontic treatment. (Courtesy J. M. Ney Co., Hartford, Conn.)

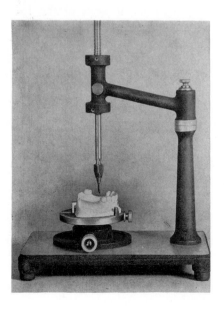

Fig. 10-2. Jelenko surveyor. Note the spring-mounted paralleling tool and the swivel at the top of the vertical arm. The horizontal arm may be fixed in any position by tightening the nut at the top of the vertical arm. (Courtesy J. F. Jelenko & Co., Inc., New York, N. Y.)

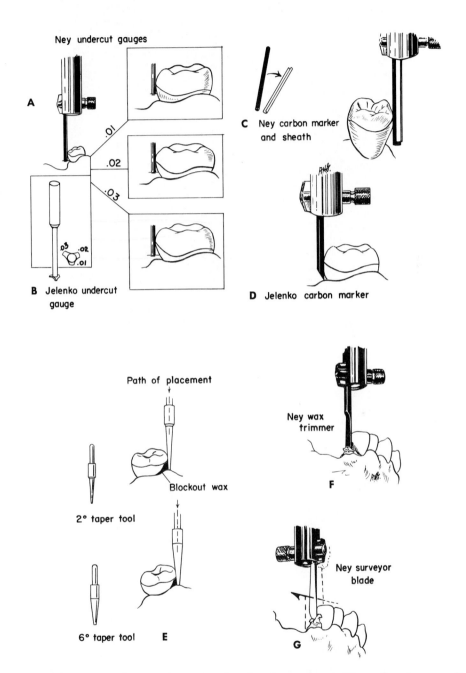

Fig. 10-3. Various tools that may be used with a dental surveyor. **A,** Ney undercut gauges. **B,** Jelenko undercut gauge. **C,** Ney carbon marker with metal reinforcement sleeve. **D,** Jelenko carbon marker. **E,** Tapered tools, 2- and 6-degree, for trimming blockout when some non-parallelism is desired. **F,** Ney wax trimmer for paralleling blockout. **G,** Surveying blade being used for trimming blockout.

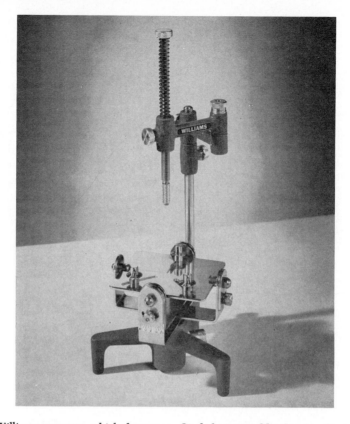

Fig. 10-4. Williams surveyor, which features a Gimbal stage table that is adjustable to any desired anterior, posterior, or lateral tilt. The degree of inclination can be recorded for repositioning of the cast at any time. A distinct advantage of this table over the universal tilt table is that the center of rotation always remains constant. The superstructure of this surveyor consists of a jointed arm and spring-supported survey rod, all components of which can be locked in a fixed position if desired. This surveyor is perhaps best suited for the placement of internal attachments, rather than for cast analyzing and other purposes. (Courtesy Williams Gold Refining Co., Buffalo, N. Y.)

both the Ney and Jelenko surveyors. This feature permits the vertical arm to be moved to scribe the survey lines without moving the cast.

Another difference in the Ney and Jelenko surveyors is that the vertical arm on the Ney surveyor is retained by friction within a fixed bearing. The shaft may be moved up or down within this bearing but remains in any vertical position until again moved. The shaft may be fixed in any vertical position desired by tightening a set screw. In contrast, the vertical arm of the Jelenko surveyor is spring mounted and returns to the top position when released. It must be held down against spring ten-

sion while in use, which to some is a disadvantage. The spring may be removed, but the friction of the two bearings supporting the arm does not hold it in position as securely as does a bearing designed for that purpose. These minor differences in the two surveyors lead to personal preference on the part of the operator but do not detract from the effectiveness of either surveyor when properly used.

Since the shaft on the Ney surveyor is stable in any vertical position, yet may be moved vertically with ease, it lends itself well for use as a drill press when a handpiece holder is added (Fig. 10-5). The handpiece may thus be used to cut recesses

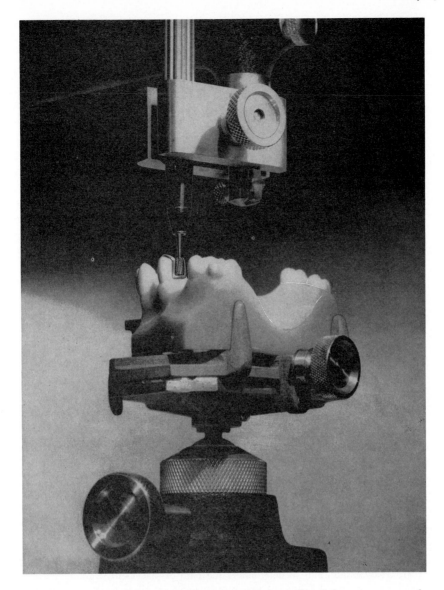

Fig. 10-5. Ney handpiece holder attached to the vertical spindle of the surveyor may be used as a drill press to cut internal rests and recesses in wax patterns and/or gold castings and to establish lingual surfaces above a ledge, which are parallel to the path of placement in abutment restorations. (Courtesy J. M. Ney Co., Hartford, Conn.)

in gold restorations with precision by using burs or carborundum points of various sizes in a dental handpiece.

Several other surveyors have been designed and are in use today (Figs. 10-6 to 10-8). Many of these are more elaborate and costly and therefore are used primarily by larger laboratories in which volume justifies the more costly equipment. Their

main advantage lies in the incorporation of some kind of precision gauge for locating the prescribed undercut to be used with plastic patterns of standard dimensions.

An electronic surveyor was developed at the School of Aviation Medicine, Randolph Air Force Base, by Colonel Donald C. Hudson, Director, Research Dentistry Division (Fig. 10-9). The object of this surveyor is

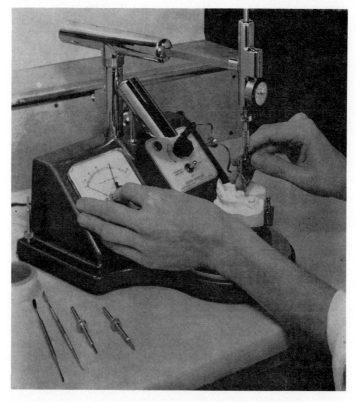

Fig. 10-6. Austenal Micro-Analyzer. Undercuts are measured electrically in millimeters in relation to selected Flexseal pre-formed clasp patterns, which are used as the standards of measurement. Micro-Analyzer also aids in determining the path of placement, marking the height of contour and relieving or blocking out undesirable undercuts. It is equipped with a vertical gauge calibrated in hundredths of a millimeter up to 0.51. Sweep dial indicator shows the desired amount of undercut, and flashing light tells when the exact depth has been reached. (Courtesy Austenal, Inc., Chicago, Ill.)

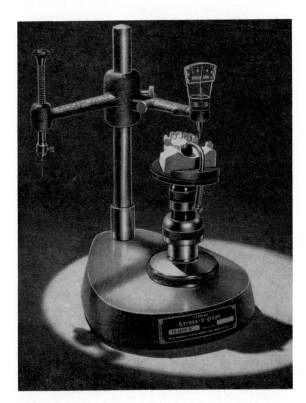

Fig. 10-7. Ticonium Stress-o-graph. Left arm contains a spring-mounted paralleling tool for performing the usual surveying and relieving operations. Right arm holds a micrometer gauge and marking pen with a vernier travel screw. Gauge is divided into hundredths of an inch up to 0.05 inch. Case-hardened, nickel-silver marking pen is used to make a fine ink line with a slow-drying ink. Gauge is used to measure the degree of tooth undercut sloping away from the height of contour. It is recommended that a clasp tip never be placed farther into the tooth undercut than the suprabulge measurement from height of contour to occlusal marginal ridge. The following reason is given: "Because the suprabulge angle of a tooth acts as a wedge, it will pass over the height of contour and close back into contact with the tooth undercut. If the clasp tip is arbitrarily placed in an undercut angle that is greater than the suprabulge angle, undue pressure can be placed on the tooth as the clasp passes over the height of contour. The result is damage to the periodontium and danger of overloading the fatigue limit of a clasp. Also, when a clasp is placed too far into an undercut, it will not be opened by the suprabulge angle of the tooth and will require relieving on the inside before it will seat on the stone cast without chipping the teeth, thus weakening the clasp arm."° (Courtesy Ticonium Division, Consolidated Metal Products Corp., Albany, N. Y.)

°From Ticonium Technique Manual, Consolidated Metal Products Corp., Albany, N. Y.

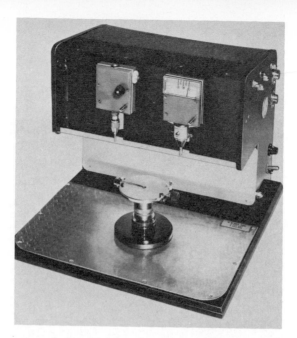

Fig. 10-8. Saddle-Lock Retentoscope, designed to be used with the Saddle-Lock principle of concealed clasp retention. In addition to a paralleling tool and a separate heated tool for paralleling blockout, a calibrated dial gauge accurately measures and marks with a carbon rod the location of the desired amount of undercut. Table may be raised and lowered in relation to a fixed vertical arm until the desired undercut area is located. (Courtesy Saddle-Lock, Inc., Brooklyn, N. Y.)

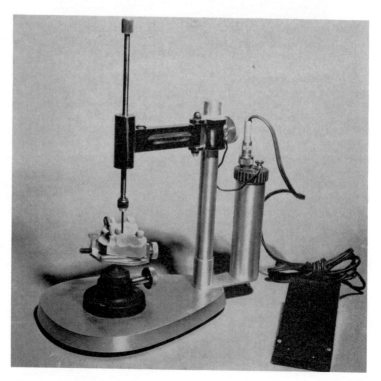

Fig. 10-9. Electronic surveyor developed at the School of Aviation Medicine, Randolph Air Force Base, Texas. Weak current passing through the paralleling tool onto the treated cast surface marks the height of contour and location of undercut areas electronically. (U. S. Air Force Photo, School of Aviation Medicine, Randolph Air Force Base, Texas.)

not so much the evaluation of the cast, which can be done just as well on a conventional surveyor, but the marking of the height of contour and a selected amount of undercut by electronic means once the relation of the cast to the vertical arm of the surveyor (that is, the path of placement) has been established.

The marking of a stone cast is accomplished by chemical change at the surface due to passage of a weak electric current through the damp cast material to the point of contact with the metal surveying tool. An indicator sensitive to pH changes (0.5% phenolphthalein in alcohol) produces the marking.

Current is supplied from two flashlight batteries in the case at the rear of the upright post and is controlled through a foot-operated switch. The movable arm of the surveying instrument is insulated from the post by means of a nonconducting bushing.

Upon closure of the switch, current flows through the post and platform, through the table holding the cast, and through the cast to the surveying tool, returning through the horizontal arm to complete the circuit. The tool is negative to the cast, attracting Ca^{++} ions to the surface at the point of contact, where recombination with moisture produces a pH change and this in turn produces a color change in the indicator.

No marking occurs unless the switch is closed to permit current flow, but upon closing the switch, the height of the contour is marked on the cast at the point of contact. Thus the location of the height of contour is accurately established without resorting to the use of a graphite marker, which is frequently too broad and is easily smeared.

The precise location of an undercut on a tooth to be clasped also may be marked by replacing the surveying tool with a Ney undercut gauge. Undercut gauges of 0.010, 0.015, and 0.020 inch are used and are selected according to the length, size, diameter, and material of the clasp arm to be used. The selected undercut gauge is used to determine the amount of undercut

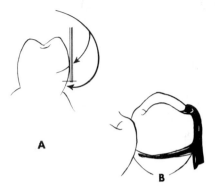

Fig. 10-10. Undercut on an abutment tooth may be located electronically through the use of an undercut gauge attached to the electronic surveyor. Simultaneous contact of the undercut gauge with the height of contour and the selected amount of tooth undercut is marked on the cast electronically as shown in **A.** As shown in **B,** this point or line is used to locate the gingival edge of the clasp tip that will engage the undercut.

that will be engaged by the tip of the clasp arm. This spot is marked on the cast electronically when the projection of the undercut gauge is allowed to contact the tooth below the height of contour simultaneous with contact of its shaft against the height of contour. This point or line represents the gingival edge of the clasp tip that will engage the undercut. (See Fig. 10-10.)

The red mark made by the electronic surveyor has been described as a *captive* mark that gradually disappears as the cast becomes dry. However, this mark can be overlayed easily with a crayon-type pencil before the captive mark disappears, rendering it permanent for future reference.

PURPOSES FOR WHICH THE SURVEYOR IS USED

The surveyor may be used for surveying the diagnostic cast, contouring wax patterns, surveying ceramic veneer crowns, placing the intracoronal retainers, placing internal rests, machining cast restorations, and surveying the master cast.

Surveying the diagnostic cast. Surveying the diagnostic cast is essential to effective diagnosis and treatment planning. The objectives are as follows:

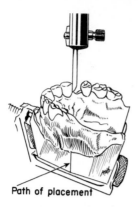

Path of placement

Fig. 10-11. Tilt of the cast on the adjustable table of the surveyor in relation to the vertical arm establishes the path of placement and removal that the partial denture will take. All mouth preparations must be made to conform to a previously determined path of placement, which has been recorded by scoring the base of the cast or by tripoding.

1. To determine the most acceptable path of placement that will eliminate or minimize interference to placement and removal (Fig. 10-11). *The path of placement is the direction in which a restoration moves from the point of initial contact of its rigid parts with the supporting teeth to the terminal resting position, with rests seated and the denture base in contact with the tissues.* The *path of removal* is exactly the reverse, since it is the direction of restoration movement from its terminal resting position of the last contact of its rigid parts with the supporting teeth. When the restoration is properly designed to have positive guiding planes, the patient may place and remove the restoration with ease in only one direction because of the guiding influence of tooth surfaces made parallel to that path of placement.

2. To identify proximal tooth surfaces that are or can be made parallel so that they act as guiding planes during placement and removal.

3. To locate and measure areas of the teeth that may be used for retention.

4. To determine whether or not tooth and bony areas of interference will need to be eliminated either by extraction or by selecting a different path of placement.

5. To determine the most suitable path of placement that will permit locating retainers and artificial teeth to the best esthetic advantage.

6. To permit an accurate charting of the mouth preparations to be made. This includes the disking of proximal tooth surfaces to provide guiding planes and the reduction of excessive tooth contours to eliminate interference and to permit a more acceptable location of reciprocal and retentive clasp arms. By marking these areas on the diagnostic cast with red pencil using an undercut gauge to estimate the amount of tooth structure that may safely (without exposing dentin) be removed, and then trimming the marked areas on the stone cast with the surveyor blade, the angulation and extent of tooth reduction may be established prior to preparing the teeth in the mouth. With the diagnostic cast on the surveyor at the time of mouth preparations, disking and reduction of tooth contours may thus be accomplished with acceptable accuracy.

7. To delineate the height of contour on abutment teeth and to locate areas of undesirable tooth undercut that are to be avoided, eliminated, or blocked out. This will include areas of the teeth to be contacted by rigid connectors, the location of nonretentive reciprocal and stabilizing arms, and the location of retentive clasp terminals.

8. To record the cast position in relation to the selected path of placement for future reference. This may be done by locating three dots or parallel lines on the cast, thus establishing the horizontal plane in relation to the vertical arm of the surveyor (Fig. 11-2).

Contouring wax patterns. The surveyor blade is used as a wax carver during this phase of mouth preparation so that the proposed path of placement may be maintained throughout the preparation of cast restorations for abutment teeth (Fig. 10-12).

All proximal surfaces of wax patterns adjacent to an edentulous area should be

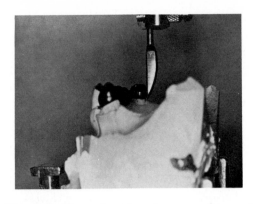

Fig. 10-12. Wax patterns have been carved to meet requirements of occlusion. After the cast has been oriented to the surveyor at the predetermined path of placement, vertical surfaces of the wax patterns are altered with the surveyor blade to meet the specific requirements for the optimum placement of framework components.

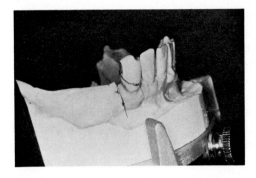

Fig. 10-13. Final glaze has not been placed on the veneer crown. Cast has been reoriented to the surveyor by indices or tripod marks on the cast and the height of contour scribed on the veneer crown. Alterations to surfaces to conform to ideal placement of components now can be performed. Final glaze is placed on the veneer crown only after necessary recontouring is accomplished.

made parallel to the previously determined path of placement. Similarly, all other tooth contours that will be contacted by rigid connectors should be made parallel when ever possible. The surfaces of restorations upon which reciprocal and stabilizing components will be placed should be contoured to permit their location well below occlusal surfaces and upon nonretentive areas. Those surfaces of the restoration that are to provide retention for clasp arms should be contoured so that retentive clasps may be placed in the cervical one third of the crown and to the best esthetic advantage. Generally, a small amount of undercut (0.015 inch or less) is sufficient for retentive purposes.

Surveying ceramic veneer crowns. Ceramic veneer crowns are often used to restore abutment teeth on which extracoronal direct retainers will be placed. The surveyor is used to contour all areas of the wax pattern for the veneer crown except the buccal or labial surface. It is unlikely that the ceramic veneer portion can be fabricated exactly to the form required for the planned placement of retentive clasp arms without some reshaping with stones. Before the final glaze is placed, the abutment crowns should be returned to the surveyor on a full arch cast to assure the correct con-

tour of the veneered portions or to locate those areas that need recontouring (Fig. 10-13). The final glaze is accomplished after the crowns have been recontoured.

Placement of intracoronal retainers (internal attachments). In the placement of intracoronal retainers, the surveyor is used as follows:

1. To select a path of placement in relation to the long axes of the abutment teeth that will avoid areas of interference elsewhere in the arch.

2. To cut recesses in the stone teeth on the diagnostic cast for estimating the proximity of the recess to the pulp (in conjunction with roentgenographic information as to pulp size and location). Also, to facilitate the fabrication of metal or resin jigs to guide the preparations of the recesses in the mouth.

3. To carve recesses in wax patterns, or to place internal attachment trays in wax patterns, or to cut recesses in the gold casting with the handpiece holder, whichever method is preferred.

4. To place the keyway portion of the attachment in the casting prior to investing and soldering, each located parallel to the other similar attachments elsewhere in the arch.

Placement of internal rests. The surveyor may be used as a drill press, with a dental handpiece attached to the vertical arm by means of a handpiece holder. Internal rests may be carved in the wax patterns and further refined with the handpiece after casting, or the entire rest may be cut in the cast restoration with the handpiece. It is best that the outline form of the rest be carved first in wax and merely refined on the casting with the handpiece.

An internal rest differs from an internal attachment in that some portion of the cast prosthesis is waxed and cast to fit into the rest rather than a matched key and keyway attachment being used. The former is usually nonretentive but provides a definite seat for a removable restoration or a cantilever rest for a broken-stress fixed partial denture. When used with fixed partial dentures, nonparallel abutment pieces may thus be placed separately.

The internal rest in partial denture construction provides a positive occlusal support that is more favorably located in relation to the rotational axis of the abutment tooth than is the conventional spoon-shaped occlusal rest. It also provides horizontal stabilization through the parallelism of the vertical walls, thereby serving the same purpose as bracing arms placed extracoronally. Due to the movement of a distal extension base, more torque may be applied to the abutment tooth by an interlocking type of rest, and for this reason its use in conjunction with a distal extension partial denture is contraindicated. The ball-and-socket, spoon-shaped occlusal, or non-interlocking rest should be used in distal extension partial denture designs. The use of the dovetailed or interlocking internal rest should be limited to tooth-borne removable restorations, except when it is used in conjunction with some kind of stressbreaker between the abutment pieces and the movable base. The use of stressbreakers has been considered in Chapter 8.

Internal rest seats may be made in the form of a nonretentive box, a retentive box fashioned after the internal attachment, or a semiretentive box. In the latter, the walls are usually parallel and nonretentive, but a recess in the floor of the box prevents proximal movement of the male portion. These are cut with dental burs of various sizes and shapes. Tapered or cylindrical fissure burs are used to form the vertical walls, and small round burs are used to cut recesses in the floor of the rest seat.

Machining cast restorations. With handpiece holder attached (Fig. 10-5), vertical surfaces of cast restorations may be refined by machining with a suitable cylindrical carborundum point. Proximal surfaces of crowns and inlays, which will serve as guiding planes, and vertical surfaces above crown ledges may be improved by machining, but only if the relationship of one crown to another is correct. Unless the seating of removable dies is accurate and held in place with additional stone or plaster, cast restorations should first be tried in the mouth and then transferred by means of a plaster index impression to a reinforced stone cast for machining purposes. The new cast is then positioned on the surveyor, conforming to the path of placement of the partial denture, and vertical surfaces are machined with a true-running cylindrical carborundum point.

Whereas machined parallelism may be considered ideal and beyond the realm of everyday application, its merits more than justify the additional steps required to accomplish it. When such parallelism is accomplished and reproduced in a master cast, it is essential that subsequent laboratory steps be directed toward the utilization of these parallel guiding plane surfaces.

Surveying the master cast. Since surveying the master cast follows mouth preparations, the path of placement, the location of retentive areas, and the location of remaining interference must be known before proceeding with the final design of the denture framework. The objectives are as follows:

1. To select the most suitable path of placement by following mouth preparations that satisfy the requirements of *guiding planes, retention, noninterference,* and *esthetics.*

2. To permit measurement of retentive

areas and to identify the location of clasp terminals in proportion to the flexibility of the clasp arm being used. Flexibility will depend upon many factors: (a) the alloy used for the clasp, (b) the design and type of the clasp, (c) whether its form is round or half-round, (d), whether it is of cast or wrought material, and (e) the length of the clasp arm from its point of origin to its terminal end. Retention will then depend upon (a) the flexibility of the clasp arm, (b) the magnitude of the tooth undercut, and (c) the depth the clasp terminal is placed into this undercut.

3. To locate areas of undesirable remaining undercut that will be crossed by rigid parts of the restoration during placement and removal. These must be eliminated by blockout.

4. To trim blockout material parallel to the path of placement prior to duplication.

USE OF THE SURVEYOR

The partial denture must be designed so that it will not stress abutment teeth beyond their physiologic tolerance, can be easily placed and removed by the patient, will be retained against reasonable dislodging forces, and will not create an unfavorable appearance. It is necessary that the diagnostic cast be surveyed with these principles in mind. Mouth preparation should therefore be planned in accordance with certain factors that will influence the path of placement and removal.

FACTORS THAT WILL DETERMINE THE PATH OF PLACEMENT AND REMOVAL

The factors that will determine the path of placement and removal are guiding planes, retentive areas, interference, and esthetics.

Guiding planes. Proximal tooth surfaces that bear a parallel relationship to one another must either be found or be created to act as guiding planes during placement and removal of the denture. Guiding planes may be compared to the valve guides in an engine and act to assure a definite path of placement as the rigid parts of the prosthesis contact parallel tooth surfaces.

Guiding planes are necessary to ensure the passage of the rigid parts of the prosthesis past existing areas of interference. Thus the denture can be easily placed and removed by the patient without strain upon the teeth contacted or upon the denture itself and without damage to the underlying soft tissues.

Guiding planes are also necessary to assure predictable clasp retention. For a clasp to be retentive, its retentive arm must be forced to flex. Hence, guiding planes are necessary to give a positive direction to the movement of the restoration to and from its terminal position.

Retentive areas. Retentive areas must exist for a given path of placement, which will be contacted by retentive clasp arms that will be forced to flex over a convex surface during placement and removal. Satisfactory clasp retention is no more than the resistance of metal to deformation. For a clasp to be retentive, its path of escapement must be other than parallel to the path of removal of the denture itself; otherwise it would not be forced to flex and thereby generate the resistance known as retention. Clasp retention is therefore dependent upon the existence of a definite path of placement and removal.

Retention at each principal abutment does not necessarily have to be balanced in relation to the tooth on the opposite side of the arch, that is, exactly equal and opposite in magnitude and relative location. This is, of course, assuming that positive reciprocation to retentive elements is present (which must be cross-arch). Retention should be sufficient only to resist reasonable dislodging forces. In other words, it should be the minimum acceptable for adequate retention against reasonable dislodging forces.

Fairly even retention may be obtained by one of two means. One is to change the path of placement to increase or decrease the angle of cervical convergence of opposing retentive surfaces of abutment teeth. The other is to alter the flexibility of the clasp arm by changing its design, its size and length, and/or the material of which it is made.

Interference. The prosthesis must be designed so that it may be placed and removed without encountering tooth or soft tissue interference. A path of placement may be selected that encounters interference only if the interference can be eliminated during mouth preparations or on the master cast by means of a reasonable amount of blockout. Interference may be eliminated during mouth preparations by surgery, extraction, disking of interfering tooth surfaces, or altering tooth contours with cast restorations.

Generally, interference that *cannot* be eliminated for one reason or another will take precedence over the factors of retention and guiding planes. Sometimes certain areas can be made noninterfering only by selecting a different path of placement at the expense of existing retentive areas and guiding planes. These must then be modified with restorations that are in harmony with the path dictated by the existing interference. On the other hand, if areas of interference *can* be eliminated by various reasonable means, this should always be done. By so doing, the contour of existing abutments may frequently be utilized with little or no alteration.

Esthetics. By one path of placement, the most esthetic location of artificial teeth is made possible, and less clasp metal and/or less base material may be displayed.

The location of retentive areas may influence the path of placement selected, and therefore retentive areas always should be selected with the most esthetic location of clasps in mind. When restorations are to be made for other reasons, they should be contoured to permit the least display of clasp metal. Generally, less metal will be displayed if the retentive clasp is placed at a more distogingival area of tooth surface, made possible either by the path of placement selected or by the contour of cast restorations.

Esthetics also may dictate the choice of

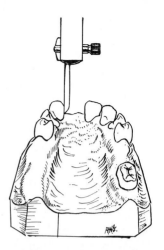

Fig. 10-14. When anterior teeth must be replaced with a partial denture, a vertical path of placement may be necessary to avoid excessively altering the adjacent abutment teeth and/or the supplied teeth.

path selected when missing anterior teeth must be replaced with the partial denture. In such situations, a more vertical path of placement is necessary so that neither the artificial teeth nor the adjacent natural teeth will have to be modified excessively (Fig. 10-14). In this instance esthetics may take precedence over other factors. This necessitates the preparation of abutment teeth to eliminate interferences and to provide guiding planes and retention in *harmony with* that path of placement dictated by esthetic factors.

Esthetics ordinarily should not be the primary factor in partial denture design. *Therefore the replacement of missing anterior teeth should be accomplished by means of fixed restorations whenever possible, rather than permit their replacement to influence the mechanical and functional effectiveness of the partial denture.* Since the primary considerations should be the preservation of the remaining oral tissues, esthetics should not be allowed to jeopardize the success of the partial denture.

STEP-BY-STEP PROCEDURES IN SURVEYING A DIAGNOSTIC CAST

Attach the cast to the adjustable surveyor table by means of the clamp pro-

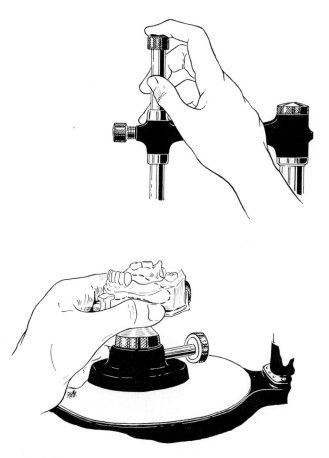

Fig. 10-15. Recommended method for manipulating the dental surveyor. Right hand is braced on the horizontal arm of the surveyor, and fingers ars used, as illustrated, to raise and lower the vertical shaft in its spindle. Left hand holding the cast on the adjustable table slides horizontally on the platform in relation to the vertical arm. Right hand must be used also to loosen and tighten the tilting mechanism as a suitable anteroposterior and lateral tilt of the cast in relation to the surveyor is being determined.

vided. Position the adjustable table so that the occlusal surface of the teeth are approximately parallel to the platform (Fig. 10-15). (This is only a tentative, but practical, way to start considering the factors that influence the path of placement and removal.)

Guiding planes. Determine the relative parallelism of proximal tooth surfaces by contacting proximal tooth surfaces with the surveyor blade or diagnostic stylus. Alter the cast position anteroposteriorly until the proximal surfaces are in a parallel relation to one another or near enough that they can be made parallel by disking. This will determine the *anteroposterior tilt*

of the cast in relation to the vertical arm of the surveyor (Fig. 10-16). Although the surveyor table is universally adjustable, it should be thought of as having only two axes, thus allowing only anteroposterior and lateral tilting.

In making a choice between having contact with a proximal surface at the cervical area only or contact at the marginal ridge only, the latter is preferred because a plane may then be established by disking (Fig. 10-17). It is obvious that when only gingival contact exists, a cast restoration is the only means of establishing a guiding plane. Therefore, if a tilt that does not provide proximal contact is accepted, the prox-

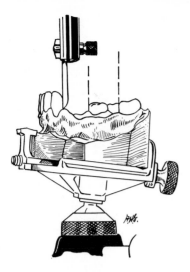

Fig. 10-16. Relative parallelism of proximal tooth surfaces will determine the anteroposterior tilt of the cast in relation to the vertical arm of the surveyor.

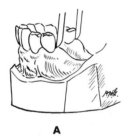

A

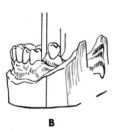

B

Fig. 10-17. In selecting the most desirable anteroposterior tilt of the cast in relation to the surveyor blade, a choice must be made between the positions illustrated in **A** and **B**. In **A** the distal surface of the left premolar abutment would have to be extended by means of a cast restoration. In **B** the right premolar could be disked slightly to provide an acceptably parallel guiding plane. Unless cast restorations are necessary for other reasons, the tilt shown in **B** is almost always preferred.

imal surface must be established with some kind of restoration. In making a choice between having a good guiding plane on one proximal surface and one on another as against having a good plane on one and disking the other, the latter is preferred, and the need for disking is indicated on the diagnostic cast with red pencil. This holds true only when cast restorations are not otherwise necessary.

The end result of selecting a suitable anteroposterior tilt should be *to provide the greatest area of parallel proximal surfaces that may act as guiding planes.*

Retentive areas. By contacting buccal and lingual surfaces of abutment teeth with the surveyor blade, the amount of retention existing below their height of convexity may be determined. This is best accomplished by directing a small source of light toward the cast from the side away from the dentist. The *angle of cervical convergence* is best observed as a triangle of light between the surveyor blade and the tooth surface being studied.

Alter the cast position by tilting it laterally until not grossly different retentive areas exist on the principal abutment teeth. If only two abutment teeth are involved, as in a Kennedy Class I partially edentulous arch, they are both principal abutments. However, if four abutment teeth are involved, as in a Kennedy Class III, modification 1, arch, they are all principal abutments and retentive areas should be located on all four. But if three abutment teeth are involved, as in a Kennedy Class II, modification 1, arch, the posterior abutment on the tooth-borne side and the abutment on the distal extension side are considered to be the principal abutments and retention is somewhat equalized accordingly. The third abutment may be considered to be secondary and less retention expected from it than from the other two. An exception is when the posterior abutment on the tooth-borne side has a poor prognosis and the denture is designed to ultimately be a Class I. In such a situation, the two stronger abutments are considered to be principal abutments.

In tilting the cast laterally to establish reasonable uniformity of retention, it is necessary that the table be rotated about an imaginary longitudinal axis without disturbing the anteroposterior tilt previously established. The resulting position is one that provides or makes possible parallel guiding planes and provides for acceptable retention on the abutment teeth. Note that we have not, as yet, taken into consideration possible interference to this tentative path of placement.

Interference. If a mandibular cast is being surveyed, check the lingual surfaces that will be crossed by a lingual bar major connector during placement and removal. Bony prominences and lingually inclined premolar teeth are the most common causes of interference to a lingual bar connector.

If the interference is bilateral, surgery and/or disking of lingual tooth surfaces may be unavoidable. If it is only unilateral, a change in the lateral tilt may be necessary to avoid an area of tooth or tissue interference. In changing the path of placement to avoid interference, previously established guiding planes, and an ideal location of retentive elements may be lost. Then the decision must be made whether to remove the existing interference by whatever means necessary or to resort to restorations on the abutment teeth, thereby changing the proximal and retentive areas to conform to the new path of placement.

In like manner, bony undercuts that will offer interference to the seating of denture bases must be studied and the decision made to remove them surgically, change the path of placement at the expense of guiding planes and retention, or design denture bases to avoid such undercut areas. The latter may be done by eliminating buccal and labial flanges and distolingual extension of denture bases. *However, it should be remembered that the maximum area available for support of the denture base should be utilized whenever possible.*

Interference to major connectors rarely

exists in the maxillary arch. Areas of interference are usually found on buccally inclined posterior teeth and those bony areas on the buccal aspect of edentulous spaces. As with the mandibular cast, the decision must be made whether to eliminate them, change the path of placement at the expense of guiding planes and retention, or design the connectors and bases to avoid them.

Other areas of possible interference to be studied are those surfaces of abutment teeth that will support or be crossed by minor connectors and clasp arms. While interference to vertical minor connectors may be blocked out, doing so may cause a resultant discomfort to the patient's tongue and may create objectionable spaces for the trapping of food. Also, it is desirable that tooth surfaces contacted by vertical connectors be utilized as auxiliary guiding planes whenever possible. Too much relief is perhaps better than too little because of the possibility of irritation to soft tissues, but it is always better that the relief be placed intentionally rather than as a blockout of interference. If possible, a minor connector should pass vertically along a tooth surface that is either parallel to the path of placement (which is considered ideal) or tapered occlusally. If tooth undercuts that would necessitate the use of an objectionable amount of blockout exist, they may be eliminated or minimized by slight changes in the path of placement or eliminated during mouth preparations. The need for such alteration should be indicated on the diagnostic cast in red pencil after final acceptance of a path of placement.

Tooth surfaces upon which reciprocal and stabilizing clasp arms will be placed should be studied to see if sufficient areas exist above the height of convexity for the placement of these components. The addition of a clasp arm to the occlusal third of an abutment tooth adds to its occlusal dimension and therefore to the occlusal loading of that tooth. *Nonretentive and stabilizing clasp arms are best located be-*

tween the middle third and gingival third of the crown rather than upon the occlusal third.

Areas of interference to more ideal placement of clasp arms usually can be eliminated by reshaping tooth surfaces during mouth preparations, and this is indicated on the diagnostic cast. Gross areas of interference to the placement of clasps may necessitate minor changes in the path of placement or changes in the clasp design. For example, a bar clasp arm originating mesially from the major connector to provide bracing might be substituted for a distally originating circumferential arm.

Areas of interference frequently overlooked are the distal line angles of premolar abutment teeth and the mesial line angles of molar abutments. These areas frequently offer interference to the origin of circumferential clasp arms. If not detected at the time of initial survey, they are not included in the plan for mouth preparations. When such an undercut exists, three alternatives may be considered:

1. It may be blocked out the same as any other area of interference. This is by far the least satisfactory method because the origin of the clasp must then stand away from the tooth in proportion to the amount of blockout used. Although this is perhaps less objectionable than its being placed occlusally, it may be objectionable to the tongue and the cheek and may create an objectionable food trap.

2. It may be circumvented by approaching the retentive area from a gingival direction with a bar clasp arm. This is frequently a satisfactory solution to the problem if other contraindications to the use of a bar clasp arm are not present, such as a severe tissue undercut or a retentive area that is too high on the tooth.

3. It may be eliminated by reducing the tooth contour during mouth preparation. This permits the use of a circumferential clasp arm originating well below the occlusal surface in a satisfactory manner. If the tooth is to be modified during mouth

preparations, it should be indicated on the diagnostic cast with red pencil.

When the retentive area is located objectionably high on the abutment tooth or the undercut is too severe, interference may also exist on tooth surfaces that are to support retentive clasps. Such areas of extreme or high convexity must be considered as areas of interference and should be reduced accordingly. These areas are likewise indicated on the diagnostic cast for reduction during mouth preparations.

Esthetics. The path of placement thus established must yet be considered from the standpoint of esthetics, both as to the location of clasps and the arrangement of artificial teeth.

Clasp designs that will provide satisfactory esthetics for any given path of placement usually may be selected. In some instances, gingivally placed bar clasp arms may be used to advantage; in others, circumferential clasp arms located cervically may be used. This is especially true when other abutment teeth located more posteriorly may bear the major responsibility for retention. In still other instances, a tapered wrought-wire retentive clasp arm may be placed to better esthetic advantage than a cast clasp arm. The location of clasp arms for esthetic reasons does not ordinarily justify altering the path of placement at the expense of mechanical factors. It should, however, be considered concurrently with other factors, and if a choice between two paths of equal merit permits a more esthetic placement of clasp arms by one path than the other, that path should be given preference.

When anterior replacements are involved, the choice of path is limited to a more vertical one for reasons previously stated. In this instance alone esthetics must be given primary consideration even at the expense of altering the path of placement and making all other factors conform. This factor should be remembered when considering the other three factors, so that compromises can be made at the time other factors are being considered.

FINAL PATH OF PLACEMENT

The final path of placement will be the anteroposterior and lateral position of the cast in relation to the vertical arm of the surveyor that best satisfies all four factors, that is, *guiding planes, retention, interference,* and *esthetics.*

All proposed mouth changes should be indicated on the diagnostic cast in red pencil, with the exception of restorations to be done. These may also be indicated on an accompanying chart if desired. Extractions and surgery are given priority to allow for healing. The remaining red marks represent the actual modifications of the remaining teeth to be done, which consists of the disking of proximal surfaces, the reduction of buccal and lingual surfaces, and, last, the preparation of rest seats. Except when they are placed in the wax pattern for a cast restoration, the preparation of rest seats should always be deferred until all other mouth preparations have been completed.

The actual location of rests will be determined by the proposed design of the denture framework. Therefore, the tentative design should be sketched on the diagnostic cast in pencil after the path of placement has been decided upon. This is done not only to locate rest areas but also to record graphically the plan of treatment prior to mouth preparations. In the intervening time between patient visits, other partial denture restorations may have been considered. The dentist should have the plan of treatment before him at each succeeding appointment to avoid confusion and to refresh his memory as to what is to be done and in what sequence.

The plan for treatment should include (1) the diagnostic cast with the mouth preparations and the denture design marked upon it, (2) a chart showing the proposed design and the planned treatment for each abutment, (3) a working chart showing the total treatment involved that will permit a quick review and a check-off of each step as the work progresses, and (4) a record of the fee quoted for each phase of treatment that can be checked off as it is recorded on the patient's permanent record.

Red pencil marks on the diagnostic cast are used to indicate the location of areas to be disked or otherwise modified, as well as the location of rests. While it is not necessary that rest areas be prepared on the diagnostic cast, it is advisable for the beginning student to have done so before proceeding to cut into the abutment teeth. Also this applies equally to crown and inlay preparations on abutment teeth. It is advisable, however, for even the most experienced dentist to have trimmed the stone teeth with the surveyor blade wherever tooth reduction is to be done. This identifies not only the *amount* to be removed in a given area but also the *plane* in which the tooth is to be cut. For example, a proximal surface may need to be disked in only the upper third or the middle third to establish a guiding plane that will be parallel to the path of placement. This is not usually parallel to the long axis of the tooth, and if the disk is laid against the side of the tooth, the existing surface angle will be maintained rather than establishing a new plane that is parallel to the path of placement.

The surveyor blade representing the path of placement may be used to advantage to trim the surface of the abutment tooth whenever a red mark appears. The resulting surface represents the amount of tooth to be removed in the mouth and indicates the angle at which the handpiece must be held. The cut surface on the stone tooth is not again marked with red pencil but is *outlined* in red pencil to positively locate the area to be disked.

RECORDING THE RELATION OF THE CAST TO THE SURVEYOR

Some method of recording the relation of the cast to the vertical arm of the surveyor must be used so that it may be returned to the surveyor for future reference, especially during mouth preparations. The same applies to the need for returning any working cast to the surveyor for shaping wax patterns, trimming blockout on the master cast, or locating clasp arms in relation to undercut areas.

Obviously, the trimmed base will vary with each cast; thus recording the position of the surveyor table is of no value. If it were, calibrations could be incorporated on the surveyor table, which would allow the same position to be reestablished. Instead, the position of each cast must be established separately, and any positional record applies only to that cast.

Of several methods, two seem to be the most convenient and accurate. One method is to place three widely divergent dots on the tissue surface of the cast with the carbon marker, having the vertical arm of the surveyor in a locked position. Preferably these dots should not be placed on areas of the cast involved in the framework design. Then the dots should be encircled with a colored pencil for easy identification. On returning the cast to the surveyor, it may be tilted until the tip of the surveyor blade again contacts the three dots in the same plane. This will produce the original position of the cast and therefore the original path of placement. This is known as *tripoding* the cast (Fig. 11-2). Some dentists prefer to make tiny pits in the cast at the location of the tripoding dots to preserve the orientation of the cast and to transfer this relationship to the refractory cast.

A second method is to score two sides and the dorsal aspect of the base of the cast with a sharp instrument held against the surveyor blade (Fig. 11-2). By tilting the cast until all three lines are again parallel to the surveyor blade, the original cast position can be reestablished. Fortunately, the scratch lines will be reproduced in any duplication, thereby permitting any duplicate cast to be related to the surveyor in a similar manner. Whereas a diagnostic cast and a master cast cannot be made interchangeable, a refractory cast being a duplicate of the master cast, can be repositioned on the surveyor at any time. The technologist must be cautioned not to trim the sides of the cast on the model trimmer and thereby lose the reference marks for repositioning.

SURVEYING THE MASTER CAST

The master cast must be surveyed as a new cast, but the prepared proximal guiding plane surfaces will indicate the correct anteroposterior tilt. Some compromises may be necessary, but the amount of guiding plane surface remaining after blockout should be the maximum for each tooth. Areas above the point of contact with the surveyor blade are not considered to be part of the guiding plane area and neither are gingival undercut areas, which will be blocked out.

The lateral tilt will be the position that provides equal retentive areas on all principal abutments in relation to the planned clasp design. Factors of flexibility and the need for extra flexibility on distal extension abutments must be considered in deciding what will provide equal retention on all abutment teeth. For example, cast circumferential or cast bar retention on the tooth-borne side of a Class II design will be balanced against the 18-gauge wrought-wire retention on a distal abutment only if the more rigid cast clasp engages a lesser undercut than the wrought-wire clasp arm. Therefore, the degree of undercut alone does not assure relatively equal retention unless clasp arms of equal length, diameter, form, and material are used.

Gross interference will have been eliminated during mouth preparation. Therefore, for a given path of placement providing guiding planes and balanced retention, any remaining interference must be eliminated with blockout. If mouth preparations have been adequately planned and executed, the undercuts remaining to be blocked out should be minimal.

The base of the cast is now scored or the cast is tripoded as described previously. The surveyor blade then may be replaced with a carbon marker and the height of convexity of each abutment tooth and soft tissue contours delineated. Similarly, any areas of interference to the rigid parts of the framework during seating and removal should be indicated with the carbon marker to locate areas to be blocked out or relieved.

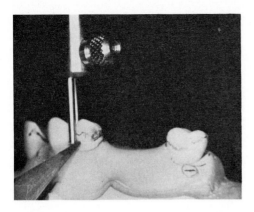

Fig. 10-18. Undercut gauge will measure the depth of undercut below the height of contour. Tip of an I bar-type direct retainer will be placed at the area being marked. The depth to which a retentive clasp arm can be placed depends not only upon its length, taper, diameter, and the alloy from which it is made, but also upon the type of clasp. A circumferential clasp arm is more flexible than is a bar-type clasp arm of the same length. (See Chapter 6.)

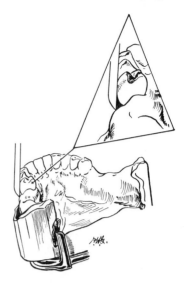

Fig. 10-19. Tooth undercut is best viewed against a good source of light passing through a triangle, which is bounded by the surface of the abutment tooth, surveyor blade, and gingival tissues.

MEASURING RETENTION

The surveyor is used with the master cast for two purposes: (1) to delineate the height of convexity of the abutment teeth for locating clasp arms and to identify both the location and magnitude of retentive undercuts, and (2) to trim blockout of any remaining interference to placement and removal of the denture. The areas involved are those that will be crossed by rigid parts of the denture framework.

The exact undercut that retentive clasp terminals will occupy must be measured and marked on the master cast (Fig. 10-18). Undercuts may be measured with the use of either an undercut gauge, such as those provided with the Ney and Jelenko surveyors, or by a dial gauge, such as is incorporated in the Saddle-Lock Retentoscope, the Ticonium Stress-o-graph, or the Austenal Micro-Analyzer. Whether an undercut gauge or a dial gauge is used, the amount of undercut is measured in hundredths of an inch, the gauges allowing measurements up to 0.03 inch. Theoretically, the amount of undercut used may vary with the clasp to be used up to a full 0.03 inch. However, many undercuts of 0.01 inch are often adequate for retention by cast retainers, an amount that can be measured with practical accuracy, whereas wrought-wire retention may safely utilize up to 0.02 inch without inducing undesirable torque on the abutment tooth provided the wire retentive arm is long enough. The use of 0.03 inch is rarely, if ever, justified with any clasp. When greater retention is required, such as when abutment teeth remain on only one side of the arch, multiple abutments should be used rather than an increase of the retention on any one tooth.

When a source of light is directed toward the tooth being surveyed, a triangle of light is visible. This triangle is bounded by the surface of the abutment tooth on one side and the blade of the surveyor on the other, the apex being the point of contact at the height of convexity and the base of the triangle being the gingival tissues (Fig. 10-19). Retention will be determined by (1) the magnitude of the angle of cervical convergence below the point of convexity, (2) the depth at which clasp terminal is placed in the angle, and (3) the flexibility of the clasp arm. The intelligent application of various clasp designs and their relative flexibility is of greater importance than the ability to measure an undercut with precise accuracy.

The final design may now be drawn upon the master cast with a fine crayon pencil, preferably one that will not come off during duplication. Graphite is usually lifted in duplication, but some crayon pencil marks will withstand duplication without blurring or transfer.* Sizing or spraying the master cast to protect such pencil marks is usually not advisable unless done with extreme care to avoid obliterating the surface detail.

BLOCKING OUT THE MASTER CAST

After the establishment of the path of placement and the location of undercut areas on the master cast, any undercut areas that will be crossed by rigid parts of the denture (which is every part of the denture framework but the retentive clasp terminals) must be eliminated by blockout.

In the broader sense the term *blockout* includes not only the areas crossed by the denture framework during seating and removal but also (1) those areas not involved that are blocked out for convenience, (2) ledges upon which clasp patterns are to be placed, (3) relief beneath connectors to avoid tissue impingement, and (4) relief to provide for later attachment of the denture base to the framework.

Ledges or shelves (shaped blockout) for locating clasp patterns may or may not be used (Fig. 10-20). However, this should not be confused with the actual blocking out of undercut areas that would offer interference to the placement of the denture framework. Only the latter is made on the surveyor, with the surveyor blade being used as a paralleling device.

Blockout material may be purchased, or

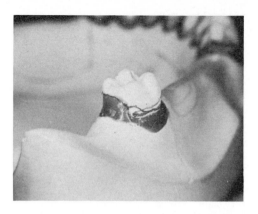

Fig. 10-20. Wax ledge on the buccal surface of the molar abutment will be duplicated in the refractory cast for the exact placement of the clasp pattern. Note that the ledge has been carved slightly below the penciled outline of the clasp arm. This will allow the gingival edge of the clasp arm to be polished and still remain in its planned relationship to the tooth when the denture is seated. It should also be noted that the wax ledge definitively establishes the planned placement of the direct retainer tip.

it may be made up according to the following formula:

Melt and mix together:
    4½ sheets of baseplate wax
    4½ sticks of temporary gutta percha stopping
    3 sticks of sticky wax
    ½ tsp. kaolin
Add ½ tube lipstick for color.

Some of the ready-made blockout materials contain a mixture of wax and clay. Pink baseplate wax also may be used satisfactorily as a blockout material. It is easily applied and is easily trimmed with the surveyor blade. Trimming is facilitated by slightly warming the surveyor blade. Whereas it is true that baseplate wax will melt more readily than a wax-clay mixture if the temperature of the duplicating material is too high, it should be presumed that the duplicating material will not be used at such an elevated temperature. If the temperature of the duplicating material is high enough to damage a wax blockout, other distortions resulting in an inaccurate duplication will also be likely.

Paralleled blockout is necessary cervical to guiding plane surfaces and over all un-

---

*Such as the Dixon Thinex pencil.

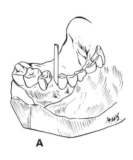

A

wax

B Blockout wax made parallel to path of placement

Fig. 10-21. All guiding plane areas must be parallel to the path of placement, and all other areas that will be contacted by rigid parts of the denture framework must at least be free of undercut if not parallel.

dercut areas that will be crossed by major or minor connectors. Other areas that are to be blocked out for convenience and to avoid difficulties in duplication should be blocked out with baseplate wax or an oil-base modeling clay (artist's modeling clay). A modeling clay that is water-soluble should not be used when duplication procedures are involved. Such areas are the labial surfaces and labial undercuts not involved in the denture design and sublingual and distolingual areas beyond the limits of the denture design. These are blocked out arbitrarily with baseplate wax or clay, but since they have no relation to the path of placement, they do not require the use of the surveyor.

Areas to be crossed by rigid connectors, on the other hand, should be trimmed with the surveyor blade parallel to the path of placement (Fig. 10-21). This imposes a considerable responsibility upon the technologist. Should he fail to trim the blockout sufficiently to expose guiding plane surfaces, the effect of these guiding planes,

which were carefully established by the dentist, will be nullified. If, on the other hand, the technician is overzealous in paralleling the blockout, the stone cast may be abraded by heavy contact with the surveyor blade. While the resulting cast framework would seat back onto the master cast without interference, interference to placement in the mouth would result. This would necessitate relieving the casting at the chair, which is not only an embarrassing and time-consuming operation but also one that may have the effect of obliterating guiding plane surfaces.

RELIEVING THE MASTER CAST

Tissue undercuts that must be blocked out are paralleled in much the same manner as tooth undercuts. The difference between *blockout* and *relief* must be clearly understood (Figs. 10-22 and 10-23). For example, tissue undercuts that would offer interference to the seating of a lingual bar connector are blocked out with blockout wax and trimmed parallel to the path of placement. This does not in itself necessarily afford relief to avoid tissue impingement. In addition to such blockout, a relief of varying thickness must sometimes be used, depending upon the location of the connector, the relative slope of the alveolar ridge, and the predictable effect of denture rotation. It must be assumed that indirect retainers, as such, or indirect retention is provided in the design of the denture to prevent rotation of the lingual bar inferiorly. A vertical downward rotation of the denture bases around posterior rests places the bar increasingly farther from the lingual aspect of the alveolar ridge when this surface slopes inferiorly toward the base of the tongue (Fig. 10-24). Adequate relief of soft tissues adjacent to the lingual bar is obtained by the initial finishing and polishing of the framework in these instances. However, excessive upward vertical rotation of a lingual bar will impinge lingual tissues if the alveolar ridge is nearly vertical or undercut from the vertical (Fig. 10-25). The region of the cast involving the pro-

Table 10-1. Differentiations between parallel blockout, shaped blockout, arbitrary blockout, and relief

Site	Material	Thickness
	Paralleled blockout	
Proximal tooth surfaces to be used as guiding planes	Hard baseplate wax or blockout material	Only undercut remaining gingival to contact of surveyor blade with tooth surface
Beneath all minor connectors	Hard baseplate wax or blockout material	Only undercut remaining gingival to contact of surveyor blade with tooth surface
Tissue undercuts to be crossed by rigid connectors	Hard baseplate wax or blockout material	Only undercut remaining below contact of surveyor blade with surface of cast
Tissue undercuts to be crossed by origin of bar clasps	Hard baseplate wax or blockout material	Only undercut remaining below contact of surveyor blade with surface of cast
Deep interproximal spaces to be covered by minor connectors or linguoplates	Hard baseplate wax or blockout material	Only undercuts remaining below contact of surveyor blade with surface of cast
Beneath bar clasp arms to gingival crevice	Hard baseplate wax or blockout material	Only undercut area involved in attachment of clasp arm to minor connector
	Shaped blockout	
On buccal and lingual surfaces to locate plastic or wax patterns for clasp arms	Hard baseplate wax	Ledges for location of nonretentive reciprocal clasp arms to follow height of convexity so that they may be placed as low as possible without becoming retentive Ledges for location of retentive clasp arms to be placed as low as tooth contour permits; point of origin of clasp to be above height of convexity, crossing survey line at terminal one third, and to include undercut area previously selected in keeping with flexibility of type of clasp being used

Arbitrary blockout

All gingival crevices	Hard baseplate wax	Enough to just eliminate gingival crevice
Gross tissue undercuts situated below areas involved in design of denture framework	Hard baseplate wax or oil-base clay	Leveled arbitrarily with wax spatula
Tissue undercuts distal to cast framework	Hard baseplate wax or oil-base clay	Smoothed arbitrarily with wax spatula
Labial and buccal tooth and tissue undercuts not involved in denture design	Hard baseplate wax or oil-base clay	Filled and tapered to within upper third of crown of teeth with spatula

Relief

Beneath lingual bar connectors or the bar portion of linguoplates when indicated (see text)	Adhesive wax sealed to cast: should be wider than width of major connector to be placed upon it	32-gauge wax if slope of lingual alveolar ridge is at right angle to occlusal plane
		32-gauge wax after parallel blockout of undercuts if slope of lingual alveolar ridge is undercut or less than right angle to occlusal plane
Areas in which major connectors will contact thin tissue, such as hard areas so frequently found on lingual of mandibular ridges and maxillary tori	Hard baseplate wax	Thin layer flowed on with hot wax spatula; however, if maxillary torus must be covered, the thickness of the relief must represent the difference in the degree of displacement of the tissues covering the torus and the tissues covering the residual ridges
Beneath framework extensions onto ridge areas for attachment of resin bases	Adhesive wax, well adapted and sealed to cast beyond involved area	20-gauge wax

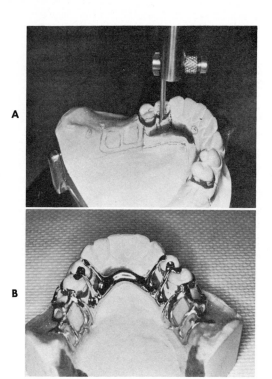

A

B

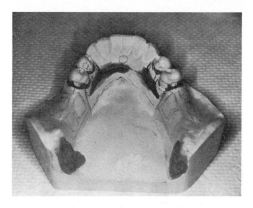

Fig. 10-23. Relief and blockout of a master cast before duplication. All undercuts involved in the denture design (except the tips of retentive clasp arms) have been blocked out *parallel* to the path of placement. Residual ridges have been relieved with 20-gauge sheet wax. Small wax window has been created adjacent to the distogingival surface of each posterior abutment. Framework will occupy this space and will definitively establish the most anterior extent of the denture bases in these regions. Severe undercuts in the retromylohyoid regions of the cast have been arbitrarily blocked out to prevent possible distortion of the duplicating mold when the master cast is removed.

Fig. 10-22. Relationship of parallel blockout and relief to the partial denture framework. A, Interproximal spaces to be occupied by minor connectors are blocked out parallel to the path of placement. In a like manner, tissue undercuts intimate to the lingual bar and minor connectors are blocked out *parallel* to the path of placement rather than using an arbitrary blockout. Arbitrary blockout in the lingual bar region creates unnecessary spaces for the entrapment of foods. Guiding planes have been prepared on the distal of the second premolar abutments. Blockout of the tissue surface inferior to the buccal surface of the right second premolar is required. Since this slight undercut coincided with the placement of a bar-type direct retainer arm, it was blocked out *parallel* to the path of placement to avoid damaging the tissue when the denture rotated or when the restoration was being removed or placed. The edentulous ridges have been covered with a 20-gauge sheet wax to provide space for the denture base to totally enclose the denture base minor connector. A 20-gauge sheet-wax relief is preferable if the residual ridges have undergone excessive vertical resorption and space available to place denture teeth is adequate. B, Finished removable partial denture framework accurately fits the blocked out master cast. Adjustment of the framework by grinding to fit the master cast is eliminated when blockout of the cast has been meticulously carried out.

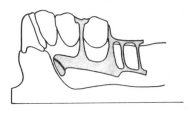

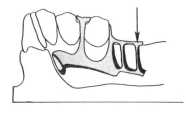

Fig. 10-24. Sagittal section of cast and denture framework. Lingual alveolar ridge slopes inferiorly toward base of tongue (upper figure). When a vertical force is directed to displace the denture base downward, the lingual bar rotates upward but does not impinge the soft tissue of the alveolar ridge (lower figure). Therefore, in such instances, adequate relief to avoid impingement is gained when the tissue side of the lingual bar is highly polished during the finishing process.

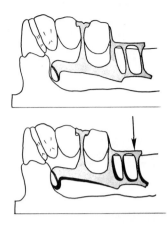

Fig. 10-25. Undercut alveolar ridge was blocked out parallel to the path of placement in fabricating the lingual bar (upper figure). Application of a vertical force to create a rotation of the lingual bar upward will cause impingement of lingual tissue on alveolar ridge (lower figure). To avoid impingement in these instances, the master cast should not only be blocked out parallel to the path of placement but an additional relief of 32-gauge sheet wax should be utilized in blocking out the cast in such undercut areas.

posed placement of the lingual bar should, in this situation be first relieved by parallel blockout and then with a 32-gauge wax strip. Low-fusing casting wax, such as Kerr's green casting wax should not be used for this purpose, for it is too easily thinned during adapting and may be affected by the temperature of the duplicating material. Pink casting wax may be used, but it is difficult to adapt uniformly. A pressure-sensitive adhesive-coated casting wax is preferable because it adapts readily and adheres to the cast surface. Any wax, even the adhesive type, should be sealed all around its borders with a hot spatula to

prevent its lifting when the cast is moistened prior to or during duplication.

Horizontal rotational tendencies of a lower distal extension denture probably account for many of the tissue irritations seen adjacent to a lingual mandibular major connector. These irritations can usually be avoided by blocking out all undercuts adjacent to the bar parallel to the path of placement, and then including adequate bracing components in the design of the framework to resist horizontal rotation. Judicious relief of the tissue side of the lingual bar with rubber wheels at the site of the irritation will most often correct the discrepancy, all other factors being equal. Under no circumstances should the rigidity of the major connector be jeopardized by grinding any portion of it.

Still other areas requiring relief are the gingival crossings and gingival crevices. All gingival areas should be protected from possible impingement due to rotation of the denture framework, and all gingival crevices should be bridged by the denture framework. Wax may be used to block out gingival crevices (Fig. 10-24).

PARALLELED BLOCKOUT, SHAPED BLOCKOUT, ARBITRARY BLOCKOUT, AND RELIEF

Table 10-1 differentiates between *paralleled blockout, shaped blockout, arbitrary blockout,* and *relief.* The same factors apply to both the maxillary and mandibular arches, except that relief is ordinarily not used beneath palatal major connectors as it is with mandibular lingual bar connectors except when maxillary tori cannot be circumvented or when resistive median palatal raphes are encountered.

CHAPTER 11

Diagnosis and treatment planning

Diagnosis and treatment planning for oral rehabilitation must take into consideration some or all of the following procedures: the restoration of individual teeth, the restoration of harmonious occlusal relationships, the replacement of missing teeth by fixed restorations, and the replacement of other missing teeth by means of removable partial dentures.

The treatment plan for the partial denture, which is too frequently the final step in an extensive and lengthy sequence of treatment, should precede earlier treatment so that abutment teeth and other areas in the mouth may be properly prepared to support and retain the partial denture. This means that diagnostic casts for designing and planning partial denture treatment must be made before definitive treatment is undertaken. The design that is drawn on the diagnostic cast, along with a detailed chart of mouth conditions and proposed treatment, is the master plan for the mouth preparations and the partial denture to follow.

Failures of partial dentures, other than structural defects, can usually be attributed to inadequate diagnosis, failure to properly evaluate the conditions present, and failure to prepare the patient and his mouth properly prior to construction of the master cast. The importance of the examination, the consideration of favorable and unfavorable aspects, and the importance of planning the elimination of unfavorable influences cannot be stressed too strongly.

VISUAL EXAMINATION

Visual examination will reveal many of the signs of dental disease. Consideration of *caries susceptibility* is of primary importance. The number of restored teeth present, signs of recurrent caries, and evidence of decalcification should be noted. Only those patients with demonstrated good oral hygiene habits and low caries susceptibility may be considered good abutment risks without resorting to such prophylactic measures as the crowning of abutment teeth.

Evidence of periodontal disease, inflammation of gingival areas, and the degree of gingival recession should be observed at the time of initial examination. In addition, the depths of periodontal pockets should be determined by instrumentation and the degree of mobility of the teeth by digital examination. Although evidence of periodontal disease is detectable visually, the *extent* of damage to the supporting structure by periodontal disease must be determined by roentgenographic interpretation and instrumentation.

The number of teeth remaining, the location of the edentulous areas, and the quality of the residual ridge will have a definite bearing upon the proportionate amount of support that the partial denture will receive from the teeth and the edentulous ridges. Tissue contours may appear representative of a well-formed edentulous residual ridge. Palpation often indicates, however, that supporting bone has been resorbed and has been replaced by displaceable, fibrous connective tissue. Such a situation is common in maxillary tuberosity regions. The removable partial denture cannot be supported adequately by tissues that are easily displaced, and this tissue should be removed surgically, unless otherwise contraindicated, in preparing the mouth. A small but stable residual ridge is preferable to a larger unstable ridge to obtain support for the denture.

The presence of tori or other bony exostoses must be detected and an evaluation of their presence in relation to framework design must be made. Failure to palpate the tissue over the median palatal raphe to ascertain the difference in its displaceability as compared to the displaceability of the soft tissues covering the residual ridges will often lead to a "rocking," unstable, uncomfortable denture and dissatisfied patient. Adequate relief of palatal major connectors must be planned and the amount of relief required is directly proportionate to the difference in displaceability of the tissues over the midline of the palate and the tissues covering the residual ridges.

During the oral examination, not only must each arch be considered separately but also its occlusal relationship with the opposing arch. A situation that looks simple when the teeth are apart may be complicated when the teeth are in occlusion. For example, an extreme vertical overlap may complicate the attachment of anterior teeth to a maxillary denture. Extrusion of a tooth or teeth into an opposing edentulous area may complicate the replacement of teeth in the edentulous area, or it may create cuspal interference, which will complicate the location and design of clasp retainers and occlusal rests. When occlusal interference cannot be adequately determined by visual examination, the interposition of wax strips of varying thickness between the teeth may assist in determining the amount of interference or clearance present. Such findings subsequently will be evaluated further by a study of mounted diagnostic casts.

Need for determining the type of man- **dibular major connector.** As discussed in Chapter 4, one of the criteria for determining the use of the lingual bar or linguoplate was the height of the floor of the patient's mouth when the tongue is elevated. Since the inferior border of both the lingual bar and linguoplate are placed at the same vertical level and since subsequent mouth preparations depend in part on the selection of the mandibular major connector, determination of the type of major connector must be made during the oral examination. This determination is facilitated by measuring the height of the elevated floor of the patient's mouth in relation to lingual gingivae with a periodontal probe and recording the measurement for later transfer to diagnostic and master casts. It is most difficult to make a determination of the type of mandibular major connector to be used solely from a stone cast that may or may not accurately indicate the active range of movement of the floor of the patient's mouth. Too many mandibular major connectors are ruined, being made flexible because subsequent grinding of the inferior border is necessary to relieve impingement of the sensitive tissues of the floor of the mouth.

Need for reshaping remaining teeth. Many failures of partial dentures can be attributed to the fact that the teeth were not reshaped properly to receive clasp arms and occlusal rests before the impression for the master cast was made. Of particular importance are the paralleling of proximal tooth surfaces to act as guiding planes, the preparation of adequate rest areas, and the reduction of unfavorable tooth contours. To neglect to plan such mouth preparations in advance is inexcusable.

The design of clasps is dependent upon the location of the retentive, bracing and supporting areas in relation to a definite path of placement and removal. Failure to reshape unfavorably inclined tooth surfaces, and, if necessary, place onlays and crowns with suitable contours not only complicates the design and location of clasp retainers but also frequently leads to failure of the partial denture because of poor clasp design.

A malaligned tooth or one that is inclined unfavorably may make it necessary to place certain parts of the clasp so that they interfere with the opposing teeth. Proximal tooth surfaces that are not parallel not only will fail to provide needed guiding planes during placement and removal but also will make excessive blockout necessary. This inevitably results in the connectors being placed so far out of contact with tooth surfaces that food traps are created. To pass lingually inclined lower teeth, clearance for a lingual bar major connector may have to be so great that a food trap will result when the restoration is fully seated, and the lingual bar will be located so that it will interfere with tongue comfort and function. These are only some of the objectionable consequences of inadequate mouth preparations.

Reduction of unfavorable tooth contours. Slight reduction of unfavorable tooth contours will greatly facilitate the design of the partial denture framework. The need for modification of tooth contours must be established during the diagnosis and treatment planning phase of partial denture service.

The amount of reduction of tooth contours should be kept to a minimum, and all modified tooth surfaces should not only be repolished after reduction but also should be subjected to fluoride treatment to lessen the incidence of caries. If it is not possible to produce the contour desired without perforating the enamel, inlays or crowns must be used. The age of the patient, caries activity evidenced elsewhere in the mouth, and the apparent oral hygiene habits all must be taken into consideration when deciding between reducing the enamel or modifying tooth contours with protective restorations.

Some of the areas frequently needing correction are the lingual surfaces of mandibular premolars, the mesial and lingual surfaces of mandibular molars, the distobuccal line angle of maxillary premolars,

and the mesiobuccal line angle of maxillary molars. The actual degre of inclination of teeth in relation to the path of placement and the location of retentive and supportive areas are not readily interpretable during visual examination. These are established during a comprehensive survey of the diagnostic cast with a cast surveyor, which should follow the visual examination.

DENTAL CAST SURVEYOR

The cast surveyor (Fig. 11-1) is a simple enough instrument but *is most essential to planning partial denture treatment.* Its main working parts are the vertical arm and the adjustable table that holds the cast in a fixed relation to the vertical arm. This represents that path of placement that the partial denture will ultimately take in the mouth.

The adjustable table may be tilted in relation to the vertical arm of the surveyor until a path that best satisfies all the factors involved can be found. A cast in a horizontal relationship to the vertical arm represents a vertical path of placement; a cast in a tilted relationship represents a path of placement toward the side of the cast that is tilted upward. The vertical arm, when brought in contact with a tooth surface, will indicate the areas available for retention and those available for support, as well as the existence of tooth and other tissue interference to the path of placement.

If conditions are found that are not favorable for the particular path of placement being considered, the conditions produced by a different path of placement should be studied. The cast is merely tilted in relation to the vertical arm until the most suitable path is found. Then mouth preparations are planned with a definite path of placement in mind.

The path of placement also must take into consideration the presence of tissue undercuts that will interfere with the placement of major connectors, the location of vertical minor connectors, the origin of bar clasp arms, and the denture bases.

Recording the path of placement. Once

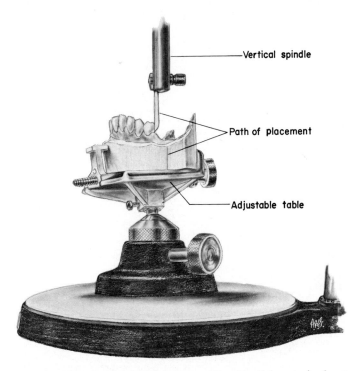

Vertical spindle

Path of placement

Adjustable table

Fig. 11-1. Most essential parts of a dental surveyor (Ney Parallelometer), showing the vertical arm in relation to the adjustable table.

the path of placement for all factors involved has been ascertained, the base of the cast can be scored or tripod marks can be placed on the cast to record the relation of the cast to the surveyor for future reference (Fig. 11-2, *A* to *C*). Then a guideline may be scribed on the surfaces of the abutment teeth by means of a graphite marker, replacing the diagnostic stylus (Fig. 11-2, *D*). This guideline will graphically locate the division between retentive and supportive areas, as well as areas of interference. Modification of tooth contours and clasp designs then may be planned with accuracy and mouth preparations planned accordingly. The cast surveyor is an indispensable instrument in surveying the cast of the mouth prior to preparing the mouth to receive a partial denture. Only by its use can the dentist ascertain the mechanical factors upon which the success or failure of the partial denture will depend. The dental cast surveyor and its uses have been discussed in detail in Chapter 10.

ORAL EXAMINATION

A complete oral examination should precede any mouth rehabilitation procedures. An oral examination should be complete—not limited to only one arch. It should include, in addition to a visual and digital examination of the teeth and surrounding tissues with mouth mirror, explorer, and periodontal probe, a complete intraoral roentgenographic survey, a vitality test of critical teeth, and an examination of casts correctly oriented on an adjustable articulator.

During the examination, the objective to be kept foremost in mind should be the consideration of the possibilities for maintaining the remaining oral structures in a state of health for the longest period of time. In addition to the elimination of infection, the primary objectives should be the prevention of tooth migration and the correction of traumatic influences. Secondarily should be the consideration of the best method for restoring lost function

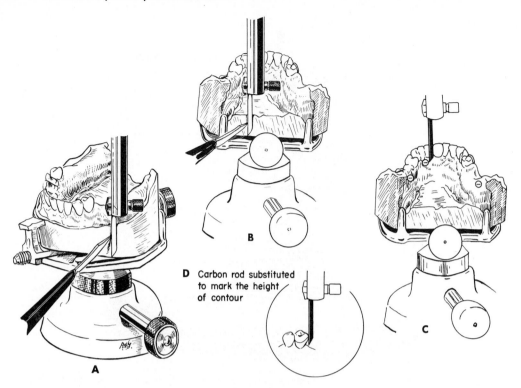

Fig. 11-2. A and **B,** Path of placement having been determined, the base of the cast is scored to record its relation to the surveyor for future repositioning. **C,** Alternate method to record the relation of the cast to the surveyor is known as *tripoding.* A carbon marker is placed in the vertical arm of the surveyor, and the arm is adjusted to a height by which the cast can be contacted in three divergent locations. Vertical arm is locked in position and the cast is brought into contact with the tip of the carbon marker. Three resultant marks are encircled with a colored lead pencil for ease of identification. Reorientation of the cast to the surveyor is accomplished by tilting the cast until the plane created by three marks is at a right angle to the vertical arm of the surveyor. **D,** The height of contour is then delineated by a carbon marker.

within the limits of tissue tolerance of the patient. Third, and not before, the decision should be made as to how best to maintain or improve upon the appearance of the mouth. As the first two objectives are satisfied, so will the requirement of a comfortable and esthetically pleasing restoration also be satisfied.

Objectives of prosthodontic treatment. The objectives of any prosthodontic treatment may be stated as (1) the elimination of disease, (2) the preservation of the health and relationship of the teeth and the health of the remaining oral tissues, and (3) the restoration in part of lost teeth and function in an esthetically pleasing manner.

Patients with missing teeth may specifi-

cally request their replacement, especially when anterior teeth are missing and they are concerned only with the cosmetic implications. On the other hand, they may seek diagnosis and advice, the result of which is frequently the recommendation that the missing teeth be replaced with either fixed or removable restorations. In many instances the patient is usually concerned only with the replacement of the missing teeth. The dentist's primary obligation to the patient is to emphasize the importance of restoring the total mouth to a state of health and of preserving the remaining teeth and surrounding tissues. Incident to this is the functional and esthetically acceptable replacement of missing teeth in a

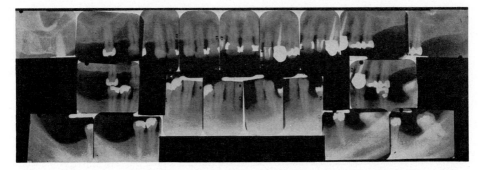

Fig. 11-3. Complete intraoral roentgenographic survey of the remaining teeth and adjacent edentulous areas reveals much information vital to effective diagnosis and treatment planning. The response of bone to previous stress is of particular value in establishing the prognosis of teeth that are to be used as abutments.

harmonious relation with the remaining teeth and surrounding structures.

In many instances restoration of lost function must be modified and minimized to avoid overloading the supporting structures. The prevention of tooth migration, the healthful stimulation of oral tissues, and the preservation of the remaining teeth are of greater importance. The amount that lost masticatory function can be restored depends upon the tissue tolerance of the individual, as influenced by his age, his general health, and the health of the oral tissues.

Sequence for oral examination. An oral examination should be accomplished in the following sequence:

1. *A thorough and complete oral prophylaxis.* An adequate examination can be accomplished best with the teeth free of accumulated calculus and debris. Also, accurate diagnostic casts of the dental arches can be obtained only if the teeth are clean; otherwise, the teeth reproduced on the diagnostic casts are not a true representation of tooth and gingival contours. Cursory examination may precede an oral phophylaxis, but a thorough oral examination should be deferred until the teeth have been thoroughly cleaned.

2. *The placement of individual temporary restorations.* This is advisable not only to relieve discomfort arising from tooth defects but also to determine as early as possible the extent of caries and to arrest further caries activity until definitive treatment can be instituted. By restoring tooth contours with temporary restorations, the impression will not be torn in removal from the mouth, and a more accurate diagnostic cast may be obtained.

3. *A complete intraoral roentgenographic survey* (Fig. 11-3). The objectives of a roentgenographic examination are (a) to locate areas of infection and other pathosis that may be present; (b) to reveal the presence of root fragments, foreign objects, bone spicules, and irregular ridge formations; (c) to reveal the presence and extent of caries and the relation of carious lesions to the pulp; (d) to permit evaluation of existing restorations as to evidence of recurrent caries, marginal leakage, and overhanging gingival margins; (e) to reveal the presence of root canal fillings and to permit their evaluation as to future prognosis (the design of the partial denture may hinge upon the decision to retain or extract an endodontically treated tooth); (f) to permit an evaluation of periodontal conditions present and to establish the need and possibilities for treatment; and (g) to evaluate the alveolar support of abutment teeth —the number, supporting length, and morphology of their roots, the relative amount of alveolar bone loss suffered through pathogenic processes, and the amount of alveolar support remaining.

4. *Vitality tests of remaining teeth.* These tests should be given particularly to those

PARTIAL DENTURE DIAGNOSIS AND TREATMENT RECORD

Patient:_____ Reg. No._____

Student:_____ Date:_____

Pertinent Radiographic Findings:_____

	UPPER	LOWER
Kennedy Classification		
Initial	Class_____, Mod._____	Class_____, Mod._____
Final	Class_____, Mod._____	Class_____, Mod._____
Abutment Teeth		
Teeth to be Extracted and Reason		
Surgical Preparation of Ridges		
Abutment Restorations		
(Tooth No. & Type Restorations)		
Final Mouth Preparations:		
Guiding Planes		
Reduction of Tooth Contours		
Occlusal Rests		
Date above completed		
Impression Materials Used:		
For Master Cast		
For Correction of Supporting Ridges		
Denture Base Materials		
Tooth Selection		
Occlusal Registration; Methods Used		
Drawing of Partial Denture Design:		
Metal framework in blue,		
Resin bases or attachments in red,		
Wrought retentive clasp arms in red.	MAXILLARY OCCLUSAL VIEW	MANDIBULAR OCCLUSAL VIEW
Placement Date:		
Post-Placement Notes:		

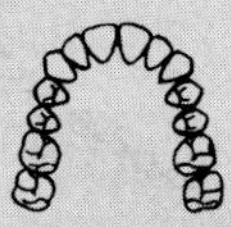

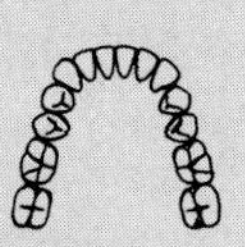

Fig. 11-4. Diagnosis and treatment record chart for recording the treatment plan and pertinent data.

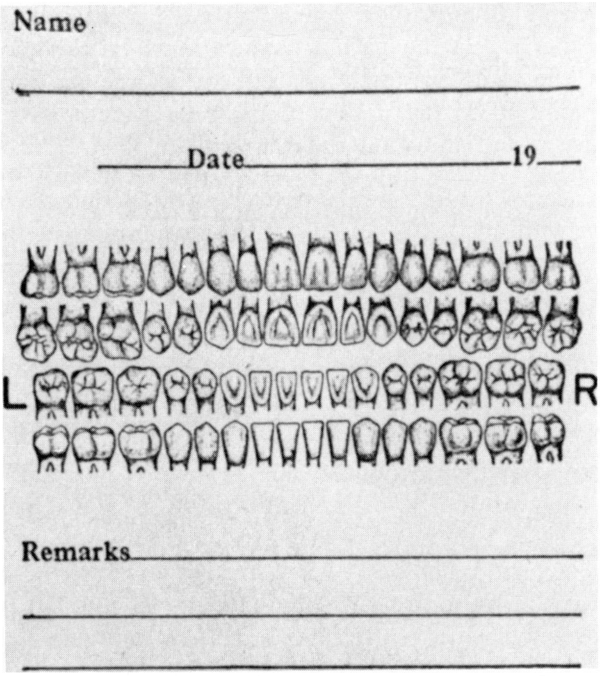

Name

Date_____19___

Remarks

Fig. 11-5. Simple working chart. Restorations for individual teeth, crowns, and fixed partial dentures to be made may be marked on the chart and checked off as completed during mouth preparations.

teeth to be used as abutments and those having deep restorations or deep carious lesions. This may be done either by thermal or by electronic means, whichever the dentist has learned best to interpret.

5. *The exploration of teeth and investing structures.* These can be explored by instrumentation and visual means. This should include a determination of tooth mobility and an examination of occlusal relationships. At this time the presence of tori and other bony protuberances should be noted and their clinical significance evaluated. Also history and diagnosis charts should be filled out at this time, as well as a simple working chart for future reference (Figs. 11-4 and 11-5). The latter does not become part of the patient's permanent record but registers the nature and sequence of treatment, and it can be used by the dentist as a checklist during treatment. A breakdown of the fee may be recorded on the back of this chart for easy reference if adjustments or substitutions become nec-

essary by changes in the diagnosis as the work progresses.

6. *Determining the height of the floor of the mouth to locate inferior borders of lingual mandibular major connectors.* Mouth preparation procedures are influenced by a choice of the major connectors. This determination must precede altering contours of abutment teeth.

7. *Impressions for making accurate diagnostic casts.* The casts, preferably, will be articulated on a suitable instrument. The importance of accurate diagnostic casts and their use will be discussed later in this chapter.

• • •

The fee for examination, which should include the cost of the roentgenographic survey and the examination of articulated diagnostic casts, should be established prior to the examination and should not be related to the cost of treatment. It should be understood that the fee for examination is based upon the time involved and the service rendered and that the material value of the roentgenographs and diagnostic casts is incidental to the effectiveness of the examination.

The examination record should always be available in the office for future consultation. If consultation with another dentist is requested, modern respect for the hazards of unnecessary radiation justifies the dentist loaning the roentgenograms for this purpose. Preferably, however, double-film packs should be used so that one copy may be retained in the dentist's files.

ROENTGENOGRAPHIC INTERPRETATION

Many of the reasons for roentgenographic interpretation during oral examination are outlined herein and are considered in greater detail in other texts. The aspects of such interpretation that are the most pertinent to partial denture construction are those relative to the prognosis of remaining teeth that may be used as abutments.

The quality of the alveolar support of an abutment tooth is of primary importance because the tooth will be called upon to withstand greater stress loads when supporting a dental prosthesis. Abutment teeth providing total abutment support to the prosthesis, be it either fixed or removable, will have to withstand a greater vertical load than before and, to some extent, greater horizontal forces. The latter may be minimized by establishing a harmonious occlusion and by distributing the horizontal forces among several teeth through the use of rigid connectors. Bilateral stabilization against horizontal forces is one of the attributes of a properly designed tooth-borne removable prosthesis. In many instances abutment teeth may be aided more than weakened by the presence of a bilaterally rigid partial denture.

In contrast, abutment teeth adjacent to distal extension bases are subjected not only to vertical and horizontal forces but to torque as well because of the movement of the tissue-supported base. Vertical support and stabilization against horizontal movement with rigid connectors are just as important as they are with a tooth-borne prosthesis, and the partial denture must be designed accordingly. In addition, the abutment tooth adjacent to the extension base will be subjected to torque in proportion to the design of the retainers, the size of the denture base, the tissue support received by the base, and the total occlusal load applied. With this in mind, each abutment tooth must be evaluated carefully as to the alveolar support present and the past reaction of that bone to occlusal stress.

The value of interpreting bone density. The quality and quantity of bone in any part of the body is often evaluated by roentgenographic means. A detailed treatise concerning the bone support of the abutment tooth should include many considerations not possible to include in this text because of space limitations. The reader should realize that subclinical variations in bone may exist but may not be observed because of the limitations inherent in technical methods and equipment.

Of importance to the prosthodontist when evaluating the quality and quantity of the alveolar bone are the height and the quality of the remaining bone. In estimating bone height, care must be taken to avoid interpretive errors resulting from angulation factors. Technically, when making an exposure, the central ray should be directed at right angles to both the tooth and the film. The most commonly used roentgenographic technique, that is, the short-cone technique, does not follow this principle; instead, the ray is directed through the root of the tooth at a predetermined angle. This technique invariably causes the buccal bone to be projected higher on the crown than is the lingual or palatal bone. Therefore, when interpreting bone height, it is imperative to follow the line of the lamina dura from the apex toward the crown of the tooth until the opacity of the lamina materially decreases. At this point of opacity change, a less dense bone extends farther toward the tooth crown. This additional amount of bone represents false bone height. Thus the true height of the bone is ordinarily where the lamina shows a marked decrease in opacity. At this point the trabecular pattern of bone superimposed upon the tooth root is lost. The portion of the root between the cementoenamel junction and the true bone height has the appearance of being bare or devoid of covering.

Roentgenographic evaluation of bone quality is hazardous but is often necessary. It is essential to emphasize that changes in bone calcification up to 25% often cannot be recognized by ordinary roentgenographic means. Optimum bone qualities are ordinarily expressed by normal-sized interdental trabecular spaces that usually tend to decrease slightly in size as examination of the bone proceeds from the root apex toward the coronal portion. The normal interproximal crest is ordinarily shown by a relatively thin white line crossing from the lamina dura of one tooth to the lamina dura of the adjacent tooth. Considerable variation in the size of trabecular spaces may exist within the limits of normal, and the roentgenographic appearance of crestal alveolar bone may vary considerably, depending upon its shape and the direction that the x-ray takes as it passes through the bone.

Normal bone usually responds favorably to ordinary stresses. Abnormal stresses, however, may create a reduction in the size of the trabecular pattern, particularly in that area of bone directly adjacent to the lamina dura of the affected tooth. This decrease in size of the trabecular pattern (that is, *so-called bone condensation*) is often regarded as a favorable bone response, indicative of an improvement in bone quality. This is not necessarily an accurate interpretation. Such bone changes usually indicate stresses that should be relieved, because if the resistance of the patient decreases, the bone may exhibit a progressively less favorable response in future roentgenograms.

An increased thickness of the periodontal space ordinarily suggests varying degrees of tooth mobility. This should be evaluated clinically. Roentgenographic evidence coupled with clinical findings may suggest to the prosthodontist the inadvisability of utilizing such a tooth as an abutment. Furthermore, an irregular intercrestal bone surface should make the prosthodontist suspicious of active bone deterioration.

It is essential that the prosthodontist realize that roentgenographic evidence shows the *result* of changes that have taken place and may not necessarily represent the present condition. For example, periodontal disease may have progressed beyond the stage visibly demonstrated in the roentgenograms. As was pointed out earlier, roentgenographic changes are not observed until approximately 25% of the calcific content has been depleted. On the other hand, bone condensations probably do represent the present situation.

Roentgenographic findings should serve the prosthodontist as an adjunct to his clinical observations. Too often the roentgenographic appearance alone is used in arriving at a diagnosis. Roentgenographic interpretation also will serve an important function if used periodically *after* the prosthesis has been placed. Future bone changes of *any type* suggest traumatic interference from some source. The nature of such interference should be determined and corrective measures taken.

Index areas. Index areas are those areas of alveolar support that disclose the reaction of bone to additional stress. Favorable reaction to such stress may be taken as an indication of future reaction to an added stress load. Teeth that have been subjected to abnormal loading due to the loss of adjacent teeth or that have withstood tipping forces in addition to occlusal loading may be better risks as abutment teeth than those that have not been called upon to carry an extra occlusal load (Fig. 11-6). If occlusal harmony can be improved and unfavorable forces minimized by the reshaping of occlusal surfaces and the favorable distribution of occlusal loading, such teeth may be expected to support the pros-

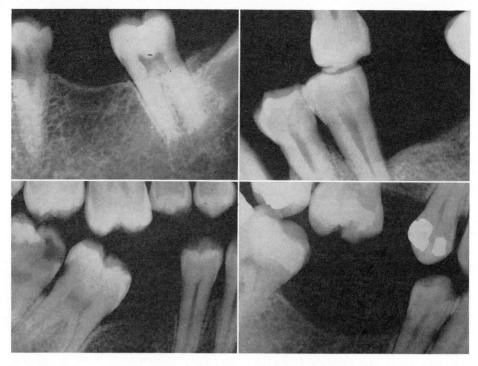

Fig. 11-6. Reaction of bone adjacent to teeth that have been subjected to abnormal stress serves as an indication of the probable reaction of that bone when such teeth are used as abutments for fixed or removable restorations. Such areas are called *index areas.*

thesis without difficulty. At the same time, other teeth, although not at present carrying an extra load, may be expected to react favorably because of the favorable reaction of alveolar bone to abnormal loading elsewhere in the same arch.

Such index areas are those around teeth that have been subjected to abnormal occlusal loading, those that have been subjected to diagonal occlusal loading due to tooth migration, and those that have reacted to additional loading, such as around existing fixed partial denture abutments. The reaction of the bone to additional stresses in these areas may be either positive or negative, with evidence of a supporting trabecular pattern, a heavy cortical layer, and a dense lamina dura, or the reverse response. With the former the patient is said to have a *positive bone factor,* meaning the ability to build additional support wherever needed. With the latter he is said to have a *negative bone factor,* meaning inability to respond favorably to stress.

Alveolar lamina dura. The alveolar lamina dura is also considered when making a roentgenographic interpretation of abutment teeth. The lamina dura is the thin layer of hard cortical bone that normally lines the sockets of all teeth. It affords attachment for the fibers of the periodontal membrane, and, like all cortical bone, its function is to withstand mechanical strain. In a roentgeongram the lamina dura is shown as a *radiopaque* white line around the radiolucent dark line that represents the periodontal membrane.

When a tooth is in the process of being tipped, the center of rotation is not at the apex of the root but is in the apical third. Resorption of bone occurs where there is pressure, and apposition occurs where there is tension. Therefore, during the active tipping process, the lamina dura is uneven, with evidence of both pressure and tension on the same side of the root. For example, in a mesially tipping lower molar, the lamina dura will be thinner on the coronal mesial and apical distal aspects and thicker on the apical mesial and coronal distal aspects because the axis of rotation is not at the root apex but above it. When the tooth has been tipped into an edentulous space by some change in the occlusion and becomes set in its new position, the effects of leverage are discontinued. The lamina dura on the side to which the tooth is sloping becomes uniformly heavier, which is nature's reinforcement against abnormal stresses. The bone trabeculations are arranged at right angles to the heavier lamina dura.

Thus it is possible to say that, for a given individual, nature is able to build support where it is needed and on this basis to predict future reaction eleswhere in the arch to additional loading of teeth used as abutments. However, since bone is approximately 30% organic, and this mostly protein, and since the body is not able to store a protein reserve in large amounts, any change in body health may be reflected in the patient's ability to maintain this support permanently. When systemic disease is associated with faulty protein metabolism and when the ability to repair is diminished, bone is resorbed and the lamina dura is disturbed. Therefore the loading of any abutment tooth must be kept to a minimum inasmuch as the patient's future health status and the eventualities of aging are unpredictable.

Root morphology. The morphologic characteristics of the roots determine, to a great extent, the ability of prospective abutment teeth to resist successfully additional rotational forces that may be placed upon them. Teeth with multiple and divergent roots will resist stresses better than will teeth whose roots are fused and conical, since the resultant forces are distributed through a greater number of periodontal fibers to a larger amount of supporting bone (Fig. 11-7).

Third molars. Unerupted third molars should be considered as prospective future abutments to eliminate the need for a distal extension removable partial denture (Fig.

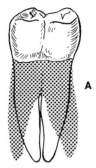
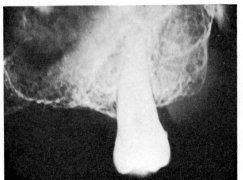

Fig. 11-7. **A,** Prognosis for abutment service is more favorable for the molar with divergent roots (shaded) than for the same tooth if its roots were fused and conical. **B,** Evidence that a prospective abutment has conical and fused roots indicates the necessity for formulating a framework design that will minimize additional stresses placed on the tooth by abutment service.

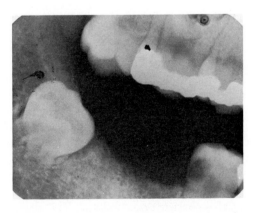

Fig. 11-8. First and second molars have been lost by this 18-year-old patient. A distal extension removable partial denture may be constructed until the third molar erupts and is fully formed. A toothborne restoration can then be constructed.

11-8). The increased stability of a tooth-borne denture is most desirable to enhance the health of the oral environment.

DIAGNOSTIC CASTS

A diagnostic cast should be an *accurate* reproduction of the teeth and adjacent tissues. In a partially edentulous arch this must include the edentulous spaces, since these also must be evaluated in determining the type of denture base to be used and the extent of available denture-supporting area.

A diagnostic cast is usually made of dental stone because of its strength and the fact that it is less easily abraded than is dental plaster. Generally, the improved dental stones (die stones) are not used for diagnostic casts because of their cost. Their greater resistance to abrasion does, however, justify their use for master casts.

The impression for the diagnostic cast is usually made with an irreversible hydrocolloid (alginate) in a perforated partial denture impression tray. The size of the arch will determine the size of the tray to be used. The tray should be sufficiently oversize to assure an optimum thickness of impression material to avoid distortion or tearing upon removal from the mouth. The technique for the making of impressions will be covered in more detail in Chapter 14.

Purposes for which the diagnostic casts are used. Diagnostic casts serve several purposes as an aid to diagnosis and treatment planning. Some of these are as follows:

1. Diagnostic casts are used to supplement the oral examination by permitting a view of the occlusion from the lingual as well as from the buccal aspect. Analysis of the existing occlusion is made possible when opposing casts are occluded, as well as a study of the possibilities for improvement either by occlusal adjustment or occlusal reconstruction, or both. The degree of overclosure, the amount of interocclusal space needed, and the possibilities of interference to the location of rests also may be determined.

As stated previously, possibilities for improvement of the occlusal scheme either by occlusal adjustment or occlusal reconstruction or both are made possible by the use of mounted diagnostic casts. Such procedures often include "diagnostic waxing" to determine the possibility of enhancing the occlusion before definitive treatment is begun (Fig. 11-9). In other words, diagnostic casts permit the dentist to "plan ahead" and avoid undesirable compromises in the treatment being rendered a patient.

2. Diagnostic casts are used to permit a topographic survey of the dental arch that is to be restored by means of a removable partial denture. The cast of the arch in question may be surveyed individually with a cast surveyor to determine the parallelism or lack of parallelism of tooth surfaces involved and to establish its influence of the design of the partial denture. The principal considerations in studying the parallelism of tooth and tissue surfaces of the dental arch are (a) proximal tooth surfaces, which can be made parallel to serve as guiding planes, (b) retentive and nonretentive areas of the abutment teeth, and (c) areas of interference to placement and removal. From such a survey a path of placement may be selected that will satisfy requirements for parallelism and retention to the best mechanical, functional, and esthetic advantage. Then mouth preparations may be planned accordingly.

3. Diagnostic casts are used to permit a logical and comprehensive presentation to the patient of his present and future restorative needs, as well as the hazards of future neglect. Occluded and individual diagnostic casts can be used to point out to the patient (a) evidence of tooth migration and the existing results of such migration, (b) effects of further tooth migration, (c) loss of occlusal support and its consequences, (d) hazards of traumatic occlusal contacts, and (e) cariogenic and periodontal implications of further neglect.

Treatment planning actually may be accomplished with the patient present, so that economic considerations may be dis-

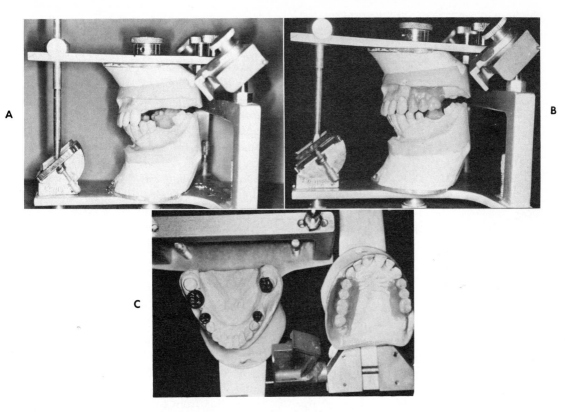

Fig. 11-9, **A**, Diagnostic casts have been mounted and the articulator has been adjusted by intraoral, eccentric, maxillomandibular records. **B**, Lower stone abutment teeth for prospective fixed partial dentures have been reduced so that diagnostic occlusal waxing may be performed. Maxillary artificial teeth have been arranged in conjunction with the waxing of the lower occlusal surfaces to satisfy the demands of the proposed occlusal scheme. **C**, Anterior stone teeth have also been altered to satisfy the occlusal scheme. With such guides developed on diagnostic casts, like oral preparatory procedures can be accomplished for a predetermined end result. (**C**, From Morris, A. L., and Bohannon, H. M., editors: Dental specialties in general practice, Philadelphia, 1969, W. B. Saunders Co.)

cussed also. Such use of diagnostic casts permits a justification of the proposed fee through the patient's understanding of the problems involved and the treatment needed. Inasmuch as mouth rehabilitation procedures are frequently protracted, there must be complete accord between dentist and patient before beginning extensive treatment, and financial arrangements must be consummated during the planning phase.

4. Individual impression trays may be fabricated upon the diagnostic casts, or the diagnostic cast may be used in selecting and fitting a stock impression tray for the final impression. If wax blockout is to be used in the fabrication of individual trays,

a duplicate cast made from an irreversible hydrocolloid (alginate) impression of the diagnostic cast should be used for this purpose. The diagnostic cast is too valuable for future reference to risk damage resulting from the making of an impression tray. On the other hand, if only a wet asbestos blockout is used, the diagnostic cast may be used without fear of damage.

Since essential areas will be known in advance of making the final impression, the tray may be selected or made with these in mind. Such areas as recorded in the final impression may then be examined critically for possible artifacts.

5. Diagnostic casts may be used as a

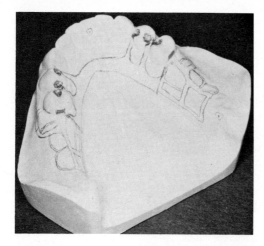

Fig. 11-10. Proposed mouth changes and design of the partial denture framework are indicated in pencil on diagnostic cast in relation to a previously determined path of placement.

constant reference as the work progresses. Penciled marks indicating the type of restorations, areas of tooth surfaces to be modified, location of rests, and the design of the partial denture framework, as well as the path of placement and removal, all may be recorded on the diagnostic cast for future reference (Fig. 11-10). Then these steps may be checked off the work sheet as they are completed.

Areas of abutment teeth to be modified may first be changed on the diagnostic cast by trimming the stone cast with the surveyor blade. A record is thus made of the location and degree of modification to be done in the mouth. This must be done in relation to a definite path of placement. Any mouth preparations to be accomplished with new cast restorations require that wax patterns be shaped in accordance with a previously determined path of placement. Even so, the shaping of abutment teeth on the diagnostic cast serves as a guide to the form of the abutment pattern. This is particularly true if the contouring of wax patterns is to be delegated to the technician, as it may be in a busy practice.

6. *Unaltered diagnostic casts should become a permanent part of the patient's record because records of conditions ex-*isting *before treatment are just as important as are preoperative roentgenograms. Therefore, diagnostic casts should be duplicated, one cast serving as a permanent record and the other cast being used in situations that may require alterations to the cast.*

Mounting diagnostic casts. Although some diagnostic casts may be occluded by hand, occlusal analysis is much better accomplished when they are mounted on an adjustable articulator. By definition, an articulator is "a mechanical device that represents the temporomandibular joints and jaw members, to which maxillary and mandibular casts may be attached." Since the dominant influence on mandibular movement in a partially edentulous mouth is the cusps of the remaining teeth, an anatomic reproduction of condylar paths is probably not obtainable. Still, movement of the casts in relation to one another as influenced by the cusps of the remaining teeth, when mounted at a reasonably accurate radius from the axis of condylar rotation, permits a relatively valid analysis of occlusal relationships. This is much better than a simple hinge mounting.

It is probably still better that the casts be mounted in relation to the axis-orbital plane to permit better interpretation of the plane of occlusion in relation to the horizontal plane. Whereas it is true that an axis-orbital mounting has no functional value on a non-arcon instrument, since that plane ceases to exist when opposing casts are separated, the value of such a mounting lies in the orientation of the casts in occlusion. (An *arcon* articulator is one in which the condyles are attached to the lower member as they are in nature, the term being a derivation coined by Bergström from the words *ar*ticulation and *con*dyle [Fig. 11-11]. All the more widely used articulators such as the Hanau [H series], Dentatus, and improved Gysi have the condyles attached to the upper member and are therefore non-*arcon* instruments.)

Mounting the upper cast to the axis-orbital plane. The face-bow is a relatively

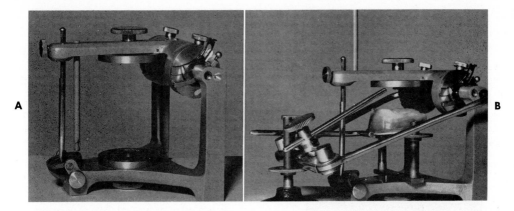

Fig. 11-11. A, Bergström arcon articulator showing the condyle attached to the lower arm of the articulator and the condyle path to the upper arm. B, Bergström face-bow attached to the articulator prior to mounting the upper cast. (Courtesy Dr. H. O. Beck.)

simple device used to obtain a transfer record for orienting a maxillary cast on an articulating instrument. Originally, the face-bow was used only to transfer a *radius* from condyle reference points so that a given point on the cast would be the same distance from the condyle as it is on the patient. The addition of an adjustable infraorbital pointer to the face-bow and the addition of an orbital plane indicator to the articulator make possible also the transfer of the *elevation* of the cast in relation to the axis-orbital plane. This permits the maxillary cast to be correctly oriented in the articulator space comparable to the relationship of the maxillae to the Frankfort horizontal on the patient. To accommodate a maxillary cast so oriented and still have room for the mandibular cast, the posts of the conventional articulator must be lengthened. The older Hanau model H articulator usually will not permit a face-bow transfer using an infraorbital pointer.

A face-bow may be used to transfer a comparable radius from arbitrary reference points, or it may be designed so that the transfer can be made from hinge axis points. The latter type of transfer requires that a hinge-bow attached to the mandible be used initially to determine the hinge axis points, to which the face-bow is then adjusted for making the hinge axis transfer.

A face-bow transfer of the maxillary cast, which is oriented to the axis-orbital plane, to a suitable articulator is an uncomplicated procedure. Hanau models S-M, S-M-X, and H-2, and the Dentatus model ARH will accept this transfer, since these models have the longer posts and orbital plane indicator necessary for such a transfer (Fig. 11-18). Both the Hanau face-bow model S-M and the Dentatus face-bow type AEB incorporate the infraorbital pointer, which permits transfer of the infraorbital plane to the articulator. Neither of these is a hinge axis bow but is used instead at an arbitrary point.

The location of this arbitrary point or axis has long been the subject of some controversy. Gysi and others have placed it 11 to 13 mm. anterior to the upper one third of the tragus of the ear on a line extending from the upper margin of the external auditory meatus to the outer canthus of the eye (Fig. 11-12). Others have placed it 13 mm. anterior to the posterior margin of the center of the tragus of the ear on a line extending to the corner of the eye. Bergström has located the arbitrary axis 10 mm. anterior to the center of a spherical insert for the external auditory meatus and 7 mm. below the Frankfort horizontal plane.

In a series of experiments reported by Beck, it was shown that the arbitrary axis suggested by Bergström falls consistently closer to the kinematic axis than do the other two. It is, of course, desirable that an arbitrary axis be placed as close as is possible to the kinematic axis. Although most authorities agree that any of the three axes will permit a transfer of the maxillary cast with reasonable accuracy, it would seem that the Bergström point compares most favorably with the kinematic axis.

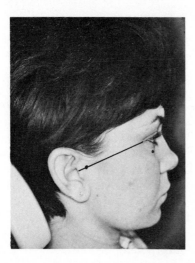

Fig. 11-12. Location of an arbitrary axis 11 to 13 mm. anterior to the upper one third of the tragus of the ear from a line extending from the upper margin of the external auditory meatus to the outer canthus of the eye. The lowest point on the inferior orbital margin is marked as the third point of reference for establishing the axis-orbital plane.

The lowest point on the inferior orbital margin is taken as the third point of reference for establishing the axis-orbital plane. Some authorities use the point on the lower margin of the bony orbit in line with the center of the pupil of the eye. For the sake of consistency, the right infraorbital point is generally used and the face-bow assembled in this relationship. All three points (right and left axes and infraorbital point) are marked on the face with an ink dot before making the transfer.

Casts are prepared for mounting on an articulator by placing three index grooves in the base of the cast. Two V-shaped grooves are placed in the posterior section of the cast and one groove in the anterior portion (Fig. 11-13).

An occlusion rim should be utilized in face-bow procedures involving the transfer of casts representative of the Class I or II partially edentulous situations. Without occlusion rims, such casts cannot be located accurately in the imprints of the wax covering the face-bow fork. Tissues covering the residual ridges may be displaced grossly when the patient closes into the wax on the face-bow fork. Therefore the wax imprints of the soft tissues are not true negatives of the edentulous regions of the diagnostic casts.

The face-bow fork is covered with a roll of softened baseplate wax with the wax

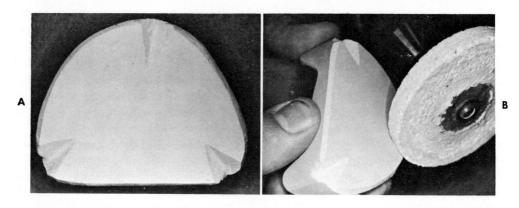

Fig. 11-13. **A,** Base of the cast has been prepared for mounting. **B,** Triangular grooves can be conveniently and quickly cut in the base of the cast by using a 3-inch stone mounted in a laboratory lathe.

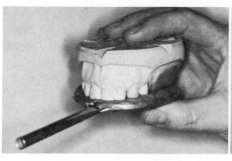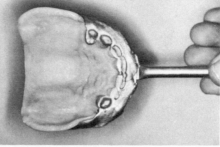

Fig. 11-14. Orienting the face-bow fork to the maxillary cast and occlusion rims will avoid displacing the occlusion rim in the mouth when the patient closes to maintain the face-bow fork in position. The face-bow fork illustrated here is a Whipmix type. When an offset type of face-bow fork (Hanau) is used, the offset handle must be on the patient's left.

distributed equally on the top and on the underneath side of the face-bow fork. Then the fork should be pressed lightly on the diagnostic cast with the midline of the face-bow fork corresponding to the midline of the central incisors (Fig. 11-14). This will leave imprints of the occlusal and incisal surfaces of the maxillary cast and occlusion rim on the softened baseplate wax and is an aid in correctly orienting the face-bow fork in the patient's mouth. The face-bow fork is placed in position in the mouth, and the patient is asked to close the lower teeth into the wax to stabilize it in position. It is removed from the mouth and chilled in cool water and then replaced in position in the patient's mouth.

With the face-bow fork in position, the face-bow toggle is slipped over the anterior projection of the face-bow fork and positioned so that the calibrations on the shaft on either side read the same as they rest lightly on the two dots located anterior to the external auditory meatuses. The calibrated shafts are then locked in this bilaterally equal position. The face-bow may have to be removed to accomplish this. It is then returned to position and locked to the face-bow fork while being held with equal contact over the dots on either side of the face. This accomplishes the *radius* aspect of the face-bow transfer.

With the infraorbital pointer on the extreme right side of the face-bow, it is angled toward the infraorbital point previ-

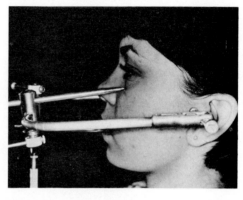

Fig. 11-15. Hanau S-M face-bow is positioned on the face so that calibrations on the shaft on either side read the same as they rest lightly on the two dots located anterior to the external auditory meatus. The infraorbital pointer is adjusted to rest lightly on the infraorbital point previously marked on the face.

ously identified with an ink dot. It is then locked into position with its tip lightly touching the skin at the dot (Fig. 11-15). This establishes the *elevation* of the face-bow in relation to the axis-orbital plane. Extreme care must be taken to avoid any slip that might damage the patient's eye.

With all elements tightened securely, the patient is asked to open the mouth, and the entire assembly is removed intact, rinsed with cold water, and set aside. The face-bow records not only the radius from the condyles to the incisal contacts of the upper central incisors but also the angular

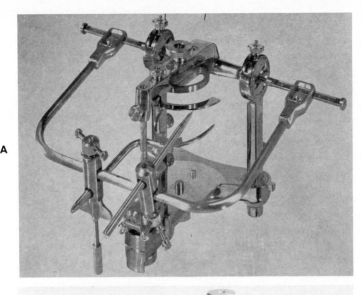

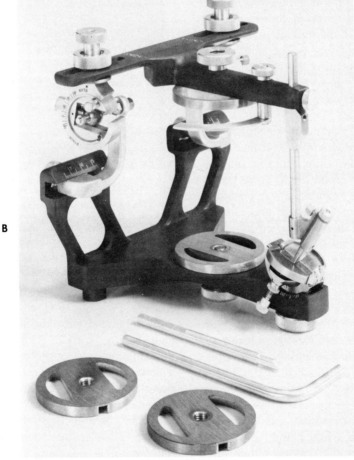

Fig. 11-16. **A,** Model H-2 Hanau articulator with S-M face-bow attached. Note the orientation of the face-bow to the orbital plane indicator, supported by the adjustable screw on the face-bow. **B,** Hanau University articulator, model 130-28, a model of the new Hanau articulator series. S-M face-bow is used on the 130-28 in the same manner as illustrated in **A.** (Courtesy Hanau Engineering Co., Buffalo, N. Y.)

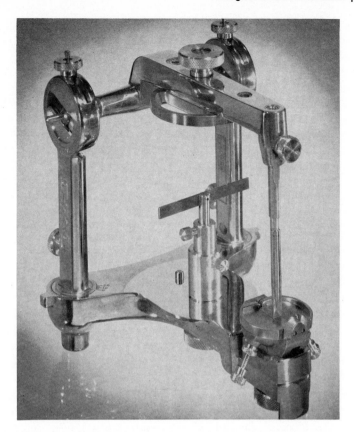

Fig. 11-17. Face-bow fork support attached to the lower arm of the Hanau H-2 articulator. This device is used to support the face-bow fork and maxillary cast at the determined elevation while it is being attached to the upper arm of the articulator with mounting stone. The orbital pointer and orbital plane indicator may then be removed to facilitate mounting the maxillary cast. (Courtesy Hanau Engineering Co., Buffalo, N. Y.)

relationship of the occlusal plane to the axis-orbital plane.

The face-bow must be positioned on the articulator in the same axis-orbital relation as on the patient (Figs. 11-16 and 11-18). The calibrated condyle rods of the face-bow ordinarily will not fit the condyle shafts of the articulator unless the width between the condyles just happens to be the same. With a Hanau model C face-bow the calibrations must be reequalized when in position on the articulator. For example, they might have read 7.4 (mm.) on each side of the patient but must be adjusted to read 6.9 (mm.) on each side of the articulator. With some later model articulators having adjustable condyle rods, these may instead be adjusted to fit the face-bow. It

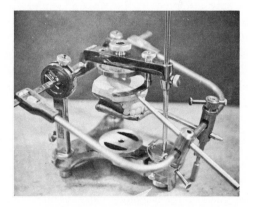

Fig. 11-18. Hanau face-bow model S-M attached to the articulator prior to mounting the maxillary cast. Note the elevation of the face-bow with the orbital plane indicator. The handle of the offset face-bow fork must be on the patient's left side, otherwise the two face-bow toggles as used here would interfere with each other.

is necessary that the face-bow be centered in either case.

The third point of reference is the orbital plane indicator, which must be swung to the right so that it will be above the tip of the infraorbital pointer. The entire face-bow with maxillary cast in place must be raised until the tip of the pointer contacts the orbital plane indicator (Figs. 11-16 and 11-18). The elevation having thus been established, for all practical purposes the orbital plane indicator and pointer may now be removed because they may interfere with placing the mounting stone.

An auxiliary device called a *cast support* is available*; it is used to support the face-bow fork and the maxillary cast during the mounting operation (Fig. 11-17). With this device the weight of the cast and the mounting stone is supported separately from the face-bow, thus preventing possible downward movement resulting from their combined weight. The cast support is raised to supporting contact with the face-bow fork after the face-bow height has been adjusted to the level of the orbital plane. Use of some type of cast support is highly recommended as an adjunct to face-bow mounting. Figure 11-20, *C*, demonstrates a simple and inexpensive method.

The keyed and lubricated maxillary cast is now attached to the upper arm of the articulator with mounting stone, thus completing the face-bow transfer (Fig. 11-19). Not only will the face-bow have permitted the upper cast to be mounted with reasonable accuracy, but it also will have served as a convenient means of supporting the cast during mounting. The ease and speed with which a face-bow transfer can be effected makes ridiculous the frequently expressed objection to its use on the basis of time involved. Once mastered, its use becomes a great convenience rather than a time-consuming nuisance.

It is preferable that the upper cast be mounted while the patient is still present, thus eliminating a possible reappointment

*Hanau Engineering Co., Buffalo, N. Y.

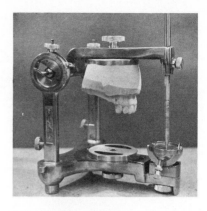

Fig. 11-19. Maxillary diagnostic cast mounted by a face-bow transfer. Note that the cast has been keyed prior to mounting and may be removed for repositioning on the surveyor.

if the face-bow record is unacceptable for some reason. Not too infrequently the face-bow record has to be redone with the offset type face-bow fork repositioned to avoid interference with some part of the articulator.

The use of an ear face-bow to orient the maxillary cast to an articulator is used by many dentists (Fig. 11-20). Although the use of such an instrument was described by Dalbey in 1914, its use has been rather limited until recently.

In an investigation by Teteruck and Lundeen it was demonstrated that by the ear face-bow method the maxillary cast could consistently be oriented more accurately to the hinge axis than by the method utilizing an arbitrary mark on the tragus-canthus line. The ear face-bow is a simple instrument to use, does not require measurements or marks on the face, consumes less time for its use, and is as accurate, if not more so, than are other arbitrary methods of face-bow transfer.

Jaw relationship records for diagnostic casts. One of the first critical decisions that must be made in a removable partial denture service involves the selection of the horizontal jaw relation to which the removable partial denture will be constructed—centric relation or centric occlusion. All mouth preparation procedures depend on this analysis. Failure to make this decision

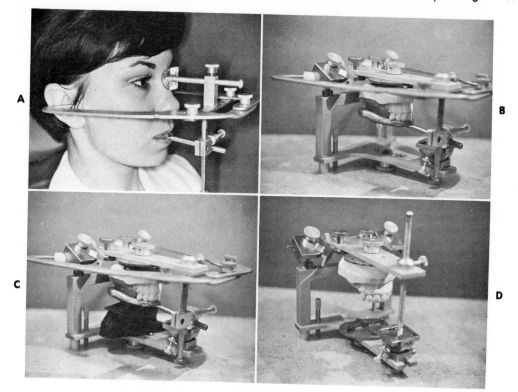

Fig. 11-20. A, Whipmix ear face-bow and face-bow fork are assembled on the patient. A *nasion* relator forms the anterior third point of reference in establishing the *axis-orbital plane.* **B,** The face-bow assembly and cast are transferred to the Whipmix articulator (an arcon instrument). **C,** Two wedge-shaped, rubber door stops are used to support the face-bow fork and cast during mounting procedures. **D,** Mounting of the maxillary cast is completed. The plane of occlusion as observed on the articulator is the same as that in the mouth when the Frankfort plane of the patient is parallel to the floor.

correctly may result in the destruction of the residual ridges and supporting structures of the teeth.

Almost all dentists agree that deflective occlusal contacts in centric occlusion and eccentric positions must be corrected as a preventive measure. Not all dentists agree that centric relation and centric occlusion must be harmonious in the natural dentition. Apparently there are many dentitions that function satisfactorily with the opposing teeth maximally intercusped or interdigitated in an eccentric position without either diagnosable or subjective indications of temporomandibular joint dysfunction, muscle dysfunction, or disease of the supporting structures of the teeth. In many such situations no attempt should be made

to alter the occlusion. It is not required to interfere with an occlusion simply because it does not completely conform to a relationship that is considered ideal.

If most natural posterior teeth remain and there is no evidence of temporomandibular joint disturbances, neuromuscular dysfunction, or periodontal disturbances related to occlusal factors, the proposed restoration may safely be constructed in centric occlusion (maximum interdigitation of remaining teeth). The proposed restoration, however, should be constructed so that centric occlusion is in harmony with centric relation when most natural centric stops are missing. By far the greater majority of removable partial dentures should be constructed in the horizontal jaw relationship of centric relation. In most instances in which edentulous spaces have not been restored, the remaining posterior teeth will have assumed malaligned positions through drifting, tipping, or extrusion. Correction of the natural occlusion to create a coincidence of centric relation and centric occlusion is indicated in such situations.

Regardless of the method employed in creating a harmonious functional occlusion, an evaluation of the existing relationships of the opposing natural teeth must be made. This evaluation is in addition to and in conjunction with other diagnostic procedures that contribute to an adequate diagnosis and treatment plan.

Diagnostic casts provide an opportunity to evaluate the relationship of remaining oral structures when correctly mounted on an adjustable articulator by using a face-bow transfer and interocclusal records. Diagnostic casts are mounted in centric relation (most retruded relation of the mandible to the maxillae) so that deflective occlusal contacts can be correlated with those observed in the mouth. Involuntary premature contacts of opposing teeth are usually destructive to the supporting structures involved and should be eliminated. Diagnostic casts demonstrate the nature and location of such interfering tooth contacts and indicate the direction that must be followed for their correction. Necessary alteration of teeth to harmonize the occlusion initially can be performed on the mounted diagnostic casts to act as guides for similar necessary corrections in the mouth. In many instances the degree of alteration required will indicate the need for crowns or onlays to be fabricated or for the recontouring, repositioning, or the elimination of extruded teeth.

The maxillary cast is correctly oriented to the opening axis of the articulator by means of the face-bow transfer and becomes spatially related to the upper member of the articulator in the same relationship that the maxillae are related to the hinge axis and the Frankfort plane. Sim-

ilarly, when a centric relation record is made at an established vertical dimension, the mandible is in its most retruded relation to the maxillae. Therefore, when the maxillary cast is correctly oriented to the axis of the articulator, the lower cast automatically becomes correctly oriented to the opening axis, with an accurate centric relation record.

It is necessary to prove that the relationship of the mounted casts is correct. This can be done simply by making another interocclusal record, fitting the casts into the record, and checking to see that the condylar elements of the articulator are snug against the condylar housings. If this is not seen, it can be assumed that the original record was incorrect or that the record was correct and the mounting procedure faulty or that the last record made was incorrect. Since centric relation is the only jaw position that can be routinely repeated by the patient, mountings in this position can be verified for correctness.

A straightforward protrusive record is made to adjust the horizontal condylar inclines on the articulator. Lateral eccentric records are made so that the lateral condylar inclinations can be properly adjusted. All interocclusal records should be made as near the vertical relation of occlusion as possible. Opposing teeth or occlusion rims must not be allowed to contact when the records are made. A contact of the inclined planes of opposing teeth will invalidate an interocclusal record.

In some instances a mounting of a duplicate diagnostic cast in centric occlusion also may be desirable to definitively study this relationship on the articulator. Since articulators only simulate jaw movements, it is not unreasonable to assume that the relationship of the casts mounted in centric relation may differ minutely in the centric occlusion that is seen on the articulator and that is observed in the mouth. When diagnostic casts are hand related by maximum interdigitation for purposes of mounting on an articulator, it is essential that three (preferably four) positive contacts of opposing posterior teeth are present, having molar contacts on each side of the arch. If occlusion rims are necessary to correctly orient casts on an articulator, centric relation should usually be the choice of the horizontal jaw relationship to which the removable partial denture will be constructed.

Materials and methods for recording centric relation. Materials available for recording centric relation are (1) wax, (2) modeling plastic, (3) quick-setting impression plaster, and (4) metallic oxide impression paste. Of these, wax is the least satisfactory material because it may not be uniformly softened when introduced into the mouth and it does not remain rigid and dimensionally stable after removal.

Modeling plastic is a satisfactory record medium because it can be flamed and tempered until uniformly soft before placing it into the mouth. After chilling, it is sufficiently stable to permit the mounting of casts with accuracy. For these reasons it is a satisfactory medium for recording occlusal relations for either complete or partial dentures. It also can be used with opposing natural teeth.

Impression plaster has advantages of softness when introduced and rigidity when set, which makes it a satisfactory material for recording jaw relations. However, it is too friable and too brittle for use between an opposing natural dentition in some instances. Its use is highly recommended when occlusion rims are indicated to mount casts correctly or to adjust articulators with interocclusal eccentric records.

Impression paste offers many of the advantages of plaster, with less friability. Although not strong enough to be used alone, when supported by a gauze mesh, it is a satisfactory recording medium. Also it may be used on occlusion rims.

The adjustable frame* was devised for use with those materials that have the combined advantage of offering no resistance when the patient closes and of being firm and stable when set. It consists of an adjustable wire frame to which gauze bibs are added to support the impression paste (Fig. 11-21). Pastes that set rapidly to a hard state are the most satisfactory, although any metallic oxide impression paste may be used.

The frame is adjusted to fit the lower cast. Each gauze bib has incorporated into it a tube, which may be slid over the lingual extension on each side of the arch. These bibs are placed so that a space remains distal to the gauze so that the dentist can see to place the frame beyond the last tooth; otherwise the patient might close on the cross bar of the frame. The gauze is then attached to the buccal wing of the frame with sticky wax.

An impression paste is mixed according to the manufacturer's directions and is applied on both sides of the gauze bibs. The frame is then placed in the mouth while the patient is guided into centric relation. When edentulous bases with wax occlusion rims are being used to support the occlusion in those areas, the wax must have been trimmed and adjusted previously so that it does not contact either the opposing natural dentition or an opposing occlusion rim. The cross bar of the frame must be placed posterior to any occlusion rims or any remaining posterior teeth.

After the paste has set, the frame is removed from the mouth and the buccal side of the gauze released where it has been secured with sticky wax. The tube on the lingual side may then be slid off the lingual extension of the frame. The frame is not needed when mounting casts with this type of registration, since the tube alone lends sufficient support to the interocclusal record.

The lower cast should be mounted on the lower arm of the articulator with the articulator inverted. The articulator is first locked in centric position and the incisal pin is adjusted so that the anterior distance between the upper and lower arms of the

---

*Kerr Manufacturing Co., Detroit, Mich.

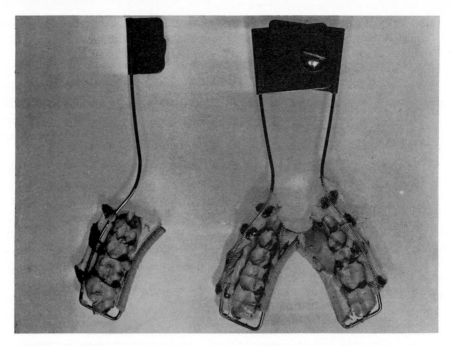

Fig. 11-21. Adjustable frame may be used either bilaterally or unilaterally but is always used bilaterally in a removable partial denture procedure. Each gauze bib is made with a tube that is slid over the open lingual portion of the frame and attached to its buccal portion with sticky wax. For bilateral use the frame must be adjusted to the mouth or cast to avoid interference distal to the last teeth in occlusion. A metallic oxide impression paste is applied to both sides of the gauze, the frame is oriented in the mouth, and the patient's lower jaw is closed into a rehearsed horizontal jaw relation until the paste hardens. After the set record is removed from the mouth, the sticky wax is released from the frame and the tube is slid off the frame. Gross excess and any sharp projections into interproximal spaces and into deep sulci are trimmed with a sharp knife before the record is placed between the casts for mounting on the articulator.

articulator will be increased 2 to 3 mm. greater than the normal parallel relationship of the arms. This is done to compensate for the thickness of the interocclusal record so that the arms of the articulator will again be parallel when the interocclusal record is removed and the opposing casts contact. The projection of the pin on the Dentatus articulator serves most conveniently as the third leg of a tripod for supporting the articulator while mounting the lower cast, whereas the Hanau articulator, when inverted, must be supported by other means. A mounting stand for this purpose is available (Fig. 11-22).

The base of the cast should be keyed and lightly lubricated for future removal. With the articulator inverted, the dentist's thumbs should be pressed through the soft mounting stone onto the base of the cast to reseat it into the interocclusal record. This is done to prevent a faulty mounting if the angle of closure into the mounting stone has caused the cast to be displaced slightly. The articulator is then propped up in the inverted position until the stone has set.

An articulator mounting thus made will have related the casts in centric relation. The dentist then can proceed to make an occlusal analysis by observing the influence of cusps in relation to one another after the articulator has been adjusted by using eccentric interocclusal records.

After an occlusal analysis has been made, the casts may be removed from their

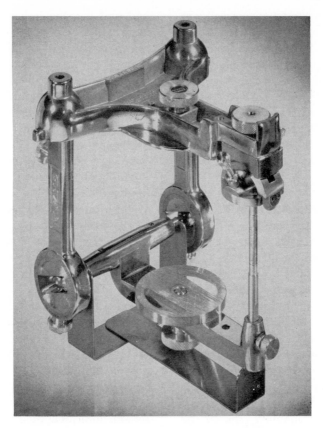

Fig. 11-22. Hanau stand is used to support any model H or SMX articulator in an inverted position while the mandibular cast is being mounted. (Courtesy Hanau Engineering Co., Buffalo, N. Y.)

mounting for the purpose of surveying them individually and for other purposes as outlined previously. The indexed mounting ring record also should be retained throughout the course of treatment in the event that further study should be needed. It is advisable that the mounting be identified with the articulator used, so that it may always be placed back onto the *same articulator.*

Factors involved in occlusal analysis. From the occlusal analysis made from mounted diagnostic casts, the dentist must decide whether it is best to accept and maintain the existing occlusion or to attempt to improve upon it by means of occlusal adjustment and the restoration of occlusal surfaces. *It must be remembered that*

the partial denture can only supplement the occlusion that exists at the time that the prosthesis is constructed. The dominant force dictating the occlusal pattern will be the cuspal harmony or disharmony of the remaining teeth and their proprioreceptal influence on kinematic movement. At best, the supplied teeth can only be made to harmonize with the cause and effect of the existing occlusion.

Improvements in the natural occlusion must be accomplished prior to the construction of the denture, not subsequent to it. The objective of occlusal reconstruction by any means should be occlusal harmony of the restored dentition in relation to the natural forces already present or established. Therefore, one of the earliest decisions in planning reconstructive treatment must be whether to accept or reject the existing occlusion. If occlusal adjustment is indicated, cuspal analysis always should precede any corrective procedures in the mouth by selective grinding. On the other hand, if reconstruction is to be the means of correction, the manner and sequence should be outlined as part of the overall treatment plan.

EXAMINATION DATA

As a result of the oral examination and diagnosis, certain data should be recorded, much of which is based upon decisions that are the result of the diagnosis. These are as follows:

1. *Patient's present and predictable future health status.*

2. *Periodontal conditions present* throughout the mouth in general and around abutment teeth in particular. This includes the amount of alveolar support remaining and the past and predictable future reaction to additional occlusal stress. Evidence of tooth mobility should be noted, as well as suggestions as to its cause and the corrective measures to be employed. This may involve simple correction of occlusal disharmony, or it may involve extensive periodontal treatment and, in some instances, splinting of periodontally weakened teeth.

3. *Oral hygiene habits* of the patient and the likelihood of patient cooperation in this regard, as well as the likelihood that the patient will return periodically for maintenance after reconstruction. The teeth remaining will need attention no less after placement of a partial denture and perhaps more so. Denture bases may need relining to compensate for changes in the supporting tissues. Therefore the patient must be willing to share with the dentist the responsibility for maintaining the health of the mouth after restorative treatment.

The most decisive evidence of oral hygiene habits is the condition of the mouth prior to the initial prophylaxis. Good or bad oral hygiene is basic to the patient's nature, and although it may be influenced somewhat by patient education, the long-range view must be taken. It is reasonably fair to assume that the patient will do little better in the long-term future than he has done in the past. In making decisions as to the method of treatment based upon oral hygiene, *the future in years*, rather than in weeks and months, must be considered. Probably in this instance it is better not to give the patient the benefit of any doubt as to future oral hygiene habits. Rather, the benefit should come from protective measures where any doubt exists as to future oral hygiene habits.

4. *Caries activity* in the mouth, past and present, and the need for protective restorations. The decision to use full coverage is based upon the age of the patient, evidence of caries activity, and the patient's oral hygiene habits. Occasionally, three-quarter crowns may be used where buccal or lingual surfaces are completely sound, but intracoronal restorations (inlays) are seldom indicated in any mouth with evidence of past extensive caries or precarious areas of decalcification, erosion, or exposed cementum.

5. *Need for surgery or extractions.* The same criteria apply to surgical intervention in the partially edentulous arch as in the completely edentulous arch. Grossly displaceable soft tissues covering basal seat areas and hyperplastic tissue should be removed to provide a firm denture foundation. Mandibular tori should be removed if they will interfere with the placement of a lingual bar connector or a favorable path of placement. Any other areas of bone prominence that will interfere with the path of placement should be removed also. The path of placement will be dictated primarily by the tooth guidance of the abutment teeth. Therefore, some areas may present interference to the path of placement of the partial denture by reason of the fact that other unalterable factors such as retention and esthetics must take precedence in selecting that path.

Extraction of teeth may be indicated for one of the following three reasons:

(a) If the tooth cannot be restored to a state of health, extraction may be unavoidable. Modern advancements in the treatment of periodontal disease and in restorative procedures, including endodontic therapy, have resulted in the saving of teeth that were once considered untreatable. *All avenues of treatment should be considered both from a prognostic and an economic standpoint before recommending extraction.*

(b) A tooth may be removed if its absence will permit a more serviceable and less complicated partial denture design. Teeth that are in extreme malposition, such as lingually inclined mandibular teeth, buccally inclined maxillary teeth, and mesially inclined teeth posterior to an edentulous space, may be removed if an adjacent tooth in good alignment and with good support is available for use as an abutment. Justification for extraction lies in the decision that a suitable crown, which will provide satisfactory contour and support, cannot be fabricated or that orthodontic treatment to realign the tooth is not feasible. An exception to the arbitrary removal of a malposed tooth is when by so doing a distal extension partial denture base would have to be made rather than the more desirable tooth-supported base through the use of the tooth in question. If alveolar support is adequate, a posterior abutment should be retained if at all possible in preference to a tissue-supported extension base.

Teeth that are deemed to have insufficient alveolar support may be extracted if their prognosis is poor and if other adjacent teeth may be used to better advantage as abutments. The decision to extract such a tooth should be based upon the degree of mobility and other periodontal considerations and upon the number, length, and shape of the roots contributing to its support.

(c) A tooth may be extracted if it is so unesthetically located as to justify its removal to improve appearance. In this regard a veneer crown should be considered in preference to removal. If removal is advisable because of unesthetic tooth position, the biomechanical problems involved in replacing anterior teeth with a removable partial denture must be weighed against the problems involved in making an esthetically acceptable fixed restoration. Admittedly, the removable replacement is frequently the more esthetic of the two, despite modern advancements in retainers and pontics. Yet, the mechanical disadvantage of the removable restoration frequently makes the fixed replacement of missing anterior teeth preferable.

6. *Need for fixed restorations for tooth-bounded spaces* rather than include them in the partial denture to the detriment of isolated abutment teeth. The advantages of splinting must be weighed against the total cost, with the weight of experience always in favor of utilizing fixed restorations for tooth-bound spaces. One of the least successful of partial denture designs is where multiple tooth-bounded areas are replaced with the partial dentures in conjunction with isolated abutment teeth and distal extension bases. Biomechanical considerations and the future health of the remaining teeth should be given preference over economic considerations where such a choice is possible.

7. *Need for occlusal correction,* either by selective grinding of teeth or by occlusal restorations, or both.

8. *Need for periodontal consultation and treatment.*

9. *Need for orthodontic treatment of malposed and disarranged teeth.* Occasionally, orthodontic movement of teeth fol-

lowed by retention through the use of fixed restorations makes possible a better partial denture design, mechanically and esthetically, than could otherwise be used.

10. *Need for restorations elsewhere in either arch,* including individual restorations, fixed partial dentures, and/or splinted abutments.

11. *Selection of the type of mandibular major connector* since the selection is influenced by the height of the floor of the patient's mouth during normal physiologic activity.

DIFFERENTIAL DIAGNOSIS: FIXED OR REMOVABLE PARTIAL DENTURES*

Total oral rehabilitation is the objective in treating the partially edentulous patient. The replacement of missing teeth by means of fixed restorations is the method of preference; a removable restoration should be used only where a fixed restoration is contraindicated.

Indications for use of fixed restorations

Tooth-bounded edentulous regions. Generally, any unilateral edentulous space bounded by teeth suitable for use as abutments should be restored with a fixed partial denture cemented to one or more abutment teeth at either end. The length of the span and the periodontal support of the abutment teeth will determine the number of abutments required.

Lack of parallelism of the abutment teeth may be counteracted with copings or locking recesses to provide parallel sectional placement. Sound abutment teeth make possible the use of more conservative retainers such as inlays rather than full crowns. The age of the patient, evidence of caries activity, oral hygiene habits, and soundness of remaining tooth structure must be considered in any decision to use less-than-full coverage for abutment teeth.

Economics should not be allowed to dic-

tate the use of a unilateral, tooth-supported removable restoration when a fixed partial is indicated. The dentist must follow the best procedure for the welfare of his patient. The patient is always free to seek more than one opinion if he so desires, but the responsibility for the choice of dental treatment becomes the patient's. In most instances, when a removable unilateral restoration is made for such a patient, it should be considered primarily as a space maintainer and an interim denture until more permanent treatment is possible.

There are two specific contraindications for the use of unilateral fixed restorations. One is a long edentulous span and abutment teeth that would not be able to withstand the trauma of horizontal and diagonal occlusal forces. The other is abutment teeth, weakened by periodontal disease, that would benefit from the bracing effect of cross-arch stabilization. In either situation a bilateral removable restoration can be used more effectively to replace the missing teeth.

Modification spaces. A removable partial denture for a Class III arch is better supported and stabilized when a modification area on the opposite side of the arch is present. Such an edentulous area need not be restored by a fixed partial denture, since it may be essential to the design of the removable partial denture. Additional modification spaces, however, particularly those involving single missing teeth, are better restored separately by means of a fixed denture. Not only is a lone-standing abutment thus stabilized by the splinting effect of a fixed restoration, but also a possible teeter-totter effect of the denture is avoided and the denture is made less complicated by not having to include other abutment teeth for the support and retention of an additional edentulous space or spaces.

When an edentulous space that is a modification of either a Class I or Class II arch exists anterior to a lone-standing abutment tooth, this tooth is subjected to trauma by the movements of a distal extension partial denture far in excess of

---

*Paraphrased from McCracken, W. L.: Differential diagnosis; fixed or removable partial dentures, J. Am. Dent. Assoc. 63:767-775, 1961.

its ability to withstand such stresses. The splinting of the lone abutment to the nearest tooth is mandatory. Splinting is best accomplished in such a situation by means of a fixed partial denture uniting the two teeth on either side of the edentulous space. The abutment crown should be contoured for support and retention of the partial denture, and, in addition, a means of supporting a stabilizing component on the anterior abutment of the fixed partial denture or on the occlusal surface of the pontic usually should be provided.

Anterior modification spaces. Usually any missing anterior teeth in a partially edentulous arch, except in a Kennedy Class IV arch in which only anterior teeth are missing, are best replaced by means of a fixed restoration. There are exceptions. Sometimes a better esthetic result is obtainable when the anterior replacements are supplied by the removable partial denture. This is also true when excessive tissue and bone resorption necessitates the placement of pontics too far posteriorly for good esthetics and for an acceptable relation with the opposing teeth. However, in most instances, from both a mechanical and a biological standpoint, anterior replacements are best accomplished with fixed restorations. The replacement of missing posterior teeth with a removable partial denture is then made much less complicated and with more satisfactory results.

Nonreplacement of missing molars. Frequently the decision of whether to replace unilaterally missing molars must be made. To do so with a removable denture necessitates the making of a distal extension restoration with the major connector joining the edentulous side to retentive and stabilizing components located on the nonedentulous side of the arch. Leverage factors are always unfavorable and the retainers that must be used on the nonedentulous side are frequently unsatisfactory. Several factors, therefore, will influence the decison to make a unilateral, distal extension partial denture.

First, the opposing teeth must be considered. If they are to be prevented from extrusion and migration, some opposing occlusion must be provided. This would influence the replacement of the missing molars far more than any improvement in masticating efficiency that might result. The replacement of missing molars on one side is seldom necessary for reasons of mastication alone.

Second, the future of a maxillary tuberosity must be considered. Left uncovered, the tuberosity frequently will seem to drop and increase in size. However, covering the tuberosity with a partial denture base, in combination with the stimulating effect of the intermittent occlusion provided, helps to maintain the normalcy of the tuberosity. This is of considerable importance in any future denture replacements. In such an instance it may be better to make a unilateral removable partial denture than to leave a maxillary tuberosity uncovered.

A third consideration is the condition of the opposing second molar. If this tooth is missing, or can logically be ignored or eliminated, then only first molar occlusion need be supplied by utilizing a cantilever-type fixed restoration. Occlusion need be only minimal to maintain occlusal relations between the natural first molar in the one arch and the prosthetic molar in the opposite arch. Such a pontic should be narrow buccolingually and need not occlude with more than one half to two thirds of the opposing tooth. Frequently such a restoration is the preferred method of treatment. However, unless three abutments are used to support a cantilevered molar opposed by a natural molar, only limited success should be anticipated.

Indications for removable partial dentures

While a removable partial denture should be considered only when a fixed restoration is contraindicated, there are several specific indications for the use of a removable restoration.

Distal extension situations. Except in situations in which the replacement of missing second (and third) molars is either inadvisable or unnecessary, or in which unilateral replacement of a missing first molar can be accomplished by means of a cantilevered fixed restoration, replacement of missing posterior teeth without the assistance of a posterior abutment must be accomplished with a removable partial denture. The most common partially edentulous situations are the Kennedy Class I and Class II. With the latter, an edentulous space on the opposite side of the arch is often conveniently present, or can be effected, to aid in the required retention and stabilization of the partial denture. If no space is present, embrasure clasps or intracoronal retainers generally must be used. As previously stated, all other edentulous areas are best replaced with fixed partial dentures.

After recent extractions. The replacement of teeth after recent extractions cannot be accomplished satisfactorily with a fixed restoration. When relining will be required later or when a fixed restoration will be constructed later, a temporary removable partial denture must be used. If an all-resin denture is used rather than a more elaborate partial denture, the immediate cost to the patient is much less and the resin denture lends itself best for future temporary modifications.

A tooth-bounded edentulous area in which, because of recent extractions, some change is anticipated in the residual ridge, is also best restored with a removable partial denture. Although the relining of a tooth-supported resin denture base thus is made possible, this is usually done only to improve esthetics, oral cleanliness, or patient comfort. Support for such a restoration is supplied by occlusal rests on the abutment teeth at each end of the edentulous space.

Long span. A long span may be totally tooth supported if the abutments and the means of transferring the support to the denture are adequate and if the denture framework is rigid. There is little, if any, difference between the support afforded a removable partial denture and that afforded a fixed restoration by the adjacent abutment teeth. However, in the absence of cross-arch stabilization, the torque and leverage on the two abutment teeth would be excessive. Instead, a removable denture deriving retention, support, and stabilization from abutment teeth on the opposite side of the arch is indicated as the logical means of replacing the missing teeth.

Need for effect of bilateral stabilization. In a mouth weakened by periodontal disease, because of the lack of cross-arch stabilization, a fixed restoration may jeopardize the future of periodontically involved abutment teeth unless the splinting effect of multiple abutments is employed. The removable partial denture, on the other hand, may act as a periodontal splint through its effective cross-arch stabilizing of teeth weakened by periodontal disease. When abutment teeth throughout the arch are properly prepared and restored, the beneficial effect of a removable partial denture can be far greater than that of a unilateral fixed partial denture.

Esthetics in anterior region. When the replacement of missing anterior teeth is the primary consideration, it is sometimes advisable, for reasons of appearance, to use translucent artificial teeth on a removable resoration rather than often dull fixed partial denture pontics. This is particularly true when several anterior teeth are missing and when a better tooth arrangement, for support, contour, and phonetics, can be accomplished.

Excessive loss of residual bone. The pontic of a fixed partial denture must be related to the residual ridge in such a manner that the contact with the mucosa is gentle. Whenever excessive resorption has occurred, however, teeth supported by a denture base may be arranged in a more acceptable buccolingual position than is possible with a fixed partial denture.

Artificial teeth supported by a denture base can be located without regard to the crest of the residual ridge and more nearly in the position of the natural dentition for normal tongue and cheek contacts. This is particularly true of a maxillary denture.

Anteriorly, loss of residual bone occurs from the labial aspect. Often, the incisive papilla lies at the crest of the residual ridge. Since the central incisors are normally located anterior to this landmark, any other location of artificial central incisors is unnatural. An anterior fixed partial denture made for such a mouth will have pontics resting on the labial aspect of this resorbed ridge and will be too far lingual to provide desirable lip support. Frequently the only way the incisal edges of the pontics can be made to occlude with the opposing lower anterior teeth is to use a labial inclination that is excessive and unnatural, and both esthetics and lip support suffer thereby. Because the same condition exists with a removable partial denture in which the anterior teeth are abutted on the residual ridge, a labial flange must be utilized to permit the teeth to be located more nearly in their natural position.

The same method of treatment applies to the replacement of missing lower anterior teeth. Sometimes a lower anterior fixed partial denture is made six or more units in length, in which the remaining space necessitates either leaving out one anterior tooth or using the original number of teeth but with all of them too narrow for esthetics. In either instance the denture is nearly in a straight line because the pontics follow the form of the resorbed ridge. A removable partial denture will permit the location of the replaced teeth in a favorable relation to the lip and opposing dentition regardless of the shape of the residual ridge. When such a removable prosthesis is made, however, positive support must be obtained from the adjacent abutments.

Unusually sound abutment teeth. Sometimes the excuse for making a removable restoration is the wish to see sound teeth preserved in their natural state and not prepared for abutment retainers. The reasons for the loss of the teeth being replaced must be considered. If loss is due to caries, then it is likely that caries will occur even-

tually in the abutment teeth. If the teeth were lost because of periodontal disease, then the periodontium of the remaining teeth must be evaluated. If the teeth were lost due to neglect of minimal caries, and the caries activity seems to be arrested, the utilization of existing tooth surfaces to support a removable restoration may be justified. If the oral hygiene habits of the patient are favorable, and the abutment teeth are sound with good periodontal support, unprotected abutments may be used to support and retain a removable restoration. When this condition exists, the dentist should not hesitate to reshape and modify existing enamel surfaces to provide proximal guiding planes, occlusal rest areas, optimal retentive areas, and surfaces on which nonretentive stabilizing components may be placed.

It is only in selected instances, then, that the making of a removable prosthetic restoration on unprotected abutments can be justified.

Economic considerations. Economics should not be the sole criterion in arriving at a method of treatment. When, for economic reasons, complete treatment is out of the question, and yet replacement of missing teeth is indicated, the restorative procedures dictated by these considerations must be described clearly to the patient as being of an interim nature and not representative of the best that modern dentistry has to offer. Ordinarily, a prosthesis that is made to satisfy economic considerations alone is doomed to failure, and both professional esteem and the patient suffer thereby.

• • •

Unilateral removable partial dentures (Class III), utilizing extracoronal direct retainers, have functioned successfully for many years in some mouths without clinical evidence of harm to abutment teeth or supporting structures. Successful restorations of this type are the exceptions rather than the rule. Being unilateral in support, in retention, and without the advantages of a broad distribution of stress or cross-arch leverage control, they are usually contra-indicated and should be resorted to only under the most extenuating circumstances (Fig. 11-23).

In *specific instances,* however, the uni-laterally retained and supported removable partial denture may serve satisfactorily. Sit-uations in which it might be used must not be selected promiscuously. The great im-portance and value of modern diagnostic methods here need to be stressed. Existing conditions in the arch must be noted care-fully, and the practical results to be ex-pected from the restoration have to be me-ticulously evaluated. Further, it is a design and size of removable partial denture that must be left out of the mouth during sleep.

Accordingly, in selected situations the Class III unilateral removable partial res-toration can be used in the following in-stances:

1. Edentulous span is short (not more than two teeth missing).
2. Occlusal stress load is light (as when opposed by a complete denture).
3. Abutment teeth are without restora-tions and the patient has no appar-ent susceptibility to caries.
4. Abutment teeth have long bell-shaped clinical crowns for ideal placement of retentive and bracing components.
5. Abutment teeth have been restored previously with full or three-quarter crowns, already ideal for clasping.
6. Patient is a nervous type of individ-ual and so averse to tooth preparation as to refuse to have a fixed partial denture.
7. Bulk of soft tissue and alveolar pro-cess that has been lost would require disproportionately sized pontics if a fixed partial denture were used.
8. Cost of the fixed partial denture might be prohibitive to a patient and conditions happen to be ideal for a removable one that may cost much less.

In judiciously selected areas in which Class III unilateral removable partial den-

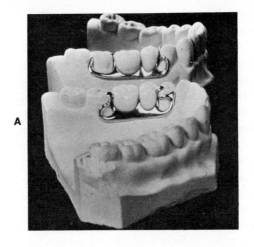

A

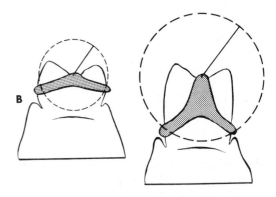

B

Fig. 11-23. A, Unilateral removable partial denture restoring a partially edentulous arch (Class III). The advantages of cross-arch stabilization and a broader distribution of forces cannot be realized with this denture. **B,** Resistance to vertical rota-tion of a tooth-supported, unilateral removable par-tial denture is enhanced by selecting those situa-tions in which the abutment teeth have long clinical crowns. A comparison of the radii of the two figures demonstrates that a longer resistance arm to rotational forces exists on the figure with the longer clinical crown.

tures can feasibly be placed, they are easily manipulated by the patient, and the re-stored area in the mouth readily lends itself to cleansing. Also the denture can be ad-justed, repaired, and altered as tissue changes result, and the cost is such as can be borne by the average individual.

THE CHOICE BETWEEN COMPLETE DENTURES AND REMOVABLE PARTIAL DENTURES

In making the diagnosis preceding prosthodontic service, the probable length of service that can be expected from a partial denture must always be weighed against the patient's economic status. A decision may have to be made between a partial denture and a complete denture, in either arch or both. One patient may prefer complete dentures to the traumatic experience of complete oral rehabilitation, regardless of his ability to pay. Another may be so determined to keep his own teeth that he will make great financial sacrifices to do so if given reasonable assurance of the success of oral rehabilitation.

The value of listening to the patient during the examination and the diagnostic procedures should not be disregarded nor treated lightly. During the presentation of pertinent facts, time should be allowed for the patient to express himself freely as to his desires in retaining and restoring his natural teeth. At this time a treatment plan may be influenced or even drastically changed to conform to the expressed and implied desires of the patient.

For example, there may be a reasonable possibility of saving teeth in both arches through the use of partial dentures. With only anterior teeth remaining, a partial denture can be made to replace the posterior teeth by utilizing good abutment support and, in the maxillary arch, utilizing full palatal coverage for retention and stability. If the patient expresses a desire to retain his anterior teeth "at any cost" and if the remaining teeth are esthetically acceptable and functionally sound, then the dentist should do his best to make successful removable dentures for both arches and thus fulfill his professional obligation to the patient.

On the other hand, if for economic or other reasons the patient believes that a complete maxillary denture would best satisfy his denture requirements, but for fear of difficulty in wearing a complete mandibular denture he would prefer restoration of that arch with a partial denture, then, all factors being acceptable, his wishes should be respected and treatment planned accordingly.

Still another patient, for economic or other reasons, may prefer to have complete dentures made for both arches rather than undergo complete rehabilitation of the partially edentulous arches. It is frequently unwise to insist on the latter course with such a patient. The professional obligation to present the facts and then do the best in accordance with the patient's expressed desires still applies.

Still another patient may wish to retain the remaining teeth for an indefinite but relatively short period of time, with eventual complete dentures a foregone conclusion. In this instance the professional obligation may be to recommend interim partial dentures without extensive mouth preparations. Such dentures will aid in mastication and/or provide esthetic replacements while at the same time serving as conditioning restorations, which will make the later transition to complete dentures somewhat easier. Such partial dentures should be designed and fabricated with care, but the total cost of partial denture service will be considerably less.

An expressed desire on the part of the patient to retain only six lower anterior teeth must be considered carefully before being agreed to as the planned treatment. The advantages to the patient are obvoius: he may retain six esthetically acceptable teeth; he does not become totally edentulous; and he has the advantage of direct retention that would not be possible if he were completely edentulous. Retaining even the lower canine teeth would accomplish the latter two objectives. These advantages cannot be denied. Yet, the disadvantages, which are less obvious to the patient, must also be considered and explained to him. These are mechanical and functional consideration; that is, the edentulous maxilla anteriorly is structurally not able to withstand the trauma of positive tooth contact against natural opposing teeth. The possible result is the loss of residual maxillary bone, loosening of the maxillary denture because of the tripping influence of the natural lower teeth, and the loss of basal foundation for the support of future prostheses However, if the maxillary anteriors are arranged to contact in eccentric positions only and the patient appreciates periodic recall, these problems are certainly minimized. The presence of inflamed hyperplastic tissue is a frequent sequel to continued loss of support and denture movement.

The prevention of this sequence of events lies in the maintenance of positive occlusal support posteriorly and the continual elimination of traumatic influence from the remaining anterior teeth. Such support is sometimes impossible to maintain without frequent relining or remaking of the lower partial denture base. On the other hand, this may cause undesirable resorption of the posterior ridges because of overloading. The results in any event are undesirable, and the patient must be made aware of the hazards involved.

Whereas some patients are able to wear a lower partial denture supported only by anterior teeth against a complete upper denture, the odds are that undesirable consequences will result unless the patient faithfully follows the instructions of the dentist. In no other situation in treatment planning is the general health of the patient and the quality of residual alveolar bone as critical as it is in this situation.

In addition to considering the age and health of the patient and his ability to build bone in response to stress, it is well to consider why the teeth being replaced were extracted. In all probability, any history of severe periodontal disease precludes the wearing of such combination dentures successfully. On the other hand, the loss of teeth due to caries or the premature loss of teeth that might have been saved justifies the conclusion that the residual bone is probably healthy and will be able to withstand stresses within reasonable limits. In such instances, combination dentures may be constucted if the patient is made aware of the need for periodic reexamination and is willing to make the transition to a complete lower denture upon the first signs of serious damage to supporting structures.

The final treatment plan should represent the best possible course for the patient after considering all physical, mental, mechanical, esthetic, and economic factors involved.

FACTORS IN SELECTING THE METAL ALLOYS FOR REMOVABLE PARTIAL DENTURE FRAMEWORKS

Practically all cast frameworks for removable partial dentures are made either from a gold alloy (Type IV) or from a chromium-cobalt alloy. The choice of the alloy from which the framework of a removable partial denture will be constructed is logically made during the treatment planning phase. Inherent differences in the physical properties of alloys presently available to the dental profession must be considered in making this choice. For example, mouth preparation procedures, especially the recontouring of abutment teeth for the optimal placement of retentive elements, depend to a large extent on the modulus of elasticity (stiffness) of a particular alloy.

It has been estimated that the chromium-cobalt alloys are utilized five times more than are the gold alloys in removable partial prosthodontics. The popularity of the chromium-cobalt alloys has been attributed to their low density (weight), high modulus of elasticity (stiffness), low material cost, and resistance to tarnish in comparison with that of gold alloys.

Use of the chromium-cobalt alloys in preference to the gold alloys continues to be somewhat controversial among members of the dental profession. This controversy stems, in part, from the necessity of using specialized equipment and techniques in the application of the chromium-cobalt alloys, which has restricted the fabrication of frameworks almost entirely to commercial dental laboratories.

Successful removable restorations may be made from either the gold or chromium-cobalt alloys. Because the cost of the alloy used for a framework is only a small part of the total cost for the service, cost alone should not justify the substitution of a base alloy for a noble alloy. The alloy chosen should show a definite superiority or an important saving in cost to justify its use for a particular patient.

Each of the alloys has advantages under certain conditions. Obviously, then, the material that is considered capable of rendering the best overall service for the patient over a period of years is the one that should be used. The choice of alloy is based on several factors: (1) weighed advantages or disadvantages of the physical properties of the alloy, (2) the dimensional accuracy with which the alloy can be cast, (3) the availabality of the alloy, (4) the versatility of the alloy, and (5) the individual clinical observation and experiences with alloys in respect to quality control and service to the patient.

The following are comparable characteristics of gold alloys and chromium-cobalt alloys: (1) each is well tolerated by oral tissues; (2) they are equally acceptable esthetically; (3) enamel abrasion by either alloy is insignificant on vertical tooth surfaces; (4) each alloy can be cast to wrought wire retentive components (this characteristic is important in overcoming the objection by some dentists to the increased stiffness of chromium-cobalt alloys for the portions of direct retainers that must engage an undercut of the abutment tooth); (5) the accuracy obtainable in casting either alloy is clinically acceptable under strictly controlled investing and casting procedures; and (6) soldering procedures for the repair of frameworks can be performed on each alloy.

Comparative physical properties. Chromium-cobalt alloys generally have a lower *yield strength* than do the gold alloys used for removable partial dentures (Table 11-1). Yield strength is the greatest amount of stress an alloy will withstand and still return to its original shape in an unweakened condition. Possessing a lower proportional limit, the chromium-cobalt alloys will deform permanently at lower loads than will gold alloys. Therefore, the dentist must design the chromium-cobalt framework so that the range of movement or degree of deformation expected in a direct retainer is less than a comparable degree of deformation for a gold component.

The *modulus of elasticity* refers to stiffness of an alloy. Gold alloys have a modulus of elasticity approximately one half of that for chromium-cobalt alloys for similar uses. The greater stiffness of chromium-cobalt alloy is advantageous but at the same

Table 11-1. Mechanical properties of representative stellite alloys[*]

Properties	Stellite alloys[†]					Hardened partial denture gold alloys
	A	B	D	E	21	
Yield strength (psi)	64,500	61,000	56,000	62,400	82,300	65,000– 90,000
Tensile strength (psi)	108,500	107,500	84,500	102,500	101,300	107,000–120,000
Elongation (%)	3.4	3.2	6.0	1.9	8.2	1.5–8
Modulus of elasticity (psi $\times$ 10^{-6})	28.0	29.5	27.5	28.5	36.0	13–15
Hardness (R[30 N])[‡]	53.0	60.0	51.0	55.0	—	—

[*]From Peyton F. A.: Dent. Clin. North Am., pp. 759-771, Nov., 1958.
[†]Data for lettered alloys from Taylor, D. F., et al.: J. Am. Dent. Assoc. **56**:343-351, 1958; for Stellite No. 21 from Metals Handbook, 1948 ed., p. 579; for gold alloys from manufacturers property charts.
[‡]Rockwell 30N hardness scale.

time offers disadvantages. Greater rigidity can be obtained with the chromium-cobalt alloy in reduced sections in which cross-arch stabilization is required, thereby eliminating an appreciable bulk of the framework. Its greater rigidity is also an advantage when the greatest undercut that can be found on an abutment tooth is in the nature of 0.005 inch. A gold retentive element would not be as efficient in retaining the restoration under such conditions as would the chromium-cobalt clasp arm.

A high yield strength and a low modulus of elasticity produce higher *flexibility*. The gold alloys are approximately twice as flexible as the chromium-cobalt alloys, which is a distinct advantage in the optimal location of retentive elements of the framework in many instances. The greater flexibility of the gold alloys usually permits location of the tips of retainer arms in the gingival third of the abutment tooth. As mentioned earlier, this problem, because of the stiffness of the chromium-cobalt alloys, can be overcome by including wrought-wire retentive elements in the framework.

The bulk of a retentive clasp arm for a removable partial denture is often reduced for greater flexibility when chromium-cobalt alloys are used as opposed to gold alloys. This, however, is inadvisable, since the grain size of the chromium-cobalt alloys is usually larger and is associated with a lower proportional limit, so a decrease in the bulk of cast clasps increases the likelihood of fracture or permanent deformation. The retentive clasp arms for both alloys should be approximately the same size, but the depth of undercut used for retention must be reduced by one half when chromium-cobalt is the choice of alloys. Chromium-cobalt alloys are reported to work harden more rapidly than gold alloys, and this, associated with coarse grain size, may lead to failure in service. When adjustments by bending are necessary, they must be executed with extreme caution and limited optimism.

Chromium-cobalt alloys have a lower *density* than do gold alloys in comparable

sections and are therefore about one half as heavy as the gold alloys. Weight of the alloy in most instances is not a valid criterion for selection of one metal over another, since after placement of a partial denture, the patient seldom notices the weight of the restoration. The comparable lightness of the chromium-cobalt alloys, however, is an advantage when full-palatal coverage is indicated for the bilateral distal extension denture. Weight is a factor that must be considered when the force of gravity must be overcome so that usually passive direct retainers will not be activated constantly to the detriment of abutment teeth.

The hardness of chromium-cobalt alloys offers a disadvantage when a component of the framework, such as a rest, is opposed by a natural tooth or one that has been restored. We have observed what is believed to be excessive wear of natural teeth opposed by some of the various chromium-cobalt alloys as contrasted to the type IV gold alloys.

It has been observed that gold frameworks for removable partial dentures are more prone to produce uncomfortable galvanic shocks to abutment teeth restored with silver amalgam than are frameworks made of chromium-cobalt alloy. This may not be a valid criterion for the selection of a particular alloy when the dentist has complete control over the choice of restorative materials. It may, however, be a consideration in some institutional dental services in which silver amalgam restorations must, of necessity, be placed rather than gold restorations.

In making a selection of materials, it must be remembered that fundamentals do not change. These are inviolable. It is only methods, procedures, and substances—by which the dentist effects the best possible end result—that change. The responsibility of decision still rests with the dentist, who must *evaluate all factors* in relation to the *results* that he hopes to achieve. In any instance, therefore, the dentist must weigh the problems involved, compare and evaluate the characteristics of different potential materials, and then honestly and judiciously chose the road leading to the greatest possible service to the patient. Such an approach will exclude a preference of materials based on friendship, convenience, franchise, or prejudiced patronage.

After the dentist makes his choice of alloy to be used in rendering a service to his patient, he should prescribe only those alloys that conform to the specifications set forth by the American Dental Association for the particular type of alloy.

It is to the lasting credit of those interested in biomaterials that continual research is being conducted to incorporate as many desirable characteristics in the chromium-cobalt alloys used in prosthodontics as possible. Efforts are being made to simplify casting procedures while obtaining greater accuracy and to make these alloys available to the profession at reasonable cost. There is little doubt in our mind but that a chromium-cobalt alloy will be developed, retaining the desirable characteristics that these alloys presently possess—plus many of the physical characteristics of our type IV gold alloys. Such an alloy could surely be made universally available to the dental profession and within the economy of all nations to utilize. Unfortunately, this is not presently true of precious metal alloys.

Up to the present time, we have found that the gold alloys available have helped accomplish to a greater extent our objectives in treating patients than the use of the chromium-cobalt alloys.

CHAPTER 12

Preparation of the mouth for removable partial dentures

The preparation of the mouth is fundamental to a successful removable partial denture service. Thorough mouth preparation, perhaps more than any other single factor, contributes to the philosophy that the prescribed prosthesis must not only replace what is missing but, of perhaps even greater importance, must also preserve what is remaining.

Mouth preparation follows the preliminary diagnosis and the development of a tentative treatment plan. Final treatment planning may be deferred until the response to the preparatory procedures can be ascertained. In general, mouth preparation includes procedures in three categories: oral surgical preparation, periodontal therapy, and preparation of abutment teeth. The objectives of the procedures involved in all three areas are to return the mouth to optimum health and to eliminate any condition that would be detrimental to the success of the partial denture.

Naturally, mouth preparation must be accomplished prior to the impression procedures that will produce the master cast upon which the denture will be constructed. Oral surgical and periodontal procedures should precede abutment tooth preparation and should be completed far enough in advanced to allow for the necessary healing period. If at all possible, a period of *at least* six weeks and preferably three months should be provided between surgical and restorative dentistry procedures.

ORAL SURGICAL PREPARATION*

As a rule, surgical treatment of all types should be completed as early as possible for the removable partial denture patient. By their very nature the surgical procedures generally indicated include the manipulation of both hard and soft tissues, which introduces the necessary for adequate healing time prior to the fabrication of the prosthesis. When possible, necessary endodontic surgery, periodontal surgery, and oral surgery should be planned so that they can be completed at the same sitting. The longer the interval between the surgery and the impression procedure, the more complete the healing and, consequently the more stable is the denture bearing area.

A variety of oral surgical techniques can prove beneficial to the clinician in preparing the patient for prosthetic replacements. However, it is not the purpose of this section to present the details of surgical correction. Rather, attention is called to some of the more common oral conditions or

---

*Revision by Emmett R. Costich, Department of Oral Surgery, College of Dentistry, University of Kentucky, Lexington, Ky., and Raymond P. White, Jr., Department of Oral Surgery, School of Dentistry, Virginia Commonwealth University, Richmond, Va.

changes in which surgical intervention is indicated as an aid to denture design and construction and to its successful function in contributing further to the health and well-being of the patient. Additional information concerning the actual techniques employed is available in a standard oral surgery text.* It is important to emphasize, however, that the dentist providing the partial denture treatment bears the responsibility for seeing that the necessary surgical procedures are accomplished. Measures to control apprehension, including the use of intravenous and inhalation agents, have made the most extensive surgery acceptable to patients. Whether he chooses to perform these himself or elects to refer the patient to someone else, perhaps more qualified, is immaterial. The important consideration is that the patient not be deprived of any treatment that would enhance the success of the partial denture.

Extractions

Planned extractions should occur early in the treatment regimen but not before a careful and thorough evaluation of each remaining member of the dental arch is completed. Regardless of its condition, each tooth must be evaluated concerning its strategic importance and its potential contribution to the success of the removable partial denture. With the knowledge and technical capability available in dentistry today, *almost any tooth may be salvaged if its retention is sufficiently important to warrant the procedures necessary*. On the other hand, heroic attempts to have seriously involved teeth or those of doubtful nature whose retention would contribute little, if anything, even if successfully treated and maintained, are contraindicated. The extraction of *nonstrategic* teeth that present complications or those whose presence may be detrimental to the design of the partial denture thus becomes not an

admission of defeat but a valuable asset to treatment and an integral part of the overall treatment plan.

Removal of residual roots

Generally, all retained roots or root fragments should be removed. This is particularly true if they are in close proximity to the tissue surface or, of course, if there is evidence of associated pathology. Residual roots adjacent to abutment teeth may contribute to the progression of periodontal pockets and compromise the results to be expected from subsequent periodontal therapy. The removal of root tips can be accomplished from the facial or palatal surfaces without resulting in a reduction of alveolar ridge height or endangering adjacent teeth (Figs. 12-1 and 12-2).

Impacted teeth

All impacted teeth should be considered for removal. This applies equally to impactions in edentulous areas as well as to those adjacent to abutment teeth. The periodontal implications of the latter are similar to those for retained roots. These teeth are often neglected until there are serious periodontal implications.

The skeletal structure of the body changes with age. Alterations that affect the jaws frequently result in minute exposures of impacted teeth to the oral cavity via sinus tracts. Resultant infections cause much bone destruction and serious illness for persons who are elderly and not physically able to tolerate the debilitation. Early elective removal of impactions prevents later serious acute and chronic infection with extensive bone loss. Any impacted teeth that can be reached with a periodontal probe must be removed to treat the periodontal pocket and prevent more extensive damage (Fig. 12-3).

Cysts and odontogenic tumors

Panoramic radiographs of the jaws are recommended to survey the jaws for unsuspected pathology. When a suspicious area appears on the survey film, a periapical

---

*See Costich, E. R., and White, R. P., Jr.: Fundamentals of oral surgery, Philadelphia, 1971, W. B. Saunders Co.

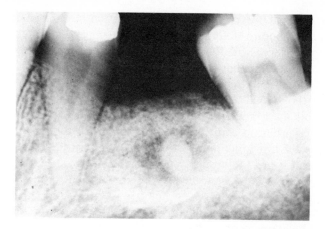

Fig. 12-1. Retained root with associated bone resorption. (From Costich, E. R., and White, R. P., Jr.: Fundamentals of oral surgery, Philadelphia, 1971, W. B. Saunders Co.)

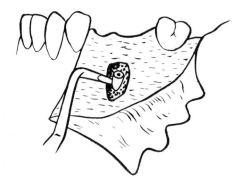

Fig. 12-2. Root tip in an edentulous area should be removed from the buccal aspect in order to preserve the crest of the residual ridge. (From Costich, E. R., and White, R. P., Jr.: Fundamentals of oral surgery, Philadelphia, 1971, W. B. Saunders Co.)

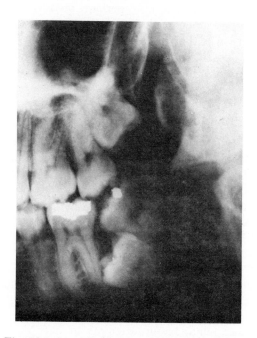

Fig. 12-3. Lateral oblique radiograph showing an unerupted maxillary third molar and impacted mandibular second and third molars. The maxillary third molar and mandibular second molar could be contacted by a periodontal probe. (From Costich, E. R., and White, R. P., Jr.: Fundamentals of oral surgery, Philadelphia, 1971, W. B. Saunders Co.)

radiograph should be taken to confirm or deny the presence of a lesion. All radiolucencies or radiopacities observed in the jaws should be investigated by biopsy. Although the diagnosis may appear obvious from clinical and radiographic examinations, the dentist should confirm his impression through submission of biopsy specimens to the pathologist for microscopic study. The patient should be assured of the diagnosis as well as the successful resolution of the abnormality as confirmed by the pathologist's report.

Exostoses and tori

The existence of abnormal bony enlargements should not be allowed to compromise the design of the removable partial denture. Although modification of denture design can, at times, accommodate for exostoses, more frequently this results in additional stress to the supporting elements and compromised function. The removal of exostoses and tori is not a complex procedure, and the advantages to be realized from such removal are great in contrast to the deleterious effects their continued presence can create. Ordinarily, the mucosa covering bony protuberances is extremely thin and friable. Partial denture components in proximity to this type of tissue may cause irritation and chronic ulceration. Also, tori approximating gingival margins may complicate the maintenance of periodontal health and lead to the eventual loss of strategic abutment teeth.

The air-turbine handpiece is ideal for removing bony irregularities and is much easier to control than a mallet and chisel. The lower speeds (20,000 to 50,000 rpm) provide more torque and thus a better sense of feel for what is being cut. All handpieces used in surgery should be vented outside the mouth to prevent the complication of emphysema. In addition, the assistant should provide copious irrigation to assure against thermal damage to the bone.

Hyperplastic tissue

Hyperplastic tissues are seen in the form of fibrous tuberosities, soft flabby ridges, folds of redundant tissue in the vestibule or floor of the mouth, and as palatal papillomatosis. All these forms of excess tissue should be removed to provide a firm base for the denture. This will result in a more stable denture and reduce stress and strain on the supporting teeth and tissues. The appropriate surgical approaches should not reduce vestibular depth. Hyperplastic tissue can be removed using any preferred combination of scalpel, curette, or electrosurgery. Some form of surgical stent should always be considered for these patients so that the period of healing will be more comfortable for the patient. An old denture modified properly can serve as a surgical

stent. Although hyperplastic tissue has no great malignant propensity, all such excised tissue should be sent to an oral pathologist for microscopic study.

Muscle attachments and freni

As a result of the loss of alveolar bone height, muscle attachments may insert on or near the alveolar crest. The mylohyoid, buccinator, mentalis, and genioglossus muscles are those most likely to introduce problems of this nature. In addition to the problem of the attachments of the muscles themselves, the mentalis and genioglossus muscles occasionally produce bony protuberances that may also interfere with denture design. Appropriate ridge extension procedures can reposition attachments and remove bony spines, which will facilitate the comfort and function of the removable partial denture.

Repositioning of the mylohyoid muscle is successfully achieved using several methods. The genioglossus muscle is more difficult to reposition but careful surgery can reduce the prominence of the genial tubercles, as well as provide some sulcus depth in the anterior lingual area.

Surgical procedures using skin or mucosal grafts have largely replaced secondary epithelialization procedures for the mandibular labial anterior region. Mucosal grafts using the palate as a donor site offer the best possibility for success.

The maxillary labial and mandibular lingual freni are probably the most frequent sources of frenum interference with denture design. These can be modified easily with any of several surgical procedures. Under no circumstances should a frenum be allowed to compromise the design or comfort of a removable partial denture.

Bony spines and knife-edge ridges

Sharp bony spicules should be removed and knifelike crests gently rounded. These procedures should be carried out with a minimal amount of bone loss. If, however, the correction of a knife-edge alveolar crest results in insufficient ridge support for the denture base, then vestibular deepening should be resorted to for correction of the deficiency.

Polyps, papilloma, and traumatic hemangiomas

All abnormal soft tissue lesions should be excised and submitted for pathologic examination prior to the fabrication of a removable partial denture. Even though the patient may relate a history of the condition having been present for an indefinite period, its removal is indicated. New or additional stimulation to the area introduced by the prosthesis may result in discomfort or even malignant changes in the tumor.

Hyperkeratoses, erythroplasia, and ulcerations

All abnormal, white, red, and/or ulcerative lesions should be investigated, regardless of their relationship to the proposed denture base or framework. Incisional biopsy of areas larger than 5 mm. should be completed, and, if the lesions are large (over 2 cm. in diameter), multiple biopsies should be taken. The biopsy report will determine whether the margins of the excised tissue can be wide or narrow. The lesions should be removed and healing accomplished before the denture is constructed. On occasion the denture design will have to be radically modified to avoid areas of possible sensitivity such as post irradiation for malignancy or the excoriations of errosive lichen planus.

PERIODONTAL PREPARATION*

The periodontal preparation of the mouth usually follows, or is performed simultaneously with the oral surgical procedures employed in the treatment of the conditions described in the previous discussion. Ordinarily, tooth extraction and

---

*Revision by Harry M. Bohannan, Dean, and Donald K. Carman, Department of Periodontics, College of Dentistry, University of Kentucky, Lexington, Ky.

removal of impacted teeth or retained roots or fragments are accomplished prior to definitive periodontal therapy. The elimination of exostoses, tori, hyperplastic tissue, muscle attachments, and freni, on the other hand, can be incorporated with periodontal surgical techniques. In any situation, periodontal therapy should be completed before restorative dentistry procedures are begun for any dental patient. This is particularly true when a removable partial denture is contemplated because the ultimate success of this restoration rests directly upon the health and integrity of the supporting structures of the remaining teeth. The periodontal health of the remaining teeth then, especially those to be utilized as abutment teeth, must be evaluated carefully by the dentist and corrective measures instituted prior to partial denture construction.

This discussion will attempt to demonstrate how periodontal procedures affect diagnosis and treatment planning in a denture service rather than how the procedures are actually accomplished. For technical details, the reader is referred to any of several excellent textbooks on periodontics.

Objectives of periodontal therapy

The overall objective of periodontal therapy is the return of health to the supporting and investing structures of the teeth so that the remaining dentition may be maintained in health, function, and comfort. The specific criteria by which the satisfaction of this objective is measured are as follows:

1. Removal of all etiologic factors responsible for periodontal changes
2. Elimination of all pockets with the establishment of gingival sulci of minimal depth—as near 0 mm. as possible
3. Restoration of a physiologic gingival and osseous architecture
4. Establishment of a harmonious, functional occlusion
5. Maintenance of the result achieved by oral physiotherapy procedures and periodic recall visits to the dentist

At the very least, the dentist considering

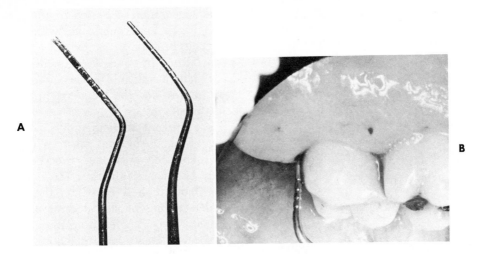

Fig. 12-4. **A,** Fox-Williams double-ended periodontal probe. The probe is graduated in millimeters (1, 2, 3, 5, 7, 8, 9, 10). **B,** The probe inserted into the distal sulcus parallel to the long axis of a terminal tooth.

partial denture construction should be certain that these criteria have been satisfied prior to proceeding with impression procedures for the master cast.

Sequence of periodontal therapeutic procedures

Diagnosis. The diagnosis of periodontal disease results from a *clinical* procedure in which the dentist systematically and carefully inspects the periodontium for deviations from normal. It follows the procurement of the health history of the patient and is performed using direct vision, palpation, periodontal probe, mouth mirror, and other auxiliary aids such as curved explorers, diagnostic casts, and radiographs.

In the diagnostic procedure nothing is so important as the careful exploration of the gingival sulcus with a suitably designed instrument—the periodontal probe (Fig. 12-4). Under no circumstances should partial denture construction begin without an accurate appraisal of sulcus depth as provided by the use of the probe. The probe is inserted gently but firmly between the gingival margin and the tooth surface, and the depth of the sulcus is explored circumferentially around each tooth. Particular attention should be given to sulcular

depth on the direct distal surface of each terminal tooth and on both the mesial and distal surfaces of isolated teeth. All depth in excess of 3 mm. is considered to be significant and an indication for treatment.

Dental radiographs are used to supplement the clinical examination but cannot be used as a substitute for it. The extent and pattern of bone loss can be estimated from radiographs, and this information serves to substantiate the impression gained from the clinical diagnosis.

Each tooth should be tested carefully for mobility (Fig. 12-5). The degree of mobility present coupled with a determination of the etiologic factor responsible provides additional information, which is invaluable in planning for the removable partial denture. If the etiologic factor can be removed, many mobile teeth will become stable and can be used successfully to help support and retain the partial denture. Mobility is not, in itself, an indication for extraction. If the cause cannot be removed or if teeth remain mobile after treatment, they should be immobilized by splinting or should be supported by the partial denture.

Dependent upon the extent and severity of the periodontal changes present, a variety of therapeutic procedures ranging from simple to relatively complex may be indicated. As was the case with the oral surgical procedures discussed, it is the responsibility of the dentist rendering the removable partial denture service to see that the required periodontal care is accomplished for his patient.

Oral physiotherapy instruction. Ordinarily, dental treatment should be introduced to the patient through instruction in a carefully devised oral physiotherapy regimen.

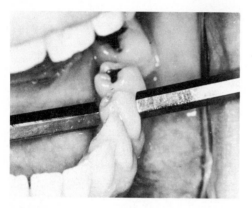

Fig. 12-5. Mobility can be visualized best when pressure is exerted on the tooth through instrument handles. If the fingers are used for this purpose, the movement of the soft tissue may mask the accurate determination of mobility.

The cooperation witnessed by the patient's acceptance and compliance with the prescribed procedure, as evidenced by improved oral hygiene, will provide the dentist with a valuable means of evaluating his interest and the long-term prognosis of treatment.

For the oral physiotherapy routine to be successful, the patient must be motivated to follow the prescribed procedure regularly and conscientiously. The most effective motivation is based on the patient's understanding of dental disease and the benefits to be derived from the procedures advocated. Hence, an explanation of dental disease, its etiology, initiation, and progression, is an important component of oral physiotherapy instruction. After this discussion the patient should be instructed in the use of disclosing wafers, soft nylon toothbrush, and unwaxed dental floss (Fig. 12-6). At subsequent appointments oral hygiene can be evaluated carefully and further treatment should be withheld until a satisfactory level has been achieved (Fig. 12-7). This is a particularly critical point for the patient requiring extensive restorative dentistry or a removable partial denture. Without good oral hygiene, any den-

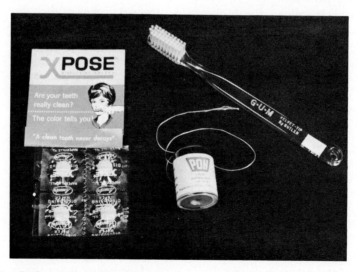

Fig. 12-6. Standard oral physiotherapy armamentarium prescribed includes disclosing wafers; soft, nylon toothbrush; and unwaxed dental floss. Supplementary hygiene aids may be recommended for those patients with special needs.

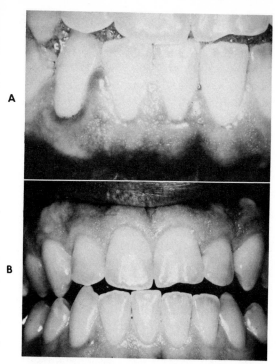

Fig. 12-7. **A,** Tissue response to poor oral hygiene procedures. Note bulbous papillae in interproximal areas of mandibular anterior teeth. **B,** Favorable tissue response in same patient to effective oral hygiene procedures only (one month). Especially noticeable is reduction of the inflamed and edematous interdental papillae.

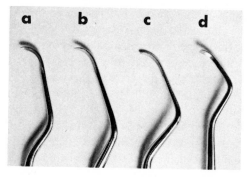

Fig. 12-8. Basic set of curettes for calculus removal includes the following: a, Gracey 5-6 for anterior teeth; b, Columbia 2R-2L for premolar teeth; c, Columbia 4R-4L for molar teeth; d, Columbia 13-14 as a universal instrument.

tal procedure, regardless of how well it is performed, is ultimately doomed to failure. The wise dentist insists that acceptable oral hygiene be demonstrated and maintained prior to embarking on an extensive restorative dentistry treatment plan.

Scaling and root curettage. One of the most important services rendered to the patient is the removal of calcareous deposits from the coronal and root surfaces of the teeth. Scaling and root curettage comprise the definitive treatment for periodontal disease. Without meticulous calculus removal, no other form of periodontal therapy can be successful.

Although some of the new ultrasonic instruments may be helpful in calculus removal, hand instrumentation remains the treatment of choice. The curette is the best designed hand instrument for scaling and root curettage (Fig. 12-8). Thorough calculus removal precedes other forms of periodontal therapy that must be completed prior to impression procedures for the removable partial denture.

Elimination of local irritating factors other than calculus. Overhanging margins of amalgam alloy and inlay restorations, overhanging crown margins, and open contacts leading to food impaction should be corrected prior to beginning definitive prosthetic treatment. Although periodontal health predisposes to a much better environment for restorative correction, it is not always possible to delay all restorative procedures until complete periodontal therapy and healing have occurred. This is especially true for patients with deep-seated carious lesions, for whom pulpal exposures are a possibility. Excavation of these areas and placement of adequate restorations must be incorporated early in treatment. Amalgam restorations are far superior to the cements in treating these patients, since the margins can be controlled and the possibility of washouts is eliminated. The placement of temporary or treatment fillings must not, in itself, become a local etiologic factor.

Elimination of gross occlusal interferences. Oral accretions and poor restorative dentistry cause damage to the periodontium as also may poor occlusal relationships. Although occlusal interferences may be eliminated by a variety of techniques, at this stage of treatment selective grinding is the procedure generally applied. Particular attention is directed to the occlusal relationships of mobile teeth. Traumatic cuspal interferences are removed by a judicious grinding procedure. An attempt is made to establish a positive centric occlusion that coincides with centric relation. Prematurities in the centric path of closure are removed eliminating mandibular displacement from the closing pattern. After this, the relationship of the teeth in the various excursive movements of the mandible are observed with special attention to cuspal contact, wear, mobility, and radiographic changes in the periodontium. Interferences on both the working and nonworking sides should be observed and, if present, removed. Narrowing of buccolingual diameters to bring occlusal forces within the range of root structure is included if excessive wear has produced abnormally wide occlusal surfaces.

The mere presence of occlusal abnormalities in the absence of demonstrable pathologic change, associated with the occlusion, does not necessarily constitute an indication for the grinding procedure. The indication for occlusal adjustment is based on the presence of pathology rather than on a preconceived articular pattern. In the natural dentition the attempt to create bilateral balance, in the prosthetic sense, has no place in the occlusal adjustment procedure. Not only is balanced occlusion impossible to obtain on natural dentition but it is also apparently unnecessary in view of its absence in most normal healthy mouths. Occlusion on natural teeth needs to be perfected only to a point at which cuspal interference within the patient's functional range of contact is eliminated and normal physiologic function can occur.

Guide to occlusal adjustment. Schuyler has provided the following guide to occlusal adjustment by selective grinding:

In the study or evaluation of occlusal disharmony of the natural dentition, accurately mounted diagnostic casts are extremely helpful, if not essential, in determining static cusp to fossae contacts of opposing teeth and as a guide in the correction of occlusal anomalies in both centric and eccentric functional relations. Occlusion can be coordinated only by selective spot grinding. Ground tooth surfaces should be subsequently smoothed and polished.

1. A static coordinated occlusal contact of the maximum number of teeth when the mandible is in centric relation to the maxillae should be our first objective.

 A. A prematurely contacting cusp should be reduced only if the cusp point is in premature contact in both centric and eccentric relations. If a cusp point is in premature contact in the centric relation only, the opposing sulcus should be deepened.

 B. When anterior teeth are in premature contact in centric, or in both centric and eccentric relations, corrections should be made by grinding the incisal edge of the lower teeth. If premature contact occurs only in the eccentric relation, correction must be made by grinding the lingual incline of the upper teeth.

 C. Usually, premature contacts in the centric relation are relieved by grinding the buccal cusps of the lower teeth, the lingual cusp of upper teeth, and the incisal edges of the lower anterior teeth. In deepening the sulcus of a posterior tooth or the lingual contact area in centric of an upper anterior tooth, we change and increase the steepness of the eccentric guiding inclines of the tooth; and so while we relieve trauma in the centric relation, we may predispose the tooth to trauma in eccentric relations.

2. After establishing a static, even distribution of stress over the maximum number of teeth in the centric relation, we are ready to evaluate opposing tooth contact or lack of contact in eccentric functional relations. Our attention is directed first to

balancing side contacts. In extreme cases of pathological balancing contacts, relief may be needed even before the corrective procedures in the centric relation. Where balancing contacts exist, it is extremely difficult to differentiate the harmless from the destructive because we can not visualize the influence of these fulcrum contacts upon the functional movements of the condyle in the articular fossa. Subluxation, pain, lack of normal functional movement of the joint, or loss of alveolar support of the teeth involved may be evidence of excessive balancing contacts. Balancing side contacts receive less frictional wear than working side contacts and premature contacts may develop progressively with wear. A reduction in the steepness of the guiding tooth inclines on the working side will increase the proximity of the teeth on the balancing side and may contribute to destructive prematurities. In all corrective grinding to relieve premature or excessive contacts in eccentric relations, care must be exercised to avoid the loss of a static supporting contact in the centric relation. This static support in centric may exist between the lower buccal cusp fitting into the central fossae of the upper tooth and/or the upper lingual cusp fitting into the central fossae of the lower tooth. While both the upper lingual cusp and the lower buccal cusp may sometimes have a static centric contact in the sulcus of the opposing tooth, often only one of these cusps has this static contact. In such instances the contacting cusp must be left untouched to maintain this essential support in centric occlusion, and all corrective grinding to relieve premature contacts in eccentric positions would be done on the opposing tooth inclines. The lower buccal cusp is in a static central contact in the upper sulcus more often than the upper lingual cusp is in a static contact in its opposing lower sulcus. Therefore, corrective grinding to relieve premature balancing contacts is more often done on the upper lingual cusps.

3. To obtain maximum function and the distribution of functional stress in eccentric positions on the working side, necessary grinding must be done on the lingual surfaces of the upper anterior teeth. Corrective grinding on the posterior teeth at this time should always be done on the buccal cusp of the upper premolars and molars and on the lingual cusp of the lower premolars and molars. The grinding of lower buccal cusps or upper lingual cusps at this time would rob these cusps of their static contact in the opposing central sulcul in the centric relations.

4. Corrective grinding to relieve premature protrusive contacts of one or more anterior teeth should be accomplished by grinding the lingual surface of the upper anterior teeth. Anterior teeth should never be ground to bring the posterior teeth into contact in either protrusive position or on the balancing side. In the elimination of premature protrusive contacts of posterior teeth neither the upper lingual cusps nor the lower buccal cusps should be ground. Corrective grinding should be done upon the surface of the opposing tooth upon which these cusps function in the eccentric position leaving the centric contact undisturbed.

5. Any sharp edges left by grinding should be rounded off.*

Temporary splinting. Teeth that are mobile at the time of the initial examination frequently present a diagnostic problem for the dentist. Their response to temporary immobilization may be helpful in establishing a prognosis for them and may lead to a rational decision as to whether they should be retained or sacrificed. Mobility due to the presence of an inflammatory lesion may be reversible if the disease process has not destroyed too much of the attachment apparatus. Mobility caused by occlusal interference also may disappear after selective grinding. In some cases, however, the teeth must be stabilized to allow the healing process to occur. In these situations temporary splinting provides a distinct advantage.

*Courtesy Dr. C. H. Schuyler, Montclair, N. J.

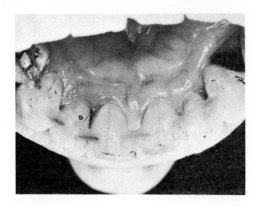

Fig. 12-9. An **A** splint used to stabilize a mobile anterior segment. Markley pins embedded in plastic filling material in dovetail preparations on the lingual surfaces. (Courtesy Dr. Daniel R. Trinler, Lexington, Ky.)

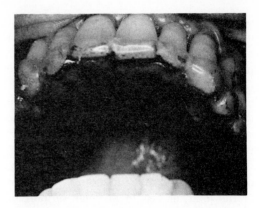

Fig. 12-10. Removable acrylic resin splint with flat occlusal plane can be used effectively as a form of temporary stabilization and as a means of eliminating excessive lateral forces created by clenching and grinding habits.

Teeth may be immobilized during periodontal treatment by interdental wiring with acrylic resin splints, with cast removable splints, or with intracoronal attachments (Fig. 12-9). The latter, an example of which is the A splint, necessitates cutting tooth surfaces and imbedding a ridge connector between adjacent teeth. This is to be avoided unless the patient is committed to a permanent restorative dentistry program allowing its replacement or unless there is no other alternative.

After periodontal treatment, splinting may be accomplished with cast removable restorations or cast cemented restorations. The most preferred form of permanent splinting is with two or more cast restorations soldered or cast together. They may be cemented with either permanent (zinc oxyphosphate or resin) cements or temporary (zinc oxide–eugenol) cements. A properly designed removable partial denture can also stabilize mobile teeth if provision for such immobilization is planned as the denture is designed.

Use of the nightguard. The removable acrylic resin splint, originally designed as an aid in eliminating the deleterious effects of nocturnal clenching and grinding, has been used to advantage for the removable partial denture patient. The nightguard may be helpful as a form of temporary splinting if worn at night when the partial denture has been removed. The flat occlusal surface prevents the interdigitation of the teeth, which eliminates lateral occlusal forces, and the immobilization provided aids the repair process (Fig. 12-10).

The nightguard is particularly useful prior to the fabrication of a partial denture when one of the abutment teeth has been unopposed for an extended period of time. The periodontium of a tooth without an antagonist undergoes deterioration characterized by a loss of orientation of periodontal ligament fibers, loss of supporting bone, and narrowing of the periodontal membrane space. If such a tooth is suddenly returned to full function when it is carrying an increased burden, pain and prolonged sensitivity may result. If, however, a nightguard is used to return some functional stimulation to the tooth, the periodontal changes are reversed and an uneventful course is experienced when the tooth is returned to full function.

Minor tooth movement. The increased utilization of orthodontic procedures in conjunction with restorative and prosthetic dentistry has contributed to the success of many restorations by altering the periodontal climate in which they are placed.

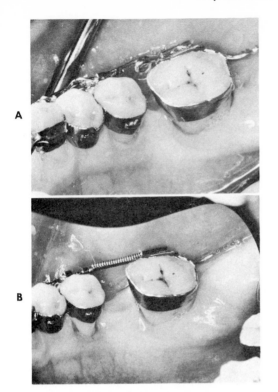

Fig. 12-11. Tooth movement used to upright a tilted molar tooth to prepare the segment for the receipt of a pontic. **A,** Placement of orthodontic appliance. **B,** Space gained after 3 months' active movement.

Malposed teeth that were once doomed to extraction should be considered now for repositioning and retention. The additional stability provided for a removable partial denture from uprighting a tilted or drifted tooth may mean much in terms of comfort to the patient. The techniques employed are not difficult to master, and the rewards in terms of a better restorative dentistry service are great (Fig. 12-11).

Periodontal surgery

A variety of periodontal surgical techniques can be employed to advantage in satisfying the objectives of periodontal therapy for the removable partial denture patient. These are largely directed at the elimination of the periodontal pocket, the lesion pathognomonic of periodontal disease, and at a return of physiologic architecture to the area.

Pocket elimination may be achieved by shrinkage, surgical excision, and new attachment procedures. Of these, surgical excision presents the therapist with the most predictable result. Surgical procedures also afford the opportunity for recreating a physiologic architectural pattern, and, hence, much periodontal therapy is surgical in nature.

Gingivectomy. Perhaps the basic surgical procedure in periodontics can be said to be the gingivectomy. It certainly is one of the oldest excision-type procedures and is one that has been used widely for years. When the gingivectomy is indicated, it satisfies the objectives previously stated for periodontal therapy. However, as periodontics has experienced greater refinement in recent years and as the requirements for successful treatment have expanded, situations in which the gingivectomy alone will suffice have been greatly reduced.

The gingivectomy is indicated when the following conditions are present (Fig. 12-12):

1. Suprabony pockets of fibrotic tissue
2. Absence of deformities in the underlying bony tissue
3. Pocket depth confined to the band of attached gingiva

If osseous deformities are present or if pocket depth traverses or approximates the mucogingival junction, the gingivectomy is *not* the procedure of choice. The gingivectomy technique is best accomplished with appropriate cutting instruments, and the use of chemicals or electric cautery should be avoided.

Because the greatest majority of patients with moderate to advanced periodontal disease have experienced various degrees of bone loss, the gingivectomy alone can only rarely reestablish the desired physiologic architecture. For that reason, more complex forms of treatment, including osseous and mucogingival surgery, have been developed as periodontics has entered an era of plastic and reconstructive surgery.

Repositioned flap. Today the apically repositioned flap is the periodontal surgical

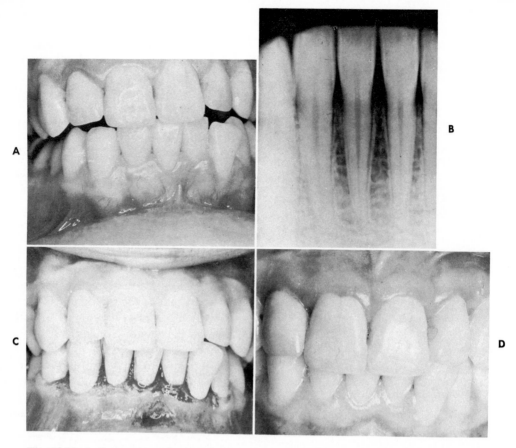

Fig. 12-12. **A,** Preoperative photograph of patient with pocket depth in anterior segment. Tissue is fibrotic and pocket depth is confined within the band of attached gingiva. **B,** Radiograph confirms clinical impression of minimal bone loss and acceptable bony topography. **C,** Immediate gingivectomy view of mandibular anterior segment. Frenectomy included in the operative procedure. **D,** Appearance of maxillary and mandibular anterior segments approximately 3 months after gingivectomy procedures.

procedure of greatest versatility and, consequently, is widely applied in the treatment of periodontal disease (Fig. 12-13). Several healing studies have contributed to a greater understanding of periodontal therapy and because of these, emphasis is currently placed on the closure of the surgical area for which is provided flap techniques.

Indications for the repositioned flap are as follows:

1. Pocket depth traversing the mucogingival junction
2. Presence of osseous deformities that must be corrected to eliminate the

pocket and restore physiologic architecture
3. Muscle or frenum attachment at the gingival margin

Adjunctive procedures. In addition to the apically repositioned flap, other adjunctive mucogingival surgical techniques have added to the armamentarium of the therapist in eliminating periodontal disease and in the preparation of the mouth for restorative and prosthetic dentistry. Among these are lateral sliding flaps, pedicle grafts (Fig. 12-14), and free gingival grafts (Fig. 12-15). These procedures have particular application in the reestablishment of an ade-

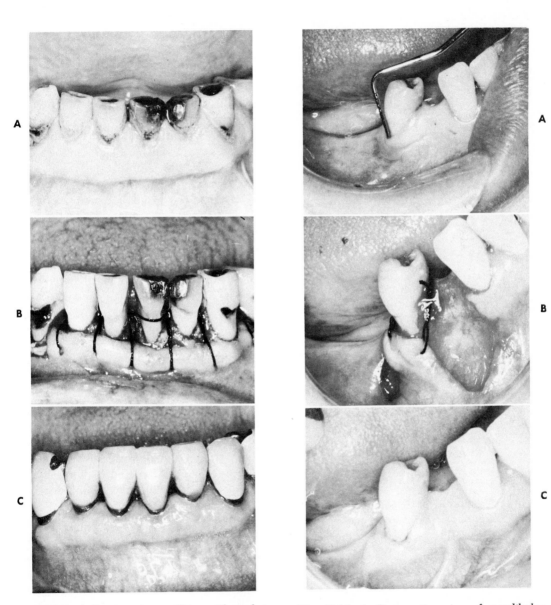

Fig. 12-13. **A,** Preoperative condition with pocket depth traversing the mucogingival junction, osseous deformities and carious lesions extending beneath the gingival margin. **B,** Gingival flap repositioned after osseous correction and crown-lengthening procedure on mandibular right canine tooth. **C,** Permanent splint with provision for removable partial denture. (Courtesy Dr. Keith Brooks, Lexington, Ky.)

Fig. 12-14. **A,** Preoperative view of mandibular second premolar with inadequate zone of attached gingiva and pocket depth traversing the mucogingival junction. **B,** Pedicle graft sutured into position. **C,** Postoperative view showing new zone of attached gingiva with no pocket depth present.

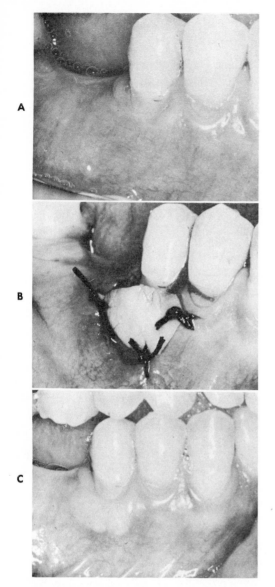

Fig. 12-15. A, Preoperative condition showing patient with no attached gingiva on buccal of mandibular second premolar. **B,** Operative site with free gingival graft in place. **C,** New zone of attached gingiva 9 weeks postoperatively.

quate zone of attached gingiva and in the elimination of gingival clefts.

Advantages of periodontal therapy

Periodontal therapy prior to the fabrication of a removable prosthesis has several advantages. First, the elimination of periodontal disease removes a primary etiologic factor in tooth loss. The long-term success of dental treatment is dependent upon the maintenance of the remaining oral structures, and periodontal health is mandatory if further loss is to be avoided. Second, a periodontium free of disease presents a much better environment for restorative correction. The elimination of periodontal pockets with the associated return of a physiologic architectural pattern establishes a normal gingival contour at a stable position on the root surface. Thus the optimum position for gingival margins of individual restorations can be established with accuracy. The coronal contours of these restorations also can be developed in correct relationships to the gingival margin assuring the proper degree of protection and functional stimulation to the gingival tissues. Third, the response to strategic but questionable teeth to periodontal therapy provides an important opportunity for reevaluating their prognosis before the final decision to include (or exclude) them in the partial denture design. And last, the overall reaction of the patient to periodontal procedures provides the dentist with an excellent indication of the degree of cooperation to be expected in the future.

Even in the absence of periodontal disease, periodontal procedures may be an invaluable aid in partial denture construction. Through periodontal surgical techniques the environment of potential abutment teeth may be altered to the point of making an otherwise unacceptable tooth a most satisfactory retainer for a partial denture. The lengthening of a clinical crown through the removal of gingival tissue and bone is a common example of the application of periodontal surgical techniques as an aid in partial denture construction (Fig. 12-16).

ABUTMENT TEETH

Abutment restorations. Equipped with the diagnostic casts upon which a tentative partial denture design has been drawn, the dentist is able to accomplish preparation of abutment teeth with accuracy. The infor-

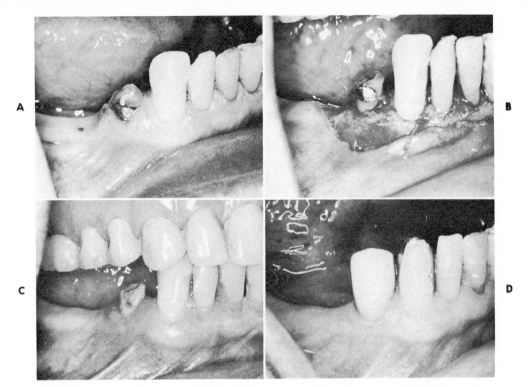

Fig. 12-16. A, Fractured first premolar tooth after endodontic therapy. **B,** Periodontal flap retracted for access for bone removal and apical repositioning of the gingival margin. **C,** Appearance of tooth after healing and preparation to receive crown. **D,** Restoration in place, splinted to canine tooth, to act as an abutment for a removable partial denture.

mation at hand should include the proposed path of placement, the areas of teeth to be disked and tooth contours to be changed, and the location of rests.

During examination and subsequent treatment planning, in conjunction with a survey of diagnostic casts, each abutment tooth is considered individually as to whether or not full coverage is indicated. Abutment teeth presenting sound enamel surfaces in a mouth in which good oral hygiene habits are evident may be considered a fair risk for use as partial denture abutments. One should not be misled, however, by a patient's promise to do better, so far as oral hygiene habits are concerned. Good or bad oral hygiene is a habit of long standing, and is not likely to be changed appreciably because a partial denture is being worn. Therefore, one must be conservative in evaluating the oral hygiene habits of the

patient in the future. It is well to remember that clasps as such do not cause teeth to decay, and if the individual will keep the teeth and the partial denture clean, one need not condemn clasps from a cariogenic standpoint. On the other hand, more partial dentures have been condemned as cariogenic because the dentist did not provide for the protection of abutment teeth than because of inadequate care on the part of the patient.

The full cast gold crown is objectionable from an esthetic standpoint and therefore the veneer-type of full crown must be resorted to when a canine or premolar abutment is to be restored or protected. Less frequently does the molar have to be treated in such a manner, and the full gold crown is usually acceptable except for maxillary first molars.

When there is proximal caries on abutment teeth with sound buccal and lingual enamel surfaces, in a mouth exhibiting average oral hygiene and low caries activity, a gold inlay is usually indicated. Silver amalgam for the restoration of proximal caries should not be condemned, however, although one must admit that an inlay cast of a hard-type gold will provide the best possible support for occlusal rests, at the same time giving an esthetically pleasing restoration. But an amalgam restoration, properly condensed, is capable of supporting an occlusal rest, without appreciable flow, over a long period of time.

The most vulnerable area on the abutment tooth is the proximal gingival area, which lies beneath the minor connector of the partial denture framework and is therefore subject to the lodgment of debris in an area most susceptible to caries attack. Even when the partial denture is removed for cleaning the teeth, these areas, especially those on the distal surface of an anterior abutment, are often missed by the toothbrush, and bacterial plaques and debris are allowed to remain for long periods of time. Except in a caries-immune mouth or in a mouth in which the teeth are subjected to meticulous brushing, decalcification and caries frequently occur in this region. It is necessary, therefore, that this area of the tooth be fully protected by whatever restoration is used. When an inlay restoration is used, the preparation should be carried to or beneath the gingival margin and well out onto the buccal and lingual surfaces to afford the best possible protection of the abutment tooth. Even the full crown can be deficient in this most vulnerable area, which lies at and just above the gingival margin. The full crown, which is cast short of this area will not afford protection where it is most needed.

All proximal tooth surfaces that are to serve as guiding planes for the partial denture should be disked so that they will be made as nearly as possible parallel to the path of placement. This is accomplished on sound enamel or on existing restoration by disking those tooth surfaces parallel to the path of placement, and the same can be done

for the recently placed full crown or inlay.

Contouring wax patterns. Modern indirect techniques using hydrocolloid or rubber base impression materials permit the contouring of wax patterns on the stone abutments with the aid of the surveyor blade. All abutment teeth to be restored with castings can be prepared at one time and an impression made that will provide an accurate stone replica of the prepared arch. Wax patterns may then be refined on separated individual dies or removable dies. All tooth surfaces facing edentulous areas should be made parallel to the path of placement by the use of the surveyor blade. This will provide proximal tooth surfaces that will be parallel without any further disking in the mouth, will permit the most positive seating of the partial denture along the path of placement, and will provide the least amount of undesirable space beneath minor connectors for the lodgment of debris.

Rest seats. After the proximal surfaces of the wax patterns have been made parallel, and buccal and lingual contours have been established, which will satisfy the requirements of retention with the best possible esthetic placement of clasp arms, the occlusal rest seats should be prepared in the wax pattern rather than in the finished gold restoration. The placement of occlusal rests should be considered at the time that the teeth are prepared to receive cast restorations so that there will be sufficient clearance beneath the floor of the occlusal rest seat. Too many times we see a completed gold restoration cemented in the mouth for a partial denture abutment without any provision for the occlusal rest having been made in the wax pattern. The dentist then proceeds to cut an occlusal rest seat in the gold restoration, being ever conscious of the fact that he may perforate the gold during the process of forming the rest seat. The unfortunate result is usually a poorly formed rest seat that is too shallow and one that does not incline toward the center of the tooth in the desired manner.

If tooth structure has been removed to provide for the placement of the occlusal rest seat, the rest seat may be ideally placed in the wax pattern by using a No. 8 round bur to lower the marginal ridge and establish the outline form of the rest, and then using a No. 6 round bur to deepen slightly the floor of the rest seat inside this lowered marginal ridge. This provides for an occlusal rest that best satisfies the requirements that the rest be placed so that any occlusal force will be directed toward the center of the tooth and that there will be the least possible interference to occlusion with the opposing teeth.

Perhaps the most important function of a rest is the division of stress loads coming upon the partial denture to provide for greatest efficiency with the least damaging effect to the abutment teeth. For a distal extension partial denture, the rest must be able to transmit occlusal forces to the abutment teeth in a vertical direction only, thereby permitting the least possible lateral stresses to be transmitted to the abutment tooth.

For this reason, the floor of the rest seat should incline toward the center of the tooth so that the occlusal forces, in so far as possible, are centered over the root apex. Any other form but that of a spoon shape permits a locking of the occlusal rest and the transmission of tipping forces to the abutment tooth. A ball-and-socket type of relationship between occlusal rest and abutment tooth is the most desirable. At the same time the marginal ridge must be lowered so that the angle formed by the occlusal rest with the minor connector will stand above the occlusal surface of the abutment tooth as little as possible and avoid interference with the opposing teeth. Simultaneously, sufficient bulk must be provided for to prevent a weakness in the occlusal rest at the marginal ridge. The marginal ridge must be lowered and yet not be the deepest part of the rest preparation. To permit occlusal stresses to be directed toward the center of the abutment tooth, the angle formed by the floor of the occlusal rest with the minor connector should be less than 90 degrees. In other words, the floor of the occlusal rest should

incline slightly from the lowered marginal ridge toward the center of the tooth.

This proper form can be readily accomplished in the wax pattern if care is taken during crown or inlay preparation to provide for the location of the rest. If an amalgam restoration is used, sufficient bulk must be present in this area to allow proper occlusal rest seat form without weakening the restoration. When the rest seat is placed in sound enamel, it is best accomplished by the use of round diamond points of approximately Nos. 4, 6, and 8 sizes in the following sequence. First, the larger of the diamonds is used to lower the marginal ridge and at the same time create the relative outline form of the rest seat. The result is a rest seat preparation with marginal ridge lowered and gross outline form established but without sufficient deepening of the rest seat preparation toward the center of the tooth. The smaller diamond points or a carbide bur of approximately No. 4 or 6 size may then be used to deepen the floor of the rest seat to a gradual incline toward the center of the tooth. Enamel rods are then smoothed by the planning action of a round bur revolving with little pressure. Abrasive rubber points, followed by the use of wet flour of pumice on a stiff bristle brush, are sufficient to complete the polishing of the rest seat preparation.

Rest seat preparations in existing restorations or on abutment teeth where no restorations are to be placed should always follow, not precede, the disking of proximal tooth surfaces. The disking of proximal tooth surfaces should be done first because if the occlusal portion of the rest seat is placed first and the proximal tooth surface is disked later, the outline form of the rest seat is sometimes irreparably altered.

The success or failure of a removable partial denture may well depend upon how well the mouth preparations were accomplished. It is only through intelligent planning and competent execution of mouth preparations that the denture can satisfactorily restore lost dental functions and contribute to the health of the remaining oral tissues.

CHAPTER 13

Preparation of abutment teeth

After surgery, periodontal treatment, and any endodontic treatment of the arch involved, the abutment teeth then may be prepared to provide support, stabilization, bracing, and retention for the partial denture.

Endodontic treatment of any teeth elsewhere in the arch, as well as abutment teeth, should precede the making of the partial denture, so that the success of treatment can be reasonably well established before proceeding. Similarly, favorable response to any deep restorations and the results of periodontal treatment should be established prior to construction of the denture, since if the prognosis of a tooth under treatment becomes unfavorable, its loss can be compensated by a change in the denture design. The condemned tooth or teeth may then be included in the original denture design, whereas if they are lost subsequently, the partial denture must be added to, remade, or replaced. Many partial denture designs do not lend themselves well to later additions, although this eventuality should be remembered when designing the denture.

Particularly when the tooth in question will be used as an abutment, every diagnostic aid should be used to determine the success of previous treatment. It is usually not so difficult to add a tooth or teeth to a partial denture as it is to add a retaining unit when the original abutment is lost and the next adjacent tooth must be used for that purpose.

It is sometimes possible to design a removable partial denture so that a single posterior abutment about which there is some doubt can be retained and utilized as one end of a tooth-supported base. Then, if that posterior abutment is lost, it can be replaced with a distal extension base. Such a design will include provision for future indirect retention and flexible clasping on the future terminal abutment. Anterior abutments, which are considered to be poor risks, may not be so freely used because of the problems involved in adding a new abutment retainer when the original one is lost. It is better that such questionable teeth be condemned in favor of a better abutment, even though the original treatment plan must be modified accordingly.

CLASSIFICATION OF ABUTMENT TEETH

The subject of abutment preparations may be grouped as follows: (1) those abutment teeth that are to be used in their present state, (2) those that are to have cast inlays, and (3) those that are to have cast crowns. The latter group includes abutments for fixed partial dentures, since inlay retainers are not commonly used for such restorations.

Abutment teeth to be used in their present state include teeth with sound enamel, those having small restorations not involved in the denture design, those having acceptable restorations that will be involved in the denture design, and those having existing crown restorations. The latter may exist either as an individual crown or as the abutment of a fixed restoration.

The use of unprotected abutments has been discussed previously. Although full protection of all abutments is desirable, it is not always possible nor practical to do so. The decision to use unprotected abutments involves certain risks of which the patient must be advised, including his own responsibility for maintaining oral hygiene and caries control. The making of crown restorations to fit existing denture clasps is an art in itself, which will be covered later in this chapter, but the fact that it is possible to do so may influence the decision to use uncrowned but otherwise sound teeth as abutments.

Preferably, silver amalgam alloy should not be used for the support of occlusal rests because of its tendency to flow. Although cast gold will provide the best possible support for occlusal rests, an amalgam alloy restoration, properly condensed, is capable of supporting an occlusal rest without appreciable flow over a long period of time. If the patient's economic status or other factors beyond the control of the dentist prevent the use of cast restorations, any existing silver amalgam alloy fillings about which there is any doubt should be replaced with new amalgam restorations. This should be done far enough in advance of disking and the preparation of occlusal rest seats to permit aging and polishing of the restoration.

SEQUENCE OF ABUTMENT PREPARATIONS ON SOUND ENAMEL OR EXISTING RESTORATIONS

Abutment preparations on either sound enamel or existing restorations should be done in the following order:

1. The disking of proximal surfaces parallel to the path of placement to provide guiding planes (Fig. 13-1, A). The term *disking* is used in a broad sense and refers

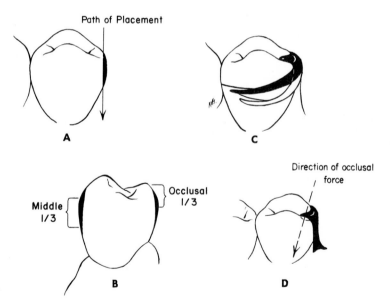

Fig. 13-1. Abutment contours should be altered during mouth preparations in the following sequence. **A,** The proximal surface is disked parallel to the path of placement to create a guiding plane. **B,** The height of contours on the buccal and lingual surface is lowered when necessary to permit the retentive clasp terminus to be located within the gingival third of the crown and the reciprocal clasp arm on the opposite side of the tooth to be placed no higher than the middle third of the crown. **C,** The area of the tooth at which a retentive clasp arm originates should be altered if necessary to permit more direct approach to the gingival third of the tooth. **D,** An occlusal rest preparation that will direct occlusal forces along the long axis of the tooth should be the final step in mouth preparations.

to the paralleling of proximal surfaces by the use of abrasive instruments. With ultra speeds parallelism can frequently be accomplished as well or better by the use of cylindrical diamond points moved buccolingually across the proximal surface. The term disking may ultimately be replaced by terminology descriptive of modern cutting methods.

2. The reduction of excessive tooth contours (Fig. 13-1, *B* and *C*), thereby lowering the height of contours so that (a) the origin of circumferential clasp arms may be placed well below the occlusal surface, preferably at the junction of the gingival and middle thirds; (b) retentive clasp terminals may be placed in the gingival third of the crown, for better esthetics and better mechanical advantage; and (c) reciprocal clasp arms may be placed on and above a height of contour that is no higher than the middle third of the crown of the abutment tooth.

3. The preparation of occlusal rest areas that will direct occlusal forces along the long axis of the abutment tooth (Fig. 13-1, *D*).

Mouth preparation should follow a plan that was outlined on the diagnostic cast in red pencil at the time the cast was surveyed and also follow the design of the partial denture outlined. Better still, proposed changes to abutment teeth actually may be made on the diagnostic cast and *outlined* in red pencil to indicate not only the area but also the *amount* and *angulation* of the disking to be done (Chapter 11). Although occlusal rests also may be prepared on the diagnostic cast, indication of their *location* in red pencil is usually sufficient for the experienced dentist, since rest preparations follow a definite pattern (Chapter 5).

ABUTMENT PREPARATIONS USING CAST INLAYS

Inlay preparations on teeth to be used as removable partial denture abutments differ from conventional inlay preparations in the amount of protection afforded the tooth, the width of the preparation at the occlusal rest, and the depth of the preparation beneath the occlusal rest.

Conventional inlay preparations are permissible on the proximal surface of the tooth not to be contacted by a minor connector of the partial denture. On the other hand, proximal and occlusal surfaces supporting minor connectors and occlusal rests require somewhat different treatment than the conventional inlay preparation. The extent of occlusal coverage (that is, whether or not cusps are capped) will be governed by the usual factors, such as the extent of caries, the presence of unsupported enamel walls, and the extent of occlusal abrasion and attrition.

Of primary consideration in the preparation of proximal inlays that will lie beneath minor connectors is the amount of protection afforded vulnerable areas by the inlay. The most vulnerable area on the abutment tooth is the proximal gingival area lying beneath the minor connector of the partial denture, because of accumulation of debris and the difficulty of keeping this area clean.

Except in a caries-immune mouth or in a mouth in which the teeth are kept meticulously clean, some decalcification and caries attack in this region is inevitable. Even the most conscientious toothbrushing may miss the distal surfaces of abutments because they cannot be seen. It is always important that the patient be instructed, with casts and before a mirror, in the significance of brushing these areas and the correct use of dental floss.

It is necessary that these areas be fully protected by the cast restoration, whether it be an inlay or a partial or full crown. Even the full crown can be deficient in this most vulnerable area, which lies at or just above the gingival margin. A full crown that is short or becomes short because of gingival recession does not afford protection where it is most needed.

When an inlay is the restoration of choice for an abutment tooth, certain modifications of the outline form are necessary. To prevent the buccal and lingual proximal

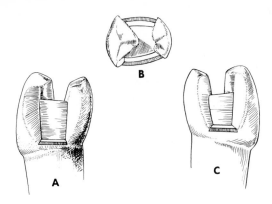

Fig. 13-2. MOD inlay preparation for a lower left, second premolar to be used as a partial denture abutment. **A,** View of the distal surface showing the broad extension of the box, well beyond the area that will be covered by the minor connector of the partial denture. **B,** Occlusal view showing that the axial wall is curved to conform with the external proximal curvature of the tooth. **C,** View of the mesial surface where normal tooth contact occurs, being extended into a free-cleansing area but not as broadly as the distal surface.

margins from lying at or near the minor connector or the occlusal rest, these margins must be extended well beyond the line angles of the tooth. This additional extension may be accomplished by slicing the conventional box preparation. However, the gold margin produced by such a preparation may be quite thin and may be damaged by the clasp during placement or removal of the partial denture. This hazard may be avoided by extending the outline of the box beyond the line angle, thus producing a strong gold-to-tooth junction. (See Fig. 13-2.)

In this type of preparation the pulp is particularly vulnerable unless the axial wall is curved to conform with the external proximal curvature of the tooth. When caries is of minimal depth, the gingival seat should have an axial depth at all points about the width of a No. 559 fissure bur. It is of utmost importance that the gingival seat be placed below the free gingival margin. The proximal contour necessary to produce the proper guiding plane surface and the close proximity of the minor connector render this area particularly vulnerable to

future caries attack. Every effort should be made to provide the restoration with maximum resistance and retention as well as clinically imperceptible gold margins. The first requisite can be satisfied by preparing opposing cavity walls 5 degrees or less from parallel and producing flat floors and sharp, clean line angles. Through the use of modern impression materials and casting technique, the second requisite is not nearly as difficult as it was a few years ago.

The extended box provides the broad occlusoproximal area necessary to accommodate an occlusal rest. Care should be exercised to place the rest area in such a manner that an adequate amount of gold is allowed in both buccal and lingual directions. The proposed depth of the rest must be determined prior to preparing the tooth to ensure an adequate thickness of gold in the axiopulpal area. Additional depth in this area may be obtained by rounding the axiopulpal line angle of the preparation. In most instances, if the preparation is well into dentin at this point, adequate thickness of gold will be ensured. However, in problem situations, a careful study of the roentgenogram will give some indication regarding the depth to which the pulpal floor can be carried with safety.

It is sometimes necessary to use an inlay on a lower first premolar for the support of an indirect retainer. The narrow occlusal width buccolingually and the lingual inclination of the occlusal surface of such a tooth often complicates the two-surface inlay preparation. Even the most exacting occlusal cavity preparation often results in a thin and weak lingual cusp remaining.

Fig. 13-3 illustrates a modification of the two-surface extended-box inlay preparation, which lends support to a weak lingual cusp. Enough of the tip of the lingual cusp must be removed to allow for sufficient thickness of gold to withstand occlusal forces. Tooth structure should be removed in the direction of the enamel rods, and the cut is terminated with a bevel just lingual to the proximal embrasure. A short bevel

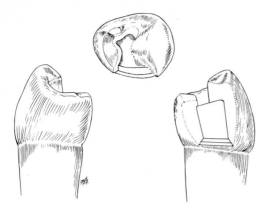

Fig. 13-3. MO inlay preparation on a lower left, first premolar to be used for the support of a mesially placed occlusal rest. The weak lingual cusp is protected by an extension of the inlay margin lingually.

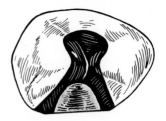

Fig. 13-4. Occlusal view of a Class II inlay properly designed to support an occlusal rest. The inlay preparation has been made with sufficient width to accommodate the occlusal rest without jeopardizing the inlay margins.

is then placed along the lingual surface of the reduced cusp. A modified inlay preparation such as this permits adequate coverage of a potentially weak cusp and eliminates the necessity of resorting to some type of more extensive restoration such as an MOD inlay or three-quarter crown.

An inlay preparation should be wide enough that the margins will be well beyond the occlusal rest area (Fig. 13-4). Since the rest seat will be carved in the wax pattern with round burs, the margins of the inlay should not be jeopardized by their proximity to the rest seat. Generally, there should be at least 1 to 1.5 mm. of gold between the occlusal rest and the inlay margin. The refinement of the margins, which is the final step in creating an inlay wax pattern, should not infringe upon the outline form of the rest seat. The depth of the occlusal rest seat should be provided for in the preparation. If there is any doubt, the axiopulpal line angle should be beveled or made concave to accommodate the occlusal rest.

One of the advantages of making cast restorations for abutment teeth is that mouth preparations that would otherwise have to be done in the mouth may be done on the surveyor with far greater accuracy.

It is extremely difficult, and many times impossible to make several proximal surfaces parallel to one another by disking them intraorally. The opportunity of paralleling and contouring wax patterns on the surveyor in relation to a path of placement should be utilized to the fullest advantage whenever cast restorations are being made.

Although it is not always possible, it is best that all wax patterns be made at the same time. A cast of the arch with removable dies may be used if they are sufficiently keyed for accuracy (Fig. 13-5). If preferred, the paralleling and contouring of wax patterns may be done on a solid cast of the arch, using supplementary individual dies to refine margins. Modern impression materials and indirect techniques make either method equally satisfactory.

The same sequence for preparing teeth in the mouth applies to the contouring of wax patterns, differing only in that it may be done with greater accuracy and precision when indirect methods are used. After the cast has been placed on the surveyor to conform to the selected path of placement, and the wax patterns have been carved for occlusion and contact, proximal surfaces that are to act as guiding planes then may be carved parallel to the path of placement with a surveyor blade. This usually will be extended to the junction of the middle and gingival thirds of the tooth surface involved but not to the gingival margin, since the minor connector must be

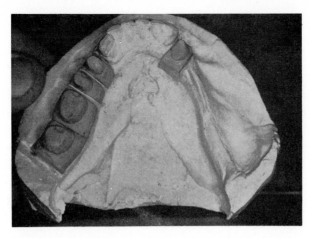

Fig. 13-5. Full arch with removable dies for five abutment crowns. Note the depressions in the preparations to accommodate occlusal rests.

relieved when it crosses the gingivae. A guiding plane that includes the occlusal two thirds or even one half of the proximal area is usually adequate without endangering gingival tissues.

After the paralleling of guiding planes and any other contouring, occlusal rest seats are carved in the wax pattern with suitable round burs, thus lowering the marginal ridge and inclining the floor of the rest preparation toward the center of the tooth. This has been outlined in Chapter 5.

It should be emphasized that critical areas thus prepared in wax should not be destroyed by careless spruing or polishing. The wax pattern should be sprued to preserve paralleled surfaces and rest areas. Polishing should consist of little more than burnishing. Rest areas should need only refining with round finishing burs of the same sizes that were used to carve the rest seat originally. If some interference by spruing is unavoidable, the casting should be returned to the surveyor for the refinement of proximal surfaces. However, this can only be done accurately with the aid of a handpiece holder attached to the vertical arm of the surveyor or some similar maching device. Need for later corrections to the casting can be avoided by carving the wax pattern with care and spruing and polishing with equal care.

ABUTMENT PREPARATIONS USING CAST CROWNS

Much that has been said in the preceding paragraphs about the preparation of inlays for partial denture abutments applies equally to cast-crown restorations. These may be in the form of three-quarter or full cast gold crowns or resin or porcelain veneer crowns. The latter are, of course, used for esthetic reasons only, but consideration for esthetics must not be allowed to jeopardize the success of the partial denture design. Retentive contours, therefore, must be provided on veneer crowns the same as on full cast crowns.

The ideal crown restoration for a partial denture abutment is the full cast gold crown, which can be carved to satisfy ideally all requirements for support, stabilization, and retention without compromise for cosmetic reasons. Porcelain and resin veneer crowns can be made equally satisfactory but only by the added step of contouring the veneered surface on the surveyor. If this is not done, retentive contours may be excessive or inadequate. The full cast crown is preferable as an ideal abutment piece whenever esthetics will allow its use.

The three-quarter crown does not permit the creating of retentive areas as does the full crown. However, if buccal or labial

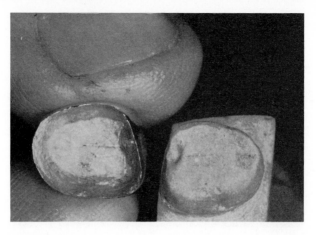

Fig. 13-6. Close-up view of a full crown abutment preparation with depression to accommodate the depth of the occlusal rest.

surfaces are sound and retentive areas are acceptable or can be made so by slight modification of tooth surfaces, the three-quarter crown is a conservative restoration of merit. The same criteria apply in the decision to leave a portion of an abutment unprotected, as in the decision to leave any tooth unprotected that is to serve a partial denture abutment.

Regardless of the type of crown used, the preparation should be made to accommodate the depth of the occlusal rest seat. This is best accomplished by creating a depression in the prepared tooth at the occlusal rest area (Fig. 13-6). Since the location of any occlusal rests will have been established previously during treatment planning, this will be known in advance of any crown preparations. If, for example, double occlusal rests are to be used, this will be known so that the tooth can be prepared to accommodate the depth of both rests. It is almost as bad to find, when waxing a pattern, that a rest seat has to be made more shallow than is desirable because of lack of foresight as it is to have to make a rest seat shallow in an existing crown or inlay because its thickness is not known. Here, the opportunity for creating an ideal rest seat depends only upon the few seconds it takes to create a space for it.

LEDGES ON ABUTMENT CROWNS

In addition to providing abutment protection, more nearly ideal retentive contours, definite guiding planes, and optimal occlusal rest support, crown restorations on teeth used as partial denture abutments offer still another advantage not obtainable on natural teeth. This is the crown ledge or shoulder, which provides effective reciprocation and stabilization.

The functions of the reciprocal clasp arm have been stated in Chapter 6. Briefly, these are reciprocation, stabilization, and auxiliary indirect retention. Any rigid reciprocal arm may provide horizontal stabilization. To a large extent, since it is placed about the height of convexity, a rigid reciprocal arm may also act as an auxiliary indirect retainer. However its function as a reciprocating arm against the action of the retentive clasp arm is limited only to stabilization against possible orthodontic movement when the denture framework is in its terminal position. Only when the retentive clasp produces an active orthodontic force, because of accidental distortion or improper design, is such reciprocation needed. Reciprocation is most needed when the restoration is being placed or when a dislodging force is applied, to prevent transient horizontal forces

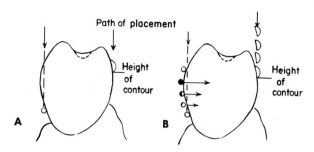

Fig. 13-7. A, Relationship of a retentive and a reciprocal clasp arm to each other when the partial denture framework is fully seated. As the retentive clasp arm flexes over the height of contour during placement and removal, the reciprocal clasp arm cannot be effective because it is not in contact with the tooth until the denture framework is fully seated. **B,** The horizontal forces that are applied to an abutment tooth as a retentive clasp flexes over the height of contour during placement and removal. The open circle at the top and bottom illustrates that the retentive clasp is only passive at its first contact with the tooth during placement and when in its terminal position with the denture fully seated. During placement and removal a rigid clasp arm placed on the opposite side of the tooth cannot provide resistance against these horizontal forces.

that may be detrimental to abutment stability. Perhaps the term *orthodontic force* is incorrect, since the term signifies a slight but continuous influence that would logically reach equilibrium as soon as the tooth is orthodontically moved. Instead, the transient forces of placement and removal lead to periodontal destruction and eventual instability rather than to orthodontic movement followed by consolidation.

True reciprocation is not possible with a clasp arm that is placed upon an occlusally inclined tooth surface because it does not become effective until the prosthesis is fully seated. Immediately, when a dislodging force is applied, the reciprocal clasp arm, along with the occlusal rest, breaks contact with the supporting tooth surfaces and they are no longer effective. Thus, as the retentive clasp flexes over the height of contour, thereby exerting a horizontal force on the abutment, reciprocation is nonexistent just when it is needed most. (See Fig. 13-7.)

True reciprocation can be obtained only by creating a path of placement for the reciprocal clasp arm that is paralled to other guiding planes. In this manner, the inferior border of the reciprocal clasp makes contact with its guiding surface before the

retentive clasp on the other side of the tooth begins to flex (Fig. 13-8). Thus, reciprocation exists during the entire path of placement and removal. The presence of a ledge on the abutment crown acts as a terminal stop for the reciprocal clasp arm, as well as augmenting the occlusal rest and providing some indirect retention for a distal extension partial denture.

A ledge on an abutment crown has still another advantage. Although the usual reciprocal clasp arm is half-round, and therefore convex, and is superimposed upon an already convex surface, a reciprocal clasp arm built on a crown ledge is actually inlayed into the crown and reproduces more nearly normal crown contours (Fig. 13-8). The patient's tongue then contacts a continuously convex surface rather than the projection of a clasp arm. Unfortunately, the enamel cap is neither thick enough nor is the tooth so shaped that an effective ledge can be created on an uncrowned tooth. Narrow enamel shoulders are sometimes used as rest seats on anterior teeth, but these do not provide the parallelism that is essential to reciprocation during placement and removal.

The crown ledge may be used on any full or three-quarter crown restoration that

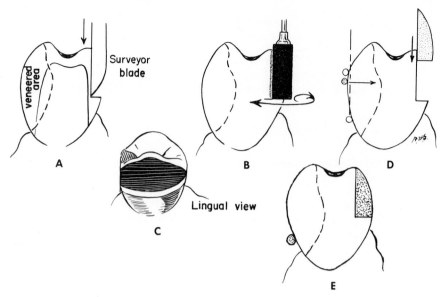

Fig. 13-8. **A,** The preparation of a ledge on a wax pattern with the surveyor blade parallel to the path of placement. **B,** The refinement of the ledge on a gold casting, using a suitable carborundum stone in a handpiece attached to a dental surveyor or a specialized drill press for the purpose. **C,** The approximate width and depth of the ledge formed on an abutment crown, which will permit a reciprocal clasp arm to be inlayed within the normal contours of the tooth. **D,** The true reciprocation throughout the full path of placement and removal that is possible when a reciprocal clasp arm is inlayed onto a ledge on an abutment crown. **E,** Direct retainer assembly is fully seated. The reciprocal arm restores the lingual contour of the abutment.

covers the nonretentive side of an abutment tooth. It is used most frequently on premolars and molars but also may be used on canine restorations. It is not ordinarily used on buccal surfaces for reciprocation against lingual retention because of the excessive display of metal, but it may be used just as effectively on posterior abutments when esthetics is not a factor.

The fact that a crown ledge is to be used should be known in advance of crown preparation to assure sufficient removal of tooth structure in this area. Although a shoulder or ledge is not included in the preparation itself, adequate space must be provided so that the ledge may be made sufficiently wide and the surface above it may be made parallel to the path of placement. The ledge should be placed at the junction of the gingival and middle third of the tooth, curving slightly to follow the curvature of the gingival tissues. On the side of the tooth at which the clasp arm will originate, the

ledge must be kept low enough to allow the origin of the clasp arm to be wide enough for sufficient strength and rigidity.

In forming the crown ledge, which is usually located on the lingual surface, the wax pattern of the crown is completed except for refinement of the margins before the ledge is carved. After the proximal guiding planes and the occlusal rests and retentive contours are formed, the ledge is carved with the surveyor blade so that the surface above is parallel to the path of placement. Thus, a continuous guiding plane surface will exist from the proximal around the lingual surface, the difference being only that the lingual portion ends in a definite ledge and the proximal does not.

The full effectiveness of the crown ledge cannot be had with a crown that is not returned to the surveyor for refinement after casting. To afford true reciprocation, the crown casting must have a surface above

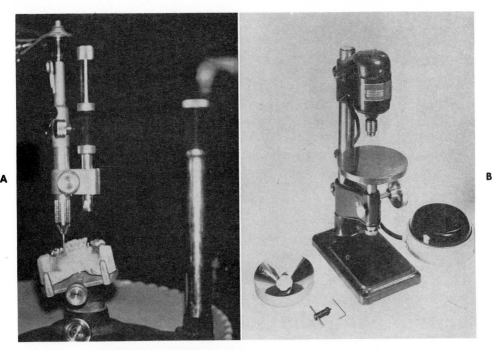

Fig. 13-9. A, Faro laboratory handpiece attached to a Ney surveyor by means of a handpiece holder. With the use of a bur or stone, the lingual surface and ledge are machined in relation to the previously established path of placement. **B,** Austenal Micro-Drill used to mill internal rest seats and lingual grooves and ledges in cast gold restorations. Such a device permits more precise milling than is possible with a dental handpiece attached to a dental surveyor. To be effective, the cast must be positioned on the Micro-Drill in such a manner that the previously established path of placement is maintained. The movable stage or base, therefore, should be adjustable until the relation of the cast to the axis of the drill has been made the same as that obtained when the cast was on the dental surveyor. (**B** courtesy Austenal, Inc., Chicago, Ill.)

the ledge that is parallel to the path of placement. This can be accomplished with precision only by machining the casting parallel to the path of placement with a handpiece holder in the surveyor or some other suitable machining device (Fig. 13-9). Similarly, the parallelism of proximal guiding planes needs to be perfected after casting and polishing. Although it is possible to *approximate* parallelism and, at the same time, form the crown ledge on the wax pattern with a surveyor blade, some of its accuracy is lost in casting and polishing. The use of suitable burs such as Nos. 557, 558, and 559 fissure burs and true cylindrical carborundum stones in the handpiece holder permits the paralleling of all guiding planes on the finished casting with the accuracy necessary to the effectiveness

of those guiding plane surfaces (Figs. 13-10 to 13-12).

The reciprocal clasp arm is ultimately waxed on the investment cast so that it is continuous with the ledge inferiorly and contoured superiorly to restore the crown contour including the tip of the cusp. It is obvious that polishing must not be allowed to destroy the form of the shoulder that was prepared in wax nor destroy the parallelism of the guiding plane surface. It is equally vital that the denture casting must be polished with great care so that the accuracy of the counterpart is not destroyed. Modern investments, casting alloys, and polishing techniques make this degree of accuracy possible. Only the human element, by carelessness or lack of understanding, may fail to produce a crown

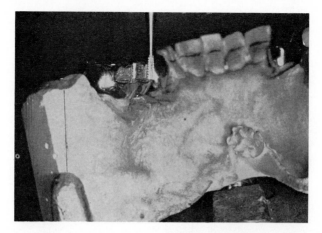

Fig. 13-10. Lingual ledges on cast gold crowns are machined, using a No. 558 dental bur. Experience has shown that in the absence of a rigid jig for holding the cast, a bur is difficult to use. Therefore, it is best that the ledge be formed as accurately as possible in the wax pattern and that machining of the finished casting be done with a cylindrical carborundum point. Note the scratch line on the left posterior portion of the cast, indicating the path of placement.

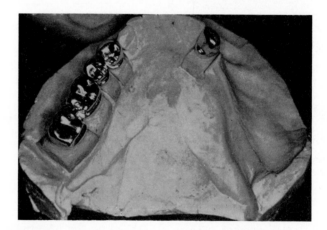

Fig. 13-11. Lingual ledges after machining and polishing. Note that embrasures for clasping are also machined parallel to the path of placement and that occlusal rests are used in addition to the supporting ledges. These are to prevent tooth separation and to shunt food away from interproximal areas.

and counterpart with the desired accuracy. It is just as necessary for the technician to understand the purpose of the crown ledge as it is for the dentist who designs and plans for its use.

VENEER CROWNS FOR THE SUPPORT OF CLASP ARMS

Resin and porcelain veneer crowns are used for cosmetic reasons on abutment teeth that would otherwise display an objectionable amount of metal. They may be in the form of porcelain veneers retained by pins and cemented to the crown, porcelain fused directly to a cast crown, or acrylic resin processed directly to a cast crown.

The retentive clasp terminal should rest on metal when an acrylic resin veneer crown is utilized as an abutment restora-

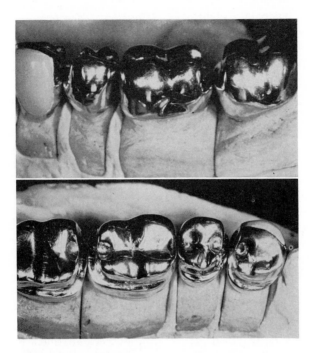

Fig. 13-12. Buccal and lingual views of abutment crowns designed to accept embrasure clasps and lingual reciprocal arms resting on prepared ledges. All surfaces above the ledges are made parallel with the path of placement. Note the size and form of the occlusal rests on either side of the embrasure ledges.

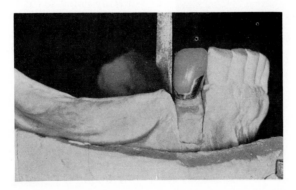

Fig. 13-13. Close-up view of the relation of the surveyor blade to the distal surface of an abutment crown. Note that this guiding plane is made parallel to the path of placement as indicated by the scratch line on the base of the cast. Note also the gold surface on the veneer crown where the retentive terminus of the clasp arm will rest.

tion (Fig. 13-13). In this instance, the crown is contoured to be retentive in the desired area, and that area is not included in carving the space for the veneer. Whereas the suprabulge portion of the clasp arm crosses the surface of the veneer, the portion that crosses the height of contour and engages an undercut in which abrasion could occur is supported by the metal of the crown itself. The only disadvantage of a veneer crown so prepared is the display of metal, which, more often than not, is on the mesial side of the abutment tooth and therefore is cosmetically objectionable.

If the veneer crown is not contoured to provide retention on metal, suitable retention does not exist until the veneer has been added. This means that the veneer must be slightly overcontoured and then shaped to provide the desired undercut for the location of the retentive clasp arm (Fig. 13-14). If the veneer is of procelain, this procedure must precede glazing, and if of resin, before final polishing. If this most important step in the making of veneered abutments is neglected or omitted, excessive or inadequate retentive contours may result, to the detriment of effective clasp design.

The flat underside of a cast clasp makes sufficient contact with the surface of the

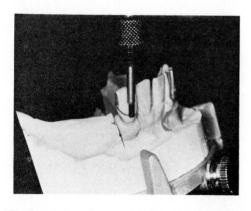

Fig. 13-14. Porcelain veneer crown is resurveyed prior to glazing. At this stage the veneered portion can be recontoured by grinding to achieve the optimal height of contour to place the bracing and retentive portion of the planned clasp assembly.

veneer so that abrasion of a resin veneer may result. Although the underside of the clasp may be polished (with some loss in accuracy of fit), abrasion results from the trapping and holding of food debris against the tooth surface as the clasp moves during function. *Therefore, unless the retentive clasp terminal rests on metal, glazed porcelain should be used to assure the future retentiveness of the veneered surface.* Present-day acrylic resins, being cross-linked copolymers, are much harder than formerly and will withstand abrasion for considerable time but not to the same degree as porcelain. Therefore acrylic resin veneers are used best in conjunction with exposed metal supporting the half-round clasp terminal.

SPLINTING OF ABUTMENT TEETH

Frequently a tooth is deemed too weak to use alone as a partial denture abutment because of the short length and/or excessive taper of a single root or because of bone loss resulting in an unfavorable crown-root ratio. In such instances, splinting of weak abutment teeth to the adjacent tooth or teeth is utilized as a means of gaining *multiple abutment support.* Thus two single-rooted teeth may be used as a multirooted abutment.

Splinting should not be used to retain a tooth that would otherwise be condemned for periodontal reasons, in the futile hope that by doing so the tooth may be retained. Such a gamble may be justified when, if successful, the need for a prosthetic restoration would be avoided. However, when the length of service of a restoration may depend upon the serviceability of an abutment, any periodontally questionable tooth should be condemned in favor of using an adjacent healthy tooth as the abutment, even though the span is increased one tooth by doing so.

The most frequent application of the use of multiple abutments is the splinting of two premolars or a first premolar and a canine. Mandibular premolars generally have round and tapered roots, which are easily loosened by rotation as well as by tipping. They are the weakest of posterior abutments. But maxillary premolars also often have tapered roots, which make them also poor risks as abutments, particularly when they will be called upon to resist the leverage of a distal extension base. Such teeth are best splinted by casting or soldering two crowns or inlays together. When a first premolar to be used as an abutment has poor root form or support, it is best that it be splinted to the stronger canine in a similar manner.

Anterior teeth upon which lingual rests are to be placed frequently need to be splinted together to avoid orthodontic movement of individual teeth. Mandibular anterior teeth are seldom so used, but if they are, splinting of the teeth involved is advisable. When such splinting is impossible for one reason or another, individual lingual rests on cast restorations may be inclined slightly toward the center of the tooth to avoid possible tooth displacement, or lingual rests may be used in conjunction with incisal rests, engaging slightly the labial surface of the teeth.

Lingual rests should always be placed as low on the cingulum as possible, and single anterior teeth, other than canines, should not ordinarily be used for occlusal support. Where lingual rests are employed on central and lateral incisors, as many teeth as possible should be included to distribute the load over several teeth, thereby minimizing the force on any one tooth. Even so, some movement of individual teeth is likely to occur, particularly when they are subjected to the forces of indirect retention. This is best avoided by splinting several teeth with united cast restorations. The condition of the teeth and cosmetic considerations will dictate whether full veneer crowns, three-quarter crowns, or pinledge inlays will be used for this purpose.

Splinting of molar teeth for multiple abutment support is less frequently used, because they are generally multirooted teeth to begin with and a two- or three-rooted tooth that is not strong enough

alone is probably a poor abutment risk. There may be exceptions, however, that are notable when, because of fused and conical roots, the abutment would benefit from the effect of splinting.

USE OF ISOLATED TEETH AS ABUTMENTS

Although splinting is advocated for any abutment teeth that are considered too weak to risk using alone, a single anterior abutment standing alone in the dental arch generally requires the splinting effect of a fixed partial denture if a distal extension base will extend from it. Even though the form and length of the root and the supporting bone seem to be adequate for an ordinary abutment, the fact that the tooth lacks proximal contact endangers the tooth when it is used to support a distal extension base.

The average abutment tooth is subjected to some distal tipping, to rotation, and to horizontal movement, all of which must be held to a minimum by the design of the denture and the quality of tissue support for the distal extension base. The isolated abutment tooth, however, is subjected also to mesial tipping because of lack of proximal contact. Despite indirect retention, some lifting of the distal extension base is inevitable, causing torque to the abutment as the fulcrum of a teeter-totter.

In a tooth-borne prosthesis an isolated tooth may be used as an abutment by using a fifth abutment for additional support. Thus, rotational and horizontal forces are resisted by the additional stabilization obtained from the fifth abutment. When two such isolated abutments exist, that is, two second premolars with first premolars missing, the sixth abutment should be used. Thus the two canines, the two isolated premolars, and two posterior teeth are used as abutments.

In contrast, an isolated anterior abutment adjacent to a distal extension base usually should be splinted to the nearest tooth by means of a fixed partial denture. The effect is twofold: (1) the anterior edentulous segment is eliminated, thereby creating an intact dental arch anterior to the space; and (2) the isolated tooth is splinted to the other abutment of the fixed partial denture, thereby providing multiple abutment support. Here, also, splinting should be used only to gain multiple abutment support rather than to support an otherwise weak abutment tooth.

The economic aspect of using fixed restorations as part of the mouth preparations for a partial denture is essentially the same as that for any other splinting procedure: the best design of the partial denture that will assure the longevity of its service makes the additional procedure and expense necessary. Although it must be recognized that economic considerations, combined with a particularly favorable prognosis of an isolated tooth, may influence the decision to forego the advantages of using a fixed partial denture, the original treatment plan should include this precautionary measure even though the alternative method is accepted for economic reasons.

A second factor may also influence the decision to use an isolated tooth as an abutment; this is the esthetic consideration for an otherwise sound anterior tooth that would have to be used as an abutment for a fixed restoration. However neither esthetics nor economics should deter the dentist from recommending to the patient that an isolated tooth that will be used as a terminal abutment be given the advantage of splinting by means of a fixed partial denture. Then, if compromises are necessary, the patient must share a measure of the responsibility for using the isolated tooth as an abutment.

MISSING ANTERIOR TEETH

When a partial denture is to replace missing posterior teeth, especially in the absence of distal abutments, any additional missing teeth anteriorly are best replaced by means of fixed restorations rather than by being added to the denture. In any distal extension situation, some teeter-totter

action will inevitably result from the adding of an anterior segment to the denture. Here again, the ideal treatment plan that treats the anterior edentulous space separately comes in conflict with economic and esthetic considerations. Each situation must be treated according to its own merits. Frequently, the best esthetic result can be obtained by replacing missing anterior teeth with the partial denture rather than with a fixed restoration. From a biomechanical standpoint, however, a partial denture should replace only the missing posterior teeth, *after* the remainder of the arch has been made intact by means of fixed restorations.

Although the occasional need for compromises is recognized, the decision to include an anterior segment on the denture will depend largely upon the support available for that part of the denture. The greater the number of natural anterior teeth remaining, the better the support that will be available for the edentulous segment.

If definite rests are obtainable, the anterior segment may be treated as any other tooth-bounded modification space. Sound principles of rest support apply just as much as elsewhere in the arch. *Inclined tooth surfaces should not be used for occlusal support, nor should rests be placed upon unprepared lingual surfaces.* The best possible support for an anterior segment is multiple support extending, if possible, posteriorly across prepared lingual rest seats on the canine teeth to mesial occlusal rest seats on the first premolars. Such support will permit the missing anterior teeth to be included in the denture, frequently with some cosmetic advantages over fixed restorations.

In some instances the replacement of anterior teeth by means of a partial denture cannot be avoided. However, without adequate tooth support, any such prosthesis will lack the stability that would exist from replacing only the posterior teeth with the partial denture and the anterior teeth with fixed restorations. When anterior teeth have been lost through accident or have been missing for some time, resorption of the anterior ridge may have progressed to the point that neither fixed nor removable pontics may be butted to the residual ridge. In such instances, for esthetic reasons, the missing teeth must be replaced with a denture base supporting teeth that are more nearly in their original position, considerably forward from the residual ridge. Although such teeth may be positioned to better cosmetic advantage, the contouring and coloring of a denture base to be esthetically pleasing requires the maximum artistic effort of both the dentist and the technologist. Such a partial denture, both from an esthetic and a biomechanical standpoint, is one of the most difficult of all prosthetic restorations. However, a splint bar, connected by abutments on both sides of the edentulous space, will provide much-needed support to the anterior segment of the removable partial denture. Since the splint bar will act as an occlusal rest, rest seats on abutments adjacent to the edentulous area need not be prepared, thus simplifying an anterior restoration to some extent.

TEMPORARY CROWNS AND TEMPORARY FIXED PARTIAL DENTURES

Each time a tooth is prepared for a full crown, a temporary crown must be placed for the protection and comfort of the exposed dentin. Ideally, this crown will restore occlusion and contact, although not necessarily so.

Most inlay preparations may be filled with a thick mix of white WondrPak cement. Occasionally, this may suffice also for a three-quarter crown preparation when only the deeper grooves need to be filled. However, for most three-quarter crown preparations and for large inlay preparations, a temporary acrylic resin crown is used in preference to the WondrPak alone. In any case, WondrPak is the preferred cementing medium.

Individual full crown preparations, when esthetics does not prevent their use, may be satisfactorily covered with fitted aluminum crowns. Contact and occlusion may be less than ideal, but the length of time the crown will be worn is usually short. Temporary crowns should be trimmed short of the gingival tissues and should be smoothed and contoured to eliminate rough edges. The temporary crown should protect the tooth, yet should not interfere with gingival healing nor induce inflammation that might cause gingival pathology or recession.

For esthetic reasons, anterior temporary crowns should be made of a rapid-curing acrylic resin of a matching tooth shade or polycarbonate crowns should be used. Anterior temporary fixed partial dentures may also be made of resin, and even posterior fixed partial dentures when better esthetics or occlusion is desirable. Single acrylic resin crowns may be made by filling a contoured copper band with the tooth-shade resin and pressing onto the prepared tooth that has been coated with petrolatum (Fig. 13-15). On anterior teeth the copper band may be pinched labiolingually to form a more natural tooth contour. *In any direct application of tooth-shade resin for temporary purposes, the crown must be removed and reseated while the material is still plastic, to make sure that the hardened crown will withdraw.* After hardening, the crown is removed and the copper band is slit on the lingual side and stripped away. The crown may then be ground to resemble the tooth being restored, polished, and cemented with temporary cement. Such a temporary crown provides excellent esthetics and fit and will serve for an indefinite period if necessary.

Individual acrylic resin crowns may also be made by the same methods as those used for making a temporary fixed partial denture. Once a technique has been adopted, acrylic resin temporary crowns are quickly made and are preferable because of their appearance and the fact that their natural contours are much more comfortable to the patient. Several methods for making acrylic resin temporary crowns

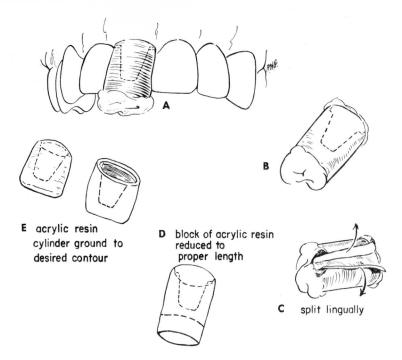

Fig. 13-15. Making of a single anterior resin temporary crown. **A,** A contoured copper band that has been flattened labiolingually is filled with acrylic resin of the correct shade and pressed onto the prepared tooth that has been coated with petrolatum. **B,** When the acrylic resin has reached a leathery consistency, the copper band is removed from the tooth momentarily and then reseated onto the tooth until the resin has hardened. This is necessary to assure the withdrawal of the hardened acrylic resin without difficulty. **C,** As soon as the acrylic resin has hardened, the copper band is slit longitudinally with a carborundum disk and peeled off. **D,** The acrylic resin coping, which will be shaped in the form of a temporary crown, is placed back onto the tooth and marked with a pencil where excess thickness and occlusal interference is to be reduced. This is repeated until a temporary crown of acceptable contours has been formed. At the same time, any flash extending beyond abutment shoulders must be removed. **E,** The acrylic resin crown is then polished and temporarily cemented to the abutment tooth.

and temporary fixed restorations are outlined as follows:

1. a. An impression is made of the mouth before the tooth or teeth are prepared. This impression may be made in alginate hydrocolloid or with baseplate wax in a fixed partial denture impression tray. The use of baseplate wax is expedient, inexpensive, does not require special handling during the interlude, and is rigid enough to permit compression molding. It is easily carved to create teeth to be added and is easily trimmed to increase the thickness of temporary crowns when little tooth structure has been removed, such as in the gingival one third.

Prior to making this impression, missing tooth contours should be restored with inlay wax so that an impression of intact tooth surfaces can be made. If missing teeth are to be replaced, they may be waxed into the space or a denture tooth may be fitted into each space before the impression is made. An alternate method is to carve the tooth form of the tooth or teeth to be replaced into the impression, which is then filled and shaped along with adjacent crowns. By placing some of the impression material on the opposite side of the tray and having the patient close into it, a means of stabilizing the tray in the mouth later is established. The patient then may close into the impression, thus making it unnecessary for the dentist to hold it while the plastic resin material is setting.

b. Rather than making an impression of the mouth before the preparations are begun, the dentist or assistant may make an impression of a previous diagnostic cast, after artificial tooth replacements have been waxed in to form the temporary pontics.

Whether method a or b is used, the impression should be trimmed to eliminate undercut areas and projections into interproximal spaces, which would interfere with reseating. If the impression is of alginate hydrocolloid, it must be wrapped in a wet towel and set aside while the teeth are being prepared. A baseplate wax impression may be set aside without any special precautions.

2. a. After the preparations are completed and impressions for working casts and jaw relations have been made, the prepared teeth are dried and coated with petroleum jelly. If the original impression was made with alginate hydrocolloid, it is now removed from the wet towel and dried with compressed air.

The portion of the impression involving the crowns is now filled with a self-curing acrylic resin of the desired shade. Although powder and liquid may be mixed to form a dough, a sprinkling method is preferred. At the time of this writing, a material known as Jet repair acrylic resin is available in New-Hue shades and has proved to be a nearly ideal material for making temporary crowns and temporary fixed partial dentures. The powder is packaged in a flexible container that permits dispensing without waste and is therefore both economical and convenient to use for filling tooth molds by sprinkling. Sprinkle some powder into the mold first and then wet with liquid from a medicine dropper. This is repeated until the mold is filled, tapping the impression on the bench each time to facilitate absorption. After the crown area is filled, any excess that has flowed into other areas should be removed with a pledget of cotton. The material must then be allowed to

reach a soft, rubbery state before it is seated onto the petrolatum-coated teeth.

Using the unprepared teeth as a guide, the impression is reseated into the mouth and held until sufficient time has elapsed for the material to reach a stiff rubbery consistency. Unfortunately, this must come from experience with the particular resin material being used. It is necessary that the crowns be removed once before the material has hardened, to assure their withdrawal. Preferably, the rubbery plastic will remain in the impression at this time. It then may be removed from the impression, excess material trimmed away with fine scissors, and reseated in the impression. The impression is then reseated in the mouth to finish compression molding of the plastic resin while it hardens. After time has elapsed for hardening, the impression is removed. This time the hardened resin will remain on the teeth, but having been removed once, it may easily be tapped off, trimmed, and polished. Parallelism of abutment teeth is an absolute necessity when temporary fixed partial dentures are made by this method. Otherwise, serious difficulty may be encountered in attempting to remove the rigid, temporary resin restoration. To avoid this hazard, the rubbery plastic resin may be allowed to harden in the impression out of the mouth. If the material has reached a stiff rubbery state before removal from the mouth, this does not seem to materially affect its accuracy. (Even a well-fitting temporary crown should be reamed slightly to accommodate the temporary cement and make its subsequent removal less difficult.) After the material has hardened, it is removed from the impression, the excess trimmed away, and then polished, taking care to preserve the accuracy of the gingival margins.

b. Rather than forming the temporary crowns or temporary fixed partial denture in the mouth, the following alternate method may be used: As soon as the preparations are completed, an alginate hydrocolloid impression of the prepared teeth is made and poured immediately in stone.

The making of this impression should precede the making of other impressions, which may then be made while the stone cast is hardening. Retraction of tissues is not necessary for this impression, and if some of the alginate hydrocolloid is first smeared onto the prepared teeth with the finger, the impression will be relatively free of defects.

As soon as the cast can be separated from the hydrocolloid impression of the prepared teeth, any small air bubbles are removed and the cast is then painted with a tin-foil substitute. The original impression is filled with tooth-shade resin as in 2a, but rather than being placed back into the mouth, it is seated onto the cast of the prepared teeth. It is removed while rubbery, as before, the excess trimmed with scissors, and then reseated until it hardens. This method differs from method 2a only in that the prepared teeth are made more accessible and the danger of damage to the mouth during removal of the hardened resin is avoided. If the stone teeth fracture during removal, no harm has been done, and the stone may be removed from the hardened resin crowns.

The alginate hydrocolloid impression of the prepared teeth may be poured in low-fusing metal rather than stone and thus separated immediately rather than waiting for the stone to set. Although some cooling shrinkage of the metal occurs, temporary crowns made on such a die can be reamed slightly if necessary. This usually should be done anyway to allow for the thickness of the temporary cement and to make removal of the crowns easier. The impression should be dried thoroughly with compressed air before pouring the low-fusing metal (such as Dialoy) into it. The molten metal should be poured from the ladle when just slightly above the congealing point rather than immediately after removal from the flame. This avoids sizzling and results in a more accurate cast.

Low-fusing metal may also be used to advantage in other ways when an immediate cast is desired. For example, during the preparation of abutment teeth, there may be some question as to the parallelism of the preparation or of two or more fixed partial denture abutments. An alginate hydrocolloid impression of the prepared and adjacent teeth may be poured in low-fusing metal and separated immediately. In this way the dentist may see what further modifications are necessary before proceeding. Since the low-fusing metal is reusable, little time and material are used, and the possibility of making final impressions of inadequate preparations is thus eliminated.

TEMPORARY CROWNS WHEN A PARTIAL DENTURE IS BEING WORN

Occasionally, an existing removable partial denture must remain serviceable while the mouth is being prepared for a new denture. In such situations, temporary crowns that will support the old denture and not interfere with its placement and removal must be made. Only rarely can an aluminum crown be made to serve this purpose. Instead, an acrylic resin temporary crown that duplicates the original form of the abutment tooth must be made (Fig. 13-16).

The technique for making temporary crowns to fit the inside of direct retainers is similar to that given for other types of acrylic resin temporary crowns. The principal difference is that an alginate hydrocolloid impression must be made of the entire arch with the existing partial denture in place. This is wrapped in a wet towel and set aside while the tooth or teeth are being prepared for new crowns.

After the preparations are completed and the impressions and jaw relation records have been made, the prepared teeth are dried and coated with petroleum jelly. The original alginate hydrocolloid impression is trimmed to eliminate any excess, undercuts, and interproximal projections that would interfere with its replacement in the mouth.

The tooth-shade resin is sprinkled into the impression in those areas that are to be temporary crowns, and any excess is removed with a pledget of cotton. When the material reaches a soft rubbery state,

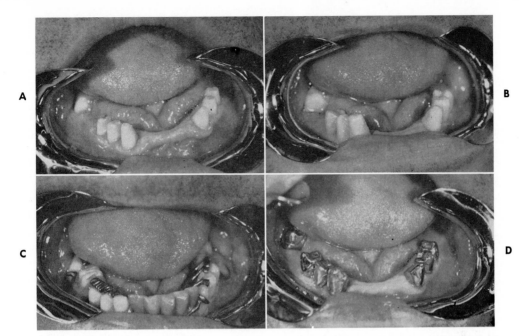

Fig. 13-16. Sequence of mouth preparations with temporary crowns formed to support an existing partial denture while a new one is being made. **A,** Several abutment teeth have been prepared to receive full coverage crowns. **B,** Acrylic resin temporary crowns duplicating the original tooth contour. An impression of the teeth before preparation was begun was used to establish the shape of the temporary crowns. **C,** The existing partial denture, seated onto the temporary crowns. These are then removed as often as necessary during succeeding appointments. **D,** Gold castings are tried in, prior to soldering and adding veneers. The temporary crowns and existing partial denture are then returned to the mouth until the abutment pieces are ready for cementation.

the impression is seated into the mouth, where it is held by the dentist until time has elapsed for it to reach a stiff rubbery stage. This again must be based on experience with the particular plastic material being used. At this time, the impression is removed, the crowns remaining in the impression. These are then stripped out of the impression; all excess is trimmed away with scissors, and the crowns are reseated on the prepared abutments. The partial denture is then removed from the alginate impression and reseated in the mouth onto the plastic crowns, which are at this time in a stiff rubbery state. The patient may bring the teeth into occlusion to reestablish the former position and occlusal relationship of the existing partial denture.

After the plastic crown or crowns have hardened, the partial denture is removed,

the crowns remaining on the teeth. These are then tapped off, trimmed, polished, and temporarily cemented. The result is a temporary crown that restores the original abutment contours and allows the partial denture to be placed and removed without interference, at the same time providing the same support temporarily to the denture that existed before the teeth were prepared. This service, made possible by modern materials, should be routine for all patients requiring such service.

Cementation of temporary crowns. Cementation of acrylic resin temporary crowns differs from the cementation of aluminum crowns in that the plastic crowns fit closely and do not require cementation for retention. Since little or no space exists for the temporary cement, the crowns may need to be reamed slightly to accommodate the temporary cement and to facilitate removal. The temporary cement should be thin and applied only to the inside rim of the crowns to assure complete seating. As soon as the temporary cement has hardened, the occlusion may be checked and relieved accordingly.

Regardless of the type of temporary cement used, any excess that might be irritating to the gingivae should be removed. Too frequently, the final act before dismissing the patient is the cementation of the temporary crowns. Instead, two considerations are necessary. One is the removal of excess cement after it has hardened. The second is the application of some medication to the lacerated gingivae to facilitate healing and to prevent discomfort to the patient. Topical application of some antibacterial agent is, at best, a transient treatment that does little to prevent discomfort. Hydrocortisone acetate, 0.5%, in a denture adhesive powder, when applied topically to a freshly lacerated surface, both facilitates healing and prevents after-pain. It should be applied to the lacerated gingivae around each temporary crown and the patient dismissed without further rinsing of the mouth. Tissue response to this treatment has been so favorable that it is included here as a specific treatment. Apparently, it is effective only on fresh wounds and is of little value as a follow-up treatment.

THE MAKING OF CROWNS AND INLAYS TO FIT EXISTING DENTURE RETAINERS

It is frequently necessary that an abutment tooth be restored with a full crown (and occasionally with an inlay) that will fit the inside of the clasp of an otherwise serviceable partial denture. The technique for doing so is simple enough but requires that an indirect-direct-indirect pattern be made and therefore justifies a fee for service above that for the usual full crown.

The technique for making a crown to fit the inside of a clasp is as follows: An alginate hydrocolloid impression of the mouth is made with the partial denture in place.

This impression, which is used to make the plastic temporary crown, is wrapped in a wet towel and set aside while the tooth is being prepared. Even though several abutment teeth are to be restored, it is usually necessary that each one be completed before beginning the next. This is necessary so that the original support and occlusal relationship of the partial denture can be maintained as each new crown is being made.

The abutment tooth is then prepared, during which time the partial denture is replaced frequently enough to ascertain that sufficient tooth structure is being removed to allow for the thickness of the gold casting. When the preparation is completed, a copper band impression of the tooth is obtained, from which a stone die is made.

An acrylic resin temporary crown is then made in the original alginate hydrocolloid impression as outlined in the preceding paragraphs. It is trimmed, polished, and temporarily cemented, and the denture is returned to the mouth. The patient is dismissed after removing excess cement and treating the traumatized gingiva, as mentioned previously.

Upon the stone die made from the copper band impression, a thin self-curing resin coping will be formed with a brush technique. The stone die should first be trimmed to the finishing line of the preparation, which is then delineated with a pencil, and the die painted with a tin-foil substitute. A material such as Al-Cote tin-foil substitute should be used, which will form a thin film on a cold, dry surface. Not all tin-foil substitutes are suitable for this purpose.

With self-curing acrylic resin powder and liquid in separate dappen dishes and a fine sable brush, a coping of acrylic resin of uniform thickness is painted onto the die. This should extend not quite to the pencil line representing the limit of the crown preparation. After hardening, the resin coping may be removed, inspected, and trimmed if necessary. The thin film of foil

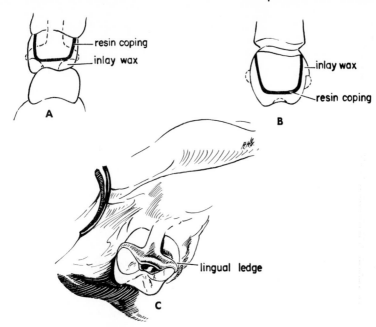

Fig. 13-17. Making of a cast crown to fit an existing partial denture clasp. **A,** A thin resin coping is first made on an individual die of the prepared tooth. Inlay wax is then added and the coping placed onto the prepared tooth when occlusal surfaces and contact relations are established directly in the mouth. The clasp assembly is warmed with a needle-point flame only enough to soften the inlay wax, and the partial denture is placed in the mouth where it is guided gently to place by the opposing occlusion. This step must be repeated several times and excess wax removed or wax added until full supporting contact with the underside of the clasp assembly has been established, with the denture fully seated. Usually the wax pattern withdraws with the denture and must be gently teased out of the clasp each time. **B,** The wax pattern is then placed back onto the individual die to complete occlusal anatomy and refine the margins. Excess wax remaining below the impression of the retentive clasp arm must be removed, but a wax ledge may be left below the reciprocal clasp arm. **C,** The finished casting in the mouth. The terminus of the retentive clasp is then readapted to engage an undercut. It is frequently necessary to remove some interference from the casting, as indicated by articulating paper placed between the clasp and the crown, until the clasp is fully seated.

substitute should be removed before re-seating the coping onto the die.

The wax pattern is usually not begun until the patient returns, at which time it is built up at the chair. First, the occlusal portion of the wax pattern is established by having the patient close and carve excursive paths in the wax (Fig. 13-17, *A*). Dull areas are added to until a smooth occlusal registration has been obtained. Except for narrowing the occlusal surface and the carving of grooves and spillways, this will be the occlusal anatomy of the finished restoration.

The second step is the adding of suffi-cient wax to establish contact relations with the adjoining tooth. At this time, the occlusal relation of the marginal ridges also must be established.

Next, wax is added to buccal and lingual surfaces where the clasp arms will contact the crown, and the pattern is again reseated in the mouth. The clasp arms, minor connectors, and occlusal rests involved on the partial denture are warmed with a needle-point flame, being careful to avoid flaming any adjacent resin, and the denture is positioned in the mouth and onto the wax pattern (Fig. 13-17, *B*). Several attempts may be necessary until the denture is fully seated and the components of the clasp clearly recorded in the wax pattern. Each time the denture is removed, the pattern will draw with it and must be teased out of the clasp.

When contact with the clasp arms and the occlusal relation of the denture has been established satisfactorily, the temporary crown may be replaced and the patient dismissed. The crown pattern is completed on the die by narrowing the occlusal surface buccolingually, adding grooves and spillways, and refining the margins.* Any wax ledge remaining below the reciprocal clasp arm may be left to provide some of the advantages of a crown ledge described earlier in this chapter. Excess wax remaining below the retentive clasp arm, however, must be removed to permit the adding of a retentive undercut later (Fig. 13-17, *C*).

If an acrylic resin veneer is to be added, the veneer space must now be carved in the wax pattern. In such case, the contour of the veneer may be recorded by making a stone matrix of the buccal surface, which can later be replaced onto the completed casting for waxing in the veneer. This stone matrix is then invested with the casting when the acrylic resin veneer is being processed.

The wax pattern must be sprued with care so that essential areas on the pattern are not destroyed. After casting, the crown should be subjected to a minimum of polishing, since the exact form of the vertical and occlusal surfaces must be maintained.

Since it is impossible to withdraw a clasp arm from a retentive undercut on the wax pattern, the casting must be made without any provision for clasp retention. After

trying the crown in the mouth, with the denture in place, the location of the retentive clasp terminal is identified by scoring the crown with a sharp instrument. Then the crown may be ground and polished slightly in this area to create a retentive undercut. The clasp terminal then may be carefully adapted into this undercut, thereby creating clasp retention on the new crown.

The technique for making inlay patterns to fit the inside of denture clasps is essentially the same as for full crowns, except that it may be done entirely in wax. However, patterns for larger inlays that might be distorted during placement of the denture are best supported also by an acrylic resin foundation. In such cases, the pattern is started by brushing in the acrylic resin until a supporting frame has been established. The wax pattern is then completed in the mouth as for a full crown.

Ideally, all abutment teeth would best be protected with full crowns before the partial denture is constructed. Except for the possibility of recurrent caries because of defective crown margins or gingival recession, abutment teeth so protected may be expected to give many years of satisfactory service in the support and retention of the partial denture. Economically, a policy of insisting on full coverage for all abutment teeth may well be justified from the long-term view point. It must be recognized, however, that in practice full coverage of all abutment teeth is not always possible nor at the time indicated. Many factors act to influence the future health status of an abutment tooth, some of which cannot be foreseen. It is necessary, therefore, that the dentist be able to treat abutment teeth that become defective at some later date in such a manner that their service as abutments may be restored and the serviceability of the partial denture maintained. Although it is not part of the original mouth preparations, this service accomplishes much the same objective by providing the denture with support, stability, and retention, and the dentist must be techni-

---

*Margins on all crown and inlay wax patterns are refined with S. S. White red casting wax, which contrasts with the blue or green wax used for the pattern and permits the carving of delicate margins with accuracy. The preferred wax for the body of crown and inlay patterns is Maves inlay wax. This wax is available in both cone and stick form and has excellent carving properties and color.

cally equipped to provide this service when it becomes necessary.

CEMENTATION FOR FIXED RESTORATIONS

Final cementation of fixed restorations should be deferred until evidence of the success of the restoration can be evaluated. Single crowns may be cemented permanently more often than fixed partial dentures. It seems that nonpermanent cementation of fixed restorations has many advantages and few disadvantages. Zinc oxide and eugenol temporary cements will adequately retain the restoration and protect the abutment teeth, yet may be removed without difficulty for future inspection of the abutments and the adjacent tissues. The restoration then may be cemented permanently or again only semipermanently. Restorations have been removed after intervals as long as five years without evidence of leakage or deterioration of zinc oxide–eugenol cements.

Advantages of semipermanent cementation of fixed restorations. Some of the advantages of semipermanent cementation are as follows:

1. By cementing the restoration temporarily at first, the dentist can be sure that the crowns are fully seated and that the margins are satisfactory.

2. Less postoperative discomfort generally results from cementation with a temporary cement. Temporary cements are sedative, while zinc oxyphosphate cements are irritating to a pulp suffering already from trauma caused by operative procedures.

3. Restorations may be removed to inspect the tooth beneath and to take roentgenograms. The hazard of a single leaking abutment piece causing destruction of the tooth before it is detected can thus be eliminated.

4. Restorations may be removed to inspect and treat gingival and subjacent tissues. Future periodontal treatment is thus facilitated.

5. If root canal therapy becomes necessary, treatment may be accomplished without cutting through a cemented restoration.

6. Porcelain or acrylic resin pontics may be extended when needed to compensate for changes in the residual ridge.

7. Acrylic resin veneers may be replaced if they are lost or if they have become discolored or the shade no longer matches the aging enamel on adjacent teeth.

8. Fractured porcelain veneers or pontics may be more satisfactorily replaced.

9. Solder joints may be reinforced if they become weakened by attrition.

10. Future addition of another abutment for increased support is made possible.

11. Patient is encouraged to return at recommended intervals for inspection and maintenance. In this way the dentist has an opportunity at reasonable intervals to inspect both the fixed restorations and any removable partial dentures present and to recommend relining or the reestablishment of occlusion of partial dentures when needed. Also oral hygiene habits may be noted and the patient advised accordingly.

Patients seem quick to appreciate the value of semipermanent cementation, particularly for fixed partial dentures, and are prone to request a continuation of the practice. To the patient, as to the dentist, permanent cementation appears to be an irrevocable act that has fewer advantages than cementation with a reliable, semipermanent material.

CHAPTER 14

Impression materials and procedures for removable partial dentures

Impression materials used in the various phases of partial denture construction may be classified as being rigid, thermoplastic, or elastic substances. Rigid impression materials are those that set to a rigid consistency. Thermoplastic impression materials are those that become plastic at higher temperatures and resume their original form when the temperature has again been lowered. Elastic impression materials are those that remain in an elastic or flexible state after removal from the mouth.

Most impression materials used in prosthetic dentistry may be included in the following classification:

> Rigid materials
> > Plaster of Paris
> > Metallic oxide pastes
> Thermoplastic materials
> > Modeling plastic
> > Impression waxes and resins
> Elastic materials
> > Reversible hydrocolloid (agar-agar)
> > Irreversible hydrocolloid (alginate)
> > Mercaptan rubber-base materials (Thiokol)
> > Silicone materials

Although rigid impression materials may be capable of recording tooth and tissue details accurately, they cannot be removed from the mouth without fracture and reassembly. Thermoplastic materials cannot record minute details accurately because they undergo distortion during withdrawal from tooth and tissue undercuts. Elastic mate-rials are the only ones that can be withdrawn from tooth and tissue undercuts without permanent deformation and are therefore the only ones that are suitable for impressions of irregular contours of oral tissues. Whereas the rigid and thermoplastic impression materials are most frequently used in various combinations in the making of impressions for complete dentures, the elastic impression materials are most generally used for the making of impressions for removable partial dentures, immediate dentures, and crowns and fixed partial dentures when tooth and tissue undercuts and surface detail must be recorded with accuracy.

RIGID MATERIALS*

Plaster of Paris. One type of rigid impression material is plaster of Paris, which has been used in dentistry for over 200 years. Although all plaster-of-Paris impression materials are handled in approximately the same manner, the setting and flow characteristics of each manufacturer's product will vary. Some are pure, finely ground plaster of Paris with only an accelerator added to expedite setting within reasonable

---

*Much of this discussion has been quoted or paraphrased from McCracken, W. L.: Impression materials in prosthetic dentistry, Dent. Clin. North Am., pp. 671-684, Nov., 1958.

working limits. Others are modified impression plaster in which binders and plasticizers have been added to permit limited border molding while the material is setting. These do not set as hard or fracture as clean as pure plaster of Paris and therefore cannot be reassembled with as much accuracy if fracture occurs. However, they are preferred by some dentists because of their setting characteristics.

Plaster of Paris was once the only material that could be used for partial denture impressions, but now elastic materials have completely replaced the impression plasters in this phase of prosthetic dentistry. It is still widely used for making accurate transfers of abutment castings or copings in the fabrication of fixed restorations and internal attachment dentures and for making rigid indexes and matrices for various purposes in prosthetic dentistry.

Metallic oxide pastes. A second type of "rigid impression materials is that classified as metallic oxide pastes, these usually being some form of a zinc oxide–eugenol combination. A number of these pastes are available today and they are probably more widely used than any other secondary impression material." They are not used as primary impression materials and are not used in stock impression trays.

Metallic oxide pastes are manufactured with a wide variation of consistencies and setting characteristics. For convenience, most of them are dispensed from two tubes, an arrangement that enables the dentist to mix the correct proportion from each tube onto a glass or paper mixing slab. The previously prepared tray is loaded and positioned in the mouth with or without any attempt at border molding. Generally, border molding of metallic oxide impression pastes is not advisable, as wrinkles will occur if movement is permitted at the time the material reaches its setting state. Therefore, as in most modern impression techniques, the accuracy of the primary impression and of the impression tray has a great influence upon the final impression. Some metallic oxide pastes remain fluid for a longer period of time than others, and some manufacturers claim that border molding is possible. In general, however, all metallic oxide pastes have one thing in common with plaster of Paris impression materials; this is that they all have a setting time during which they should not be disturbed and after which no further border molding is effective.

Although metallic oxide pastes, being rigid substances, are widely used as secondary impression materials for complete dentures, they are also used for secondary impressions in removable partial denture techniques. One widely used removable partial denture impression technique utilizes a paste impression of the edentulous ridge made in a resin or shellac impression tray, which is then finger-loaded through an opening in a stock perforated tray while an overall alginate hydrocolloid impression is taken of the entire arch. This technique attempts to relate the zinc oxide impression of the edentulous ridge to the rest of the arch in a relationship similar to that which will be assumed when an occlusal load is applied. (See Chapter 15.)

Metallic oxide pastes are also used as an impression material for relining denture bases and may be used successfully for this purpose if the original denture base has been relieved sufficiently to allow the material to flow without displacement of either the denture or the underlying tissues.

THERMOPLASTIC MATERIALS*

Modeling plastic. Like plaster of Paris, modeling plastic is among the oldest of the impression materials used in prosthetic dentistry. It is manufactured "in several different colors, each color being an indication of the temperature range at which the material is plastic and workable. A common error in the use of modeling plastic is that it is subjected to higher temperatures than intended by the manufacturer. It then

*Much of this discussion has been quoted or paraphrased from McCracken, W. L.: Impression materials in prosthetic dentistry, Dent. Clin. North Am., pp. 671-684, Nov., 1958.

becomes too soft and loses [some of] its favorable working characteristics. If a controlled water bath is not used, a thermometer should be used routinely to maintain a temperature within limits that will not cause a weakening of the material or influence its working characteristics. If modeling plastic is softened at a temperature above that intended by the manufacturer, the material becomes brittle and unpredictable. Also, there is the ever-present danger of burning the patient when the temperature used in softening the modeling plastic is too high."

The most commonly used modeling plastic is the red material that, in cake form, softens at about 132° F. It should never be softened at temperatures much above this. Neither it nor any other modeling plastic should be immersed in the water bath for an indefinite period of time. Rather, it should not leave the dentist's fingers during the softening period for more than a few seconds. It should be dipped and kneaded until soft, and it should be subjected to no more heat than necessary before loading the tray and positioning it in the mouth. Then it may be flamed with an alcohol torch for the purpose of border molding but should always be tempered by being dipped back into the water bath before its return to the mouth to avoid burning the patient. The modeling plastic then may be chilled before removal from the mouth, although this is not necessary if care is used in removing the impression. During sectional flaming and border molding, it should be chilled in ice water after each placement. Then it may be trimmed with a sharp knife without danger of fracture or distortion.

The red, gray, and green modeling plastics are obtainable in stick form, for use in border molding an impression or an impression tray. The green material is the lowest fusing of the modeling plastics. The red and gray sticks have a higher and broader working range than do the cakes of like color so that they may be flamed without harming the material. Because of its con-

trasting lighter color, the gray material in stick form is preferred by some dentists for border molding. The choice between the use of green and gray sticks is purely optional and entirely up to the dentist.

Although modeling plastic has been used in past years as an impression material for diagnostic casts, it has now been replaced by the elastic materials. Some dentists still prefer to use modeling plastic as a secondary impression material for the recording of edentulous ridges in partial denture construction, but, when this is done, the limitations and disadvantages are the same as for making a full modeling plastic impression for complete dentures. Similarly, modeling plastic is sometimes used as a reline impression material for partial denture bases. It is generally used, however, only as a means of building up the underside of the denture prior to recording the tissues with some secondary impression material. (See Chapter 15.)

Impression waxes and resins. "A second group of thermoplastic impression materials is those impression waxes and resins commonly spoken of as 'mouth-temperature waxes.' The most familiar of these are the Korecta waxes and the Iowa wax, both of which were developed for specific techniques. One must be cognizant of the characteristics of mouth-temperature waxes and use them knowingly."

The Iowa impression wax, for example, was designed to be used as a wax impression over a modeling plastic correction in an acrylic resin tray. The Korecta waxes were developed to record the supporting form of the edentulous areas, which provide support for a distal extension partial denture base. Although four Korecta waxes are available, the No. 4 wax is the most fluid and is quite similar to the Iowa formula in most respects. In fact, the two waxes may be used interchangeably without any detectable difference in results. The No. 1 Korecta wax is not an impression wax, but is instead a supporting wax that is unaffected by mouth temperature. Therefore, it is used as a means for supporting the impression of the border during the making of fluid wax impressions. The No. 2 and No. 3 Korecta waxes, although developed to provide a broader range of flow characteristics, are not generally used today as impression waxes.

The No. 4 Korecta wax was developed for use in recording the functional or supporting form of an edentulous ridge beneath a distal extension partial denture base. It may be used either as a secondary impression material or as an impression material for rebasing the finished partial denture to obtain support from the underlying tissues. "The mouth-temperature waxes lend themselves well to all rebasing techniques as they will flow sufficiently in the mouth to avoid overdisplacement of tissues. As with any rebasing technique, it is necessary that sufficient relief be provided. In addition, escapement slots or holes in the original base must be used, to avoid locking the impression material against the tissues without opportunity for escape." Given an opportunity to flow, the fluid waxes record the tissues without overdisplacement and assure uniformity of support for the partial denture base.

The difference between impression wax and modeling plastic is that the impression waxes have the ability to flow as long as they are in the mouth and thereby permit equalization of pressure and prevent overdisplacement; whereas the modeling plastics flow only in proportion to the amount of flaming and tempering that can be done out of the mouth, and this does not continue after the plastic has approached mouth temperature. The principal advantage of mouth-temperature waxes is that, given sufficient time, they permit a rebound of those tissues that have been over-displaced.

The impression waxes also may be used to correct the borders of impressions made of more rigid materials, thereby establishing optimal contact at the border of the denture. All mouth-temperature wax impressions have the ability to record border detail accurately and at the same time es-

tablish the correct width of the denture border. They have the advantage of being correctable, and if the dentist will take sufficient time in the making of the correction, he may record accurately not only surface detail but also all border areas that are available for support and retention of the denture.

Some mouth-temperature waxes vary in their working characteristics from those mentioned herein. Among these are the Jelenko Adaptol impression material and the Stalite impression material. Both of these seem to have a more resinous base. They are designed primarily for impression techniques that attempt to record the tissues under an occlusal load. In such techniques the occlusion rim or the arrangement of artificial teeth is completed first. Mouth-temperature wax is then applied to the tissue side of the denture base, and the final impression is made under functional loading, using various movements simulating functional activity. However, these mouth-temperature materials also may be used successfully in open-mouth impression techniques.

The Iowa wax and the Korecta wax will not distort after removal from the mouth at ordinary room temperatures, but the more resinous waxes must be stored at much lower temperatures to avoid flow out of the mouth. Resinous waxes are not ordinarily used in partial denture impression techniques, their use being limited to specific techniques for complete denture impressions.

ELASTIC MATERIALS*

Reversible hydrocolloids. Reversible (agar) hydrocolloids, which are fluid at higher temperatures and gel upon a reduction in temperature, are used primarily as impression materials for fixed restorations. They are unsurpassed for accuracy when

---

*Much of this discussion has been quoted or paraphrased from McCracken, W. L.: Impression materials in prosthetic dentistry, Dent. Clin. North Am., pp. 671-684, Nov., 1958.

properly used. However, the reversible hydrocolloid impression materials offer few advantages over the irreversible, or alginate, hydrocolloids when used as a partial denture impression material. Present-day alginate hydrocolloids are sufficiently accurate for the making of master casts for partial dentures. However, border control of impressions made with these materials is difficult.

Irreversible hydrocolloids. The irreversible (alginate) hydrocolloids are used for the making of diagnostic casts, orthodontic treatment casts, and master casts for removable partial denture procedures. Since they are a colloidal material, an alginate hydrocolloid impression cannot be stored for any length of time but must be poured immediately. The same precautions in handling apply equally to both the reversible and irreversible hydrocolloid impression materials.

Mercaptan rubber-base impression materials. The mercaptan rubber-base (Thiokol) impression materials are not as widely used for removable partial denture impressions as in crown and fixed partial denture procedures because of their cost and because an individual impression tray is required. To be accurate, the impression must have a uniform thickness not exceeding ⅛ inch. This necessitates the use of a carefully made individual impression tray of acrylic resin or some other material possessing adequate rigidity and stability. It is doubtful that the accuracy of a mercaptan rubber-base impression exceeds that of a properly made alginate hydrocolloid impression, and as with the hydrocolloid impression materials, certain precautions must be taken to avoid distortion of the impression. The mercaptan rubber-base impression materials do have an advantage over the hydrocolloid materials in that the surface of an artificial stone poured against them is of a smoother texture and therefore appears to be smoother and harder than one poured against a hydrocolloid material. This is probably due to the fact that the rubber material does not have the ability to retard or etch the surface of the setting stone. De-

spite their accuracy, this has always been a disadvantage of all hydrocolloid impression materials. A cast made from a mercaptan rubber or silicone impression possesses a smoother surface that may possibly lead to a more accurate dental casting. The fact that a smoother surface results does not, however, preclude the possibility of a grossly inaccurate impression and stone cast resulting from other causes.

Another use of the mercaptan rubber-base impression materials is in the making of stabilized bases for recording jaw relations. The elasticity of the rubber material offers comfort to the patient during the recording of jaw relations. However, there is some question as to how this jaw relation record then may be accurately transferred back onto a rigid cast.

Silicone impression materials. The silicone impression materials are similar in their accuracy and convenience to the rubber-base impression materials. They are used primarily as impression materials for crown and fixed partial denture procedures and require the same precautions as do the rubber-base materials. However, they are more delicate to handle in the laboratory, and because of their cost and delicate nature, they are not widely used as impression materials for removable partial denture master casts. They require the same precautions as do the mercaptan rubber materials. They are somewhat more delicate to handle in the laboratory and at the present time are a little more costly than Thiokol materials. In general, however, they possess many of the same advantages and disadvantages and may be similarly used when handled with care.

IMPRESSIONS OF THE PARTIALLY EDENTULOUS ARCH

An impression of the partially edentulous arch must record accurately the anatomic form of the teeth and surrounding tissues. This is necessary so that the prosthesis may be designed to follow a definite path of placement and removal and also that support and retention on the abutment teeth may be precise and accurate.

Materials that could be permanently deformed by removal from tissue undercuts may not be used. This excludes the use of the thermoplastic impression materials for recording the anatomic form of the dental arch. The rigid materials such as plaster of Paris are capable of recording tissue detail accurately, but they must be sectioned for removal and subsequently reassembled.

Before the advent of the elastic hydrocolloid materials, plaster of Paris and modeling plastic were the only impression materials available for impressions of the partially edentulous arch. Modeling plastic was used for making preliminary impressions for diagnostic casts, despite its distortion upon removal from undercuts. Such diagnostic casts were grossly inaccurate and permitted only approximate evaluation of tooth contours. Impressions for master casts were made of plaster of Paris, which was scored and sectioned for removal and then reassembled. This was time-consuming and discomforting to the patient.

Plaster of Paris is accurate and dimensionally stable, is inexpensive, and requires no special equipment for its use. Its main disadvantages are its inflexibility and the fact that some separating medium must be used prior to pouring the cast to prevent the cast material, which is usually also a gypsum product, from adhering to it. Damage to the resulting cast can easily occur during removal of the impression from the cast. Since it must be removed from the mouth sectionally, small pieces from essential areas may be lost, and reassembly of the pieces may take considerable time.

The introduction of hydrocolloids as impression materials was a long step forward in dentistry. For the first time impressions could be made of undercut areas with a material that was elastic enough to be withdrawn from those undercuts without permanent distortion. It permits the making of a one-piece impression, which does not require the use of a separating medium, and it is an extremely accurate material when handled properly.

Phillips has reduced the complicated chemistry of the hydrocolloid impression materials to its simplest form in the following paragraphs:

Hydrocolloids can be classified into two general types: reversible and irreversible. These materials are suspensions of aggregates of molecules in a dispersing medium of water, the water being held by capillary action. Gelation of the reversible hydrocolloids is primarily a physical change in which a latticework of fibrils forms as the temperature is lowered. This gel can be readily dispersed by merely heating the material—thus the term reversible. An example of a reversible hydrocolloid is ordinary gelatin. When gelatin is dissolved in boiling water, it forms a colloidal sol which gels upon cooling. This gel can be returned to the liquid sol by heating, formed again by cooling, etc.

The base for dental reversible hydrocolloids is agar-agar, a material that can be liquefied at temperatures compatible to oral tissues and then solidified to a firm, yet elastic, gel at temperatures slightly above 100° F. This gelation is accomplished by means of water-cooled impression trays. Such factors as ability to secure routinely accurate reproductions of cavity preparation with one impression, reproductions of minor undercuts without rupture or distortion, and actual saving in chair time have been instrumental in the successful adaptation of this material for use in the indirect inlay technique. It is unexcelled when used in this procedure.

The irreversible hydrocolloids, or alginates, are not thermally reversible and their gelation is induced by an actual chemical reaction rather than by physical means. The powder is essentially sodium alginate and calcium sulphate which when mixed with water react to form a latticework of fibrils of insoluble calcium alginate. These materials have been used extensively in prosthetics and orthodontia. . . .

In general it can be said that the alginates approach the accuracy of reversible hydrocolloid but, due to the greater number of variables both in their manufacture and use, they are not routinely quite as accurate.*

The principal differences between agar and alginate hydrocolloids are as follows:

1. Agar converts from the gel form to a

---

*From Phillips, R. W.: The physical properties of hydrocolloids and alginates and factors influencing their work qualities and accuracy, Fortn. Rev. Chic. Dent. Soc. **26:**9-12, 1953.

sol by the application of heat. It may be reverted to gel form by a reduction in temperature. This physical change is reversible.

2. Alginate hydrocolloid becomes a gel via a chemical reaction as a result of mixing alginate powder with water. This physical change is irreversible.

Agar hydrocolloid does have some disadvantages. It must be introduced into the mouth while warm enough to be a sol, converting to an elastic gel upon cooling. Therefore, there is an ever-present danger of burning the tissues of the mouth, a burn that is painful and slow to heal. It requires warming and tempering equipment that is thermostatically controlled and necessitates the use of water-jacketed impression trays for cooling.

All hydrocolloids are dimensionally stable only during a brief period after removal from the mouth. If exposed to the air, they rapidly lose water content, with a resulting shrinkage and other dimensional changes. If immersed in water, they imbibe water, with an accompanying swelling and dimensional changes. All hydrocolloid impressions should be poured immediately, but if they must be stored for a brief period of time, it should be in a saturated atmosphere rather than in water. This is accomplished simply by wrapping the impression in a wet towel.

All hydrocolloids also exhibit a phenomenon known as syneresis, which is associated with the giving off of a mucinous exudate. This mucinous exudate has a retarding effect on any gypsum material, which results in a soft or chalky cast surface. Sometimes this is less obvious and only detected by a close examination of the impression after removal from the cast. Nevertheless, such a cast surface is inaccurate, and an inaccurate denture casting ultimately results in proportion to the inaccuracy of the master cast. This can only be prevented by pouring the cast immediately and using some chemical accelerator such as potassium sulfate to counteract the retarding effect of the hydrocolloid.

Agar hydrocolloid impressions should be immersed in a 2% solution of potassium sulfate for five to ten minutes prior to pouring the cast even though some accelerator may have been incorporated by the manufacturer. Most all modern alginate hydrocolloid impression materials have an accelerator incorporated into the powder and no longer need to be treated with a "fixing solution" unless it is supplied by the manufacturer. However, an alginate hydrocolloid impression material that is compounded to require a "fixing solution" consistently gives a smoother cast surface than those that do not require immersion in such a solution. It is probably because of the popular demand for alginate impression materials that do not require fixing that the suppliers have all but abandoned the manufacture of those requiring a "fixing solution."

Since no heat is employed in the preparation of alginate hydrocolloid, there is no danger of burning the patient. For this reason, the patient will be more relaxed and cooperative during the positioning of the tray. However some disadvantages are associated with the use of alginate hydrocolloid. This material gels by means of a chemical reaction that is accelerated by the warmth of the tissues; whereas agar hydrocolloid gels from the tray in toward the tissues, because of the cooling action of the water circulating through the tray. In the former, gelation takes place first next to the tissues, and any movement of the tray during gelation of the remote portions results in internal stresses that are released upon removal of the impression from the mouth. A distorted and therefore inaccurate impression results from an alginate hydrocolloid impression that is not held immobile during gelation.

Another disadvantage of alginate hydrocolloid is that it must be introduced into the mouth at approximately 70° F., which causes an immediate increase in the viscosity and surface tension of the saliva. Air bubbles are therefore harder to dispel and it is inevitable that more air will be trapped in an alginate impression than in an agar impression. Every precaution must be taken to avoid the entrapment of air in critical areas.

Important precautions to be observed in the handling of hydrocolloid. Some important precautions to be observed in the handling of hydrocolloid are as follows:

1. Impression should not be exposed to air because some dehydration will inevitably occur, resulting in shrinkage.

2. Impression should not be immersed in water for long periods because some imbibition will inevitably result, with an accompanying expansion.

3. Impression should be protected from dehydration by placing it in a humid atmosphere or wrapping it in a wet towel until a cast can be poured. To avoid volume change, this should be within fifteen minutes after removal from the mouth.

4. Exudate from hydrocolloid has a retarding effect on the chemical reaction of gypsum products and results in a chalky cast surface. This can be prevented by pouring the cast immediately and by first immersing the impression in a solution of accelerator.

Step-by-step procedure for making a hydrocolloid impression. The step-by-step procedure and important points to observe in the making of a hydrocolloid impression are as follows:

1. Select a suitable perforated impression tray that is large enough to provide a 4 to 5 mm. border thickness of the impression material.

2. If the maxillary arch has a high palatal contour, build up the tray with beeswax to prevent the hydrocolloid from sagging away from the palatal surface (Fig. 14-1, A). If gelation occurs next to the tissues while the deeper portion is still fluid, a distorted impression of the palate may result, which cannot be detected in the finished impression. This may result in the major connector of the finished casting not being in contact with the underlying tissues. The maxillary tray frequently has to be extended posteriorly to include the tuberosities and vibrating line region of the palate. Such an extension also aids in cor-

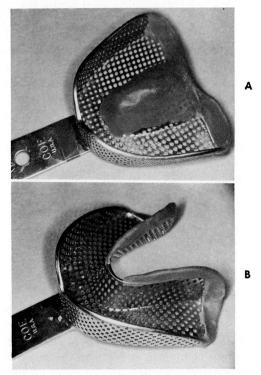

Fig. 14-1. A, Maxillary impression tray with the palatal portion built up with beeswax to prevent the impression material from sagging away from the palatal surface. Beeswax is also added across the posterior border of the tray to cover the maxillary tuberosities and to prevent impression material from being expelled posteriorly when the impression is made. B, Mandibular impression tray with beeswax added to the lingual flanges to prevent the tissues of the floor of the mouth from rising inside the tray. The posterior end of the tray is extended with beeswax to cover the retromolar pad regions.

rectly orienting the tray in the patient's mouth when making the impression.

3. The lingual flange of the mandibular tray may need to be lengthened with beeswax in the retromylohyoid area or to be extended posteriorly but rarely ever needs to be lengthened elsewhere. Beeswax may need to be added *inside* the distolingual flange to prevent the tissues of the floor of the mouth from rising inside the tray (Fig. 14-1, B).

4. Place the patient in an upright posi-

tion, with the involved arch nearly parallel to the floor.

5. When using alginate hydrocolloid, place the measured amount of water (at 70° F.) in a clean, dry, rubber mixing bowl (600 ml. capacity). Add the correct measure of powder. Spatulate rapidly against the side of the bowl with a short, *stiff* spatula (Kerr laboratory spatula No. 1 or Buffalo dental spatula No. 11R). This should be accomplished in less than one minute.

6. In placing the material in the tray, try to avoid entrapping air. Have the first layer of material lock through the perforations of the tray to prevent any possible dislodgment after gelation.

7. After loading the tray, quickly place (rub) some material with the finger on any critical areas such as rest preparations and abutment teeth. If an upper impression is being made, place material in the highest aspect of the palate and over the rugae.

8. Use a mouth mirror or index finger to retract the cheek on the side away from you as the tray is being rotated into the mouth from the near side.

9. Seat the tray first on the side away from you, next on the anterior area while reflecting the lip, and then on the near side, using the mouth mirror or finger for cheek retraction. Finally, make sure that the lip is draping naturally over the tray.

10. Be careful not to seat the tray too deeply, leaving room for a thickness of material over the occlusal and incisal surfaces.

11. Hold the tray immobile for three minutes with light finger pressure over left and right premolar areas. Do not allow the tray to move during gelation to avoid internal stresses in the finished impression.

12. After releasing the surface tension, remove the impression quickly in line with the long axis of the teeth to avoid tearing or other distortion.

13. Rinse the impression free of saliva with gently running, room temperature tap water and examine critically. Cover the impression immediately with a wet towel.

A cast should be poured immediately into a hydrocolloid impression to avoid dimensional changes and syneresis. Circumstances often necessitate some delay, but this time lapse should be kept to a minimum. A fifteen-minute delay is not deleterious if the impression is kept in a humid atmosphere.

Step-by-step procedure for making a stone cast from a hydrocolloid impression. The step-by-step procedure for making the stone cast from the impression is as follows:

1. Have the measured dental stone at hand, along with a measured quantity of water, as recommended by the manufacturer. For most laboratory stones, 28 ml. of water for each 100 gm. is recommended; for improved stones the proportion is 24 ml. of water for each 100 gm. A clean 600 ml. mixing bowl, a stiff spatula, and a vibrator complete the preparations. A No. 7 spatula also should be within reach.

2. First pour the measure of water into the mixing bowl and then add the measure of stone. Spatulate thoroughly for one minute, remembering that a weak and porous stone cast may result from insufficient spatulation. *Mechanical spatulation or vacuum spatulation if such facilities are available may be used to advantage.* After any spatulation other than in a vacuum, place the mixing bowl on the vibrator and knead the material to permit the escape of any trapped air.

3. The hydrocolloid impression material used may require a fixing solution. If so, follow the manufacturer's instructions. Any fixing is done just prior to pouring the cast and is not meant to be used as a storing medium. After removing the impression from the damp towel or fixing solution, gently shake out surplus moisture and hold the impression in the left hand over the vibrator with the impression side up. The impression material must not be placed in contact with the vibrator because of possible distortion of the impression.

4. With a small spatula, add the first cast material to the distal area away from you. Allow this first material to be vibrated around the arch from tooth to tooth toward

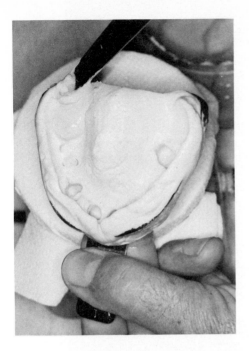

Fig. 14-2. Small portions of mechanically spatulated stone are applied at a posterior section of the impression and vibrated around the arch, pushing moisture and diluted stone ahead of the mass. Stone is applied at this point only until the impressions of the teeth are filled and the diluted stone is discarded at the opposite end. Only then is the remainder of the impression filled with larger portions, using a larger spatula. Only the handle of the impression tray should be allowed to touch the vibrator so that distortion of the impression material will be avoided. (Note that the vibrator is protected with a paper towel as the impression is being filled.)

the anterior part of the impression (Fig. 14-2). Continue to add small increments of material at this same distal area, each additional portion of added stone pushing the mass ahead of it. This avoids the entrapment of air. The weight of the material causes any excess water to be pushed around the arch and to be expelled ultimately at the opposite end of the impression. Discard this fluid material. When the impressions of all teeth have been filled, continue to add artificial stone in larger portions until the impression is completely filled.

5. Then the filled impression should be placed on a supporting jig and the base

of the cast completed with the same mix of stone (Fig. 14-3). The base of the cast should be ⅝ to ¾ inch at its thinnest portion and should be extended beyond the borders of the impression so that buccal, labial, and lingual borders will be recorded correctly in the finished cast. *A distorted cast may result from an inverted impression.*

6. As soon as the cast material has developed sufficient body, trim the gross excess from the sides of the cast. Wrap the impression and cast in a wet paper towel or place it in a humidor until the initial set of the stone has taken place. The impression is thus prevented from losing water by evaporation, which might in turn deprive the cast material of sufficient water for crystallization. Chalky cast surfaces around the teeth are often the result of the hydrocolloid acting as a sponge and robbing the cast material of its necessary water for crystallization.

7. After the cast and impression have been in the humid atmosphere for thirty minutes, separate the impression from the cast. Thirty minutes is sufficient for initial setting. Any stone interfering with separation must be trimmed away with a knife.

8. Clean the impression tray immediately while the used impression material is still elastic.

9. The trimming of the cast should be deferred until final setting has occurred. The sides of the cast then may be trimmed to be parallel, and any blebs or defects due to air bubbles in the impression may be removed. If this is a diagnostic cast or a cast for a permanent record, it may be trimmed to orthodontic specification to present a neat appearance for demonstration purposes. Master casts and other working casts are ordinarily trimmed only to remove excess stone.

Possible causes of an inaccurate cast of a dental arch. The possible causes of an inaccurate cast are as follows:

1. Distortion of the hydrocolloid impression (a) by partial dislodgment from tray, (b) by shrinkage due to dehydration, (c)

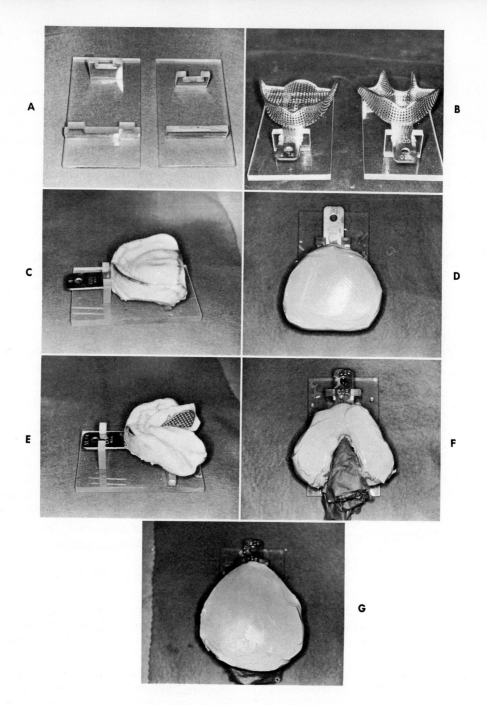

Fig. 14-3. A, Homemade plastic jigs are used to support the impressions. The handle of the tray is placed in slotted portion and the posterior end of the tray is supported by the elevated cross-members. The jig used to support the mandibular impression is on the left. B, Note that the impression trays are elevated and contact the jigs at only three points. C, An impression could be easily distorted when the cast is being poured if the tray was placed on the laboratory bench. Since the impression is elevated by the jig, distortion of the impression is minimized. D, After the impression is filled with stone, as previously demonstrated, it is placed in the jig and additional stone is added to form the base of the cast. E, The mandibular impression placed in the jig to demonstrate support by the jig. Note that the impression is supported by contact of the tray only at the handle and on either side posteriorly. F, The impression is returned to the supporting jig after being filled with stone. Wet paper is placed in the tongue space to support the stone base in this region and to avoid locking the impression tray to the cast. G, Additional stone is added to the impression to form a base for the cast.

by expansion due to imbibition (this will be toward the teeth and will result in an undersize rather than an oversize cast), (d) by attempting to pour the cast with stone that is too resistant.

2. A ratio of water to powder that is too high. While this may not cause volumetric changes in the size of the cast, it will result in a weak cast.

3. Improper mixing. This also results in a weak cast or one with a chalky surface.

4. Trapping of air, either in the mix or in pouring, because of insufficient vibration.

5. Soft or chalky cast surface due to the retarding action of the hydrocolloid or the absorption of necessary water for crystallization by the dehydrating hydrocolloid.

6. Premature separation of the cast from the impression.

7. Failure to separate the cast from the impression for extended periods of time.

Pouring of working casts upon which abutment restorations are to be fabricated. The pouring of casts into hydrocolloid, mercaptan rubber, or silicone impressions to make removable dies is adequately covered in crown and fixed partial denture textbooks. However, five methods will be given here for the making of working casts upon which the contours of wax patterns may be refined to satisfy the requirements of *noninterference to placement, parallelism, and retention* for the partial denture. They are as follows:

1. The use of a double-pour technique, with separation of removable dies by means of a fine (No. 2) jeweler's saw blade (such as a Herkules saw for hard metals, No. 2). The removable portion of the die must have keyed dowel pins for handling and for accuracy in seating back in the cast (Fig. 14-4, *A*). If a metal die surface is preferred, mercaptan and silicone impressions may be electroplated prior to pouring dies, which are then separated by sawing (Fig. 14-4, *B* and *C*).

2. The use of thin stainless steel separators in hydrocolloid impressions. Keyed dowel pins are placed in each removable segment. This method accomplishes the same objective as does the previous method without the necessity of sawing the cast and may provide greater accuracy in reseating the dies. By removing the separators prior to pouring the remainder of the cast and by using a suitable liquid separator, removable dies may be made that will seat accurately without any space for possible rotation such as is caused by a saw cut. This method may be used only with hydrocolloid impressions, and extreme care must be taken to avoid distortion of gingival margins in the placement of the thin metal separators. Two metal strips acting as coffer dams must be so placed for each tooth involved that a tapered die seat results.

3. The pouring of the entire cast without provision for separating individual dies. The margins of each prepared tooth are then exposed by carefully trimming away the surrounding stone in much the same manner as the trimming of an individual or removable die. Interproximally this is a particularly meticulous procedure since these areas are not readily accessible. A sharp knife, such as a No. 11 Bard-Parker surgical blade, and some means of working under magnification facilitate accurate trimming of nonremovable dies.

After all margins of prepared teeth have been exposed, the cast is duplicated, following the duplication procedure outlined in Chapter 17. A second stone cast is thus obtained, which is used as a working cast to be mounted on the articulator. (In this method a cast of the entire arch is always used rather than a unilateral or anterior segment. This facilitates the transfer of jaw relations with greater accuracy.)

The original cast is then cut into segments, using separating disks applied to the base of the cast between each prepared tooth. Individual dies are thus obtained upon which final waxing and finishing may be done. Wax patterns and finished castings then may be transferred to the nonremovable dies on the articulator for perfecting the occlusion and contact. This method de-

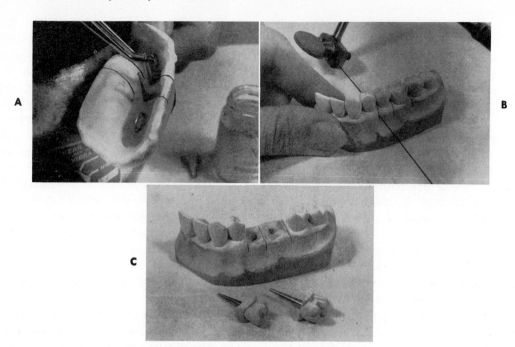

Fig. 14-4. A, Placement of dowel pins in an impression of prepared teeth is guided by indelible pencil or pen lines previously drawn buccally and lingually at the center of the long axis of those teeth. After the impression is filled above the level of the prepared teeth, it is supported between two pieces of clay and the dowel pins are placed between and parallel to the pencil lines. Lock washers then may be partially embedded into portions where separation is not desired. If the impression is of prepared fixed partial denture abutments, a lock washer is also placed in the edentulous space between the abutments. After the stone has set, areas to be separated are treated with a solution of sodium silicate or a commercial separating fluid such as Super-Sep. The impression may be boxed with wax if desired, and the ends of the dowel pins should be covered with a piece of utility wax so that they may be located after pouring the remainder of the cast. B, After the remainder of the cast is poured, preferably in stone of a different color, the sides of the cast should be trimmed and then allowed to dry overnight. With a No. 2 jeweler's saw blade in a saw frame, the cast is cut throughout the interproximal spaces, down to the junction with the second pour of stone. The saw cuts are made vertical unless a single die is involved; in such case, they are made converging. The dowel pin will not be encountered if it was placed perpendicular in the center of the prepared tooth. The utility wax is removed from the ends of the dowel pins, and each die is gently tapped out of its seat. C, The dies are now removed and are trimmed to expose precise gingival margins. The margins are lightly marked with pencil to facilitate accurate waxing and later finishing operations. The gingival thickness below the margins should be as in the die on the left rather than too close to the margin as on the right. (Courtesy Kerr Manufacturing Co., Detroit, Mich.)

mands precise technical skill but has the advantage of eliminating the possibility of removable stone dies becoming inaccurate because of abrasion of the die or its seat.

4. The replacement of electroformed dies into the original mercaptan rubber or silicone impression before pouring the remainder of the cast. Although this may not be done with hydrocolloid impressions, if the careful person can reseat electroformed

dies with accuracy, it is an acceptable method for making removable dies.

The method for making an electroformed die is as follows: After electroplating the impression with silver or copper, the inside of the plated impression of each tooth involved is painted with a flux made of equal parts of concentrated hydrochloric acid, water, and glycerine. Into this fluxed concavity low-fusing metal alloy (Dialoy or

Cerrosafe metal) is poured to the top of each impression. A keyed dowel pin for each tooth is fluxed and dipped into the ladle of low-fusing alloy to tin the portion to be embedded in the impression. The metal in the impression is then melted on the surface with a needle-point frame and the tinned dowel pin inserted and held until the metal has solidified. Then each die may be removed and trimmed without fear of separation of the electroformed surface from the core of the die.

5. The use of individual dies from copper band impressions combined with an accurate solid cast for surveying and contouring the wax patterns. The stone at the gingival margin on the solid cast must be cut away to expose the full length of the preparation. The wax pattern is begun on the individual die, then placed on the solid cast on which critical areas are carved with the surveyor blade, retentive contours are established, and contact and occlusion are perfected. The pattern is then returned to the individual die to finish the margins. It is always sprued from the individual die and returned to it for polishing. If marginal interference has been cut away on the solid cast, the casting may be returned to it to check and refine contours or to establish the contours of veneered surfaces.

Regardless of the method used, the individual die, whether or not it is a removable die, must be trimmed to expose all margins of the preparation (Fig. 14-5). This is done as illustrated, thereby facilitating both the waxing and polishing of precise gingival margins. If the die is not so trimmed, the location of gingival margins will be less exact, resulting in an overextended or, more often, an underextended restoration.

Copper band impressions. Although it is possible to record subgingival portions of a prepared tooth with hydrocolloid, mercaptan, or silicone impression materials at times those areas are not as sharply defined as might be desired. Unquestionably, a copper band impression is capable of recording subgingival areas better than any

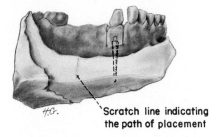

Scratch line indicating
the path of placement

Fig. 14-5. Trimmed removable die for an abutment crown. The working cast is placed on the surveyor in relation to the path of placement and the wax pattern formed with proximal guiding plane and with retentive and nonretentive contours in conformity with this path of placement.

technique that calls for the injection of the impression material and subsequent removal from subgingival areas. For this reason, the use of copper band impressions continues to have a place in restorative dentistry.

The object of the copper band impression is to make an individual die for use with, or in place of, a removable die. It is used frequently to supplement the latter when subgingival areas are not sharply defined. In this application modeling plastic may not be used because of its lack of flexibility. Withdrawal of such an impression from undercut areas apical to the preparation inevitably results in fracture of the impression. Therefore, some elastic material must be used. Mercaptan rubber or silicone may be used, or the older but respected Dietrich's impression material. Believing that this is a dependable material for copper band impressions of prepared teeth, the step-by-step procedure for its use is as follows (Fig. 14-6):

1. Select a copper band one size larger than would be used for a modeling plastic impression. Score it on the buccal side with a sharp instrument to identify its position, contouring it so that it extends beneath the gingivae in all areas except where buccal or lingual surfaces have not been prepared, as in a three-quarter crown or inlay preparation. Here the band is contoured above the height of convexity of the unprepared tooth surfaces.

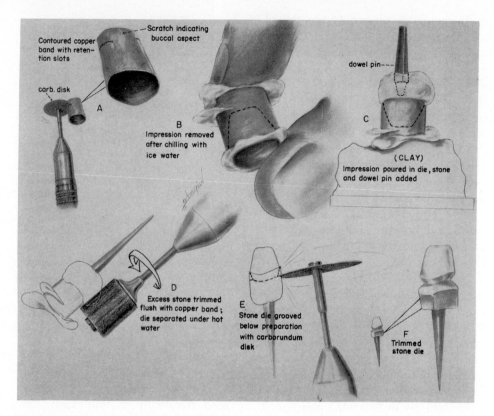

Fig. 14-6. Steps in making an individual stone die from a copper band impression, using Dietrich's elastic impression material.

2. With a carborundum disk, make two slots in the upper portion of the band at right angles to the long axis of the band. This is done to secure the chilled impression in the copper band.

3. Place sufficient Dietrich's material in a small amount of water in a test tube and bring to a boil. Dump this into a plaster bowl containing hot water. Fill the contoured copper band with the soft material, taking care to avoid wrinkles and voids. Again place the filled band in the test tube with a small amount of water and again bring to a boil. Again dump the material into the bowl containing hot water and immediately remove it and carry it to the mouth.

4. Place the filled band on the tooth, using the scratch line on its buccal aspect to identify its original position. Seat it be-

neath the gingivae and then use the butt end of an instrument as a plunger to force the impression material beneath the gingivae and out the slots in the band, which were placed there for retention. Then hold the band securely with a finger on the open end while three or more syringefuls of *iced* water are emptied slowly upon it. (Chilling is essential to the accuracy of such an impression. After removal from the mouth, it remains stable at room temperature but should be poured as soon as possible.)

5. Remove the chilled band by applying the edge of a chisel blade to one side of the band while stabilizing with the finger on the other. Since it is an elastic material, squeezing removal must be avoided. Then check the impression for accuracy. A portion of the tooth below the preparation

must be recorded, clearly identifying the margin of the preparation. The copper band should not be visible at any point.

6. Being elastic, gingival excess may not safely be trimmed away for fear thin areas may pull away and distort. The impression band may be boxed lightly with lead backing from a roentgenogram, wax, or gummed paper. However, the preferred method is to overfill slightly the unboxed band with the die stone, place it on a ball of clay, and then add a dowel pin. After the stone has set, any excess is cut back to the limits of the copper band with a stone or arbor band, which simplifies removal and trimming. Separation of the die from the impression is then accomplished under hot water.

This technique has been given as a respected and time-proved method of obtaining individual dies. Other elastic materials may be used if preferred, the only difference being the method of preparing the impression material and the use of heavier-gauge band materials and of adhesives for securing the material to the band.

An alternate method of using a copper band is the use of a loosely fitted band that is filled with rubber-base impression material and seated subgingivally before making an overall impression with a mass of the same material. In this method, the band is trimmed almost to the height of the prepared tooth and must be formed with a rim that is crimped outward to ensure its being engaged by the overall impression. This method recognizes the need for a subgingival record of crown preparations beyond that ordinarily obtained by the usual retraction and injection techniques and may serve to eliminate the necessity for individual impressions in difficult situations.

A modification of this method is to make an acrylic resin coping of each abutment tooth upon a cast made in quick-setting stone from a wax impression of the prepared teeth. If fixed partial denture abutments are involved, the resin copings are connected by a span of resin that is relieved of any tissue contact. The copings are reamed slightly, and after the gingiva has been retracted and the teeth dried, the copings are filled with the rubber-base or silicone impression material and seated on the teeth, thus forcing the impression material subgingivally. An overall impression is then made of the same material, using a suitable metal or resin tray, which had been treated with adhesive. A syringe for applying the impression material subgingivally is ordinarily not necessary when the impression is made in this manner. Upon removal, the copings are not visible, being embedded in the overall impression, but they will have carried the impression material beneath the gingivae without the use of a syringe, thus eliminating the need for a second mix of injectable material.

INDIVIDUAL IMPRESSION TRAYS

This chapter has dealt previously with the making of an impression in a stock tray of the anatomic form of a dental arch for making either a diagnostic cast, a working cast for restorations, or a master cast. There are times, however, when a stock tray is not suitable for the making of the final anatomic impression of the dental arch. Most tooth-borne partial dentures may be made upon a master cast from such an impression. Some maxillary distal extension partial dentures with broad palatal coverage, particularily those for a Kennedy Class I arch, may also be made upon an anatomic cast, but usually these necessitate the use of an individually made tray.

Unless a stock tray can be found that will fit the mouth with about ¼-inch clearance for the impression material, yet without interference with bordering tissues, an individual tray made of some resin tray material should be used for the final anatomic impression.

Most partial denture trays are either of the rim-lock or perforated varieties. Both are made in a limited selection of sizes and shapes. One manufacturer in particular has gone to considerable length to provide a wide selection of perforated trays, including trays for both bilateral and unilateral edentulous areas, trays with built-in oc-

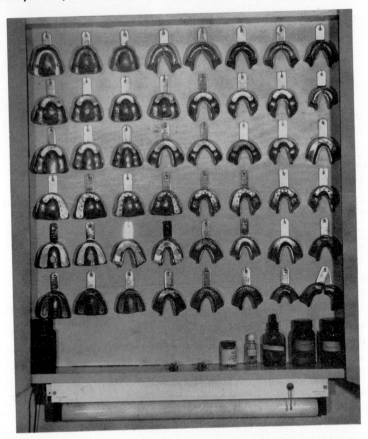

Fig. 14-7. Impression tray cabinet with doors open, exposing a wide selection of perforated impression trays for alginate hydrocolloid impressions. Beginning at the top can be seen trays for completely edentulous mouths, depressed anterior trays, trays with unilateral occlusal stops, Hindels trays for use with a double impression technique, and the more commonly and regularly used perforated trays.

clusal stops, and trays for particular techniques.* (See Fig. 14-7.)

All these trays have reinforced borders. Although a complete denture impression tray is, or should be, made of material that permits trimming and shaping to fit the mouth, the existence of a beaded border and the rigidity of a stock partial denture tray allows no trimming and little shaping. The resulting impression is often a record of border tissues distorted by an ill-fitting tray rather than an impression of tissues draping naturally over a slightly underextended impression tray.

An individual acrylic resin tray, on the other hand, can be made with sufficient clearance for the impression material and can be trimmed just short of the vestibular reflections to allow the tissues to drape naturally without distortion. The partial denture borders may then be made as accurate as complete denture borders with equal advantages.

Although techniques have been proposed for the making of individual impression trays that incorporate plastic tubing for water-cooling agar hydrocolloid impressions, the final anatomic impression usually will be made with alginate hydrocolloid, mercaptan rubber, or silicone impression materials.

---

*Nevin, J. J.: Tray selection for partial denture impressions, Cal **26:**10-16, July, 1963.

Technique for making individual acrylic resin impression trays. The diagnostic cast is often adequate for the preparation of the individual tray. However, if extensive surgery or extractions were performed after the making of the diagnostic cast, a new impression in a stock tray and a new cast must be made. The procedures for making the new cast are identical with those described previously.

A duplicate of the diagnostic cast should be made upon which the individual tray can be fabricated. The cast upon which an individual tray is made is often damaged or must be mutilated to separate the tray from the cast. Obviously, the original diagnostic cast must be retained as a permanent record in the patient's file.

The technique for making an individual, maxillary acrylic resin tray is as follows:

1. Outline the extent of the tray on the cast with a pencil. The tray must include all teeth and tissues that will be involved in the removable partial denture. Adequate space must be provided for frenal attachments. Mark the area of the posterior palatal seal on the upper cast and cut a 1 mm. × 1 mm. groove following the line designating the posterior extent of the tray (Fig. 14-8, A).

2. Adapt one layer of baseplate wax over the tissue surfaces and teeth of the cast to serve as a spacer for impression material. The wax spacer should be trimmed to the outline drawn on the diagnostic cast. Wax covering the posterior palatal seal area should be removed so that intimate contact of the tray and tissue in this region may serve as an aid in correctly orienting the tray when making the impression. (See Fig. 14-8, B.)

3. Adapt an additional layer of baseplate wax over the teeth if the impression is to be made in irreversible hydrocolloid (alginate). This step is not necessary if the choice of impression material is a rubber-base or silicone type of material.

4. Expose portions of the incisal edges of the central incisors to serve as anterior stops when placing the tray in the mouth.

Bevel the wax so that the completed tray will have a guiding incline that will help position the tray on the anterior stop.

5. Paint the exposed surfaces of the cast that may be contacted by the acrylic resin tray material with a tin-foil substitute (Alcote) to facilitate separation of the cured tray from the cast.

6. Mix the correct proportions of quick-setting acrylic resin monomer and polymer (8 ml. of monomer to 24 ml. of polymer) in a mixing jar or paper cup. When the resin mix is no longer stringy and can be handled without adhering to the fingers, form it into a wafer the size and thickness of a cake of modeling plastic or use special stone templates to form the wafer. (See Fig. 14-8, C-E.)

7. Carefully transfer the resin wafer to position on the cast and adapt the resin with the fingers, covering the wax spacer and palatal seal area and maintaining a uniform thickness. Remove the gross excess with a sharp knife while the resin is still soft.

8. Form a handle with the excess resin. The handle should be about ½ inch in width, about ¼ inch in thickness, and about 2 inches long.

9. Attach the handle to the tray over the region of the central incisors and shape it to extend ½ inch downward and 1 inch outward. (See Fig. 14-8, F.) It is usually necessary to place additional monomer on the handle and the tray to provide a satisfactory union.

10. Allow the resin to cure and remove the tray from the cast. The wax spacer can be removed from the tray with any suitable instrument.

11. Perfect the borders of the tray with rotary instruments (vulcanite burs, acrylic resin trimmers) and roughly polish the external surface of the tray (Fig. 14-8, G).

12. Place perforations (No. 8 bur size) in the resin tray at ³⁄₁₆-inch intervals, with the exception of the alveolar groove areas, if an irreversible hydrocolloid impression material is to be used (Fig. 14-9).

13. The tray must be tried in the mouth

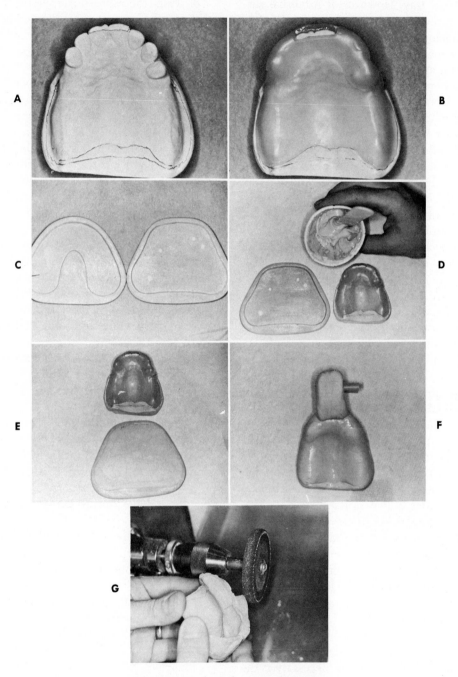

Fig. 14-8. For legend see opposite page.

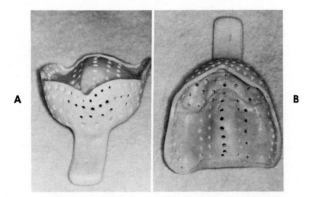

Fig. 14-9. **A,** Holes are drilled through the tray being spaced approximately ³⁄₁₆ inch apart. These holes will serve to lock the impression material in the tray. In addition, excess impression material is forced out of the holes when the impression is made, thereby minimally displacing the soft oral tissues. **B,** Note the elevated posterior palatal seal region of the tray and the incisal stop. These two features will assist in correctly orienting the individualized impression tray in the mouth.

Fig. 14-8. **A,** Desired outline of the tray is drawn on a duplicate diagnostic cast. The postpalatal seal region and a portion of the incisal edges of the central incisors are outlined. **B,** One thickness of baseplate wax is adapted to the cast and is trimmed to the penciled outline. The postpalatal seal region is not covered by the wax but will be included in the finished tray. Two thicknesses of baseplate wax cover the teeth. A window is created in the wax spacer over the incisal edges. A tinfoil substitute is painted on the stone surfaces of the cast that will be contacted by autopolymerizing acrylic resin. **C,** Stone templates are used to form uniform wafers of acrylic resin dough about ⅛ inch thick. The left template is used in making mandibular impression trays. These templates may be made by imbedding a double thick shellac baseplate form in a ½-inch thick patty of stone. They are lightly lubricated with petroleum jelly so that the soft tray material will not adhere to the stone when the acrylic resin wafer is being made. **D,** Tray resin is mixed in a paper cup with a wooden tongue depressor. The tray material is spatulated onto the stone template when it reaches a "nontacky" stage. **E,** A uniform acrylic resin wafer is made on the stone template by using the tongue depressor as a trowel to fill the mold and to remove excess tray material. **F,** The resin wafer is carefully removed from the template and adapted over the cast with the fingers. Excess tray material is removed from the borders of the cast with a sharp knife while the resin is still doughy. The excess material is used to shape a handle, which is attached over the incisal edges of the anterior teeth. It is supported by a piece of baseplate wax until the resin has become hard. **G,** As soon as the tray material has hardened, the tray is removed from the cast and the wax spacer is removed from the rough tray. An acrylic resin trimmer in a lathe is used to rough finish the **tray.**

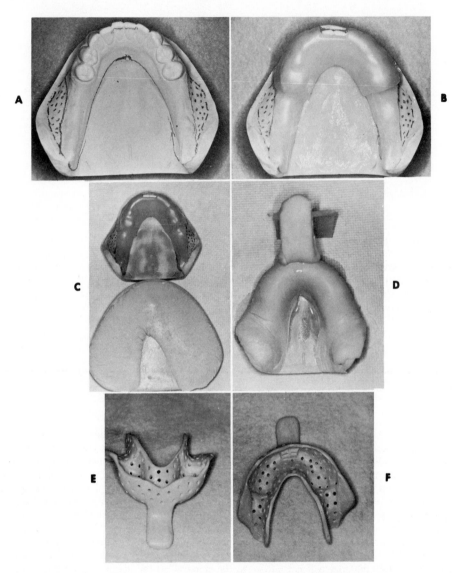

Fig. 14-10. A, An outline of the tray is penciled on a duplicate lower diagnostic cast. The buccal shelf region is outlined on each side of the cast (dotted portion). **B,** A single sheet of baseplate wax is adapted to the outline of the tray and another sheet of baseplate wax is adapted over the teeth. The buccal shelves are uncovered and a window is cut in the spacer to expose the incisal edges of the lower central incisors. **C,** An acrylic resin wafer is formed in a stone template as described in Fig. 14-8. **D,** The tray material wafer is adapted over the cast and spacer, and a handle is formed with excess tray material as previously described. **E** and **F,** Multiple holes are placed throughout the tray with the exception of the buccal shelf regions of the tray and also the elevated incisal stop in the tray. The buccal shelf region of the tray on either side and the incisal stop will assist in correctly orienting the tray in the patient's mouth.

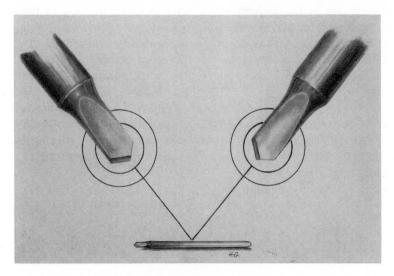

Fig. 14-11. Bi-beveled drill used for making holes in resin impression trays. Such a drill will not clog and facilitates the making of a perforated impression tray for use with alginate hydrocolloid, mercaptan rubber, or silicone impression materials.

so that any necessary corrections to the tray can be made before making the impression.

The technique for making an individual, mandibular acrylic resin tray follows the same procedures. The buccal shelf regions on the lower cast are left uncovered by the wax spacer to serve as posterior stops in orienting the tray in the patient's mouth (Fig. 14-10).

Perforations in a resin tray are not easily made with a round bur, because after a few revolutions the bur becomes clogged. Instead, a bi-beveled surgical drill is used, which will make the holes rapidly without clogging (Fig. 14-11). These are available in various sizes, Nos. 100 through 106, the higher number being the smaller size. The size of the perforations should be slightly larger than those in a stock tray, and only about one third as many are used. This will be sufficient to lock the impression material in the tray and thereby avoid distortion of the impression on removal from the mouth.

If mercaptan rubber or silicone is to be used, perforations are not usually necessary to lock the material in the tray as the adhesive provided by the manufacturer provides reliable retention, and some confine-

ment of these materials is desirable. However, a series of perforations are placed in the median palatal raphe area of the maxillary tray so that excess impression material will escape through them, thus providing relief of the tissues in this area. For the same reasons, perforations are placed in the alveolar groove of the mandibular tray. With the use of adhesives the impression material is not easily removed from the tray should a faulty impression have to be remade, but this is an inconvenience common to all newer elastic materials and does not prevent reuse of the impression tray.

The pouring of a cast in an alginate impression made in an individual tray presents a minor problem, since it is usually covered with the elastic material and is delicate to handle. Some of the excess material in the handle area may have to be cut away to expose enough of the rigid tray to make contact with the vibrator. The impression may then be vibrated while being filled, as any other hydrocolloid impression.

Master casts made from impressions in individual resin trays are generally more accurate than are those made in stock trays. The use of individual trays should be considered a necessary step in the making of the majority of removable partial dentures when a secondary impression technique is not to be used. Reasons and methods for the making of a secondary impression will be considered in Chapter 15.

Final impressions for maxillary tooth-borne removable partial dentures often may be made in carefully selected and re-contoured stock impression trays. However, an individual acrylic resin tray is preferred in those situations in the mandibular arch in which the floor of the mouth closely approximates the lingual gingiva of remaining anterior teeth. Recording the floor of the mouth at the elevation it assumes when the lips are licked is important in selecting the type of major connector to be used (Chapter 4). Modification of the borders of an individual tray to fulfill the requirements of an adequate tray is much easier than is the modification of a metal stock tray.

CHAPTER 15

Support for the distal extension denture base

In a tooth-supported removable partial denture, a metal base or the framework supporting a resin base is connected to and is part of a rigid framework that permits the direct transfer of occlusal forces to the abutment teeth through the occlusal rests. Even though the base of a tooth-supported (Kennedy Class III) partial denture supports the supplied teeth, the residual ridge beneath that base is not called upon to aid in the support of the denture. Therefore, the resiliency of the ridge tissues and the conformation and type of bone supporting these tissues are not factors in denture support. Regardless of the length of the span, if the framework is rigid, the abutment teeth are sound enough to carry the additional load, and the occlusal rests are properly formed, support comes entirely from the abutment teeth at either end of that span. Support may be augmented by splinting and by the use of additional abutments, but in any event, the abutments are the sole support of the removable restoration.

An impression (and resulting reproduction in stone) that records faithfully the anatomic form of the teeth and their surrounding structures and the residual ridges of a dental arch is the only impression needed in the making of a tooth-borne removable partial denture. The impression also should record the moving tissues that will border the denture in an unstrained position so that the relationship of the denture base to those tissues may be as accurate as possible, being neither overextended nor underextended. Although underextension of the denture base in a tooth-supported prosthesis is the lesser of two evils, an underextended base may lead to food impaction and inadequate contours, particularly on the buccal and labial sides. For this reason, and also to record faithfully the moving tissues of the floor of the mouth in the mandibular arch, an individual impression tray should be used rather than an ill-fitting or overextended stock tray. This has been discussed at length in Chapter 14.

DISTAL EXTENSION REMOVABLE PARTIAL DENTURE

The distal extension denture does not have the advantage of total tooth support, since one or more bases are extensions onto the residual ridge from the last available abutment. It therefore is dependent upon the residual ridge for a portion of its support.

Not only must the distal extension partial denture depend upon the residual ridge for some *support*, but it also should obtain *retention* from its base, aided by indirect *retention* to prevent the denture lifting away from the residual ridge. Whereas the tooth-supported base is secured at either end by the action of a direct retainer and supported at either end by a rest, this degree of support and direct retention are lacking in the distal extension restoration. *For this reason, a distal abutment should be preserved whenever possible.* In event of the loss or absence of a distal abutment tooth, the patient must be made aware of the movements to be expected with a distal extension partial denture and the limitations imposed upon the dentist when the residual ridge must be used for both support and retention for that part of the prosthesis.

FACTORS INFLUENCING THE SUPPORT OF A DISTAL EXTENSION BASE

Support from the residual ridge becomes greater as the distance from the last abutment increases and will depend on several factors:

1. Quality of the residual ridge
2. Extent of residual ridge coverage by the denture base
3. Type and accuracy of the impression registration
4. Accuracy of the denture base
5. Design of the partial framework
6. Total occlusal load applied

Quality of the residual ridge. The ideal residual ridge to support a denture base would consist of cortical bone covering relatively dense cancellous bone, a broad flat crest, and high vertical slopes and would be covered by firm, dense, fibrous connective tissue. Such a residual ridge would optimally support vertical and horizontal stresses placed upon it by denture bases. Unfortunately, this ideal is seldom encountered.

Easily displaceable tissue will not adequately support a denture base and tissues that are interposed between a sharp bony residual ridge and a denture base will not remain in a healthy state. Not only must the nature of the bone of the residual ridge be considered in developing optimal support for the denture base but also its positional relationship to the direction of forces that will be placed upon it.

The crest of the bony mandibular resid-

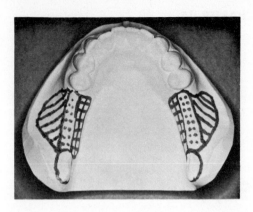

Fig. 15-1. Dotted portion outlines the crest of the residual ridge, which should be recorded in its anatomic form in impression procedures. Similarly, the retromolar pads should not be displaced by the impression. The buccal shelf regions are outlined by the herringbone pattern and selected additional pressures may be placed on these regions for vertical support of the denture base. Lingual slopes of the residual ridge (cross-hatched) may furnish some vertical support of the restoration; however, these regions principally resist horizontal rotational tendencies of the denture base and should be recorded by the impression in an undisplaced form.

ual ridge is most often cancellous in nature. Pressures placed on tissues overlying the crest of the mandibular residual ridge usually results in inflammation of these tissues accompanied by the sequelae of chronic inflammation. Therefore, the crest of the mandibular residual ridge cannot become a primary stress-bearing region. The buccal shelf region (bounded by the external oblique line and crest of alveolar ridge) seems to be more ideally suited for a primary stress-bearing role because it is covered by relatively firm, dense, fibrous connective tissue supported by cortical bone. In most instances, this region bears more of a horizontal relationship to vertical forces than does other regions of the residual ridge (Fig. 15-1). The slopes of the residual ridge then would become the primary stress-bearing region for horizontal stress.

The crest of the bone of the maxillary residual ridge may consist primarily of cortical bone and is much less cancellous in na-

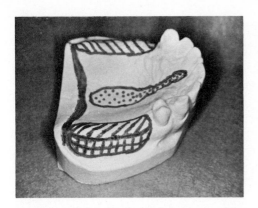

Fig. 15-2. Crest of the maxillary residual ridge (herringbone pattern) is the primary supporting region for the maxillary distal extension denture base. Buccal and lingual slopes may furnish a limited amount of vertical support of the denture base. It seems logical that their primary role is to counteract horizontal rotational tendencies of the denture base. The dotted portion outlines the incisive papilla and median palatal raphe. Relief must be provided these regions especially if the tissues covering the palatal raphe are less displaceable than the tissues covering the crest of the residual ridge.

ture than is observed in the mandible. The tissues overlying the maxillary residual alveolar bone are usually of a firm, dense nature or can be surgically prepared to support a denture base. Therefore, it seems logical to utilize the crest of the maxillary residual ridge as a primary stress-bearing region (Fig. 15-2). In each instance, the tissues covering the crest of the maxillary residual ridge must be less displaceable than are the tissues covering palatal areas, or relief of palatal tissues must be provided in the denture bases or for palatal major connectors.

Extent of residual ridge coverage by the denture base. The broader the coverage, the greater is the distribution of the load, thereby resulting in less load per unit area. Most prosthodontists agree that a denture base should cover as much of the residual ridge as possible and be extended the maximum amount within the physiologic tolerance of the limiting border structures or tissues. A knowledge of these border tissues

and the structures that influence their movement is paramount to developing broad coverage denture bases. In a series of experiments Kaires has shown that "maximum coverage of denture-bearing areas with large, wide denture bases is of the utmost importance in withstanding both vertical and horizontal stresses."

It is not within the scope of this text to review the anatomic considerations related to denture bases. The student is referred to several articles concerning this subject that are listed in Selected References.

Type of the impression registration. The residual ridge may be said to have two forms (Figs. 15-3 and 15-4). One is the *anatomic form,* which is the surface contour of the ridge when not supporting an occlusal load. It is this resting form that is recorded by a soft impression material such as plaster of Paris or a metallic oxide impression paste if the entire impression tray is uniformly relieved. Depending upon the viscosity of the particular impression material used, it is also the form recorded by mercaptan rubber and silicone impression materials. Also it is the form of the ridge recorded by a hydrocolloid impression material. Distortion and tissue displacement by pressure may result from confinement of the impression material within the tray and from insufficient thickness of impression material between the tray and the tissues, as well as from the viscosity of the impression material, but none of these factors is selective or physiologic in its action. These are accidental distortions of the tissues occurring through faulty technique.

Many prosthodontists utilize the anatomic form of the residual ridge in constructing complete dentures, believing this is the most physiologic form for support of the dentures. Such dentures are said to be made from anatomic impressions. However, many other prosthodontists believe that certain regions of the residual ridge are more capable of supporting dentures than are other regions. Their impression methods are directed to placing more stress on primary stress-bearing regions with spe-

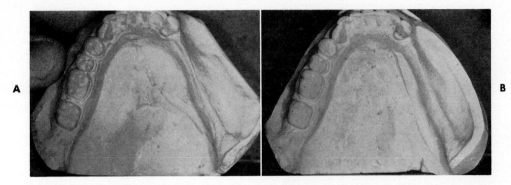

Fig. 15-3. Comparison of anatomic and functional ridge forms. **A,** The original master cast with edentulous area recorded in its anatomic form using an elastic impression material. **B,** The same cast after the edentulous area has been repoured to its functional form as recorded by a secondary impression.

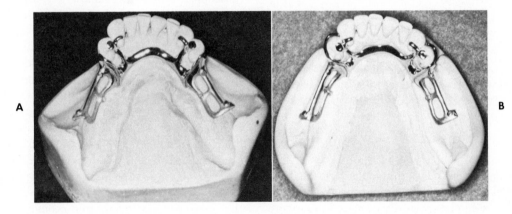

Fig. 15-4. Comparison of the functional and anatomic forms of the same edentulous ridge. **A,** The master cast with the edentulous area reproduced in its anatomic form from a hydrocolloid impression. **B,** The same master cast after the edentulous areas have been repoured in their functional, or supporting, form as recorded with a secondary impression. Note not only the difference in surface anatomy but also that the functional impression has recorded the width available for the support of the denture base. A new acrylic resin base may now be made by a sprinkling method to establish occlusal relationship on a base almost identical with that of the finished denture.

cially constructed individual trays and at the same time recording the anatomic form of the basal seat tissues, which cannot assume a stress-bearing role. Of the two rationalizations, the latter seems to be more logical.

Since there is no tooth support with which the denture base must be made compatible and since the basal seat tissues are recorded with a predominantly anatomic impression, the complete denture fits the resting form of those tissues. Presuming

that occlusion is harmonious throughout the dental arch, the complete denture may move tissueward under function until the tissues beneath assume a supporting form or a compactness that will support an occlusal load. The same principle would apply to a removable partial denture made without abutment support, differing only in that area of tissue support is less and the tissues adjacent to the remaining teeth would be impinged by tissueward movement of the denture. Without occlusal support from the natural teeth, occlusion on the tissue-supported partial denture would be negative, leaving only the remaining natural teeth to carry the masticatory load.

Several years ago, McLean and others recognized the need for recording the tissues supporting a distal extension partial denture base in their functional form or supporting state and then relating them to the remainder of the arch by means of a secondary impression. This was called a *functional impression* because it recorded the ridge relation under simulated function.

The technique consisted of making an impression of the edentulous areas in a vulcanite or denture base tray, which was provided with modeling plastic occlusion rims. Impression paste was used to record the ridge areas while under biting stress. This impression was then related to the remainder of the arch by making a hydrocolloid impression with the original impression seated in the mouth. Upon removal from the mouth, a master cast was poured in the composite impression, with the edentulous areas recorded under functional loading. Although the tray used for the overall impression was in contact with the occlusion rims, finger pressure was necessary to hold the original impression in its functional position while the hydrocolloid material gelled. Finger pressure thus applied could at best be only an approximation of the occlusal loading under which the original impression was recorded. This variable tended to nullify the advantage of making the original impression under occlusal loading.

A variation of this technique eliminated the occlusion rims as such but provided stops of modeling plastic against the underside of the hydrocolloid impression tray for finger loading the original impression. In this method, also, the impression of the edentulous areas was made with impression paste but with the tissues in their resting form. A finger load was then applied to the hydrocolloid tray for relating the edentulous areas under some loading to the remainder of the arch as the hydrocolloid gelled. The resulting master cast recorded the anatomic, or resting, form of the ridge in a pseudofunctional relationship to the rest of the arch.

More recently, Hindels and others have used with apparent success a method of finger loading the anatomic impression through a hole in the hydrocolloid impression tray. These trays are available for use with the technique and eliminate the possibility of error arising from ineffective or incorrectly placed modeling plastic stops. It does not eliminate the variable of the dentist's individual interpretation of what constitutes functional loading. The occlusal loading of McLean was unquestionably a more accurate and less variable method of recording the residual ridge beneath a distal extension base, but it became a variable finger-loading relationship in the final impression. That such methods are better than making a partial denture from a one-piece anatomic impression cannot be denied, because they recognize the need for adequate support of the distal extension base.

Any method, whether it accomplishes the recording of the *functional relationship* of the ridge to the remainder of the arch or the recording of the *functional form* of the ridge itself may provide acceptable support for the partial denture. On the other hand, those who use the static ridge form or ridge relationship for the partial denture should seriously consider the need for some mechanical stressbreaker to avoid the cantilever action of the distal extension base against the abutment teeth.

Hindels has the following to say about support for the partial denture base:

The one-piece colloidal or plaster impression will produce a cast which represents not a functional relationship between the various supporting structures of the mouth but only the hard and soft tissues at rest. With the partial denture in position in the dental arch, the occlusal rest will fit the rest seat of the abutment tooth, while the denture base will fit the surface of the mucosa at rest. When a masticatory load is applied to the extension base, the rest will act as a definite stop, which will prevent the part of the base near the abutment tooth from transmitting the load to the underlying anatomic structures. The distal end of the base, however, being able to move freely, will transmit the full masticatory load.

It is obvious that the soft tissues covering the ridge cannot by themselves carry any load applied to them. They act as a protective padding for the bone, which, in the final analysis, is the structure that receives and carries the masticatory load. Distribution of this load over a maximum area of bone is a prime requisite in preventing trauma.

A denture constructed from a one-piece impression places the masticatory load only on the abutment teeth and that part of the bone that underlies the distal end of the extension base. The balance of the bony ridge will not function in carrying the load. The result will be a traumatic load to the bone underlying the distal end of the base and to the abutment tooth, which, in turn, will result in bone loss and loosening of the abutment tooth.

Some believe that every partial denture should be relined before its final placement in the mouth. Some believe that tissue can be evenly displaced and use impression materials of heavy consistency. This process introduces traumatic stresses to the underlying tissues. Some use easy-flowing pastes that produce an impression of the soft tissues at rest. During the functioning of a partial denture so relined, the sequence of events will be similar to that of a partial denture constructed from a one-piece impression. The occlusal rest will act as a stop, preventing an even distribution of the masticatory load by the base to the edentulous ridge.

The technique as given by Hindels is as follows:

An acrylic resin tray is processed on a cast made from an impression that should include all areas of future tissue support of the partial denture. The tray is selectively relieved and, when checked in the mouth, should cover the edentulous areas up to the border tissue attachments and should include the retromolar pads. The bases of the tray should be connected with each other by means of an acrylic resin lingual bar. The bar should cover the area between the muscle attachments of the floor of the mouth and the lingual gingivae of the anterior teeth. The tray should clear the free gingivae around the abutment teeth to prevent future impingement and stripping.

This tray is loaded with an easy-flowing zinc oxide–eugenol paste and brought into position in the mouth, care being taken that the soft tissues are left in their passive state. After the material has hardened, the tray is removed and the impression examined. In a successful impression, the tissue side of the tray is fully covered with impression material, and no part of the tray itself is visible. The material that has flowed from the tray onto the abutment teeth should now be cut away and the tray reinserted in the mouth and tested for stability.

The next step is to make an impression of the teeth and to establish a relationship between the teeth and the mucosa in a displaced state. For this purpose, a perforated tray that has been provided with two circular openings of approximately ¾-inch diameter in the region of the first molars is used. The impression of the soft tissue areas is placed in the mouth. Then, while the tray is being loaded with an alginate impression material, some of this material is used to fill in the space between the soft tissue impression and the remaining teeth. The loaded metal tray is then inserted over both the teeth and the acrylic resin tray. The index fingers are passed through the openings in the perforated tray until they contact the underlying tray; then pressure is exerted upon it. This pressure should be maintained until the alginate impression material has hardened. The completed impression is then removed as one unit. The cast made in this impression will be a reproduction of both the surface of the teeth and the undistorted surface of the mucosa, but the two will be related to each other with the mucosa in a functional state as it would be found under the partial denture base during mastication. While the base is related to the occlusal rest with the mucosa in a functional state, the tissue surface of the base is actually a reproduction of the passive and undistorted mucosa as obtained with zinc oxide–eugenol paste in the individual impression tray.*

The form of the residual ridge recorded under some loading, whether by occlusal loading, finger loading, specially designed individual trays, or the consistency of the recording medium, is called the *functional form*. This is the surface contour of the ridge when supporting a functional load. How much it will differ from the anatomic form will depend upon the thickness and structural characteristics of the soft tissues overlying the residual bone. It will also differ from the anatomic form in proportion to the total load applied to the denture base.

The objective of any functional impression technique is to provide maximum support for the removable partial denture base, thereby maintaining occlusal contact to distribute the occlusal load over both natural and artificial dentition and at the same time minimize movement of the base, which would create leverage on the abutment teeth. While some tissueward movement of the distal extension base is unavoidable and dependent upon the six factors listed previously, it can be minimized by providing the best possible support for the denture base.

Steffel has classified advocates of the various methods for treating the distal extension partial denture as follows:

1. Those who believe that ridge and tooth supports can best be equalized

by the use of stressbreakers or resilient equalizers
2. Those who insist on bringing about the equalization of ridge and tooth support by physiologic basing, which is accomplished by a pressure impression or by relining the denture under functional stresses
3. Those who uphold the idea of extensive stress distribution for stress reduction at any one point

It would seem that there is little difference in the philosophy behind methods 2 and 3 as given by Steffel, for both the equalization of tooth and tissue support and stress distribution over the greatest area are objectives of the functional type of impression. Many of the requirements and advantages that may be given for the distributed stress denture apply equally well to the functionally or physiologically based denture. Some of these requirements are: (1) positive occlusal rests; (2) an all-rigid, nonflexible framework; (3) indirect retainers, whenever practical, to add stability; and (4) well-adapted, broad-coverage bases.

Those who do not accept the theory of functional basing and those who, for one reason or another, do not use some kind of secondary impression technique for partial dentures, should use some form of stressbreaker between the abutment and the distal extension base. The advantages and disadvantages of doing so have been given in Chapter 8.

Accuracy of the denture base. Support of the distal extension base is enhanced by intimacy of contact of the tissue surface of the base and the tissues covering the residual ridge. The tissue surface of the denture base must optimally represent a true negative of the basal seat regions of the master cast. Denture bases have been discussed in Chapter 8.

In addition, the denture base must be related to the partial denture framework the same as the basal seat tissues were related to the abutment teeth when the impression was made. Every precaution must be taken

---

*Paraphrased from Hindels, G. W.: Load distribution in extension saddle partial dentures, J. Prosthet. Dent. 2:92-100, 1952.

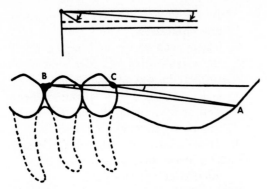

Fig. 15-5. Acute dip of a short denture base is compared with that of a long one in the upper figure. In the lower figure, when the point of rotation is changed from **C** to **B**, it can be seen that a proportionally greater area of the residual ridge is utilized to support the denture base than occurs when the fulcrum line passes through **C**. The line **AC** represents the length of the denture base.

to ensure this relationship when the altered-cast technique of making a master cast is used.

Design of the partial denture framework. Some rotation movement of a distal extension base around posteriorly placed rests is inevitable under functional loading. The greatest movement takes place at the most posterior extent of the denture base. The retromolar pad region of the mandibular residual ridge and the tuberosity region of the maxillary residual ridge therefore are subjected to the greatest movement of the denture base. *As the rotational axis (fulcrum line) of the denture is moved anteriorly, more of the residual ridge is utilized to support the denture base, thereby distributing stresses over a proportionally greater area* (Fig. 15-5). Steffel and Kratochvil have excellently demonstrated this concept in recent dental periodical literature. In many instances, occlusal rests may be moved anteriorly to utilize better the residual ridge for support without jeopardizing either vertical or horizontal support of the denture by occlusal rests and guiding planes (Fig. 15-6).

Total occlusal load applied. The total occlusal load applied is influenced by the number of supplied teeth, the width of

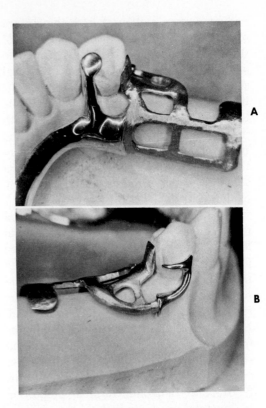

Fig. 15-6. A, Occlusal rest is placed on the mesio-occlusal surface of the lower first premolar to move the point of rotation anterior to a conventionally placed distoclusal rest. The occlusal rest is connected to the lingual bar by a minor connector, which contacts a small mesiolingual prepared guiding plane. Note the vertical extension of the denture base minor connector contacting a guiding plane surface also. The lingual guiding plane is prepared to extend from the occclusal surface inferiorly to approximately one-fourth the height of the lingual surface and is as broad as the contacting minor connector. The distal guiding plane extends from the distal marginal ridge gingivally to about two-thirds the height of the distal surface. Such preparations will not lock the tooth in a viselike grip when the denture base rotates toward the residual ridge. **B,** Buccal view of **A.** The direct retainer assembly is completed by a bar-type clasp with only the retentive tip engaging an undercut.

their occlusal surfaces, and their occlusal efficiency. Kaires conducted an investigation under laboratory conditions and concluded that "the reduction of the size of the occlusal table reduces the vertical and horizontal forces acting on the partial dentures and lessens the stress on the abutment teeth and supporting tissues."*

METHODS FOR OBTAINING FUNCTIONAL SUPPORT FOR THE DISTAL EXTENSION BASE

A thorough understanding of the characteristics of each of the impression materials leads to the obvious conclusion that no single material, of itself, can record both the anatomic form of the teeth and tissues in the dental arch and, at the same time, the functional form of the residual ridge. Therefore, some secondary impression method must be used.

This may be accomplished by several methods. Each of them seems to satisfy the two requirements for providing adequate support to the distal extension partial denture base, which are (1) that it records and relates the tissues under some loading, and (2) that it distributes the load over as large an area as possible.

FUNCTIONAL RELINING METHOD

Although there are hazards to be overcome in any relining procedure of a distal extension base, the *functional relining* method is used satisfactorily in competent hands. The principal hazard is that, unless an open-mouth technique is used whereby the original relationship of the denture framework to the supporting teeth can be positively maintained, indirect retainers may not be seated when the functional impression is made. Because any settling of the denture base will have influenced the occlusion, restoring the denture framework to its original position with indirect retainers seated will result in an elevated occlusion. For this reason, readjustment of the occlusion must be anticipated when an open-mouth relining method is used. In extreme instances, the teeth on the prosthesis will have to be reoccluded to the

---

*From Kaires, A. K.: Effect of partial denture design on bilateral force distribution, J. Prosthet. Dent. 6:373-389, 1956.

opposing dentition after relining of the denture base.

On the other hand, if a closed-mouth impression method is used, particularly with a bilateral distal extension denture, stops of self-curing resin or modeling plastic against resilient tissue may not be adequate to keep the distal extension base from settling tissueward under occlusal loading in such an event, the denture inevitably rotates about its fulcrum line and the indirect retainers lift from their terminal position. Although occlusal harmony on the relined prosthesis will have been maintained by this method, the relationship of the denture framework to the supporting teeth will not be the same as it was on the original master cast.

A second hazard of any relining procedure is the possibility of errors occurring during the reprocessing of an acrylic resin base. Relining of an acrylic resin base frequently results in an increase in vertical dimension. Although this can be minimized by careful laboratory procedures (Chapter 17), by the use of a free-flowing resin, by confirming that there is sufficient space inside the original base for the resin to flow, and by the employment of some space in the land area, some increase in dimension is always possible. Any such increase will result in a faulty relationship between the denture framework and the supporting natural teeth, as well as changes in occlusal relationships.

When a relining method for functional basing is to be used, the original denture base may be processed over a spacer of metal (No. 7 Ash's metal) that has been adapted to the anatomic ridge form. This is the form of the ridge as reproduced on the master cast from a hydrocolloid impression. The relief metal is then stripped away from the resin base, leaving a space on the tissue side for the placement of the impression material and, later, the resin reline. If this is not done, the underside of the denture base must be relieved by removing sufficient resin to accommodate the impression material. Clearance also should be

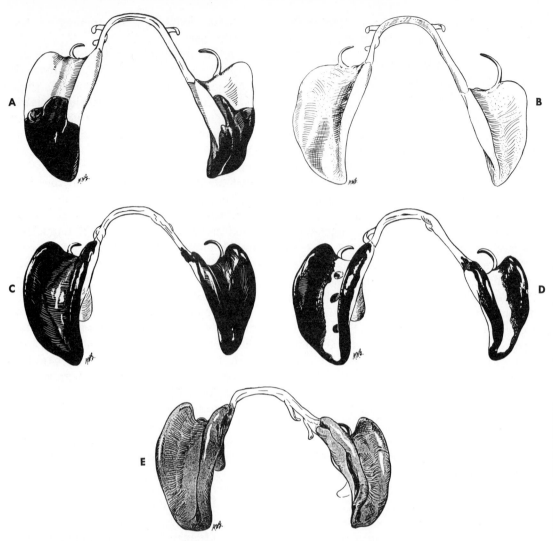

Fig. 15-7. A, Modeling plastic placed to support the distal extension bases during the correction of occlusion. **B,** The ridge surfaces of the bases prepared to receive the modeling plastic. **C,** The smooth, accurate, border-molded impression in modeling plastic. **D,** Bases prepared for the application of impression wax (Iowa formula). **E,** The finished impression made of modeling plastic and wax. Note the escape of wax through holes in the denture bases.

adequate to assure freedom for the flow of the impression material. It should be remembered that thermoplastic impression materials are sluggish and greater space for their flow is needed than when an impression paste or other fluid material is used. It also should be remembered that impression wax will not overdisplace tissue *if given sufficient space and time in which to flow.*

Following is Steffel's procedure for making a functional reline impression:

If there is an indirect retainer or additional points of contact of the framework to make tripoding or stabilization possible, it is preferred to reharmonize the positional relationship of the partial denture to teeth and tissues first, and also to correct the occlusion before proceeding with the reline impression. The procedure is as follows:

Low-fusing modeling plastic is placed in excess on the distal one third to one half of the tissue surface of the bases. The denture is now mass heated in the 140° F. water, quickly carried to the patient's mouth while the impression material is still readily moldable, and seated with firm pressure against only the framework. The material at the distal ends of the bases will have contacted the tissues and hardened so that the restoration is now reoriented in relation to its own arch, but out of harmony with the opposing arch (Fig. 15-7, A). With the modeling plastic for support distally, and accurate metal-to-tooth support anteriorly, the partial denture is stabilized and positioned, and the occlusion altered and balanced in accordance with our judgment for this specific location

After the occlusion has been corrected with the denture being supported at its proper relative elevation, the impression substance, which has now served its purpose, is removed, undercuts are eliminated, and some material is cut away from the tissue surfaces and from the borders of the denture bases to make more room for, and provide better workability of, the impression materials (Fig. 15-7, B).

An excess amount of low-fusing modeling plastic (low-fusing to prevent overdisplacement of tissues) is now applied to the bases. Excess is used so that there will always be some present wherever needed. The restoration is mass heated in the water bath and placed part way toward the tissues but not seated. The patient is not allowed to close for contact. Seating all the way at the first placement might result in too severe pressures against supporting tissues, flowing of the moldable materials into the direct retainers, and the lack of occlusal contacts in the finished denture due to overclosure. Usually about four mass heatings and placements, progressively, are necessary before allowing the patient to close natural teeth to light centric occlusion contact. For the final closure, the patient should be instructed to proceed just to the point of faint facet-to-facet or interdigita-

tive contact, not asked to close with great force. Force might result in an upward displacement of the condyloid processes. At this juncture the bases will be at their correct vertical position, occlusion will be reestablished, and because correct occlusal contacts were provided beforehand, the metal work will have accurate adaptation to the natural teeth.

The border limits are now formed by heating and tempering short sections with the torch, then manipulating the cheeks and lips for border outline.

The reline impression at this point looks acceptable, has adequate tissue coverage, rounded smooth borders, smooth impression surfaces, and a stabilized, properly repositioned composite partial denture (Fig. 15-7, C). However, the borders are really not physiologically molded, and there will be small inaccuracies in surface detail, excessive stress against the crest of the ridge, and probably against the mylohyoid ridge.

Impression substance, and even base material if necessary, is now removed all along the crest of the ridge, and usually along the mylohyoid ridge. Also, if the distal extension bases are long, escape holes are bored completely through the base material at these areas requiring relief; if they are short, their open ends provide sufficient escape ways (Fig. 15-7, D). No impression bulk is removed along the normal slopes of the ridges.

Impression wax (Iowa) is now painted over the entire impression surface, the partial denture is placed and the patient is instructed to gradually force it to place, and then to continue with the functional movements of chewing. In contrast to modeling plastic, the wax must always be well chilled before removal for examination. After a short period in the mouth, five minutes for example, excess of wax is removed and the restoration is replaced (with wax additions if necessary). The patient is again instructed to go through the functional movements of chewing together with facial and oral gymnastics for about ten minutes. The wax flows so readily that there is no danger of its remaining on any surface where its contour will not be tolerated later. Limited movement of the base extensions under the functional stresses will mold the soft wax for relief of vulnerable areas. Also, in the completed restoration, the slight movement allowed by the passive retainers will preclude the possibility of tissue strangulation.

This final step in the reline impressions (the relieving of areas and the addition of wax) does not change the previously reestablished position of the partial denture in the arch, but merely refines the impression, and specializes the fit with reference to the different types of supporting tissues. At this point, the impression is ready for accurate conversion into a permanent material (Fig. 15-17, *E*). It presents: (1) a surface that is smooth and tissue adapted, (2) a surface outline that will place additional stresses on tissues that can tolerate them, giving relief to others, and (3) borders that have a functional outline molded by physiologic muscular action and not by excessive manual manipulation.*

In executing a relining procedure three objectives generally must be remembered: (1) the repositioning of the displaced metal framework, (2) the reestablishing of lost occlusal contacts, and (3) the making of an impression that will ensure intimate tissue adaptation of the basal seat.

By this method of securing a new impression for the support of extension bases, as little or as much displacement of soft tissues as is desired can be achieved by a greater or lesser degree of heating of the impression plastic and/or wax and thereby controlling its flow. Additionally, the partial denture is placed accurately into its functional position by the *light* closure of the opposing arch of teeth into occlusion and not by questionable finger placement.

In the reline impression as advocated by Steffel, the impression wax is used as a

final correction material. Iowa formula impression wax is used in much the same manner as for a complete denture impression, except that the impression for a partial denture is coordinated with the terminal position of the cast framework.

SELECTIVE TISSUE PLACEMENT IMPRESSION METHOD

Soft tissues covering basal seat areas may be either *placed, displaced,* or recorded in their *resting* or *anatomic form.* Placed and displaced tissues differ in degree of alteration from their resting form and in their physiologic reaction to the amount of displacement. For example, the palatal tissues in the vicinity of the vibrating line can be slightly displaced to develop a posterior palatal seal for the maxillary complete denture and will remain in a healthy state for extended periods of time. On the other hand, these same tissues will develop an immediate inflammatory response when they have been overly displaced in developing the posterior palatal seal.

Oral tissues that have been overly displaced attempt to regain their anatomic form. When not permitted to do this by the denture bases, the tissues become inflamed and their physiologic functions become impaired, accompanied by bone resorption. Tissues that are minimally displaced (placed) by impression procedures respond favorably to the additional pressures placed upon them by resultant denture bases if these pressures are intermittent rather than continuous.

The selective tissue placement impression method is based on the previously stated clinical observations, the histologic nature of tissues covering the residual alveolar bone, the nature of the residual ridge bone, and its positional relationship to the direction of stresses that will be placed upon it. It is further believed that by use of specially designed individual trays for impressions, dentures bases can be developed that will utilize those portions of the residual ridge that can withstand additional stress and at the same time relieve the tis-

---

*Paraphrased from Steffel, V. L.: Relining removable partial dentures for fit and function, J. Prosthet. Dent. 4:496-509, 1954.

sues of the residual ridge that cannot withstand functional loading and remain healthy.

There are only minor variations in techniques in recording the basal seat tissues with the "functional reline method" and the "selective tissue placement impression method." The latter method is illustrated in Fig. 15-8, and is the predominant impression procedure for lower distal extension dentures in our practices.

FLUID-WAX FUNCTIONAL IMPRESSION METHOD

One must differentiate between the wax "wash," or correction impression, as originally developed by Dr. Earl S. Smith of the University of Iowa, and the fluid-wax impression, as developed by Dr. O. C. Applegate of the University of Michigan and Dr. S. G. Applegate of the University of Detroit. The latter method uses an impression wax (Korecta wax No. 4) that is slightly more fluid than the Iowa wax. Border extension is established by the impression wax and then reinforced by backing it up with a special hard wax (Korecta wax No. 1).

The Applegate method may be used for making a reline impression or for the correction of the original master cast. In either application the thickness of wax permits a greater flow of material and therefore less tissue displacement than does the wax "wash." The fluid wax impression is used with an open-mouth procedure; therefore, there is less danger of overdisplacement of tissues by the application of vertical forces. If adequate space for the flow of the material is provided and sufficient time is allowed for the escape of excess material, the fluid-wax impression will not overdisplace tissues. Only those soft tissues that can readily be displaced or made more compact by the consistency of the wax itself will be recorded in a different form from that recorded by the anatomic impression.

In addition to less displacement of tissues, the fluid wax technique records the moving border tissues physiologically, resulting in a more accurate denture border. The limits of border extension are determined by the wax alone, unencumbered by any influence from the impression tray. Both the length and the width of the border are thus established in wax and reproduced in the denture base. The harder wax (Korecta wax No. 1) is used only to back up the impression and should not be allowed to influence the impression record.

O. C. Applegate has named this method the *fluid-wax functional impression.* Although it may be used for relining purposes, it is designed primarily for the making of a secondary impression for the correcting of a master cast. The anatomic ridge form, as recorded in hydrocolloid, is thus replaced with the functional form, as recorded in fluid wax, and the denture base processed to the latter form.

Three objectives in the making of a fluid-wax impression. Three objectives must be considered in the making of a fluid-wax impression. First of these is *tissue support,* as evidenced by a glossy appearance of the wax in areas in which the tissues have reached their supporting form. No additional wax is needed in these areas, since support without overdisplacement is the primary objective of the fluid-wax impression method. It is necessary, however, that wax be added to dull areas that have not yet recorded the supporting form of the tissues.

The second objective, which is the *extension of the impression to obtain maximum coverage by the partial denture base,* is accomplished by adding wax inside the flanges of the impression until excess wax begins to turn at the border of the impression as influenced by the activity of bordering tissues. As the limits of border extension are reached, the soft wax borders are then preserved by backing them up with the hard No. 1 wax.

The third objective is the *release of any tissues that may have been overdisplaced.* This is accomplished by allowing sufficient time for the excess wax to flow to the bor-

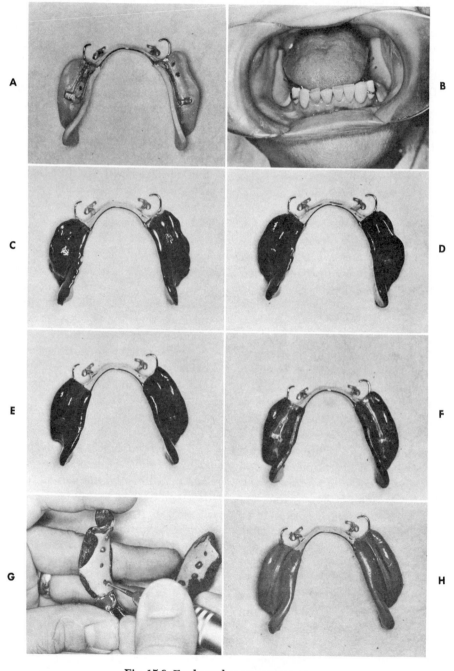

Fig. 15-8. For legend see opposite page.

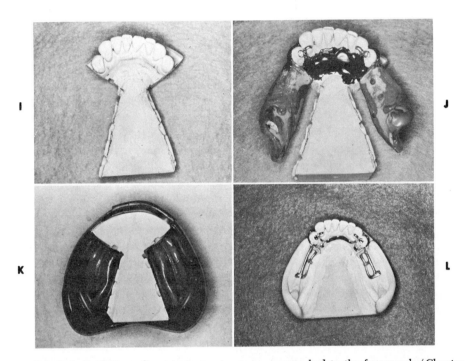

Fig. 15-8. A, Individual acrylic resin impression trays are attached to the framework (Chapter 18). Holes are placed in the tray along the alveolar groove to allow the escape of excess impression material. **B,** The framework and attached trays are tried in the patient's mouth. Borders of the tray are adjusted so that they are 2 to 3 mm. short of all reflections but cover the retromolar pads. **C,** A thin layer of red stick modeling plastic is "painted" on the tissue sides of the impression trays by first softening the modeling plastic in a flame. **D,** The modeling plastic has been softened by a flame, tempered in 135° F. water, and placed in the patient's mouth. This procedure is repeated (usually three times) until the basal seat tissues are not displaced and the framework is correctly positioned. The impression trays will be stable at this time and border-molding procedures can begin. **E,** Borders are perfected by heating individual areas, placing the tempered tray in the mouth, manipulating the cheeks, and having the patient form lingual borders by tongue movements. Note that the lingual flanges have assumed an **S** shape. This **S** shape has been formed by the action of the mylohyoid muscle. Note also that the lingual flange has been extended into the retromylohyoid fossa. There would be *no difference* in the form of the impression of the edentulous regions at this stage from a complete denture impression of the same regions if the patient was edentulous. **F,** Borders of the compound impression are shortened 1 to 1.5 mm., and the whole inside of the impression, *with the exception of the buccal shelf region,* is relieved approximately 1 mm. **G,** Modeling plastic is removed from the holes in the tray. **H,** The final impression is completed with a rubber base impression material wash. The framework must be perfectly seated and maintained in position while the impression material is setting. **I,** Edentulous regions of the cast are eliminated. The cut surfaces are grooved for additional retention of the stone poured to make the altered cast. **J,** The framework and impression are returned to the cast and are luted with sticky wax to avoid displacement during boxing and pouring procedures. **K,** A utility wax is used to box the impression. **L,** The altered master cast with the framework in position. Buccal shelf regions have been recorded in a functional form. Other regions of the basal seats have been recorded in an anatomic form.

ders where it can escape as it is turned by the action of moving border tissues. During this period, which should be about eight minutes, functional movements are repeatedly simulated to turn the excess wax as it reaches the border of the impression.

Methods of obtaining a cast of the functional ridge form. The end result of the fluid-wax impression is the making of a cast of the supporting ridge to which the partial denture base can be processed, thereby providing optimal support for that base. Although the impression technique does not vary, the manner in which the cast is corrected may be varied in accordance with the preference of the dentist and the type of prosthesis, that is, whether it is to have a metal or a resin base. These several methods of correcting the master cast are described as follows:

1. The correction of the master cast is subsequent to the making of the denture framework. The cast framework is used as a means of positioning the impression tray in the mouth and, later, back onto the master cast for repouring the ridge areas. The components of the cast framework act as a positive guide to the accurate seating of the denture, both in the mouth and on the stone cast. This method is used only when acrylic resin bases will be processed to the corrected master cast.

a. This method is identical with *1* except that the stone cast is poured against both the impression and the underside of the denture framework, thereby forming a *processing cast.* Properly done, the cast framework can then be lifted from the processing cast to remove the attached impression base and then repositioned on the processing cast with accuracy. The advantages of this method are that the master cast need not be cut, and the possibility of error in reseating the framework on the master cast is eliminated. For the first method to be done with accuracy, the denture framework must bear exactly the same relationship to the master cast as to the mouth when the impression was made. This hazard is avoided by the use of a

processing cast. When only a few natural teeth remain to aid in repositioning the cast framework, as, for example, when only six anterior teeth remain, there may not be enough tooth contact to positively establish the exact position of the framework on the master cast. In such case, the making of a processing cast is preferred over the correction of the original master cast.

b. When metal bases are to be cast separately to the functional ridge form and then attached to the original frame by soldering or with resin, the impression may be made as in *1* and the master cast corrected prior to the making of the metal bases. This method is essentially the same as *1* except that separate metal bases will be made rather than resin bases processed directly to the cast.

2. The use of an acrylic resin tray rather than the denture framework for positioning the impression in the mouth and then back onto the master cast for the correction of the ridges is a method that makes possible the correction of the master cast prior to the making of the denture framework. It was developed primarily to permit the making of a one-piece partial denture with metal bases made to functional ridge form. It may be used also to correct the master cast prior to making the cast framework for a resin-base denture, if the dentist prefers to use this method rather than method 1.

Step-by-step procedure for making a fluid-wax functional impression. The technique for making a fluid-wax functional impression is the same regardless of the method of application used for making the stone cast. The step-by-step procedure given here is for method 1, using the denture framework as a medium for carrying the impression to the mouth and then back onto the master cast for correction.

1. First outline the limits of the impression tray on the master cast with pencil. A sheet of 26-gauge wax or wet asbestos is adapted to the edentulous areas to be recorded in wax and later to be corrected to their functional form. In this way the resin impression base may be trimmed to the

limits of the spacer before its removal, thereby establishing the border limits as previously outlined.

Provide extra relief in the mandibular arch over the retromolar pad since this is easily deformed by the impression wax. A hole also may be placed in the resin base over the pad to effect the escape of confined wax and to prevent distortion of the glandular portion of the retromolar pad. If the retromolar pad is not recorded on the master cast, extend the tray onto a molded clay extension of the cast; otherwise that portion of the tray will have to be extended in the mouth with self-curing resin. Since warm wax will be used, it is best not to border mold or extend the impression base in the mouth with modeling plastic. If extension of the impression base in the mouth is necessary, use a mix of self-curing resin in a soft doughy state; wet the original base with monomer, add the soft resin dough and shape with fingers, border-mold-ing it in the mouth. After hardening, trim any excess. The base is thus extended the desired amount.

2. After painting the spacer and surrounding cast with tin-foil substitute, seat the denture framework to its terminal position on the master cast, making sure that the indirect retainers and occlusal rests are fully seated. If a wax spacer is used, slightly warm the casting to assure its seating into the wax. Then secure it anteriorly with sticky wax. Whether wax or wet asbestos is used, create some clearance around the retentive framework for the attachment of the resin impression base.

3. Sprinkle the resin tray material onto the retentive framework and beyond the limits of the spacer, sufficiently thick to assure the rigidity of the impression base.

After hardening, remove the cast framework with attached impression base(s) from the cast, trim to the limits of the spacer, and then remove the spacer.

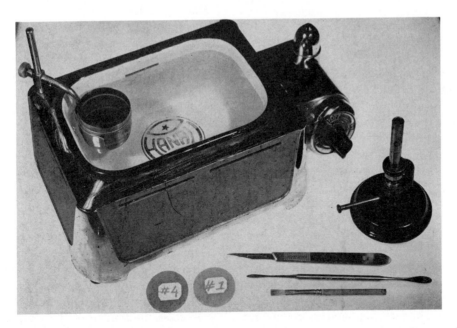

Fig. 15-9. Armamentarium for making a fluid-wax functional impression: wax cup immersed in water bath held at the medium setting, cake of No. 4 Korecta wax that is melted in the wax cup, cake of No. 1 Korecta wax used with a wax spatula to reinforce the impression wax at the borders, No. 11 Bard-Parker blade and handle used for bisecting the impression wax at the borders prior to adding the No. 1 wax for reinforcement, No. 7 wax spatula, flat bristle brush for applying the No. 4 wax, and Bunsen burner for use when applying the No. 1 wax with the wax spatula at the borders.

This is all done in the laboratory, preparatory to the appointment for the functional impression. The care with which the impression base is outlined and fabricated will do much to facilitate the impression procedure. This presumes that the dentist will have interpreted the anatomy of the master cast correctly to avoid gross overextension or underextension of the impression base, thereby avoiding the necessity of time-consuming adjustments at the chair. It is entirely possible to complete the functional impression with three placements in the mouth, as will be seen subsequently.

Equipment and materials needed. The following armamentarium should be available for making the functional impression (Figs. 15-9 and 15-10).

Bunsen burner
Air tip
Water syringe and chilled water
No. 7 spatula
Bard-Parker handle No. 3 with No. 11 blade attached
One cake Korecta wax No. 4 in a wax cup immersed in an electric compound heater
One cake Korecta wax No. 1
Rather stiff bristle brush for applying the fluid wax

4. After trying in the cast framework and adjusting the impression base for any obvious overextension or impingement, dry the base thoroughly. With broad sweeping strokes, paint the fluid wax onto the impression surface until a uniform thickness in some excess has been applied. (See Fig. 15-10.)

5. Seat the framework in the mouth and hold for about two minutes, during which time excess fluid wax will flow to the borders.

It is of utmost importance that the cast framework be seated in its original position each time and that it be held with three fingers of the working hand in the manner of a tripod. Two legs of the tripod are always the two principal occlusal rests. The third is the principal indirect retainer on the anterior portion of the major connector. In this manner, the framework is always seated in its terminal position. At no time

should finger pressure be exerted on the impression base for danger of rotating the framework away from its forward terminal position.

Now remove the impression from the mouth, chill under tap water, dry with air, and inspect. Areas of *support* will appear glossy, and all others will be dull in appearance. Ideally, the entire impression surface should show evidence of supporting tissue contact after the initial placement.

6. Paint fluid wax onto dull areas only and inside the flanges at the border. No wax should be added to the border or on the outside of the impression base.

The framework is reseated in the mouth and held as before, but this time functional border movements are begun to effect *extension of the impression to obtain maximum coverage.* These border movements are done in the following sequence:

a. Using the opposite hand, pull the mucous membrane reflection area vertically against the borders of the impression, thereby simulating the extreme position of those tissues against the denture. Do this first on one side and then the other, making sure that the denture framework remains seated at all times.

b. In the mandibular arch, to bordermold the lingual border, ask the patient to first place the tongue firmly into the left cheek, then into the right cheek, and then to press firmly against the lower anterior teeth. The first two movements mold the lingual borders and distal lingual borders of the opposite side; the third fits the floor of the mouth and brings the retromylohyoid curtain of tissue forward against the distolingual borders.

c. Ask the patient to open his mouth as wide as possible. In the mandibular arch this tenses the pterygomandibular raphe, identifies the tendon of the temporal muscle, and brings the anterior border of the masseter muscle against the distobuccal portion of the impression. On the finished impression the pterygomandibular notch should be evident. Lingual to this is the extension of the impression into the retro-

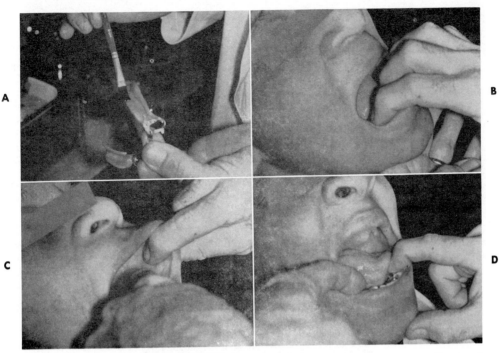

Continued.

Fig. 15-10. Nine steps in the making of a fluid-wax functional impression. **A,** Korecta wax No. 4 is painted evenly over the impression base. **B,** The denture framework is placed in the mouth and held in its terminal position with three fingers, one on each principal occlusal rest and a third in between, holding the framework forward in its terminal position with any indirect retainers fully seated. The chin is supported with the other hand. **C,** While holding the framework down, the cheek on each side is pulled vertically against the border of the impression. This limits the buccal extension to extreme positions of the limiting structures. **D,** Again keeping the framework fully seated, the patient is asked to place the tongue forcibly into each cheek. This records extreme movement of the sublingual tissues on the opposite side. **E,** Still holding the framework down, the patient is asked to press the tongue forward against the lingual surface of the anterior teeth. This limits the distolingual extension of the impression on both sides. After this movement, the patient is asked to open wide, to make the pterygomandibular raphe taut and limit the extreme distal portion of the impression. **F,** The impression is removed and examined for a glossy surface, which is evidence of tissue contact. Once this is established, the border is reinforced by bisecting the impression wax at the border with a No. 11 Bard-Parker blade, leaving unsupported the impression wax extending beyond the impression base. **G,** The hard Korecta wax No. 1 is applied with a hot No. 7 spatula to reinforce the impression wax at the border. This must be applied hot enough to effect good attachment to the impression base. Sufficient No. 1 wax is used to act as a reinforcing extension of the impression base and prevent any undesirable shifting of the impression wax at the border. **H,** More No. 4 wax is brushed on, just inside the border, to provide an excess that will then be turned at the border by a repetition of the previous movements. The wax must be hot enough that it can be brushed on with broad sweeping strokes free of brush mark. **I,** The completed functional impression. Note the border extension buccally and lingually and the thickness of the border permissible with this particular patient. This varies widely with each patient, but the border recorded by this method should always be reproduced in the finished denture.

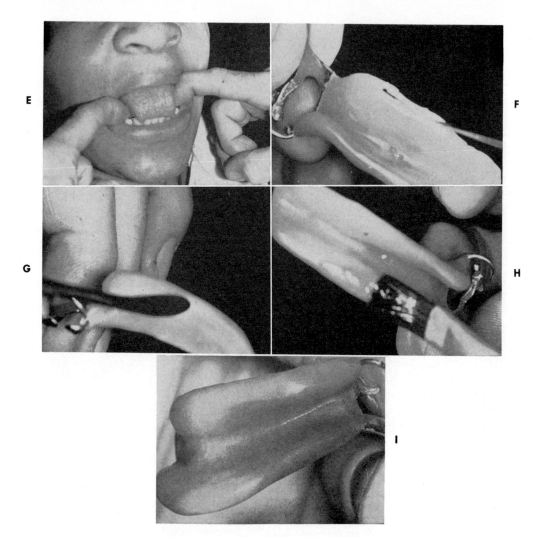

Fig. 15-10, cont'd. For legend see p. 279.

mylohyoid space. The notch or the 45-degree angle formed by the anterior border of the masseter muscle (and the external oblique ridge) should be evident at the distobuccal border of the impression.

In the maxillary arch the pterygomaxillary notch should be evident as a guide to the trimming of the denture base. Also, as a result of opening wide, the distobuccal aspect will frequently show the flattening effect of the coronoid process of the mandible.

These muscle movements are repeated at intervals of approximately one minute. In between, time is allowed for excess wax to escape to the border' at which it is turned by the next series of muscle movements.

After approximately five minutes, remove the impression, chill with tap water, then dry with air, and inspect. The length of time that the impression is left in the mouth will depend upon the size of the impression and how far the excess wax must move to reach the borders at which it may escape and be turned by the activity of bordering tissues.

This time, the entire impression surface should appear glossy, and some excess wax should be present at the border. If any dull areas remain or any of the border is deficient, brush fluid wax onto these areas in broad, sweeping strokes and return the impression to the mouth, repeating the previous step.

7. Having obtained evidence of support and border extension, the next step is to reinforce the border excess. This is done in the following manner:

Holding the impression tissue side up, use the No. 11 Bard-Parker blade to bisect the border excess back to the resin impression base. Discard that half on the side away from the tissues, as well as remove all wax that has flowed or has been accidentally applied to the outside of the impression base, leaving a wax-free surface for the attachment of the supporting No. 1 wax. The remaining half is unsupported impression wax that has flowed beyond the limits of the impression tray.

With the large end of the No. 7 spatula, apply Korecta wax No. 1 to the outside of the unsupported No. 4 wax. Apply it hot enough to be fluid and to fuse both to the impression wax and to the resin impression base, yet without melting the impression wax. Cool each application of No. 1 wax with compressed air, returning it to its original hard state. Since this wax is unaffected by mouth temperature, it becomes a stable extension of the resin base. Therefore, extend it up onto the tray for some distance. It must have been applied and smoothed with the hot spatula to become a reliable backing for the impression wax. If it is applied in layers, or if it has impression wax incorporated into it, it cannot provide stable support and will tend to move in the mouth under functional movements.

As an alternate method, the impression wax at the border may be supported with resin tray material, using a brush technique for applying. The original tray must be exposed, leaving the unsupported impression wax, which is then reinforced with the applied resin. Because time must be allowed for polymerization of the resin, this method is generally used only when gross extension of the impression tray is indicated. Minor extension is best accomplished

with No. 1 Korecta wax as outlined in the preceding paragraph.

8. Having reinforced the border extensions of the impression wax with the supporting wax, add a final application of fluid impression wax to and over the border. Up to this time, impression wax has been added only to the inside of the border. This time, not only is the border limit to be recorded under functional movements, but also border thickness. Except for the distolingual borders of the mandibular denture, which are arbitrarily thinned on the finished denture to avoid objectionable thickness in this area, the thickness of the denture border should be that recorded in the wax impression. Thus, the functional impression method provides not only support for the distal extension base but also a physiologic border thickness as established by functional movements. Support for the cheek is thus assured, and food impaction is prevented by properly contoured polished denture surfaces.

Return the functional impression to the mouth for what should be the final placement. The third objective, that of *effecting a release of any tissue that has been over-displaced,* is accomplished during this final placement. For this reason, sufficient time must elapse for the entire impression to return to its fluid state at mouth temperature and for *any excess wax to be displaced by rebounding tissues,* where it may flow to the border and be turned by functional movements. For the average impression eight minutes is usually sufficient, during which time the same sequence of functional movements is performed at intervals of approximately one minute. For a larger impression as much as twelve minutes may be necessary because the excess wax will have a greater distance to travel to the border as overdisplacement is released. During this period, as before, the denture framework must be held in its terminal position with indirect retainers fully seated.

The finished impression must not be marred during removal from the mouth, since it may not be corrected without re-

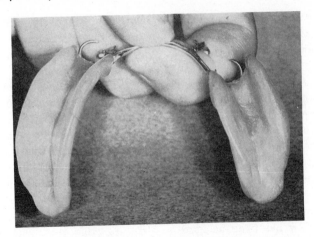

Fig. 15-11. Close view of a completed fluid-wax functional impression.

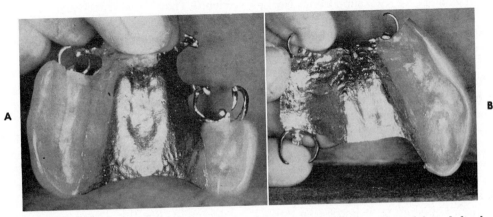

Fig. 15-12. Close view of two maxillary fluid-wax functional impressions. **A,** A bilateral distal extension denture (Class I). Note the variation in width at the borders and note that the impression wax has been trimmed flush with the palatal finishing line of the framework. **B,** A unilateral distal extension denture (Class II).

placement in the mouth (Figs. 15-11 and 15-12). For this reason, use chilled water to reduce the temperature of the wax to a more stable form. After emptying one or more syringefuls of chilled water into the mouth, which is then aspirated, remove the denture framework and attached impression. The patient should be cautioned to remain passive and allow the dentist to remove the impression unaided. After releasing the direct retainers, it is sometimes helpful to lift the framework out of the mouth with thumb forceps, although this will depend upon its accessibility and the digital dexterity of the dentist. The greatest hazard to be avoided is the cusps of the teeth nearest the impression, which may touch and mar the border during removal.

Now dry the impression with compressed air and inspect. If satisfactory, place the impression tissue side up on two cotton rolls, which preferably have been secured to the bottom of a shallow box. Although the impression need not be poured immediately and may be kept safely at normal room temperature, protect it from damage and heat.

Pouring the functional cast. This is usually done by removing the anatomic form of the residual ridge from the master cast and repouring it in its functional form as recorded by the wax impression (Figs. 15-13 to 15-16).

1. If the anatomic ridge form on the master cast is to be replaced with the functional, or supporting, form, remove and discard that portion of the master cast. This is done by sawing the cast with a spiral saw blade along lines drawn on the cast.

Beginning about 1 mm. distal to the abutment tooth, draw a line at right angles to the longitudinal axis of the ridge and down the side of the cast. Then project this line along the bottom of the cast. On the mandibular cast, draw a second line at right angles to the first, beginning just medial to the lingual sulcus and extending distally along the rim of the sulcus to the dorsal aspect of the cast and down that side. Then project this line anteriorly along the bottom of the cast to join the first line at a right angle. If a Class I cast, do this for both ridges.

With a spiral saw blade, saw the cast along these lines until the cuts meet at the anterior lingual angle. Then remove and discard the anatomic ridge form. If a Class I cast, this leaves the center portion of the cast intact.

On the maxillary cast, make the longitudinal cut on the palatal aspect to coincide with the edge of the wax impression so that a butt joint is created between the wax and the remaining cast. Otherwise, excess stone will flow beneath the denture framework. This is facilitated by scoring the cast along the wax relief at the time of blockout. Trim the palatal aspect of the relief abruptly so that a raised platform will be evident on the investment cast and a step will exist on the denture casting. This serves as a finishing line on the tissue side, first to limit the wax impression and later to establish the finishing line for the resin base. Having scored the cast previously, cut the cast longitudinally along this line. A precise junction between the impression wax and the remaining portion of the cast thus will be possible to assure a smooth junction between the new functional ridge form and the anatomic form of the palate.

After removing the anatomic ridge, roughen or undercut the fresh edges of the cast to create some mechanical retention between the new and the old stone.

2. Being sure that the denture framework and the master cast are free of any debris, seat the framework in the same terminal position as it was when in the mouth. Secure it anteriorly with sticky wax. Some wax blockout is necessary to confine the new stone, but complete boxing is neither necessary nor advisable for the fluid-wax impression.

Beginning at the base of the abutment tooth, adapt a stick of utility wax on the buccal surface down to the bottom of the cast. Seal this along its anterior border without covering the freshly cut surface to which new stone must attach. This is the only blockout on the buccal surface, and on the maxillary cast, it is the only blockout that is needed.

On the mandibular cast, adapt a sheet of soft wax, such as utility wax or adhesive wax, along the lingual sulcus. Seal this anteriorly around the lingual bar and the minor connector, all along its junction with the cast, and to the impression base some distance above the border of the impression. It is important that the hot spatula not approach the impression border as the mouth-temperature wax is easily melted.

Now the exposed remainder of the original cast should be painted with a separating film, such as tin-foil substitute, to prevent new stone from attaching to critical areas of the cast.

Place the base of the cast in a pan of water no more than ½ inch deep so that it may become saturated without immersing the impression itself. Five to ten minutes' soaking is sufficient.

3. Pour the cast with the same type of stone as the original cast or with stone of a different color for contrast. Any excess is more easily identified by using stone of contrasting colors. The object in using a separator on all but the cut surfaces

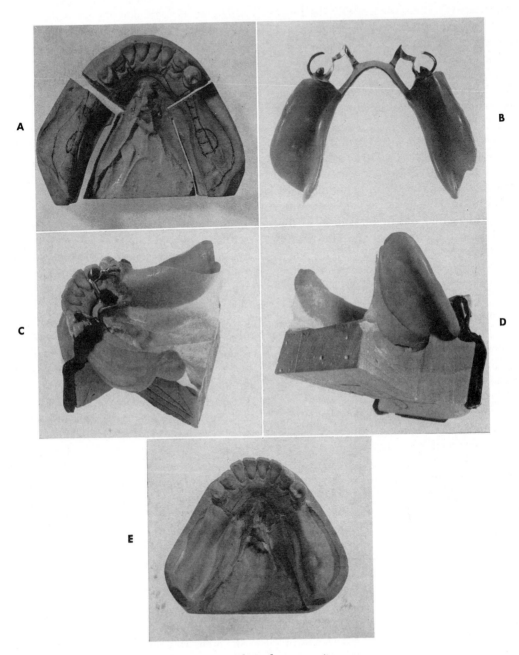

Fig. 15-13. For legend see opposite page.

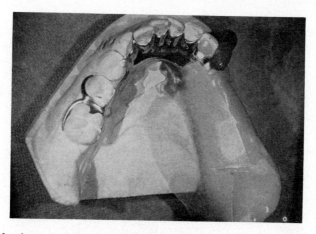

Fig. 15-14. Occlusal view of the wax blockout before repouring the edentulous area to the form recorded by the fluid-wax functional impression. The framework must be secured in position with sticky wax. Utility wax is used to limit the fresh stone on the buccal surface at the line of junction only. Adhesive sheet wax is used on the lingual surface, which is sealed anteriorly to prevent the new stone from leaking through.

Fig. 15-13. A, After the making of the resin impression base attached to the partial denture framework, the ridge areas recorded in their static or anatomic form are removed from the master cast by sawing with a spiral saw blade in two planes. One cut is made at right angles to the longitudinal axis of the ridge, 1 mm. distal to the abutment tooth. The second cut is made just lingual and parallel to the lingual sulcus as recorded in the original impression. The two are joined anteriorly and the anatomic reproduction of the ridge is removed. At this time, if the saw cuts are not rough enough, the cut surfaces of the cast should be scored with a knife to provide mechanical retention for the attachment of the new stone to the old. **B,** The completed fluid-wax functional impression. **C,** The completed wax functional impression is seated on the remainder of the master cast after the anatomic ridges have been removed. Note the scored surface for added retention. The cast metal framework is secured to the dry cast with sticky wax after first making sure that no debris interferes with seating and that all occlusal rests and indirect retainers are seated. Utility wax is placed on the original cast just anterior to the saw cut and sealed anteriorly with a hot spatula. Sheet wax of the adhesive type is placed lingually and sealed to the cast and along the side of the impression base. It must be sealed anteriorly, but the hot spatula must not come in contact with the impression. The surface of the cast anteriorly is then painted with sodium silicate or some other separator, such as Microfilm. Just prior to pouring the new ridge areas, the base of the cast is immersed in ½ inch of water for ten minutes to provide saturation of the dry stone. **D,** The wax functional impression attached to the master cast. The anatomic ridge form has been removed and the cut portion of the cast undercut to assure attachment of the new stone to the old. The cast has been saturated by placing it base downward in ½ inch of water for ten minutes prior to pouring. The only vibrating necessary in adding the new mix of stone is to prevent trapping air at the junction of the wax impression with the cut surfaces of the stone cast. **E,** The ridge areas are poured with a stone of a different color, using no more vibration than necessary, and then inverted into additional stone on a glass or ceramic slab. Stone must be brought up well around the distal ends of the impression. After the stone has hardened, the excess is trimmed away until the margins of the impression wax are exposed. The sticky wax is chilled with ice or the cast is chilled and the sticky wax flaked off. The cast is then immersed in water at 110° to 120° F., just sufficient to soften the mouth-temperature wax, and the framework with attached impression base is lifted. Usually, the impression wax remains on the impression base, leaving a clean cast as shown.

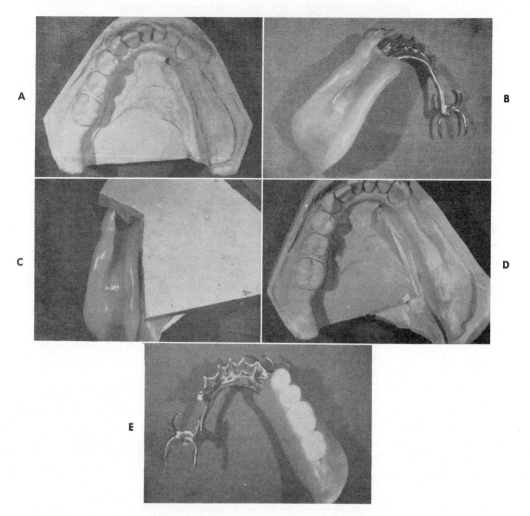

Fig. 15-15. Sequence in the correction of a lower Class II cast to functional ridge form. **A,** The master cast with anatomic ridge form as recorded from a hydrocolloid impression. The outline of the proposed impression base is drawn in pencil. **B,** The completed functional impression. **C,** The impression seated on the cut-away cast, boxed anteriorly with sticky wax and lingually with adhesive sheet wax. **D,** The corrected master cast. Compare this with **A.** **E,** An occlusal view of the completed denture showing the broad coverage made possible by this impression method. This denture base, although much larger than the denture worn previously, was accepted by the patient with no adjustment whatsoever.

is, of course, to facilitate the removal of any unwanted stone. Such excess can be prevented, however, by carefully sealing the blockout wax and by avoiding excessive vibration when filling the impression. The only reason for vibrating the impression is to avoid trapping air at acute angles at which the impression joins the cast. After this area has been filled, the remainder may be filled without vibrating. Add stone in excess, piling still more stone onto a glass slab; then invert the impression carefully onto the glass slab. Next smooth the sides of the cast with the spatula, and, as the stone stiffens, trim away the gross excess. It is not necessary to immerse the impression because by the time the stone gives off exothermic heat, the initial set has oc-

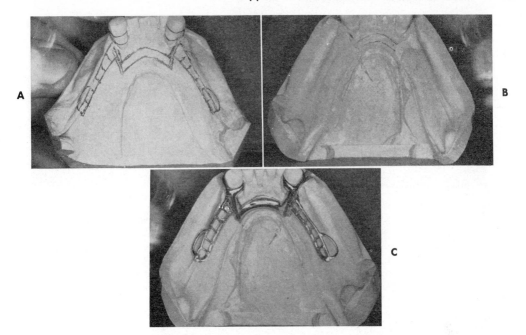

Fig. 15-16. Correction of a lower Class I master cast with only six anterior teeth remaining. A, The original master cast with edentulous areas reproduced in their anatomic form. The penciled design of the denture framework is evident. Note the positive lingual rest seats on the canines. B, The same cast with edentulous areas corrected to their functional form. Compare with A. C, The framework returned to the corrected cast for making jaw relation record bases. Tapered wrought wire was used for direct retention because a large labial tissue undercut cervical to each canine prevented the use of bar-type retainers.

curred. At this point, immersing the cast to supply additional water for crystallization may be advisable.

4. To separate the impression from the cast first chill the sticky wax and blockout wax to aid in its removal, trimming away any interfering stone around the borders and finally immersing the wax impression in water just above mouth temperature (approximately 110° F.). This latter precaution is to avoid melting the wax, which would cause wax impregnation of the cast surface and later interfere with the action of the tinfoil substitute. Failure of the tinfoil substitute to adequately act as a separating film between the cast and the denture base resin is usually due to wax contamination of the stone cast. This is particularly true when molten wax has impregnated the cast to some depth. Not only for this reason should melting of the impression wax be avoided but also because of the orange-colored pigment in the wax, which, if allowed to impregnate the stone, may cause discoloration of the resin base.

After separation of the cast from the impression, trim the corrected cast, remove any excess, and prepare for the making of a record base upon which jaw relations may be established. Since any previous base will not now fit the functional ridge form, it is necessary that new bases be made, or the original impression base corrected, before final jaw relations can be recorded.

Pouring a processing cast. Occasionally a processing cast may be preferable to a corrected master cast. This cast will then be used rather than the master cast for completion of the denture, the master cast having served its purpose for the making of the denture framework and the impression base. (See Fig. 15-17.)

The sole advantage in using a processing

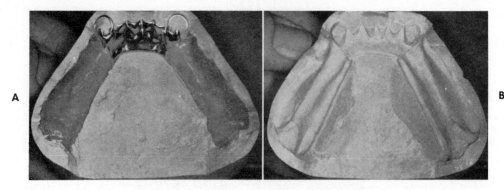

Fig. 15-17. Two steps in the making of a processing cast rather than correcting the master cast. **A,** The functional impression. This is poured completely in new stone, which is brought up anteriorly to provide a surface for reseating the denture framework. Any stone that might interfere with removal must then be trimmed away before attempting separation of the framework from the cast. **B,** The completed processing cast. Note the functional form of the edentulous areas and the index areas remaining to assure accurate repositioning of the denture framework. This method is not used when anterior tooth replacements are involved.

cast is that possible errors in returning the impression to the master cast are thus avoided. It must be created with care, however, so that the denture framework may be removed and reseated with accuracy during subsequent steps in finishing the denture. In pouring the cast, the stone must be brought up around the underside of all of the components of the denture framework to positively establish its future relation to the cast, and yet any excess that would interfere with its removal must be eliminated. For this reason, the individual pouring the cast must give it his undivided attention and trim away excess as soon as the consistency of the stone permits. If this is done, the denture framework and impression may be separated from the cast without interference, leaving an accurate imprint of the underside of the denture framework for later repositioning. Those portions of the cast lying within denture clasps should be trimmed flush with the occlusal border of the clasp arms and the occlusal rests, thereby simulating occlusal surfaces, which may be used later as vertical stops on the articulator. Those portions lying beneath major connectors and indirect retainers must remain intact to assure accurate repositioning of the framework.

Using a resin tray for the functional impression. Although the majority of distal extension partial dentures are made with acrylic resin bases, which can later be relined, there are occasions when the use of metal bases is desirable. There is good reason to believe that ridge tissues remain healthier and ridge resorption is minimized by the stimulating effect of metal bases. (See discussion under advantages of metal bases, Chapter 8.)

Since metal bases may not be satisfactorily relined, they are used only when resorption of the edentulous ridge is not anticipated. It is generally considered that when sufficient time has elapsed since extractions for a firm ridge to be established, there will be less resorption beneath the denture base. It should be remembered that the age and health of the patient and the response of the ridge to occlusal loading will influence the rapidity of tissue change beneath a denture base. It is impossible to predict with any accuracy the response of any given ridge to loading. Still, the beneficial effects of using a metal base with harmonious and moderate occlusion may prevent changes that would ordinarily occur beneath resin bases or under traumatic occlusion. In such cases, the calculated risk of using a metal base, even though it cannot be relined, may be justified.

On the other hand, a ridge that has been satisfactorily supporting a previous denture may be expected to remain constant beneath a new metal base if not subjected to excessive occlusal loading or trauma. Although disuse atrophy of an unused ridge may lead to immediate changes under loading, the fact that a ridge has been supporting a denture previously without unfavorable response leads to the obvious and valid assumption that it may do so in the foreseeable future. In such case, metal bases may be used satisfactorily and to advantage.

A metal-based distal extension denture is no different from a resin-based denture insofar as support is concerned, since any distal extension denture should have the best possible tissue support. But for the metal bases to be cast to the supporting or functional form of the ridge, the master cast must be corrected prior to the blockout and duplication of the master cast. Otherwise, the metal bases must be cast separately and attached to the supporting framework by soldering or other means. A technique for doing the latter will be given later in this chapter.

Several years ago, Applegate and Hall devised a technique for using a resin tray rather than the denture framework as a means of positioning the impression tray in the mouth and then back onto the master cast for correction. In this method three or more occlusal surfaces on natural teeth are used for tripoding the resin tray.

Originally, the tray was waxed on a duplicate master cast, reinforced with piano wire, and invested and processed in acrylic resin. Later a technique was developed for blocking out the cast with modeling clay and forming the tray with self-curing acrylic resin. The sprinkled acrylic resin tray was found to be just as accurate as was the processed tray, and the technique was thereby simplified.

A resin tray may be made on an accurate diagnostic cast or a duplicate thereof. The ridge areas to be corrected are covered with one thickness of 28-gauge wax to provide space for the impression material. The remainder of the cast, with the exception of three widely spaced occlusal seating areas, is blocked out with modeling clay. A trough of baseplate wax may be added anteriorly to provide a form for the molding of the tray handle, or a resin or wire handle may be added later. (See Fig. 15-18.)

The three occlusal stops are painted lightly with a tin-foil substitute, which is then permitted to dry. A separating medium such as Microfilm should never be used, as it may have a retarding effect on the self-curing resin tray material.

A self-curing acrylic resin is used with a sprinkling technique to form the tray. The area to be covered is first wet with monomer and then sprinkled with polymer, after which it is again wetted with monomer. This process is repeated until a tray of adequate thickness has been formed. (See Fig. 15-19.) An upper cast is treated the same as is a lower, without covering the palate. The tray is then covered to prevent too rapid evaporation of the monomer and is set aside for one hour or more. After the polymerization period, the tray is lifted and trimmed and is ready to be taken to the mouth where it should seat accurately on three occlusal legs in the manner of a tripod. The tray, when finished, should be of uniform thickness, with a handle that projects over and beyond the incisal edges of the anterior teeth. It should not contact the teeth at any points other than at the three occlusal stops. Using this tray as the impression base, a fluid-wax functional impression is then made of the edentulous areas, the same as when a cast framework is used (Fig. 15-20). The completed impression is then positioned on the cut-away master cast for the repouring of the edentulous areas.

It was mentioned previously that the tray may be formed upon an accurate diagnostic cast. This can be done only if the diagnos-

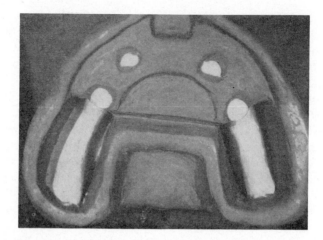

Fig. 15-18. Clay matrix for making a sprinkled acrylic resin impression tray. The ridge areas are first relieved with 28-gauge sheet wax. Three or four occlusal surfaces are left exposed for index areas for positioning the impression tray in the mouth and back onto the master cast for repouring the ridge areas. The clay is grooved from one side to the other to provide a reinforcing rib on the underside of the impression tray.

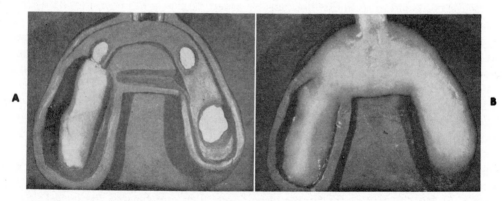

Fig. 15-19. Six steps in the correction of a master cast to functional form, using the resin tray method. **A,** The clay matrix has been formed, with the edentulous area relieved with 28-gauge sheet wax and three occlusal surfaces left exposed to form the legs of a tripod. Note the wax form for the handle extending anteriorly. **B,** Acrylic resin has been sprinkled into the clay matrix. **C,** The resin tray has been trimmed and tried in the mouth. The three bearing areas of contact are then perfected with a fresh application of self-curing resin (visible at the incisal edge of the canine teeth). Note that there is no other contact either with teeth or in the edentulous area where the impression wax will be placed. **D,** The fluid-wax impression is shown, completed. In this method, the amount of palatal area included is arbitrary, but whatever is included in the impression must be cut away from the master cast before the tray is seated upon it. Note the three bearing areas, which determine accurately the position of the tray in the mouth and when returned to the master cast. **E,** That portion of the master cast to be corrected has been cut away and undercut. The resin tray is seated accurately upon it, secured with sticky wax, and blockout placed anteriorly and palatally. The cast, only, is then soaked before repouring the edentulous portion of the cast. **F,** The corrected master cast.

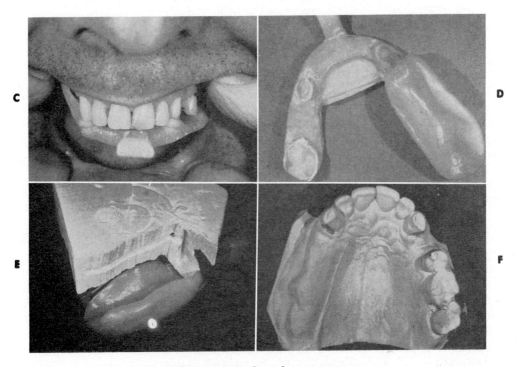

Fig. 15-19, cont'd. For legend see opposite page.

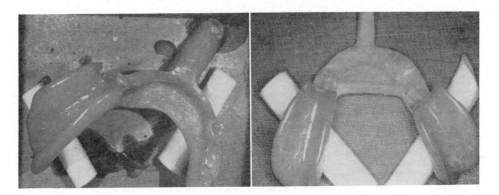

Fig. 15-20. Completed functional impression, whether with resin tray or denture framework, should be supported by cotton rolls until poured. If it must be transported to the laboratory, it may be secured to the bottom of a shallow box with sticky wax.

tic cast is made with the same care as is used in making a master cast. (Any diagnostic cast should be an accurate reproduction of the conditions present, so that diagnosis and treatment planning may be effectively accomplished.) However, whether the impression tray is made on the diagnostic cast or the master cast, the three occlusal areas should be corrected in the mouth with a thin mix of self-curing acrylic resin just prior to making the fluid-wax impression of the edentulous areas. Any change in tooth form, such as the preparation of guiding planes and occlusal rest seats, will be subtractions rather than additions to the teeth and therefore will not interfere with the seating of the impression tray. The three seating areas should be selected with the design of the partial denture framework in mind.

To conserve chair time, the appointment for the making of the wax functional impression in the previously prepared tray may be made to coincide with the making of the final hydrocolloid impression for the master cast. The wax functional impression is made first, and then the hydrocolloid impression of the anatomic form of the teeth and adjoining structures is made. In this case, the edentulous areas to be recorded in their functional form are blocked out on the hydrocolloid impression with stainless steel strips and left unpoured. After the separation of the master cast from its impression, the resin tray, with its functional wax impression, is seated onto the cast and attached to it securely with sticky wax. The edentulous areas are then poured. The resulting master cast, complete with corrected denture base areas, is then ready for the construction of either a resin or a metal partial denture base without further need for seeing the patient until the denture is ready for the recording of occlusal relationships.

Although the resin tray method was developed with metal bases in mind, it may be used regardless of the type of denture bases to be used. If the dentist prefers, he may thus send a corrected master cast to the technician rather than have the cast framework returned for making the fluid-wax impression.

Although it is basically just as accurate a method, the resin tray will not give results equal to those obtained with the denture framework unless the tray is used with considerable care to assure accurate positioning both in the mouth and upon return to the master cast. Some of the precautions to be taken when the resin tray method is used are as follows:

1. The resin tray must be made rigid and should be braced by a reinforcing cross-arch strut. It should have sufficient bulk to assure rigidity without interference to placement, removal, or functional movements.

2. The resin tray must seat in the mouth and on the master cast identically. This is facilitated by correcting the seating areas in the mouth just prior to making the impression and rechecking the accuracy of its position on the master cast. No interference or resistance to seating may exist and no instability should be present. The corrected areas should extend onto suprabulge buccal or labial surfaces of the supporting teeth for added stability. Foreign particles or folded-under pieces of resin material must be eliminated beneath all seating areas to assure accurate repositioning of the tray.

3. The tray must have three or more widely spaced seating areas. Ideally, this would be three legs of a tripod, resting on the occlusal surface of two posterior teeth and one anterior tooth. For a Class I arch two second premolars and one or both canines are best suited for stable support. For a Class II arch the distal extension abutment on one side, the most posterior tooth on the opposite side, and the canine farthest from the extension end are preferred for optimal support of the tray.

The mandibular incisors seldom should be used for support of the resin tray, but when they are, the incisal edges of two or more adjacent teeth are considered one area. The anterior support should not be located beneath the handle but should be freely visible, both in the mouth and on the master cast.

4. The resin tray must be held in the mouth during the entire impression sequence by direct finger pressure over the seating areas *only*. Since no clasps, minor connectors, and bracing components exist to help stabilize the position of the impression tray, only vertical forces may be used to stabilize the tray on the supporting teeth.

5. The master cast and the seating areas of the tray must be free of any debris when it is reseated onto the master cast. The cast must be dry so that sticky wax will adhere to it. The tray should be attached to the cast with sticky wax at places other than the seating areas. These should remain uncovered at all times so that any change in position or inaccuracy in seating may be detected.

6. Blocking out the master cast prior to pouring up the altered cast must be done with extreme caution to prevent dislodgment of the tray. The application of a separating medium, such as a tin-foil substitute, to exposed cast surfaces is important, since the tray may interfere with a complete blockout of areas not to be corrected.

7. The sticky wax should be chilled with cold water and removed before removal of the tray to prevent damage to the surfaces of the cast to which it was attached. The impression wax is then warmed in water just above mouth temperature and lifted off.

8. Any excess stone must be carefully removed and the junction between anatomic and functional cast surfaces smoothed by light scraping. The resulting master cast, with ridges corrected to functional form, can be entirely accurate if the preceding precautions are taken. The master cast is now ready for final surveying, blocking out, duplication, and the making of either a metal-base denture or a casting with retention elements for the attachment of a resin base.

Assembled metal bases. The preceding technique permits correction of the master cast for making a one-piece casting with metal bases made to the functional, or supporting, form of the edentulous ridge. This type of distal extension partial denture is not designed to be rebased; therefore, it is only used for selected patients. There has been some demand for removable partial dentures that combine the advantages of metal bases with the opportunity of replacing those bases in the event of changes in tissue support. The solution lies in replaceable metal bases attached to the denture framework with resin rather than by soldering. (See Fig. 15-21.)

In this method the denture framework is designed and cast as for a resin-base denture, except that an open retentive framework, which will fit inside the finishing line of the future metal base, is made. If, because of recent extractions or the possibility of changes due to disuse atrophy, any change in the supporting ridge is anticipated, the denture may be made first with a resin base. Such a base is preferably made to functional form, even though it is to be replaced later with a metal base. Better support and better stimulation of the residual ridge will result if the functional form is used to support reasonable occlusion. Under such conditions the amount of change in ridge form will be held to a minimum.

Although artificial teeth are usually added, the resin base alone may be used permitting stimulation as an exercise prosthesis as advocated by Applegate, who has this to say about the reconditioning of alveolar bone:

One of the most difficult situations with which the prosthodontist must deal is that existing when disuse atrophy (osteoporosis) has occurred in the edentulous area. Frequently, the missing teeth may have been extracted many years before their prosthetic replacement is accomplished. Bone is maintained only in response to the stimulation associated with its functional use. Of this, Weinmann and Sicher say, "If the loss of teeth is extensive or if the teeth bordering the edentulous area have lost their function, for instance, through the elimi-

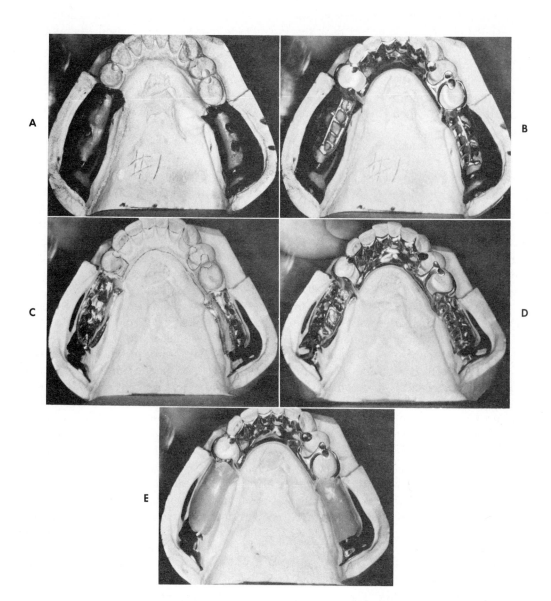

Fig. 15-21. Five steps in the making of replaceable metal bases for a bilateral distal extension partial denture. **A,** The wax patterns for the metal bases are formed on an investment cast duplicate of the corrected master cast. **B,** The original metal framework is placed over the wax pattern and the two are relieved or re-formed as needed to eliminate interference and provide retention and finishing lines for the resin attachment. **C,** The cast bases are returned to the master cast. **D,** The three pieces are assembled on the master cast. This should be done by the laboratory, at which time any remaining interference is eliminated. **E,** The pieces have been assembled with self-curing acrylic resin. Final jaw relations may now be established on this assembled denture, or this may be deferred until the patient and the tissues have become accustomed to the wearing of the prosthesis for a period of time before adding artificial teeth to the denture base. (Modified from McCracken's partial denture construction, ed. 3, St. Louis, 1969, The C. V. Mosby Co.)

nation of their antagonists, the osteoporosis is much more severe and the loss of bone substance at the alveolar ridge is much greater." One of the most common errors in prosthodontics is to assume that, because the bone is being maintained normally in the area of remaining teeth which have received greater than normal function the edentulous ridge in the same mouth also will furnish stable support immediately.

Frequently, the replacement of teeth is done in a manner to restore a nearly normal functional load to such edentulous areas, only to have a rapid resorptive change occur beneath the denture base. I make a plea for the preconditioning of the residual alveolar ridge, where there has been long disuse, before the normal stress load is restored. This can be done by one of the following procedures:

1. Supply a temporary exercise prosthesis for use over a period of a few months.

2. Construct the appliance with the base adapted to functional form and extended to maximum area, but do not replace the teeth until later.

In addition, have the patient exercise the ridge area with finger massage prior to the prosthetic service, while restorative and other mouth preparation is being done. Be certain, also, that the diet and vitamin intake is proper and that the physical condition of the patient is such as to assure the best possible metabolic function. . . .

To be of value, the ridge surfaces of the exercise bases should not only be maximum in area, but they should be related to the basal structures exactly as the bases of the finished partial denture will be. The daily two or three exercise periods of intermittent biting pressure will then direct stimuli through the base into the substructures in the same manner that work stimuli will later be induced by tooth surface contacts. Under this method of bone reconditioning, the edentulous ridge may be expected to undergo a process of reorganization which will prepare it to accept a reasonable occlusal load, at a later time, with much less resorptive change.*

Adding metal bases to the partial denture. When it may be presumed that the

residual ridge has undergone its initial changes under the load of supporting a denture, the metal bases may be added in the following manner.

The original resin base may be relieved and used as an impression base or it may be removed entirely and replaced with a resin impression base, as outlined previously in this chapter. A new functional impression is made and the original master cast or a new master cast is corrected to the existing functional ridge form as though for a resin base. The corrected master cast is then duplicated and an investment cast made.

Upon the investment cast, a metal base or bases is waxed, using 24-gauge wax over the ridge. The borders are reinforced using 14-gauge round wax and free-hand waxing. Prior to locating the finishing line for the resin attachment, the cast framework must be tried on the investment cast to see if the retentive frame will interfere. Any extension loops that were added to support resin bases are removed, leaving only the ladderlike retentive frame. The cross pieces should have been made originally far enough apart to accommodate nailhead retention on the metal base.

An undercut finishing line is added, forming a recess for the resin attachment beyond the limits of the retentive frame. The original cast framework may have to be warmed slightly to assure its seating into the wax pattern for the metal base. Within the boundaries of the retentive frame, two or more nailhead retention elements are added to secure the metal base to the resin attachment, which, in turn, will be attached to the retentive frame. Some care must be taken in waxing around the major connector to form a neat junction without interfering with separation of the cast framework from the wax pattern.

The cast framework now may be lifted and the metal base or bases sent to the laboratory for casting and polishing. The original framework and the master cast also must be sent to the laboratory so that the separate pieces may be fitted together on

---

*From Applegate, O. C.: The removable partial denture in the general practice of tomorrow, J. Prosthet. Dent. 8:609-622, 1958.

the master cast. On return from the laboratory, there must be no definite contact between the separate pieces. Rather, the metal base or bases must seat easily and the original framework go to its terminal position with clearance to spare. Since the attachment between the pieces will be with a self-curing acrylic resin, there is no need for their making contact, which could lead to errors in positioning.

Each piece should be tacked separately to the master cast with sticky wax. With the use of a brush technique first and then sprinkling, the pieces are secured to each other with sufficient acrylic resin to assure stability. Then occlusal relations may be established on this assembled denture.

Since the teeth will be attached to the metal base with resin, it is preferable that there be no line of junction between the acrylic resin attaching the separate pieces and the resin supporting the teeth. For this reason, before arranging teeth in wax the original resin should be cut back short of the finishing line. In this way, the only resin visible will be that supporting the denture teeth.

The principal advantage of this method is that the metal base or bases may be easily removed at some future date by point flaming the underside of the metal base enough to soften the resin attachment. The original metal base then may be separated from the original framework and discarded, leaving the denture framework intact to support a new metal base and new occlusion.

By this method it is possible to replace metal bases when it becomes necessary because of changes in support, accomplishing much the same objective as with the relining of resin bases but with all desirable advantages of using metal bases.

CHAPTER 16

Occlusal relationships for removable partial dentures

The fourth phase* in the construction of a partial denture is the establishment of a functional and harmonious occlusal relationship between the opposing dentitions. This has long been one of the most neglected aspects of partial denture construction.

Failure to provide and maintain adequate occlusion on the partial denture is primarily due to (1) lack of support for the denture base and (2) the fallacy of establishing occlusion to a single static jaw relation record only. Support for the jaw relation record base must be the same as for the finished prothesis, either through occlusal rests or through a combination of occlusal and tissue support. The establishment of functional occlusal records will be covered later in this chapter.

Balanced occlusion is desirable on complete dentures because occlusal stresses may cause instability of the dentures and/or trauma to the supporting structures. And yet, these stresses can reach a point beyond which movement of the dentures takes place. The stresses therefore are eliminated at the expense of denture stability and retention.

In partial dentures, however, because of the fixation to abutments, occlusal stresses are transmitted directly to the abutment teeth and other supporting structures, resulting in sustained stresses, which may be more damaging than those transient stresses found in complete dentures. Therefore, occlusal harmony between a partial denture and the remaining natural teeth is a major factor in the preservation of the health of their surrounding structures.

In the fabrication of complete dentures, only one factor, which is the inclination of the condyle path, is not within the control of the dentist. All other factors may be altered to obtain occlusal balance and harmony in eccentric positions to conform to the dentist's particular concept and philosophy of denture occlusion.

In establishing occlusion on a partial denture, the influence of the remaining natural teeth is usually such that the occlusal forms of the teeth on the denture must conform to an already established occlusal pattern. This pattern may have been improved upon by occlusal adjustment or reconstruction, but the pattern present at the time the partial denture is made dictates the occlusion on the partial denture. The only exceptions are those in which an opposing complete denture can be made to harmonize occlusally with the partial denture or in which only anterior teeth remain in both arches and the incisal relationship can be made noninterfering.

---

*See Chapter 2, under discussion on four phases of partial denture service.

In these situations, the recording of jaw relations and the arrangement of the teeth may proceed in the same manner as with complete dentures, and the same general principles apply.

With all other types of partial dentures, the remaining teeth must dictate the occlusion, unless the dentist is willing to accept nothing more than centric occlusal contacts and ignore interference in lateral movement or has reason to believe that he can achieve occlusal harmony on the partial denture by adjusting the occlusion in the mouth. Although some claim that a functional relationship of the partial denture to the natural dentition may be adjusted satisfactorily in the mouth, it is doubtful that this is or ever can be done adequately. Partial denture occlusion thus established can at best only perpetuate malocclusions that existed previously and help to maintain the existing vertical relationship, however inadequate it may be.

The establishment of a satisfactory occlusion for the partial denture patient should include the following: (1) an analysis of the existing occlusion, (2) the correction of existing occlusal disharmony as a necessary step in preparing the mouth for the partial denture, (3) the recording of centric relation or an adjusted centric occlusion, (4) the recording of eccentric jaw relationships or functional eccentric occlusion, and (5) the correction of occlusal discrepancies created in processing of the denture. An adjusted and corrected occlusion on the natural teeth is the occlusion that the dentist transfers to an instrument in such a manner that occlusal harmony on the partial denture is made possible.

Two methods are commonly used to develop an acceptable occlusion for the removable partial denture patient. The first and most common method involves the use of a semiadjustable articulator. Casts are oriented to the articulator by a face-bow and a static jaw relation record. The instrument is adjusted by additional static jaw relation records. Articulators can simulate but not duplicate jaw movement. A realization of the limitations of a specific instrument and a knowledge of the procedures that can overcome these limitations are necessary if an adequate occlusion is to be created. For example, if an occlusal discrepancy is noted in the mouth due to Bennett movement, which was not reproduced by the articulator when the occlusion was being formulated, the dentures are reoriented on the articulator in the eccentric position causing the difficulty. The discrepancy is corrected in that position, using the articulator as a simple hinge instrument.

A second method is preferred by some dentists. This method involves creating functionally generated paths of opposing teeth in a wax recording medium placed on a denture base. A positive of this record is recovered in stone and forms a template to which the artificial teeth are oriented. The template and opposing denture framework may be mounted on an articulator, using the instrument as a simple hinge. Opposing frames that slide vertically are also used to relate the casts, thus eliminating the need for an articulator in developing the final occlusion. The quality of the occlusion developed by this method is dependent on the stability of the denture base when the paths of opposing cusps are being generated. Design of the denture framework and the quality of the support of the denture bases are factors that influence stability.

A harmonious relationship of opposing occlusal and incisal surfaces, in itself, is not adequate to assure stability of distal extension removable partial dentures. In addition, the relationship of the teeth to the residual ridges must be considered. Bilateral eccentric contact of the lower distal extension denture need not be formulated to stabilize the denture. The buccal cusps may be favorably placed over the buccal turning point of the crest of the residual ridge, and in such positions the denture is not subjected to excessive tilting forces. On the other hand, the artificial teeth of the bilateral, distal extension, maxillary denture often must be placed laterally to the crest of the residual ridge. Such an unfavorable position is conducive to tipping the denture, restrained only by direct retainer action on the balancing side. To enhance the stability of the denture, it seems logical to provide simultaneous balancing and working contacts in these situations if possible.

Desirable contact relationships for removable partial dentures. The following occlusal arrangements, in different situations, are recommended to develop a harmonious occlusal relationship of partial dentures and to enhance stability of the dentures:

1. Simultaneous bilateral contacts of opposing posterior teeth must occur in centric occlusion.

2. Occlusion for tooth-borne dentures may be arranged similar to the occlusion seen in a harmonious natural dentition. Stability of the dentures is assured by direct retainers at both ends of the denture base.

3. Bilateral balanced occlusion in eccentric positions should be formulated when the partial denture is opposed by a maxillary complete denture. This is accomplished primarily to promote the stability of the complete denture. However, simultaneous contacts in a protrusive relationship do not receive priority over appearance, phonetics, and a favorable occlusal plane.

4. Working side contacts should be obtained for the mandibular distal extension denture. These contacts should occur simultaneously with working side contacts of the natural teeth to distribute the stress over the greatest possible areas. Masticatory function of the denture is improved by such an arrangement, especially if the patient chews in a teardrop or elliptical pattern.

5. Simultaneous balancing and working contacts should be formulated for the maxillary bilateral distal extension partial denture, whenever possible. Such an arrangement will compensate in part for the unfavorable position the maxillary artificial teeth must occupy in relation to the resid-

ual ridge which is usually lateral to the crest of the ridge. This desirable relationship often must be compromised, however, when the patient's anterior teeth have an excessively steep vertical overlap with little or no horizontal overlap. Even in this situation, working side contacts can be obtained without resorting to excessively steep cuspal inclinations.

6. Only working contacts need to be formulated for the maxillary unilateral distal extension denture. Balancing side contacts would not enhance the stability of the denture since it is entirely tooth supported by the framework on the balancing side.

7. In the Class IV removable partial denture situation, contact of opposing anterior teeth in centric occlusion is desirable to prevent a continuous eruption of the opposing natural incisors. Contact of the opposing anterior teeth in eccentric positions should not be developed. Such contact would be detrimental to the residual ridge and in no way enhances the stability of the denture.

8. Contact of opposing posterior teeth in a straightforward protrusive relationship is not desirable in any situation except when an opposing complete denture is placed.

9. Artificial posterior teeth should not be arranged farther distally than the beginning of a sharp upward incline of the lower residual ridge or over the retromolar pad. To do so would have the effect of shunting the denture anteriorly.

Wilson and also Osborne and Lammie have described four ways of establishing interocclusal relations for partial dentures. Five methods rather than four will be given in this chapter.

Before describing any of these, it is necessary that the use of a face-bow mounting and the pertinent factors in partial denture occlusion be considered. A description of the face-bow is found in most textbooks on prosthodontics and will not be repeated here. The technique for applying the face-bow has been described briefly in Chapter 11.

Whereas a hinge axis mounting may be

desirable for complete oral rehabilitation procedures, the common face-bow will facilitate the mounting of the upper cast in relation to the condylar axis of the articulating instrument with reasonable accuracy. As suggested in Chapter 11, it is still better that, in addition to mounting the casts at a comparable radius, the plane of occlusion be related to the orbital-axis plane. Since the dominant factor in partial denture occlusion is the remaining natural teeth and their proprioceptor influence on occlusion, a comparable radius at the oriented plane of occlusion on an acceptable instrument will allow reasonably valid mandibular movements to be reproduced. Such instruments are the Hanau models S-M and H-2, the Dentatus model ARH, the Whip-Mix articulator, and similar instruments.

METHODS FOR ESTABLISHING OCCLUSAL RELATIONSHIPS

The recording of occlusal relationships for the partially edentulous arch may vary from the simple apposition of opposing casts by occluding sufficient remaining natural teeth to the recording of jaw relations in the same manner as for a completely edentulous patient. As long as there are natural teeth remaining in contact, however, some consideration must be given the cuspal influence that those teeth will have on functional jaw movements.

The horizontal jaw relation (centric occlusion or centric relation) in which the restoration is to be constructed should have been determined during diagnosis and treatment planning. Mouth preparations also should have been accomplished based on this determination, including occlusal adjustment of the natural dentition, if such was indicated. Therefore, one of the following conditions should exist: (1) centric relation and centric occlusion coincide; (2) centric relation and centric occlusion do not coincide but the decision has been made to construct the restoration in centric occlusion; (3) posterior teeth do not contact and the restoration is to be constructed in centric relation, and (4) posterior teeth

are not present in one or both arches and the denture will be constructed in centric relation.

Then occlusal relationships may be established by utilizing the most apropos of the following methods to fit a particular partially edentulous situation.

Direct apposition of casts. The *first method* is used when there are sufficient opposing teeth remaining in contact to make the existing jaw relationship obvious and when only a few teeth are to be replaced on short denture bases. In this method, opposing casts may be occluded by hand. The occluded casts should be held in apposition with wooden sticks or wire nails attached with sticky wax to the bases of the casts until they are securely mounted on the articulator.

At best, this method can only perpetuate the existing vertical dimension and any existing occlusal disharmony present between the natural dentition. *Occlusal analysis and the correction of any existing occlusal disharmony should precede the making of such a jaw relation record.* The limitations of such a method are obvious. Yet, such a jaw relation record is better than an inaccurate interocclusal record between the remaining natural teeth. Unless a record is made that does not influence the closing path by reason of its bulk and the consistency of the recording medium, direct apposition of opposing casts at least eliminates the possibility of the patient giving the dentist a faulty jaw relationship.

Interocclusal records with posterior teeth remaining. A *second method*, which is a modification of the first, is used when sufficient teeth remain to support the partial denture (Kennedy Class III), but the relation of opposing teeth does not permit the occluding of casts by hand. In such cases, jaw relations must be established as for fixed restorations using some kind of interocclusal record.

The least accurate of these is the interocclusal wax record. The successful recording of centric relation with an interocclusal wax record will be influenced by the bulk and the consistency of the wax and the accuracy of the wax after chilling. Excess wax contacting mucosal surfaces may distort soft tissues, thereby preventing accurate seating of the wax record onto the stone casts. Distortion of wax during or after removal from the mouth may also interfere with accurate seating. Therefore, a definite procedure for making interocclusal wax records is given as follows:

A uniformly softened wafer of baseplate wax is placed between the teeth, and the patient is guided to close in centric relation. Correct closure should have been rehearsed prior to placing the wax so that there will be no hesitancy or deviation on the part of the patient. The wax is then removed and immediately chilled thoroughly in room-temperature water. It should be replaced a second time to correct the distortion resulting from chilling and again chilled after removal.

With a sharp knife, all excess wax should now be removed. It is most important at this time that all wax contacting mucosal surfaces be trimmed free of contact. The chilled wax record again should be replaced to make sure that no contact with soft tissue exists.

A wax record should be further corrected with an impression paste, which is used as the final recording medium. Some impression pastes are more suitable than others for this purpose. Generally, a material that sets quite hard is preferred.

In making such a corrected wax record, the opposing teeth (and also the patient's face and the dentist's fingers) should first be coated with petroleum jelly or a silicone preparation. The impression paste is then mixed and applied to both sides of the wax record. It is quickly placed and the patient is assisted with closing in the rehearsed path, which will this time be guided by the previous wax record. After the paste has set, the corrected wax record is removed and inspected for accuracy. Then any excess projecting beyond the wax matrix should be removed with a sharp knife.

Such a record should seat on accurate casts without discrepancy or interference and will provide an accurate interocclusal record. When an intact opposing arch is present, use of an opposing cast may be dispensed with and a hard stone be poured directly into the impression paste record to serve as an opposing cast. However, although this may be an acceptable procedure in the construction of a unilateral fixed partial denture, the advantages of having casts properly oriented on a suitable articulator contraindicates the practice. The only exception to this is when the upper cast upon which the partial denture is to be fabricated has been mounted previously with the aid of a face-bow. In such an instance, an intact lower arch may be reproduced in stone by pouring a cast directly into the interocclusal record.

An interocclusal record also may be made using an adjustable frame (Fig. 11-21). Reference to this method has previously been made in Chapter 11. The adjustable frame was devised for use with materials that offer no resistance to closure, such as zinc oxide and eugenol impression pastes.

Some of the advantages of using a metallic oxide paste over wax as a recording medium for occlusal records are as follows: (1) uniformity of consistency, (2) ease of displacement on closure, (3) accuracy of occlusal surface reproduction, and (4) dimensional stability; also (5) some modification in occlusal relationship is possible after closure, if made before the material sets, and (6) distortion is unlikely during mounting procedures.

Three important details to be observed when using such a material are as follows:

1. Make sure that the occlusion is satisfactory before making the interocclusal record.

2. Be sure that the casts are accurate reproductions of the teeth being recorded.

3. Trim the record with a sharp knife whenever it engages undercuts, soft tissues, or deep grooves.

Occlusal relations using occlusion rims on jaw relation record bases. A *third* *method* is used when one or more distal extension areas are present, when a tooth-bounded edentulous space is large, or when opposing teeth do not meet. In these instances, occlusion rims on accurate jaw relation record bases must be used. It should not be necessary to add that simple wax records of edentulous areas are never acceptable, despite the unfortunate continuation of this practice. Any wax, however soft, will displace soft tissues. It is totally impossible to seat such a wax record on a stone cast of the arch with any degree of accuracy.

In this method, the recording proceeds much the same as in the second method, except that occlusion rims are substituted for remaining teeth. It is essential that accurate bases be used to help support the occlusal relationship. Shellac bases may be adapted to the casts and then corrected with some kind of impression paste. This is best done by first burnishing tin foil onto the lubricated cast, mixing a suitable zinc oxide and eugenol impression paste and applying it to the shellac base, and then seating the shellac base onto the cast until the paste has set. The tin foil adheres to the impression paste, giving a tin-foil-lined correction of the original base. Such a corrected base is entirely acceptable for jaw relation records. Shellac bases also may be lined with some self-curing resin to accomplish the same purpose. In either case, undercuts on the cast must first be blocked out, and tin foil or, when resin is used, a tin-foil substitute must be used.

Record bases also may be made entirely of self-curing resin. Those materials used in dough form lack sufficient accuracy for this purpose unless they are corrected by relining. A resin base may be formed by sprinkling monomer and polymer into a shallow matrix of wax or clay, after blocking out any undercuts. If the matrix and blockout have been formed with care, interference to removal will not occur, and little trimming will be necessary. When the sprinkling method is used and sufficient time is allowed for progressive polymeriza-

tion to occur, such bases are the most stable and accurate obtainable short of using cast metal, vulcanite, or pressure-molded resin bases for jaw relation records.

Occlusal rest lugs may be formed of stiff wire and located where they will not interfere with the occlusion. These are first attached to the occlusal surfaces with sticky wax, with a retention loop or hook extending into the area to be filled by the sprinkled acrylic resin. The rest lug is thus attached to the record base in much the same manner as a wrought-wire clasp is attached to an interim restoration or an orthodontic retainer.

Jaw relation records made by this method accomplish essentially the same purpose as the two previous methods. The fact that record bases are used to support edentulous areas does not alter the effect. Therefore, in any of these three methods, the skill and care used by the dentist in making occlusal adjustments on the finished prosthesis will govern the accuracy of the resulting occlusion.

Methods for recording centric occlusion on record bases. There are many ways by which centric occlusion may be recorded when record bases are used. The least accurate is the use of softened wax occlusion rims. Modeling plastic occlusion rims, on the other hand, may be uniformly softened by flaming and tempering, resulting in a generally acceptable occlusal record. This method is time proved, and when competently done, it is equal in accuracy to any other method.

When wax occulsion rims are used, they should be reduced in height until just out of occlusal contact. A single stop is then added to maintain its terminal position while a jaw relation record is made in some uniformly soft material, which sets to a hard state. Quick-setting plaster of Paris, impression paste, or self-curing resin may be used. With any of these materials, opposing teeth must be lubricated to facilitate easy separation. Whatever the recording medium, it must permit normal closure into centric occlusion without resistance and must be transferable with accuracy to the casts for mounting purposes.

Relative to the third method, some mention must be made of the ridge upon which the record bases are formed. If the prosthesis is to be tooth supported or a distal extension base is to be made upon the anatomic ridge form, the bases will be made to fit that form of the residual ridge. But, if a distal extension base is to be supported by the functional form of the residual ridge, it is necessary that the recording of jaw relations be deferred until the master cast has been corrected to that functional form. Record bases must be as identical as possible to those of the finished prosthesis. Jaw relation record bases are useless unless they are made upon the same cast to which the denture will be processed, or a duplicate thereof, or are themselves the final denture bases. The latter may be either of cast alloy or a processed resin base. Therefore, for distal extension dentures that are to be made to conform to the functional form of the edentulous ridge, the making of final jaw relation records must be deferred until the functional impression has been made, the functional ridge form has been reproduced on the stone cast, and accurate record bases have been made to fit that functional form.

Jaw relation records made entirely on occlusion rims. The *fourth method* is used when no occlusal contact exists between the remaining natural teeth, such as when an opposing maxillary complete denture is to be made concurrently with a lower partial denture. It may also be used in those rare situations in which the few remaining teeth do not occlude and will not influence eccentric jaw movements. Jaw relation records are made entirely on occlusion rims when either arch has only anterior teeth present (a fixed anterior restoration is considered the same).

In either case, jaw relation records are made entirely upon occlusion rims. The occlusion rims must be built upon accurate jaw relation record bases. Here the choice of method for recording jaw relations is much the same as that for complete dentures. Either some direct interocclusal method or a stylus tracing may be used. As with complete denture construction, the use of a face-bow, the choice of articulator used, the choice of method for recording jaw relations, and the use of eccentric positional records are optional according to the training, ability, and desires of the individual dentist.

The same principles of occlusion apply to such a partial denture as to a complete denture. If the dentist believes that he can adjust occlusion adequately in the mouth, a simple hinge mounting is all that is needed. On the other hand, if he believes in the use of a fully adjustable instrument with the casts mounted to the hinge axis, then he should do so with a partial denture. In between these two extremes we find the majority of dentists who are trained in prosthodontics using a simple face-bow mounting on a semiadjustable articulator (Hanau, Whip-Mix, and so forth) and recording jaw relations to correctly orient casts and adjust the articulator by means of either static records or a stylus tracing.

Establishing occlusion by the recording of occlusal pathways. The *fifth method* of establishing occlusion on the partial denture is the registration of occlusal pathways and the use of an occluding template rather than a cast of the opposing arch. When a static jaw relation record is used, with or without eccentric articulatory movements, the denture teeth are arranged to occlude according to a specific concept of occlusion. On the other hand, when a functional occlusal record is used, the teeth are modified to accept every possible eccentric jaw movement.

These movements are made more complicated by the influence of the remaining natural teeth. Occlusal harmony on complete dentures and in complete mouth rehabilitation may be obtained by the use of modern instruments and techniques. Schuyler has emphasized the importance of establishing first the anterior tooth relation and incisal guidance before proceeding with any complete oral rehabilitation. Others have shown the advantages of establishing canine guidance as a key to functional occlusion before proceeding with any functional registration against an opposing prosthetically restored arch. This is done on the theory that the canine teeth serve to guide the mandible during eccentric movements when the opposing teeth come into functional contact. It also has been pointed out that the canine teeth transmit periodontal proprioceptor impulses to the muscles of mastication and thus have an influence on mandibular movement even without actual contact guidance. However, as long as the occlusal surfaces of unrestored natural teeth remain in contact, as in many a partially dentulous mouth, these will always be the primary influence on mandibular movement, and the degree of occlusal harmony obtainable on a fixed or removable restoration will depend upon the occlusal harmony existing between these teeth.

Regarding occlusion, Thompson has said: "Observing the occlusion with the teeth in static relations and then moving the mandible into various eccentric positions is not sufficient. A dynamic concept is necessary in order to produce an occlusion that is in functional harmony with the facial skeleton, the musculature, and the temporomandibular joints."* To this needs only be added "and with the remaining natural teeth," and we have defined the requirements for partial denture occlusion.

In the registration of occlusal pathways, an occlusion rim of a suitable hard wax, such as Peck's purple hard inlay wax, is attached to an accurate jaw relation record base. This base must be securely attached to the partial denture framework. It may be the final denture base of processed resin or metal. The occlusion rim is worn by the patient for a period of time, preferably for

twenty-four hours or more and preferably during sleep. It is removed by the patient only while eating.

Whereas some of the methods described previously may be applied to the construction of partial dentures in both arches simultaneously, this method requires that an opposing arch be intact or restored to the extent of planned treatment. If partial dentures are planned for both arches, a choice must be made as to which denture is to be made first and which is to bear a functional occlusal relation to the opposing arch. Generally, the maxillary arch is restored first and the mandibular partial denture occluded to that restored arch. Similarly, if the maxillary arch is to be restored with a complete denture or a fixed partial denture and/or crowns, this is done before establishing the occlusion on the opposing partial denture.

Regardless of the method used for recording jaw relations, when one arch is completely restored first, that arch is treated as an intact arch even though it is wholly or partially restored by prosthetic means. It is well to consider at the time of treatment planning the possible advantages of establishing the final occlusion to an intact arch.

By wearing and biting into a wax occlusion rim, a record is made of all extremes of jaw movement. The wax occlusion rim must maintain positive contact with the opposing dentition in all excursions and must be left high enough to assure that a record of the functional path of each cusp will be carved in wax. This record should include not only voluntary excursive movements but also involuntary movements and changes in jaw movement caused by changes in posture. Extreme jaw positions and habitual movements during sleep should also be recorded.

The occlusal paths, thus recorded, will represent each tooth in its three-dimensional aspect. Although the cast poured against this will resemble the opposing teeth, it will be wider than the teeth that carved it because it represents those teeth

---

*From Thompson, J. R.: In Sarnat, B. S., editor: Temporomandibular disorders: diagnosis and dental treatment in the temporomandibular joint, Springfield, Ill., 1951, Charles C Thomas, Publisher.

in all extremes of movement. The recording of occlusal paths in this manner eliminates entirely the need for attempting to reproduce mandibular movement on an instrument.

Occlusion thus established on the partial denture will have more complete harmony with the opposing natural or artificial teeth than can be obtained by adjustments in the mouth alone, because occlusal adjustment to accommodate voluntary movement does not necessarily prevent occlusal disharmony in all postural positions or during periods of stress. Furthermore, occlusal adjustment in the mouth without occlusal analysis is limited by the dentist's ability to interpret correctly occlusal markings made intraorally, whether by articulating ribbon or by other means.

The registration of occlusal pathways has still further advantages. It makes possible the obtaining of jaw relations under actual working conditions, with the denture framework in its terminal position, the opposing teeth in function, and an opposing denture, if present, fully seated. In some instances, it also makes possible the recovery of lost vertical dimension, either unilaterally or bilaterally, when overclosure or mandibular rotation has occurred, rather than perpetuating an abnormal mandibular relationship.

Step-by-step procedure for registering occlusal pathways. The technique for the registration of occlusal pathways is as follows:

1. Support the wax occlusion rim by a denture base having the same degree of accuracy and stability as the finished denture base. Ideally, this would be the final denture base, which is one of the advantages of making the denture with a metal base. Otherwise, make a temporary base of sprinkled self-curing acrylic resin, which is essentially identical to the final resin base. In any distal extension partial denture, make this base on a cast that has been corrected to the functional, or supporting, form of the edentulous ridge (Fig. 16-1).

Place a film of sticky wax upon the base before the wax occlusion rim is secured to it. The wax used for the occlusion rim should be hard enough to support biting stress and should be tough enough to resist fracture. Peck's purple hard inlay wax has proved to be suitable for the majority of patients. However, some individuals with weak musculature or tender mouths may have difficulty in reducing this wax. In such situations, use a slightly less hard wax. Make the occlusion rim wide enough to

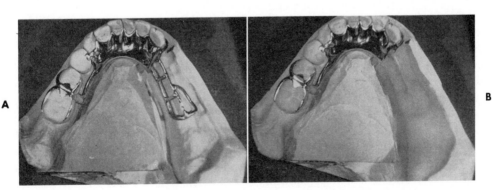

Fig. 16-1. A, After the correction of the edentulous area to functional form, the framework is reseated accurately on the corrected master cast, any undercuts are blocked out with clay, and a tin-foil substitute is applied to the surface of the cast. **B,** A new resin base is made with self-curing acrylic resin by sprinkling to form a record base that is as nearly as possible identical to the form of the finished denture base. After curing, the framework is lifted and any flash or excess is trimmed away. This base is then used to establish occlusal relations by whatever method is indicated, depending upon the opposing dentition and the dentist's preference.

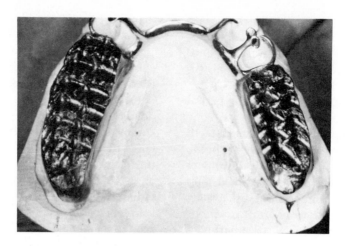

Fig. 16-2. Example of a completed occlusal registration in a hard inlay wax supported by accurate record bases. Note that the width of each cusp in all extremes of mandibular movement is recorded as a continuous glossy surface. Yet, the anatomy of each opposing tooth is well defined. The completed registration must be placed back onto the master cast without intervening debris or discrepancy and secured there with sticky wax so that the accuracy of the occlusal registration will be maintained. (Modified from McCracken's partial denture construction, ed. 3, St. Louis, 1969, The C. V. Mosby Co.)

record all extremes of mandibular movement.

2. Have the patient wear the occlusion rim for a period of twenty-four hours or longer. It should be worn constantly, including nighttime, except for removal during meals. Instruct the patient in the removal and placement of the partial denture supporting the occlusion rim and advise him that by chewing and gliding, the wax will be carved by the opposing teeth. Therefore, the opposing teeth must be cleaned occasionally of accumulated wax particles. It is necessary that the patient comprehend what is being accomplished and that he understand that both voluntary and involuntary movements must be recorded.

Before dismissing the patient, add or remove wax where indicated, to provide continuous contact throughout the chewing range. To accomplish this, repeatedly warm the wax with a hot spatula and have the patient carve the warmed wax rim with the opposing dentition, each time adding to any areas that are deficient. Support with additional wax any wax left unsupported by its flow under occlusal forces.

It is important that the wax rim be absolutely dry and free of saliva before additional wax is applied. Each addition of wax must be made homogeneous with the larger mass to avoid separation or fracture of the occlusion rim during the time it is being worn. Leave the wax occlusion rim from 1 to 3 mm. high, depending on whether or not vertical dimension is to be increased.

3. After twenty-four hours, the occlusal surface of the wax rim should show a continuous gloss, indicating functional contact with the opposing teeth in all extremes of movement (Fig. 16-2). Any areas deficient in contact should be added to at this time. The reasons for maintaining positive occlusal contact throughout the time the occlusion rim is being worn are (a) all opposing teeth may be placed in function; (b) an opposing denture, if present, will become fully seated; and (c) vertical dimension in the molar region will be increased, thus repositioning the head of the mandibular condyle and allowing temporomandibular tissues to return to a normal relationship.

On the other hand, if during this period

the wax occlusion rim has not been reduced to natural tooth contact, warm it by directing air from the air syringe through a flame onto the surface of the wax. By holding the wax rim with the fingers while warming, a gradual softening process will result, rather than a melting of the surfaces already established. Repeatedly warm the occlusion rim and replace it in the mouth until the occlusal height has been reduced and lateral excursions have been recorded. At this time, support with additional wax those areas left unsupported by the flow of the wax to the buccal or lingual surfaces. At the same time, trim the areas obviously not involved, thus narrowing the occlusion rim as much as possible. Remove also those areas projecting above the occlusal surface, which, by their presence, might limit functional movement.

Having accomplished seating of the denture and changes in mandibular position by the previous period of wear, it is possible to complete the occlusal registration at the chair. However, if all involuntary movements and those caused by changes in posture are to be recorded, the patient should again wear the occlusion rim for a period of time.

4. After a second twenty-four to forty-eight hour period of wear, the registration should be complete and acceptable. The remaining teeth serving as vertical stops should be in contact and the occlusion rim should show an intact glossy surface representing each cusp in all extremes of movement.

Not all natural teeth formerly in contact will necessarily be in contact upon completion of the occlusal registration. Those teeth that have been depressed over a period of years and those that have been moved to accommodate overclosure or mandibular rotation may not be in contact when mandibular equilibrium has been reestablished. Such teeth may possibly return to occlusal contact in the future or may have to be restored to occlusal contact after initial placement of the denture. Since the mandibular position may

have been changed during the process of occlusal registration, the cuspal relation of some of the natural teeth may be different than before. This fact must be recognized in determining the correct restored vertical dimension.

The completed registration is now ready for conversion to an occluding template. This is usually done by boxing the occlusal registration with modeling clay after it has been reseated and secured onto the master or processing cast (Figs. 16-3 to 16-6). Only the wax registration and areas for vertical stops are left exposed. It is then filled with a hard stone to form an occluding template. (See Chapter 17.)

It is necessary that stone stops be used to maintain the vertical relation rather than relying on some adjustable part of the articulating instrument, which might be changed accidentally (Fig. 16-7). Also, by using stone stops and by mounting both the denture cast and the template before separating them, a simple hinge instrument may be used.

Because of its simplicity and the accessibility it affords in arranging teeth, the Hagman Junior Balancer is preferred as an articulating instrument for use with an occluding template (Fig. 16-8). In this application, the instrument is used as a hinge only, with all other moving elements securely locked in a fixed position. However, any hinged articulator may be similarly used.

Materials for artificial posterior teeth. Modern resin teeth are preferred by some over porcelain teeth because they are more readily modified and thought to more nearly resemble enamel in their action against opposing teeth. Resin teeth with gold occlusal surfaces are preferably used in opposition to enamel and gold occlusal surfaces, whereas porcelain teeth are generally used in opposition to other porcelain teeth.

Some changes in this concept have occurred in recent years. Sears and, later, Myerson have introduced the feasibility of using porcelain and resin teeth in opposi-

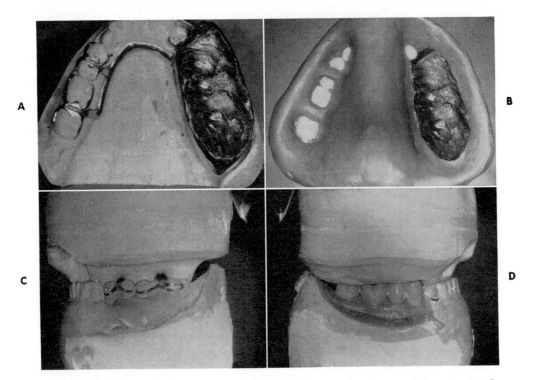

Fig. 16-3. Four views of an occlusal registration for a lower Class II partial denture. **A,** The occlusal registration in wax returned to the master cast. Note the extreme horizontal movement recorded. **B,** The same cast boxed with clay, leaving multiple occlusal surfaces exposed as vertical stops. **C,** The effect of the occlusal stops, eliminating any possible changes in vertical dimension on the articulator. **D,** The processed denture remounted for occlusal readjustment. Note the modification in the occlusal anatomy of the stock denture teeth and the slight increase in the height of the occlusal plane. This is in harmony with natural tooth contact elsewhere in the arch.

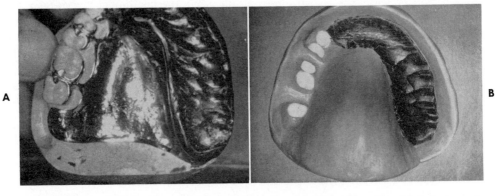

Fig. 16-4. Five views of an occlusal registration for an upper Class II partial denture. **A,** Partial view of the occlusal registration returned to the master cast. Again, note the extreme horizontal movement recorded. **B,** The same cast boxed with clay, leaving multiple occlusal surfaces exposed as vertical stops. **C,** The occlusal view of the occluding template. **D,** The processed denture remounted for occlusal readjustment. Note the modification of the teeth even to the point of disregarding interdigitation, to effect good occlusion with the template. The anterior teeth must be tried in the mouth and positioned for esthetics before arranging the posterior teeth. **E,** The occlusal stops in full contact after processing and occlusal readjustment following remounting.

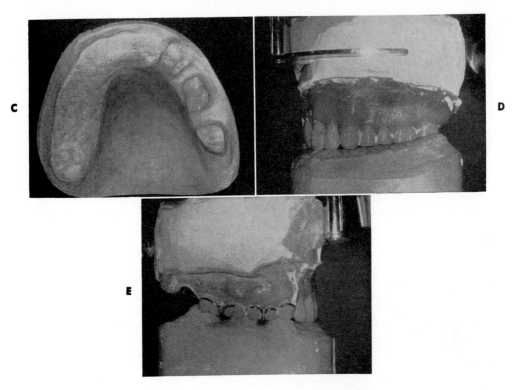

Fig. 16-4, cont'd. For legend see opposite page.

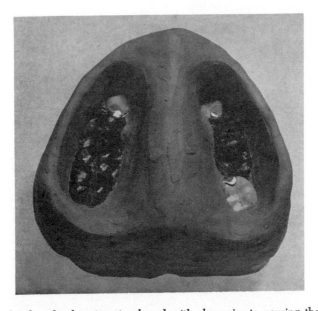

Fig. 16-5. Completed occlusal registration boxed with clay prior to pouring the template in a hard die stone. The occlusal surfaces of adjacent abutment teeth are left exposed to serve as stone-to-stone vertical stops. The clay is trimmed just to the margins of the registration and raised in the center to provide an arch for lingual access while arranging teeth to occlude with the template.

tion and the advantage of reduced frictional resistance by doing so. Myerson has compared the effect of porcelain teeth against resin teeth to that of a diamond stylus against a vinyl phonograph record, which results in less wear by friction than does the less hard sapphire stylus. For this to be truly comparable, the porcelain tooth should possess a glazed surface, but experience has shown that even a polished vacuum-fired porcelain surface causes limited wear and reduced frictional resistance when in opposition to a modern resin denture tooth.

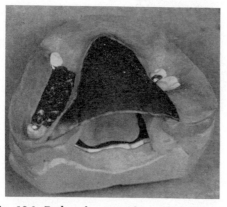

Fig. 16-6. Rather than use clay sufficient to arch across from one side to another, the same may be done with wax with less time and material. It is better that the clay form a more acute angle with the occlusal wax registration and exposed occlusal surfaces than illustrated here.

A second fact also has been recognized, which is that resin tooth surfaces may in time become impregnated with abrasive particles, thereby becoming an abrasive substance themselves. This may explain why resin teeth are sometimes capable of wearing opposing gold surfaces. *An evaluation of occlusal contact or lack of contact, however, should be meticulously accomplished at each six-months recall appointment regardless of the choice of material for posterior tooth forms.*

Although some controversy still may exist in regard to the use of porcelain or resin denture teeth, there is broad agreement that narrow occlusal surfaces are desirable. Posterior teeth that will satisfy this requirement should be selected, and the use of tooth forms having excessive buccolingual dimension should be avoided.

It has been our observation that artificial posterior resin teeth become excessively abraded in comparative short periods of time regardless of the material by which they are opposed. The attendant ills of excessive abrasion of occlusal surfaces may often be avoided by using porcelain teeth to oppose porcelain teeth, gold occlusals to oppose other gold occlusal surfaces or natural teeth, and removal of the denture upon retiring.

Acrylic resin teeth are easily modified

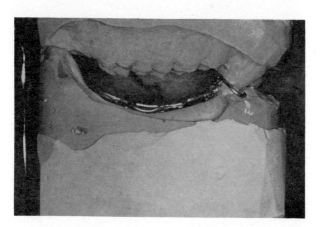

Fig. 16-7. Profile view of an occlusal template and one of its vertical stops. Despite the fact that this a record of all extremes of mandibular movement for this patient, the anatomy of the occluding teeth can easily be identified.

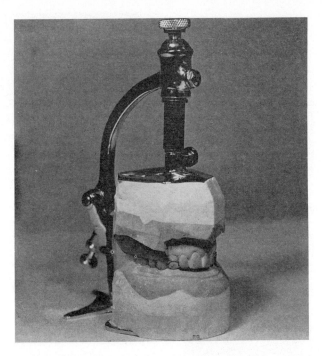

Fig. 16-8. Completed upper partial denture with artificial teeth arranged and modified to occlude with a template made from a wax occlusal registration. The Hagman Junior Balancer is used as a hinge alone, with all adjustable elements securely locked before mounting the cast and template. Stone stops are used to preserve the vertical relation. Note the notch in the upper cast for keying the cast to the articulator to facilitate accurate remounting after processing.

and readily lend themselves to construction of cast gold surfaces on their occlusal portions. A simple procedure for fabricating gold occlusal surfaces and attaching them to acrylic resin teeth is described in Chapter 17 under the heading "Posterior tooth forms."

Arranging teeth to an occluding template. The occlusal surface of the denture teeth, porcelain or resin, must be modified to occlude with the template. In this method, they are actually only raw materials from which an occlusal surface that is in harmony with an existing occlusal pattern is developed. Therefore, the teeth must be occluded too high and then modified to fit the template at the established vertical dimension.

Teeth arranged to an occluding template ordinarily should be placed in the center of the functional range. Whenever possible, the teeth should be arranged buccolin-

gually in the center of the template. When natural teeth have registered the functional occlusion, this may be considered the normal physiologic position of the artificial dentition regardless of its relation to the residual ridge. On the other hand, if some man-made occlusion in the opposing arch has been recorded, such as that of an opposing denture, the teeth should be arranged in a favorable relation to their foundation, even if this means arranging them slightly buccally or lingually from the center of the template.

The teeth are usually arranged to interdigitate with the opposing teeth in a normal cuspal relationship. As is customary, whenever possible the mesiobuccal cusps of the maxillary first molar is located in relation to the buccal groove of the mandibular first molar and all other teeth arranged accordingly. With functional occlusion, however, it is not absolutely necessary that

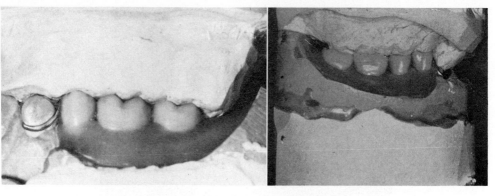

Fig. 16-9. A, View of the interdigitation sometimes possible when teeth are arranged to an occlusal template. This is possible only when gross migration of the opposing teeth has not occurred. B, View of the modification to occlusal surfaces necessary when interdigitation is not possible without leaving objectionable spaces. Note that the original cusp-to-cusp relation of the denture teeth has been altered until marginal ridges have actually become the interdigitation cusps. Such an occlusal relationship is entirely permissible and effective. (Modified from McCracken's partial denture construction, ed. 3, St. Louis, 1969, The C. V. Mosby Co.)

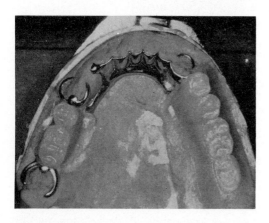

Fig. 16-10. Occlusal surfaces after remounting and final occlusal readjustment to the template. Note the functional occlusal anatomy resulting. This is an entirely different occlusal surface from that which was present on the stock artificial teeth as manufactured.

a normal anteroposterior relation be reestablished. (See Fig. 16-9.) In the first place, the opposing teeth in a broken dental arch may not be in normal alignment, and interdigitation may be difficult to accomplish. In the second place, the occlusal surfaces will be modified so that they will function favorably regardless of their anteroposterior position (Fig. 16-10). Since cusps modified to fit an occlusal template will be in harmony with the opposing den-

tition, it is not necessary that the teeth themselves be arranged to conform to the usual concept of what constitutes a normal anteroposterior relationship.

Making the occluding template of metal. Some indicator must be used to guide the alteration of occlusal surfaces to fit the template. Articulating paper has several disadvantages when used for this purpose. One is that it does not conform readily to irregular surfaces and quickly becomes perforated, giving irregular markings. Another is that the waxlike substance with which the paper is impregnated tends to accumulate on the surface of the template, changing the vertical relation somewhat and giving false marks on the teeth. An inked marking tape (silk ribbon, dental tape, or typewriter ribbon) is superior to articulating paper because it will not tear and yet will conform better to irregular surfaces, (Fig. 16-11). In this regard it also permits more accurate marking of proximal surfaces as they are being ground to fit the denture framework. An ink mark may be more reliably interpreted than may a crayon mark made with articulating paper.

The inked ribbon may be held with forceps, such as the Miller articulating paper forceps, or in a wire frame (Fig. 16-12).

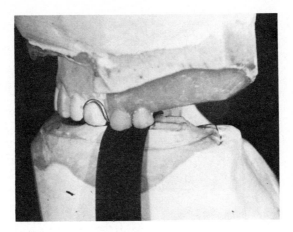

Fig. 16-11. When arranging teeth to an occluding template, marking tape should be used in positioning and modifying each tooth to fit the template. Note that at this early stage the articulator has been opened approximately 0.5 mm., as evidenced by the slight space at the vertical stop. (Modified from McCracken's partial denture construction, ed. 3, St. Louis, 1969, The C. V. Mosby Co.)

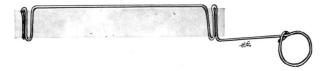

Fig. 16-12. Drawing of a wire holder for marking tape or typewriter ribbon. The wire used is 0.036-inch orthodontic wire. The ribbon is held taut at either end after passing over the inner arch (over, under, and then over).

The latter is easily made of orthodontic wire and holds the ribbon taut at all times, whereas the forceps are designed primarily for use with articulating paper.

One of the hazards of arranging teeth to a stone template is that the template becomes abraded by continuous closure against the artificial teeth as they are being adjusted to occlude with the template. It is inevitable that during the process of alternately marking and grinding occlusal surfaces the stone template is subjected to considerable abuse and wear (Fig. 16-13). This abrasion can be minimized by using the hardest dental stone available for the template and by avoiding forceful contact of the template with the occlusal surfaces of the teeth. It also can be avoided by electroplating the wax occlusal registration, thus forming a relatively indestructible occlusal template. (See Figs. 16-14 to 16-19.) The technique is as follows:

Low-fusing metal has been preferred to stone as an occluding cast material, but molten metal cannot be poured into a wax mold. Electroplating permits a metallic surface to be formed on the wax record with accuracy and with greater hardness than low-fusing metals. Electroforming with silver has proved to be the simplest and most satisfactory method.

Interest in electroplating has been revised since the advent of the Thiokol and Silicone impression materials. The change from time-honored copper dies to silver dies was made necessary by the introduction of these new impression materials when electroformed dies were preferred to stone dies.

The technique for electroplating the occlusal template is basically identical with electroplating of Thiokol and Silicone impressions. The main differences are that the vessel containing the electrolyte must be larger, the leads must be attached bilaterally in a manner that will allow the denture to be suspended in the solution, and the denture framework must be protected from the electrolytic current.

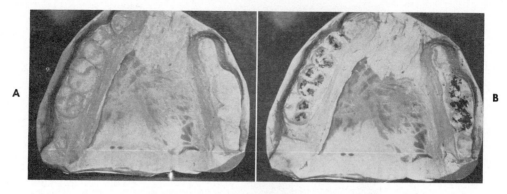

Fig. 16-13. Stone occlusal template before and after use. **A,** The occlusal surfaces are unmarred by abrasion. **B,** Evidence of abrasion through the articulating marks shows the damage and therefore the inaccuracy resulting from abrasion and crushing forces as the template is tapped against the opposing teeth. If the occlusal surfaces during remounting are readjusted to fit this altered surface, some occlusal inaccuracies are inevitable, which must then be compensated for by occlusal adjustment of the completed denture.

Ten milliamperes of current per tooth, plus 10 for the leads, is sufficient. Greater amperage would cause the electroplating to be too soft. The total area of the anode immersed in the solution should not be more than twice the area to be plated. The distance from the anode to the surface to be plated should be about 4 inches.

Since the number of teeth involved will vary, the plating machine must have a widely variable output. The machine being used is a self-made device with a variable output of from 35 to 200 Ma., although suitable machines ready for use may be purchased.

The wax occlusal registration is metallized with Staco silver lacquer, and the leads are painted down the lingual side to joint with a T-shaped wire lead. This lead is attached to the wax rims with sticky wax. It is very important that all parts of the denture framework be painted with a protective lacquer, such as Kerr's Plate Mask, to prevent the casting itself from being plated.

At 10 Ma. per tooth, the occlusal registration to be plated should be left in the solution approximately 5 hours. A uniform plate of sufficient thickness will result. A heavier plate seems to cause some curling at the edges and pulling away from the wax surface. This leads to inaccuracies and must be avoided. Since the plated surface will be backed up with stone, a thin plate is all that is needed.

The attachment of the stone backing to the silver plate was a problem at first. In some cases, the metal separated from the stone backing due to the absence of mechanical attachment. The problem has been solved by imbedding two or more wire staples into the wax surface of the occlusal registration before plating. These staples become part of the plated surface and aid in securing the metal to the stone. The small tip end of each staple projecting through the metal template can easily be ground away without marring the surfaces of the template.

The plated surface is boxed with clay, and stone is poured against it in the same manner as an unplated wax record. The articulator mounting and occluding the teeth to the template is the same, except for the advantages of the metal surface over a stone surface.

It is not expected that the silver plating of a wax occlusal record will receive wide acceptance because of the added step of electroplating. But just as there are those who prefer to work with electroformed dies, so there may be some who would prefer to arrange teeth to a metal template.*

Functional registration of occlusal surfaces for fixed partial dentures and single crowns. Many of the advantages to be found in the registration of occlusal pathways for removable partial dentures may

---

*From McCracken, W. L.: Functional occlusion in removable partial denture construction. J. Prosthet. Dent. 8:955-963, 1958.

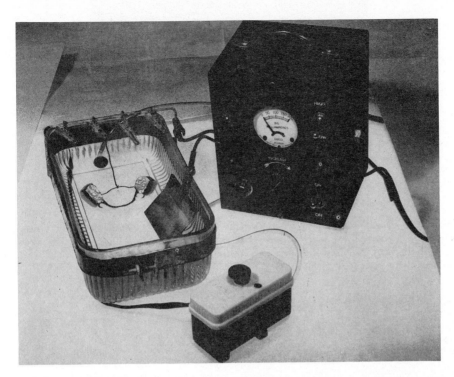

Fig. 16-14. Homemade equipment for electroplating the wax occlusal registration. Milliamperage can be varied from 35 to 200 Ma. The electrolyte in the glass container is silver potassium cyanide; the anode is pure silver. Commercial electroplating equipment may be purchased, or the equipment may be assembled as shown by the diagram in Fig. 16-15. The work is suspended in the solution from an alligator clip superstructure attached to one side of the electric circuit. The anode may be suspended or placed in a refrigerator dish as illustrated. The variable factor of the distance from anode to work may be eliminated by agitating the solution with an aquarium aerator pump, the open end of the plastic tubing being held in the solution by passing it through an egg-shaped fishing sinker.

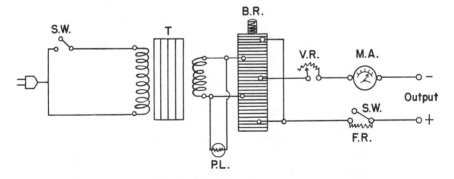

Fig. 16-15. Diagram and parts needed for making electroplating device for silver plating Thiokol and silicone impressions and wax occlusal registrations. **S.W.,** Toggle switch; **T,** small filament transformer; **P.L.,** pilot light; **B.R.,** full-wave bridge rectifier; **V.R.,** variable rheostat; **M.A.,** milliammeter; **F.R.,** fixed resistor. Parts required include 6.3-volt filament transformer, milliammeter, 1.5 Å full-wave bridge rectifier, 50-ohm, 4-watt variable rheostat, pilot light, 2 SPST switches, 10-watt, 50-ohm wire-wound resistor, and utility cabinet. (Courtesy Dr. Paul E. Hammons.)

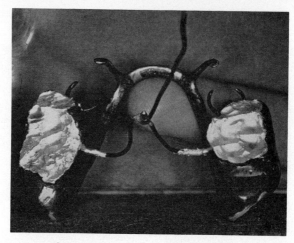

Fig. 16-16. Leads are attached below the wax occlusal registration with sticky wax, and the denture framework is coated with a protective lacquer (Kerr plate mask). The occlusal registration is then metalized with a silver lacquer, which is carried down the lingual surface to join the wire leads. (From McCracken, W. L.: J. Prosthet. Dent. 8:955-963, 1958.)

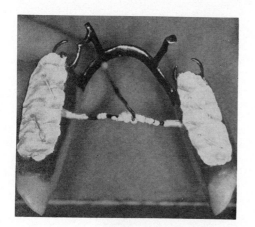

Fig. 16-17. Wax occlusal registration after electroplating. Note the wire staples added to the wax to provide retention to the stone that will be poured against the silver surface. The leads and the protective lacquer over the metal framework are now removed prior to reseating the occlusal registration onto the master cast.

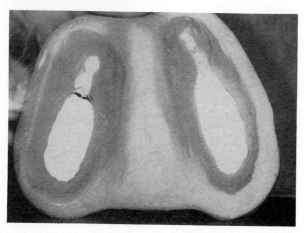

Fig. 16-18. After accurately reseating the denture framework onto the master cast and securing it there with sticky wax, a clay matrix is formed, leaving one or more occlusal surfaces on each side exposed to serve as vertical stops. The clay is made to rise from the borders of the registration at a 45-degree angle and is arched across the midline to provide lingual access when setting teeth to the template. The exposed occlusal surfaces are painted with a separator and stone is vibrated into the clay matrix to form the remainder of the occluding template.

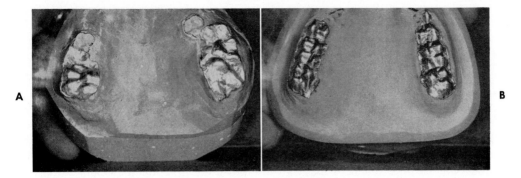

Fig. 16-19. **A,** Electroformed silver occluding template with stone stops anteriorly to preserve the vertical dimension. **B,** Another electroformed occluding template involving six opposing teeth (the functional width of each cusp is readily discernible). (**A** from McCracken, W. L.: J. Prosthet. Dent. **8**:955-963, 1958.)

be applied also to the construction of fixed restorations and individual crowns. A more harmonious occlusion results from establishing a functional relationship than when only a centric occlusal relation is recorded.

Since fixed restorations and individual crowns are often essential to adequate mouth preparations for partial dentures, it is necessary that methods for obtaining occlusal harmony on those restorations be considered in this chapter. It has been stated previously that analysis and adjustment of the natural occlusion is an essential part of mouth preparations. It is equally essential that any occlusion reconstruction be done in harmony with the accepted or corrected natural occlusion. It is doubtful that this is possible without having some record of the existing occlusal pattern.

Functional occlusion for fixed partial dentures and crowns must be established entirely at the chair, because the patient cannot be given a restoration that he can remove at mealtime. Although such a jaw relation record does not possess all the advantages of an occlusal registration made during a twenty-four-hour period, it does create an occlusion that is in harmony with the majority of jaw movements. Occlusal discrepancies on the finished restoration caused by changes in posture can be recorded and eliminated only by having the patient wear an unpolished gold restoration or one made dull by sandblasting for a pe-

riod long enough to register any remaining interference. This limitation of a functional registration done at the chair should be recognized and then corrected on the finished restoration.

Establishing functional occlusion on a single crown. The method of registering functional occlusion on a single crown was mentioned previously in conjunction with the making of a crown pattern to fit a denture clasp (Chapter 13). In this technique a thin coping of self-curing resin is made to support the wax pattern. An occlusal pattern is then established directly in the mouth with little danger of fracture or distortion. Any hard inlay wax may be used for this purpose.

Either removable dies or individual dies in conjunction with a solid cast may be used to establish vertical surfaces on the wax pattern, which will satisfy requirements for marginal contact, guiding planes, and contours for clasp retention and reciprocation. This may be done prior to establishing occlusal relations, or the occlusal aspect of the pattern may be completed first and the pattern then returned to the cast for the shaping of vertical surfaces.

When individual dies are used, occlusion is usually established first and then the pattern is placed on a solid cast of the arch to contour the crown in relation to the path of placement. This is done with the aid of a surveyor. Finally, the pattern is returned to the individual die to refine the margins. When removable dies are used, the contouring of vertical surfaces may be done first, then the occlusal relationship may be established in the mouth, and finally the pattern is returned to the die for the refinement of the margins.

When several such restorations are to be made for the same arch, it is best that as many wax patterns be made concurrently as possible. On the other hand, it may be necessary to restore only one or two teeth at a time to preserve vertical and horizontal relations. This may sometimes be facilitated by making plastic temporary crowns for all prepared teeth in harmony with the existing occlusion, and then using these temporary crowns alternately as guides while establishing a functional occlusion on the wax patterns.

As with an occlusal registration for a partial denture, the completed occlusal registration should have a glossy surface and should make contact with the opposing teeth throughout the functional range. Sufficient chewing time must be allowed for any excess wax to be eliminated, with the teeth elsewhere in the arch again in contact.

The occlusal surface thus established will be broader than will a natural tooth. In the registration for a removable partial denture or a fixed partial denture this is converted to a template and an occlusal surface of acceptable width formed to occlude with only a part of the template. The occlusal registration for a crown pattern, on the other hand, is the wax pattern that becomes the finished casting. This occlusal surface is much too wide and has too much occlusal contact to be within the toleration limits of periodontal support. The wax pattern must therefore be narrowed to reduce the width of the occlusal table. Spillways should be added to further reduce the occlusal area and to increase masticating ef-

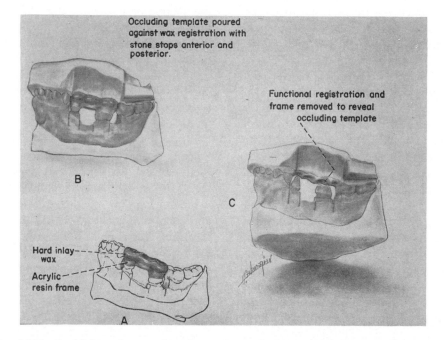

Fig. 16-20. Establishing functional occlusion for a fixed partial denture by means of an occlusal registration of the opposing teeth. **A,** The acrylic resin frame with hard inlay wax occlusal surface. **B,** The occluding template poured against the wax registration with stone stops anterior and posterior. **C,** The resulting template to which the occlusal surfaces of the restoration will be formed.

ficiency. This is generally done to conform to concepts of normal occlusal anatomy, the objective being to further reduce the area of occlusal contact and to assure maximum efficiency. A crown restoration thus formed will possess maximum efficiency without interference, in harmony with all eccentric movements and with the other teeth in the arch.

Step-by-step procedure for recording occlusal pathways for a fixed partial denture. The objectives in establishing functional occlusion on a fixed partial denture are the same as for a single crown. The method, however, is somewhat different.

Functional occlusion for a fixed partial denture is established by means of an occlusal registration on an acrylic resin or cast metal frame or platform. The technique of occlusal registration is much the same as for removable partial denture occlusion except that the frame is not removable by the patient, and therefore occlusal registration must be done entirely at the chair. (See Fig. 16-20.)

The technique for establishing functional occlusion for a fixed partial denture is as follows:

1. Although a cast metal frame may be used, one made of acrylic resin is adequate for the purpose. The frame may be made on a cast from a separate alginate hydrocolloid impression of the prepared teeth or from a second pour of a rubber-base impression. The cast containing trimmed dies is not used for making a frame, for fear of marring its surface.

Clay or utility wax is added to block out the gingival one fourth of the prepared teeth and the adjacent soft tissues and edentulous areas. This eliminates any interference to the seating of the frame onto the working cast. Any irregularities in the preparations are also blocked out. Then a wax or clay matrix is formed to confine the self-curing acrylic resin within the desired limits.

The cast is painted with tin-foil substitute, which is allowed to dry. Self-curing acrylic resin is then applied, using the sprinkling method, until a resin platform of the desired thickness has been obtained. The occlusal portion is left wide but thin.

After polymerizing at least an hour, but preferably overnight, the frame is lifted from the cast and trimmed of excess. It should be no bulkier than is necessary for strength. The only adjustment that should be necessary in the mouth is the reduction of the occlusal plane to provide space for the registration wax.

2. The resin frame must seat accurately on the abutment teeth, and there must be no contact with soft tissues. The occlusal surface should be reduced sufficiently to provide ample clearance for the registration wax. Apply a film of sticky wax to the dried frame and then add a hard inlay wax to the occlusal surface.*

While the wax is still soft, place the resin frame in the mouth and ask the patient to make centric contact and excursive movements. Add wax where deficient and support the width buccally and lingually with additional wax. Reduce excess width as well as excess height at the limits of excursive movements. Do not add to glossy areas, but only those areas in which contact is deficient. This registration differs from the partial denture registration, in which the occlusion rim is left 1 to 3 mm. high for the patient to reduce during a twenty-four-hour period. The fixed partial

---

*For an occlusal registration done entirely at the chair, any inlay wax may be used rather than the harder Peck's purple inlay wax that is used for recording occlusal pathways on a removable partial denture.

In recent years interest in the functionally generated path has led to the development of special waxes for this purpose, such as the Jelenko "Hi-Fi" wax. These waxes are suitable only for direct registration at the chair and cannot be worn by the patient away from the operatory; but then neither can a registration frame be worn outside the dental office because it must be removed by the patient during mealtime, which would leave prepared abutment teeth exposed. When this softer type of wax is used at the chair, it is best supported at its borders by a harder inlay wax to prevent distortion at the limits of excursion.

denture registration is done entirely at the chair and can only record voluntary movements at the vertical level determined by the other teeth in the arch. As mentioned repeatedly in preceding paragraphs, this should be an occlusion that is acceptable or made so by previous occlusal adjustments and/or reconstruction.

The completed registration should make contact with the opposing teeth throughout the functional range. The registration should have an intact glossy surface and will be much wider than will the occlusion on the finished restoration.

3. The completed occlusal registration is treated much the same as a registration for a removable partial denture. A hard die stone is poured against it, or it may be metallized and electroplated. In either case, seat it accurately on the working cast and secure it there with sticky wax.

Form a clay matrix at a 45-degree angle from the margins of the registration, leaving the cast exposed anteriorly and posteriorly to provide vertical stops. Pour stone directly against the wax registration or the electroplated surface. After this has set, mount the cast and opposing template on some kind of hinge articulator before the two are separated. The resulting mounting will not be dependent upon the articulator

for maintaining the vertical relation because stone-to-stone stops will have been provided for this purpose.

Patterns are waxed to occlude with the opposing template. Generally, occlusal relations with the opposing teeth will not be jeopardized from an esthetic standpoint by carving restorations to a template alone. However, when interdigitation or the correct horizontal overlap might be difficult to ascertain when a template alone is used, another procedure may be followed. In this procedure, a conventional mounting to an occluding cast is made first, using an occluding stone cast that has been poured directly into a wax or other interocclusal record (Fig. 16-21, *A*). This provides an anatomic opposing cast for the establishment of interdigitation and the desired amount of horizontal overlap. This is frequently desirable from an esthetic standpoint and to avoid a cusp-to-cusp occlusion on the completed restoration.

An occlusal registration made on an acrylic resin frame is then positioned on the working cast as described previously and a clay matrix formed around it, leaving stone exposed at either end for a vertical stop. The opposing anatomic cast is then lubricated or treated with some separating medium such as a solution of sodium sili-

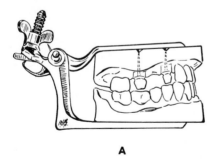
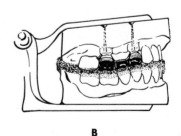

A   B

Fig. 16-21. Articulated casts providing both anatomic and functional registrations of the opposing teeth on the same articulator. **A,** A conventional mounting to an occluding cast obtained on a wax interocclusal record. The correct vertical relationship is maintained by natural tooth contact anteriorly; otherwise a stone stop should be provided rather than depend on the vertical stop of the articulator alone. **B,** An occluding stone template formed from a functional occlusal registration is interposed between the two casts to establish functional occlusal surfaces on the restorations. This removable template overlays the opposing anatomic cast and is extended anteriorly and posteriorly to provide vertical stops when the template is in use.

cate, the occlusal registration filled with stone, and the anatomic cast seated into the stone (Fig. 16-21, *B*). Sufficient thickness of stone must remain for strength.

After the occlusal template has set, it may be separated and trimmed. Two articulator mountings are thus obtained; one is an anatomic opposing cast, and the other is a removable stone template complete with vertical stops to which a functional occlusion may be perfected that will be free of eccentric interference. The same degree of occlusal harmony is possible by this method as with the functional occlusal record alone, with the added advantage of assuring an acceptable esthetic relationship with the opposing teeth. Occlusal surfaces may be made as narrow as desired, and occlusal anatomy should be added for masticating efficiency. Finished castings and the assembled fixed partial denture then should be reoccluded to the template to eliminate discrepancies caused by spruing and soldering.

Fig. 16-22 illustrates an articulator made by the Hanau Company, called the twin-stage occluder, which further facilitates the use of both a functional and an anatomic cast when occluding wax patterns to a functional record. Fig. 16-23 shows an improved version of the Verticulator made by the Jelenko Company for the use with either full arch or sectional casts, which also permits the use of dual opposing surfaces. Two upper arms are provided, both machined to fit a single lower arm. A static interocclusal record may be attached to one arm and a functional record to the other, and the two can be interchanged at will.

One disadvantage of using a simple hinge articulator as illustrated in Fig. 16-21 is the small arc of closure dictated by the proximity of the hinge to the occlusal surface. An occluding template is most effectively used when vertical or nearly vertical closure is possible. When an instrument such as the Hagman Balancer is used, the arc of closure is sufficiently great that it may be considered nearly vertical at the plane of occlusion. Otherwise it is best that an instrument such as the Jelenko Vertic-

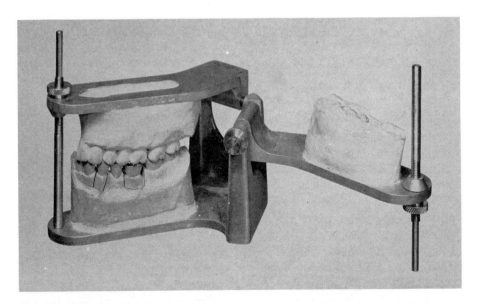

Fig. 16-22. Hanau twin-stage occluder. An anatomic occluding cast is attached to one upper arm and an occlusal template to the other. Better esthetic results are made possible by occluding the wax patterns to both a functional and an anatomic cast. (Courtesy Hanau Engineering Co., Buffalo, N. Y.)

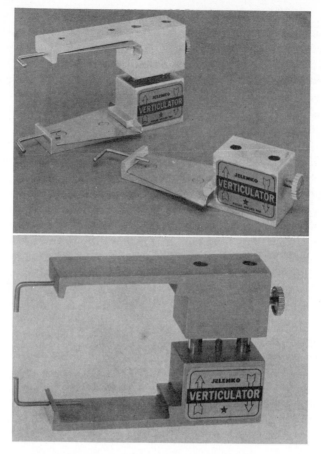

Fig. 16-23. Two models of the Jelenko Verticulator. Designed for use with the Pankey-Mann technique, they are suitable for use with either an anatomic occluding cast or a functionally generated path. However, since only vertical movement is permitted, with positive metal-to-metal vertical limitation, the instrument is best suited for use with the functionally generated path. The dual model permits an interchange between a functional cast and an anatomic cast by substituting two matched and identical upper members. (Courtesy J. F. Jelenko & Co., Inc., New York, N. Y.)

ulator (Fig. 16-23), which permits only vertical closure, be used in conjunction with an occluding template. The Verticulator has a further advantage of providing a spring-loaded metal-to-metal stop, which positively prevents possible abrasion of the occluding surfaces and loss of the established vertical dimension.

A fixed partial denture restoration made with functional occlusal surfaces should have a harmonious occlusion in centric and in all voluntary eccentric positions. As with a single crown, any remaining eccentric interference must be eliminated in the mouth. Since these are not caused by voluntary

movements, it is best that the patient wear the restorations with dull occlusal surfaces (preferably sandblasted surfaces) for a period of twenty-four hours or more. Any remaining interference may then be identified by shiny areas in eccentric position, and these may be eliminated before final polishing. Indeed, it may be esthetically desirable at times to leave occlusal surfaces unpolished, with only a satin finish created by sandblasting.

Establishing jaw relations for a mandibular removable partial denture opposing a maxillary complete denture. It is not uncommon for a mandibular removable partial denture to be made to occlude with an opposing maxillary complete denture. The maxillary denture may already be present or it may be made concurrently with the opposing partial denture. In any event, the establishment of jaw relations in this situation may be accomplished by one of several methods previously outlined.

If an existing maxillary complete denture is satisfactory and is not to be replaced, that arch is treated as an intact arch as though natural teeth were present. A face-bow transfer is made of that arch and the cast mounted on the articulator in the usual manner. Maxillomandibular relations may be recorded on accurate record bases attached to the mandibular partial denture framework, using one of the recording mediums previously outlined, such as wax, modeling plastic, quick-setting plaster, impression paste, or quick-curing acrylic resin. Centric relation is thus recorded and transferred to the articulator. Eccentric records can then be made to adjust the articulator.

In rare instances, when the mandibular partial denture replaces all posterior teeth and the anterior teeth are noninterfering, a central bearing point tracer may be mounted in the palate of the maxillary denture and centric relation recorded by means of an intraoral stylus tracing against a stable mandibular base.

If the relationship of the posterior teeth on the maxillary denture to the mandibular ridge is favorable and the complete denture is *stable,* jaw relations may be established by recording occlusal pathways in the mandibular arch the same as for any opposing intact arch. The success of this method depends upon the stability of the denture bases, the quality of tissue support, the relation of the opposing teeth to the mandibular ridge, and the interrelation of existing artificial and natural teeth.

More times than not, the existing maxillary complete denture will have been made to occlude with malpositioned mandibular teeth, which have since been lost, or the teeth will have been arranged without consideration for the future occlusal relation with a mandibular partial denture. Too frequently one sees a maxillary denture with posterior teeth arranged close to the residual ridge without regard for interarch relationship and with an occlusal plane that is too low. In such instances, the least that can be done is to reposition the posterior teeth on the maxillary denture before establishing maxillomandibular relations. This can only be justified when the maxillary denture is otherwise satisfactory as to fit, appearance, and occlusion elsewhere in the arch. Usually, however, a new maxillary denture must be made concurrently with the mandibular partial denture and jaw relations may be established in one of two ways.

If the mandibular partial denture will be tooth supported (a Kennedy Class III arch accommodating a bilateral removable prosthesis), that arch is restored first. The same applies to a mandibular arch being restored with fixed partial dentures. In either situation, the mandibular arch is completely restored first, and jaw relations are established as they would be to a full complement of opposing teeth. Thus the maxillary complete denture is made to occlude with an intact arch, and the procedure for doing so need not be included here.

On the other hand, as is more frequently the situation, the mandibular partial denture may have one or more distal extension bases. The situation then requires that either the occlusion be established on both dentures simultaneously or the maxillary denture be completed first.

After the making of final impressions, which includes the correction of the mandibular cast to establish optimal support for the bases of the partial denture (the denture framework must be made previously if a wax correction method is used), the maxillary occlusion rim is contoured, vertical relation with the remaining lower teeth is established, and a facebow transfer of the maxillary arch is made. Then maxillomandibular relations may be recorded by any one of the several methods previously outlined and the articulator mounting completed. Occlusion may be established as for complete dentures, taking care to establish a favorable tooth-to-ridge relationship in both arches, an optimal occlusal plane, and cuspal harmony between all occluding teeth.

After try-in, either of two methods may be used. Both dentures may be processed concurrently and remounted for occlusal correction, or the maxillary denture may be processed first and, after remounting, the teeth, still in wax on the partial denture, adjusted to any discrepancies occurring.

Up to the point of establishing the final occlusion on the partial denture, jaw relations, articulator mounting, and try-in are accomplished as though both dentures were to be completed at the same time. The teeth on the mandibular partial denture are arranged in wax so that a favorable ridge relationship and occlusal plane will have been established. The maxillary denture alone is then remounted to adjust the occlusion to the remaining natural teeth and is placed in the mouth as a completed restoration.

The teeth in wax are removed from the partial denture base and replaced with hard inlay wax occlusion rims secured to acrylic resin bases, which are attached to the denture framework. A functional occlusal record by registering occlusal pathways is then accomplished, treating the opposing complete denture as an intact arch. The occlusal registration thus obtained is placed back on the master cast, boxed with clay, and an occluding template formed complete with stone-to-stone vertical stops. The same articulator may be used, replacing the original upper cast with the template, or the mandibular cast and the template may be mounted on a simple hinge-type articulator.

It is necessary that the acrylic resin record base be removed by softening it over a flame before the teeth are rearranged to occlude with the template. The teeth that were formerly arranged to occlude with the maxillary denture are then modified to fit the template, and the denture bases are waxed and processed. Investing must be done in such a manner that the cast may be recovered intact and remounted for occlusal refinement to the template.

Occlusion thus established on a mandibular partial denture opposing a maxillary complete denture provides occlusal harmony. Not only does stability of both dentures result, but trauma conducive to tissue changes beneath both dentures is held to a minimum. The harmony of occlusion thus established justifies the added steps necessary to accomplish such results.

Correction of occlusal discrepancies created during processing must be accomplished before the patient is permitted to use the denture(s). Methods by which these discrepancies may be corrected are discussed in Chapter 17.

Laboratory procedures

This chapter will cover only those phases of dental laboratory procedures that are directly related to partial denture construction. Familiarity with laboratory procedures relative to the making of fixed restorations and complete dentures is presumed. Such information is already available in the numerous excellent textbooks on those subjects and will not be duplicated here. For example, the principles and techniques involved in the waxing, casting, and finishing of single inlays, crowns, and fixed partial dentures are adequately covered in lecture material and textbooks and in manuals available to the dental student, the dental laboratory technician, and the practicing dentist. Similarly, knowledge of the principles and techniques for mounting casts, articulating teeth, and waxing, processing, and polishing complete dentures is presumed as a necessary background for the laboratory phases of partial denture construction. Therefore, this chapter will be directed specifically toward the laboratory procedures involved in the making of a removable partial denture.

DUPLICATING A STONE CAST

A stone cast may be duplicated for one or two purposes. One is the duplication in stone of the original or corrected master cast to preserve the original. Upon this duplicate cast the denture framework may be fitted without danger of abrading or fracturing the surface of the original mas-

ter cast. Most of the better commercial dental laboratories have adopted a policy of doing all work on a duplicate cast, including the fitting procedures. The finished casting is then returned to the dentist after all fitting has been completed on the duplicate cast.

The student or the dentist doing his own laboratory work should likewise follow the policy of making a duplicate cast for fitting the denture framework. Although some dental laboratories also may use the duplicate cast for surveying and blockout, it is preferable to do the blockout on the master cast just prior to a second duplication rather than to use the duplicate cast for this purpose.

After blockout of the master cast, a second duplication is done for making an investment cast. Upon this investment cast the wax and/or plastic pattern is formed, and the metal framework is ultimately cast against its surface.

Although both the fitting cast and the investment cast must be an accurate reproduction of the original, the fitting cast is made of a hard stone and is not directly involved in the making of the metal framework. The investment cast, on the other hand, must possess the properties of a casting investment, such as the ability to withstand burnout temperatures while providing the necessary mold expansion. Gold alloys and also Ticonium are cast to plaster-bound silica investments, whereas the

325

higher melting stellite alloys are cast to investments containing quartz held together by a suitable binder so that they will withstand the higher casting temperatures necessary with these alloys. Although the latter are generally harder than are gypsum investments, any investment cast may be easily abraded and must be handled carefully to preserve the accuracy of its surface. The practice of treating the dried investment cast by dipping it in melted rosin and beeswax reduces considerably the danger of its becoming abraded during subsequent handling.

The use of pre-formed plastic patterns eliminates some of the danger of altering the surface of the investment cast in the process of forming the pattern. With free-hand waxing, considerable care must be taken not to score or abrade the investment cast. The student, however, needs the experience of free-hand waxing to give him a better comprehension of the bulk and contours necessary to produce an acceptable denture framework. A continuation of this practice is recommended. For the same rea-

sons, it is also recommended that the laboratory technician be experienced in the use of wax shapes and free-hand waxing before he is allowed to use pre-formed patterns.

Duplicating materials and flasks. Duplicating materials are colloidal materials, which are made fluid by heating and return to a gel upon being cooled.

The cast to be duplicated must be placed in the bottom of a suitable flask, called a duplicating flask. This flask is necessary to contain the fluid material, to facilitate cooling, to facilitate removal of the cast from the mold without permanent deformation or damage to the mold, and to support the mold while it is being filled with the cast material. Numerous duplicating flasks are on the market (Fig. 17-1). One type is a metal bell with holes in the top for pouring. Another is a simple metal ring with removable bottom and top, the latter having a center hole for pouring. Still another has the top and bottom secured with thumb screws.

More recently a new style of duplicating

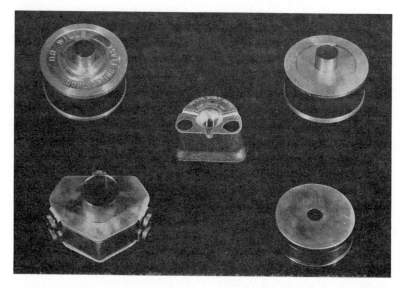

Fig. 17-1. Five types of duplicating flasks. Upper left, the Wills flask, type E; upper right, the Wills flasks, type F. Both of these flasks have a formica ring, 4-inch inside diameter and are two inches in height. The formica is used for its non-heat-conducting property and is machined with a 5-inch inside taper. In the center is a bell-shaped flask; lower left, the Kerr duplicating flask; lower right, a lightweight brass flask in common usage.

flask has been designed by Dr. N. G. Wills. To Dr. Wills is due much credit for his untiring efforts in furthering the development of accurate cast duplication equipment. Two of these duplicating flasks are illustrated in Fig. 17-1. They consist of a machined metal top and bottom fitting onto a formica ring 2 or 2¼ inches high. Formica rather than metal is used for the ring because formica acts as an insulator to prevent too rapid cooling through the sides of the flask. The center hole in the top of each type is provided with a filling reservoir, or "feeder ring." Although not all duplicating flasks provide for a filling reservoir, it is most desirable that a ring superstructure be provided to serve as a reservoir for feeding the warm material into the mold. Thus as cooling and subsequent shrinkage occur, additional fluid material is fed into the mold from the reservoir above. This is similar to the cooling of dental gold after casting. Gold requires an additional bulk of metal so that upon cooling the piece being cast can draw upon additional metal from the reservoir, which we call the *button*. Without the additional bulk of metal the casting would likely show porosity. In duplication, cooling from the bottom of the flask causes the duplicating material to shrink, which has a tendency to draw the chilling solution into closer adaptation to the cast.

The metal bottom of one of the types is provided with legs to hold it off the bottom of the cooling tank, thus allowing circulation of water beneath (Fig. 17-2). While initially the flask should not be immersed completely in running water, any depth short of the metal top is permissible because of the insulating properties of the formica ring.

The principal difference in the two types is in the disassembly of the flask to remove the cast from the mold (Fig. 17-3). One type has a lid that is machined to provide a definite undercut for securing the mold to the lid. The bottom and the formica ring may be removed to permit flexing the mold while the cast is being removed, but the mold remains securely attached to the lid at all times. Then the tapered ring may be placed back over the mold to support it while it is being filled. While this type provides support for the mold at all times, any accidental dislodgment from the undercut metal top would lead to permanent deformation of the mold. This hazard is eliminated in the second type, which permits complete disassembly of the mold from the flask to facilitate removal of the cast from the mold. The inside of the ring is tapered and every part is keyed to facilitate the return of the mold to its original relationship with the flask. This type is preferred for school use.

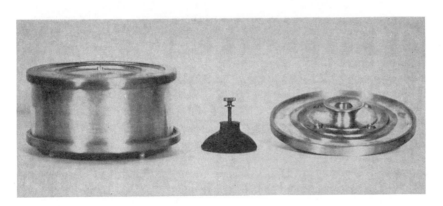

Fig. 17-2. Wills type D flask, made entirely of aluminum, with a ring 1¾ inches high. The upper portion of the top lid has a depressed surface for holding surplus duplicating material, thus serving as a reservoir. This flask is competitively priced because the costlier formica ring is not used.

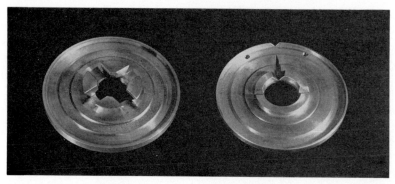

Fig. 17-3. Underside of the lids from two types of Wills duplicating flasks. Type E on the left is undercut for locking the duplicating material to the lid, whereas the type F (right) is keyed to permit complete removal of the mold from the flask and later repositioning.

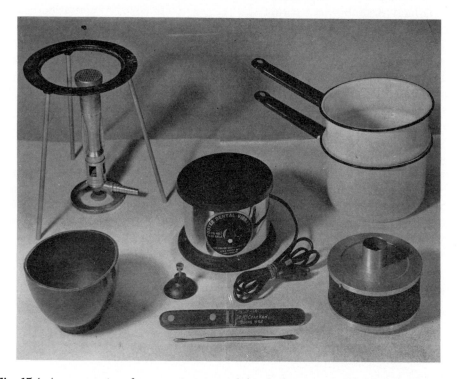

Fig. 17-4. Armamentarium for preparing material for duplicating: double boiler, ring stand, Bunsen burner, stiff laboratory spatula for stirring the duplicating material and for mixing the cast material in the plaster bowl, No. 7 wax spatula for directing the stream of fluid duplicating material over critical areas of the cast, vibrator, duplicating flask with feeder ring, and rubber suction cup for extracting the cast from the chilled mold.

The technique for duplicating is the same for any cast, whether or not blockout is present. However, if wax or clay blockout is present, the temperature of the duplicating material must not be any higher than that recommended to avoid melting and distorting the blockout material.

Any clay used for blockout prior to duplication must be of the insoluble type (Chapter 10). Therefore, only an oily base clay may be safely used for this purpose.

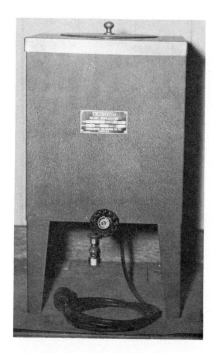

Fig. 17-5. Ready Duplicator maintains the duplicating material at a controlled temperature and ready for immediate use. The duplicating hydrocolloid flows through a rubber hose at the base of the duplicator, and the rate of flow is controlled by a manually operated shut-off valve. Its use is particularly suited when several duplications are accomplished daily. (Courtesy Ticonium Division, CMP Industries, Inc., Albany, N. Y.)

Although ordinary baseplate wax may be used for paralleled blockout and ledges, care must be taken that the temperature of the duplicating material is not high enough to melt the wax. The use of prepared blockout material may be preferred, such as Ney blockout wax or Wills undercut material. A formula has been given in Chapter 10 for those preferring to prepare their own blockout material.

Duplicating procedure. The equipment needed for duplication is as follows (Fig. 17-4):

Bunsen burner and tripod
Enamel or stainless steel double boiler (aluminum utensils should not be used, as aluminum seems to have a deleterious effect on the composition of the duplicating colloid)*

---

*"Ready Duplicator" may be used in lieu of an enamel or stainless steel double boiler (Fig. 17-5).

Duplicating flask
Plaster bowl (600 ml.)
Stiff spatula (Kerr laboratory spatula or Buffalo Dental No. 4 R)
Vibrator
Rubber suction cup
No. 7 spatula

Step-by-step procedure (Fig. 17-6). Although the procedure given describes the use of the Wills late-model flask, it applies as well to the use of any duplicating flask.

1. New hydrocolloid duplicating material is usually packaged in a semidried state. It may be in the form of a crumbled meal. In such case, further chopping is unnecessary. If in bulk form, it must be chopped into fine particles. This is greatly facilitated by running it through a kitchen food chopper. Any duplicating material being reused should similarly be reduced to small pieces before heating.

Heat the duplicating material in the top of the double boiler, stirring to dissipate lumps. New material must be diluted with water in the proportions recommended by the manufacturer; material being reused may be diluted if needed to replace water lost by evaporation. Remember that duplicating material may be further thinned with warm water during preparation as it becomes necessary, but the incorporation of dry material into a mix that is too thin is much more difficult to accomplish. Therefore, it is best that any thinning be done by adding water slowly until the right consistency has been obtained.

When a smooth, creamy mix has been obtained, remove the upper pan of the double boiler from the burner and *continue stirring* until the temperature has dropped to 125° to 130° F. At this temperature, which is just low enough not to burn a finger immersed in it, the duplicating material is ready to pour.

2. For ten minutes just prior to duplication, immerse the cast in water at about 85° F., preferably in water (slurry) that has lost its ability to etch the surface of the stone. Do this while the duplicating material is being cooled to a usable tempera-

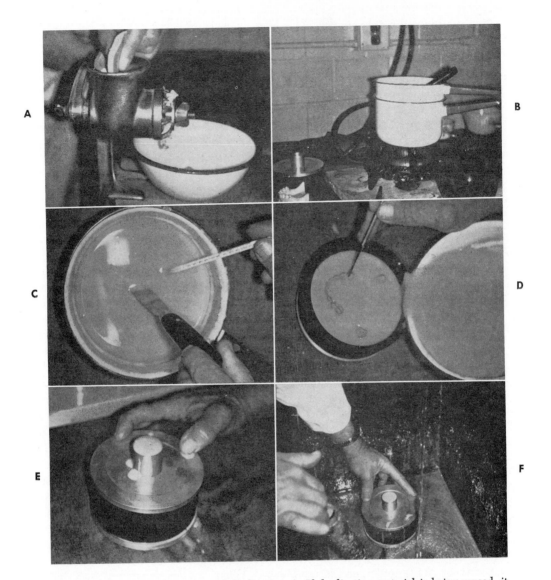

Fig. 17-6. Ten steps in the process of duplication. **A,** If duplicating material is being reused, it should be ground into small pieces before being heated, to avoid lumps and uneven consistency. **B,** The material is then placed in the top of a double boiler and stirred well with a spatula until it has reached a smooth, creamy consistency. Warm water may be added sparingly to dilute it if necessary, but avoid overdilution. **C,** Remove the pan from the double boiler and continue stirring until the temperature has dropped to about 130° F. This is a temperature at which the finger may be immersed without burning, but it is more accurately checked with a thermometer. **D,** The cast to be duplicated, which has been immersed in water just prior to duplication, is placed in the bottom of the duplicating flask, over a small pellet of clay. A small continuous stream of duplicating material is poured in at a posterior end of the cast while the material is guided over critical areas with a No. 7 spatula held in the other hand. **E,** After filling the flask, the top and feeder ring are positioned, and duplicating material is added to fill completely the feeder ring. **F,** The flask is placed in running tap water about 1 inch deep until the material in the feeder ring has completely gelled, with a depression in its center to show that shrinkage has occurred. Then the flask may be completely immersed in running tap water for an additional thirty minutes.

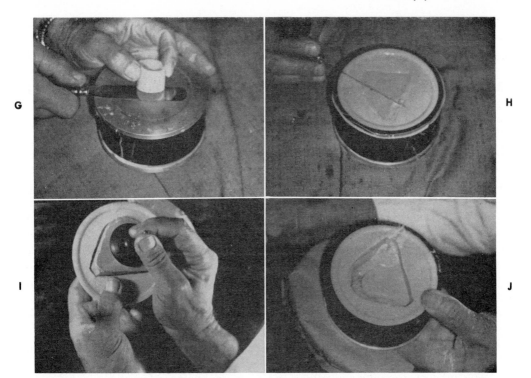

Fig. 17-6, cont'd. **G,** The feeder ring is removed and the projecting material cut off flush with the top of the flask. **H,** The flask is inverted and the bottom of the flask removed, exposing the base of the cast. In this position, the open end now becomes the top of the mold and the original top of the flask becomes the bottom. Excess duplicating material is then removed around the base of the cast. **I,** A rubber suction cup is applied to the base of the cast *under water*. The mold is then removed from the flask and flexed gently around the sides as the cast is removed with the suction cup acting as a handle. **J,** The *mold* is dried gently with compressed air and inspected for defects. It is then returned to the flask precisely in its original position, the original lid placed on the bottom for support, and the stone or investment, properly proportioned and spatulated, is slowly vibrated around the arch, tooth by tooth, to avoid trapping air or diluting the material with moisture. The mold is then completely filled and either immersed in still water or covered with a wet towel or a bell jar to prevent dehydration of the mold at the expense of the water of crystallization of the cast material. While a duplicating mold will not be poured a second time, its dimensional accuracy must be preserved until the cast material has completely set.

ture. Immerse the cast upside down to allow the escape of any air trapped beneath sheets of wax placed on the master cast for relief.

Water that has been allowed to stand for some time with pieces of dental stone or plaster in it will have lost its ability to etch the surface of a stone cast. Therefore, any soaking of a stone cast should be done in water prepared for that purpose rather than in tap water.

When pieces of plaster or stone have been previously placed in tap water, solution will occur until the water becomes saturated with calcium sulfate. Once the water has become saturated, an equilibrium occurs with no further dissolution taking place. A stone cast placed in such water will not become etched because the water already contains all of the calcium sulfate it can hold. A container of such water should be available in the laboratory for use any time a cast needs to be soaked, such as prior to duplication or prior to repouring a portion of the original cast.

The broken pieces of plaster or stone

should be small to medium in size but not fine enough to remain suspended in the water when it is agitated. These pieces should remain in the water at all times to maintain the equilibrium of the calcium sulfate. When used, the water should be clear.

Blow surface moisture off of the cast with compressed air, and center the cast in the bottom of the duplicating flask over a small pellet of clay. Press the base of the cast firmly against the bottom of the flask.

3. With one hand, slowly pour the duplicating material into the flask just behind one posterior end of the cast. A stream of duplicating material about ⅛ inch in diameter should be poured continuously at this point until the base of the cast has been completely covered. At this time, with a No. 7 spatula in the other hand, guide the material around the teeth, into interproximal spaces, and upon critical tooth surfaces. This prevents trapping air bubbles in critical areas.

After the teeth have been completely covered, fill the flask within ⅛ inch of the top. Then interrupt the pouring while positioning the metal top and feeder ring, after which completely fill the mold to the top of the feeder ring.

4. Now place the flask in about 1 inch of cold (preferably running) water. The water should cover no more than the metal base and the lower ½ inch of the formica ring, so that initial cooling will occur only through the metal bottom.

Although cooling *must* be done slowly and from the bottom to control shrinkage and avoid distortion, it is not absolutely necessary that cooling be hastened by using cold water. Time permitting, a hydrocolloid mold may be bench cooled without affecting its accuracy, whereas too rapid cooling may cause distortion. With this in mind, allow the mold to set completely in a shallow water bath. However, to facilitate early separation of the mold, when the feeder ring has gelled, immerse the flask in cold running water, where it should be left for at least thirty minutes to assure chilling throughout.

5. After thorough chilling, remove the flask from the water bath and remove the feeder ring. Cut off the hydrocolloid projecting above the lid flush with the top of the lid. Then invert the flask and remove the bottom, exposing the base of the cast. Remove any hydrocolloid covering the base of the cast and the flattened piece of clay, leaving the smooth base of the cast exposed.

The inside of the formica ring is tapered; therefore it may be removed by sliding it away from the top, leaving the mold attached only to the top. In the inverted position, the top now has become the bottom and will remain so during the subsequent procedures. The original bottom, now removed, will not be replaced on the mold, as this becomes the open end into which the cast material is poured.

If the top of the flask is undercut, the mold is not removed from it, and it becomes the base for supporting the mold. If the flask has a top that is keyed but not undercut, the mold is removed from it also to facilitate flexing as the cast is being removed from the mold. In either case, removal is best accomplished by applying a rubber suction cup to the base of the cast under running tap water and lightly flexing the mold while extracting the cast.

The suction cup is used as a convenient handle. Without it, the mold would have to be cut away to expose enough of the sides of the cast for a finger grip. After pouring and removing the duplicate cast, an excess would result where the mold has been cut away. Although this may be trimmed on the model trimmer, it must be remembered that the base of the cast has been scored in three places to facilitate repositioning on the surveyor. If the scored areas are inadvertently trimmed away, there will be no record of the path of placement on the duplicate cast to aid in positioning it on the surveyor for locating contour lines. This necessity does not exist when clasp ledges (indices) were formed on the master cast. However, when waxing is to be done in relation to a survey line only, it is necessary that the original cast position be recorded on the duplicate cast. On the other hand, such a record always must be preserved on a duplicate stone cast to be used for fitting. This is particularly true when wrought-wire clasp arms must be accurately adapted in relation to the height of contour of the abutment teeth.

6. After removing the cast, replace the mold in the flask in exactly the same position as before. This is made possible by the keyed relationship of the parts of the flask. Reposition the hydrocolloid in the tapered formica ring so that the longer of the three grooves in the hydrocolloid mold points to the centering screw on the outside of the ring. Replace the keyed top, which is to become the bottom, and invert the ring so that the open end of the mold is up. If the reassembly has been properly done, the mold is in exactly the same relation to the flask as before; otherwise distortion of the mold may result.

Remove any free moisture from the mold by inverting it and blowing it out with a gentle stream of compressed air. Care must be taken not to hold the stream of air on any area long enough to cause dehydration of that area.

With the correct amount of water in the plaster bowl, add a measured amount of stone or investment, following the manufacturer's recommendations. The correct water-powder ratio is given by the manufacturer for each 100 gm. of powder.

Mix thoroughly with a stiff spatula or a mechanical mixer. *Vacuum mixing is always preferable, to eliminate entrapped air.* If this equipment is not available, knead the mixture on the vibrator to remove as much air as will come to the surface. Many of the small air voids in a cast are due to air bubbles being carried into the mold in the mix rather than to air trapped in the mold during pouring.

Fill the hydrocolloid mold in much the same manner as an impression of a dental arch. With the No. 7 spatula, add small amounts of material only at one posterior end while using the vibrator. The material is thus made to flow around the arch by the weight of the material behind it. Add material only at the original site until all critical areas of the mold have been filled. In this manner, excess moisture is pushed ahead of the material until it reaches the extreme opposite end of the mold, where it should be expelled and discarded. This avoids any dilution of the mix by the moisture remaining in the mold, minimizes the chances of trapping air, and results in a uniformly dense cast.

7. Immediately upon filling the mold immerse it in still water and allow it to set for about forty-five minutes. Immersion supplies the cast material with needed water of crystallization, some of which may otherwise be taken up by the hydrocolloid, resulting in a chalky cast surface. On the other hand, immersion should not be for longer than approximately an hour, and never overnight, or etching of the surface of the cast may result.

After the cast material has hardened, remove the flask from the mold and *break the mold away from the cast* rather than attempt to remove the cast from the intact mold. The mold should not be poured a second time anyway, and fresh surfaces of the cast may be rubbed off in withdrawing it from the mold. Therefore, the mold should always be broken away from the cast.

Duplicating material may be washed and placed in water in a covered jar for reuse, especially when it will likely be reused in the near future. However, if any doubt exists as to its texture, it should be discarded. One should not attempt to revitalize old duplicating material by replenishing with new. Instead, any questionable material should be discarded and a new batch of material mixed as needed.

A freshly duplicated cast should not be handled unnecessarily, particularly one made of investment material, until it has been allowed to dry in air or in an oven. An investment cast should not be trimmed on a model trimmer, as this causes a slurry of investment to splash over the cast, which may not then be entirely removed by rinsing. For that matter an investment cast should not be rinsed at all. Instead, any necessary grinding should be done with a dry stone on a lathe and any powdered investment blown off with compressed air.

After initial drying and trimming, an investment cast should be dried in an oven at 180° to 200° F. for one to one and one-half hours, depending upon the size of the cast. Then it should be dipped in a rosin-beeswax preparation as follows:

Melt the beeswax in a pan to a temperature of near 300° F. or just when the beeswax begins to smoke. This temperature is approximately 100° F. above that of the cast when it is removed from the drying oven.

Remove the cast from the oven and immerse it in the beeswax for approximately ten seconds. Then remove and stand the cast on a piece of absorbent paper until it has cooled.

Some of the advantages of dipping an investment cast in a rosin-beeswax preparation are (a) it eliminates the necessity for soaking the investment cast prior to painting on the outer investment; (b) it provides a smooth dense surface on the investment cast; and (c) the combination of drying and dipping eliminates any excess moisture in the cast.

WAXING THE PARTIAL DENTURE FRAMEWORK

Experience with free-hand waxing and the use of ready-made wax shapes is recommended as a prerequisite to the use of pre-formed plastic patterns (Fig. 17-7). Unless plastic patterns are selected and used with care, they are better not used at all. The fact that they facilitate rapid production of partial denture castings has led to their widespread use in commercial laboratories, but this alone does not justify their use. Even when plastic patterns are used, parts of the denture framework must be waxed free-hand to avoid excessive bulk and to create the desired contours. (See Fig. 17-8.)

The use of ready-made wax shapes fa-

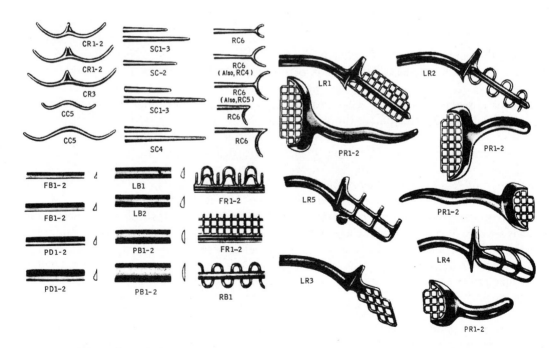

Fig. 17-7. Pre-formed plastic patterns are available in many different shapes and sizes. Being a soft plastic material, they have a tendency to regain their original carded shape after being adapted to the refractory cast unless a "tacky" liquid is first applied to the cast. (Courtesy J. F. Jelenko & Co., Inc., New York, N. Y.)

cilitates free-hand waxing to the point that an experienced dentist or dental laboratory technician can complete a wax pattern in little more time than is necessary when plastic patterns are used. Much of the speed with which a wax pattern may be produced depends upon how well the step-by-step procedure is organized to take fullest advantage of the wax shapes.

The student in the preclinical laboratory should begin his waxing experience on a stone cast rather than on the softer investment cast, so that he may be free to modify and correct his errors as they are pointed out to him. Only after having a clear understanding of the location, bulk, and contours of the various parts of the wax pattern being done should he be allowed to wax on the investment cast. Since corrections on the investment cast may result in

a rough casting, it is imperative that the waxing on the investment cast be done in a positive manner with a minimum of changes and corrections.

The same applies to the making of a removable partial denture framework in the undergraduate dental clinic. Although the typical dental student probably will not fabricate his own partial denture castings after graduation, it is essential that he has a background and experience in dental laboratory procedures that will enable him to design the denture framework and prescribe how it is to be fabricated (Fig. 17-9). *Not only this, but he must also be capable of evaluating the finished product to the end that the quality of dental laboratory services is maintained* (Fig. 17-10).

With this in mind, it is desirable that two or more partial denture frameworks be

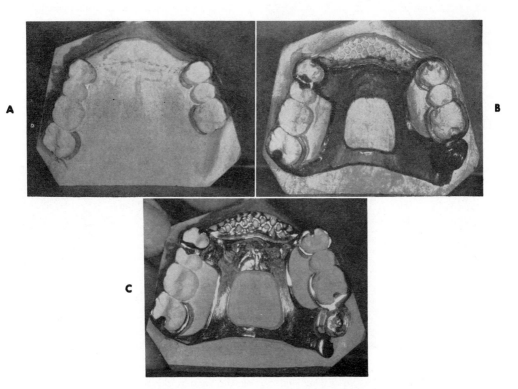

Fig. 17-8. Three steps in the making of a denture framework using blockout ledges and ready-made pattern forms. **A,** The master cast with shaped blockout ledges for the location of retentive and nonretentive clasp arms. **B,** The completed pattern using an anatomic replica pattern, plastic clasp forms resting on investment ledges, and retention mesh anteriorly. The pattern is then waxed to completion. **C,** The finished casting returned to the master cast. The blockout ledges may be seen below the three lingual clasp arms.

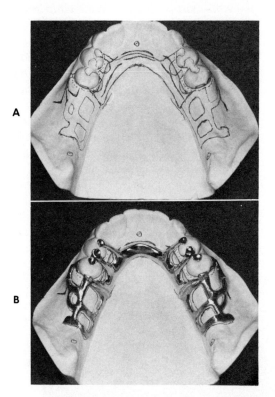

Fig. 17-9. The technician should receive from the dentist a master cast that has been surveyed and had reference lines scratched on the two sides and dorsal aspect of the base of the cast or has been marked for tripoding. Upon this cast, the outline of the denture framework should be drawn precisely, without marring the cast, where the component parts of the framework are to be placed and their dimensions be indicated. In addition, written instructions, including waxing specifications, which ideally should accompany the outlined master cast, must be included (see Fig. 18-2). From such a work authorization, the technician may be expected to return a polished casting that accurately conforms to the penciled design as in **B**.

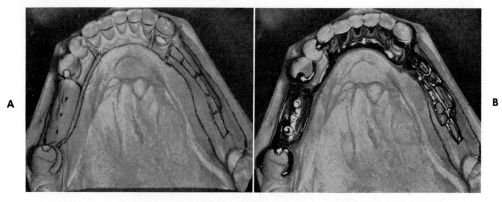

Fig. 17-10. **A,** Design of the partial denture framework is outlined on the master cast for the technician to follow in waxing and casting the framework. **B,** The cast framework as returned from the laboratory, superimposed upon the penciled design. Note the contouring of the thin lingual apron continuous with the half-pear-shaped lingual bar major connector. In the modification space a metal base is used with undercut finishing lines and nailhead retention for the attachment of artificial posterior teeth later with a resin base material. Also note the use of lingual ledges on the abutment teeth of the modification space. (From McCracken, W. L.: J. Prosthet. Dent. 8:71-84, 1958.)

waxed to completion, if not cast and finished, by the clinical student himself. To avoid discrepancies occurring as a result of inept waxing and subsequent corrections on the investment cast, it is most desirable that the student first do a practice wax pattern on a duplicate stone cast. After all corrections have been approved by his instructor, waxing on the investment cast may be done with confidence and dispatch, resulting in a casting of high quality. Although this policy may be criticized as time-consuming, the total time spent should be little more than that required when it is done on the investment cast alone with numerous corrections. A higher percentage of satisfactory castings and fewer remakes will result when this policy is followed in the undergraduate clinic. The quality of the finished product and the knowledge and experience gained by the student more than justify the additional time spent.

Forming the wax pattern for a lower Class II removable partial denture framework. One waxing exercise will be given that embodies many of the essentials of waxing a partial denture framework. This exercise includes the waxing of three types of direct retainers, namely, circumferential, combination, and bar type. A lingual bar major connector is utilized and also a cast denture base for the tooth-bound edentulous space. The adaptation of a round, 18-gauge wrought wire is required for the formation of the retentive arm of a combination-type direct retainer.

The student should be furnished two stone casts that are duplicates of the blocked-out and relieved master cast (Fig. 17-11). One of the stone casts will be utilized to adapt a wrought-wire, retentive direct retainer arm, and the other stone cast will be used to simulate a refractory cast upon which the wax pattern will be completed.

1. On one of the stone casts, outline lightly the pattern for the framework, being guided by the transfer indices (Fig. 17-12). A black lead pencil may be used to designate the outline of the framework for this exercise; however, a color-type pencil (Eagle Verithin) should be used when outlining the pattern on a refractory cast. In either instance, extreme caution must be used in this procedure to avoid the slightest abrasion of the cast.

2. *Forming the wrought-wire retentive arm.* The design for the mandibular partial denture framework calls for the use of a wrought-wire retentive direct retainer arm

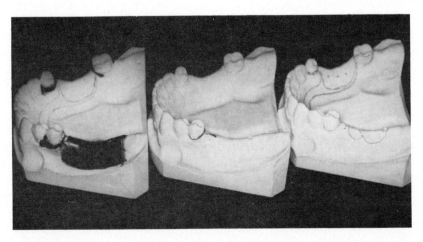

Fig. 17-11. Blocked out master cast is on the left. Wrought-wire direct retainer arm is adapted to one of the duplicate stone casts (center figure). Right figure is duplicate stone cast simulating a refractory cast upon which the outline of the framework has been lightly drawn.

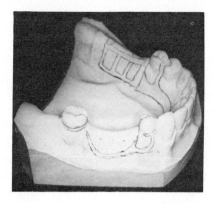

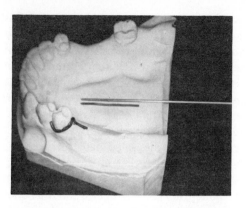

Fig. 17-12. Penciled outline of framework. Outline of major connector and borders of cast denture base was scratched lightly on the master cast and duplicated in the "refractory" cast. Ledge indices of direct retainers and outlined major connector and denture base permit exact duplication of the penciled outline on the master cast to the "refractory" cast.

Fig. 17-13. Outline for retentive wrought-wire arm is outlined on cast following the ledge index. An 18-gauge round wax strip is adapted to the penciled outline. Wax strip straightened out determines the length of 18-gauge wrought wire (Type II) required to form the direct retainer arm.

on the lower left second premolar. The wrought wire used may be either 18-gauge round, Type II wire, or Ticonium wire. Gold or cobalt-chromium alloys may be cast directly to these types of wire without appreciably changing physical characteristics of the wire.

Any wrought wire may be fatigued by repeated bending and straightening, and prolonged manipulation with pliers causes nicks in the wire. Either may result in early failure of the clasp arm through no fault of the material itself. To avoid having to correct mistakes by rebending, the student should practice first with paper-clip wire of similar gauge. When the student has learned to contour the wire with a minimum of manipulation he may then proceed to adapt the tougher 18-gauge wrought wire.

Pliers that may be used most effectively for clasp wire–contouring purposes are those designated by the numbers 53 G (Dixon), 200 (three-pronged), 107 (round nose), 115 (contouring), and 47 (flat-round). Similar pliers are available from different manufacturers. It is not inferred that all the mentioned pliers are used to contour every clasp made of a wrought

wire. However, it is doubted that any wire-bending situation will be encountered that cannot be accomplished by utilization of the above listed pliers.

Step-by-step procedure. The procedure for forming wrought-wire direct retainer arms is as follows:

a. On the second stone cast, being guided by the ledge index, outline in pencil the design of the wrought-wire retentive arm (Fig. 17-13). Extend the outline just lingual to the center of the guiding plane area on the abutment and then continue the outline downward to the gingival area. Extend the line posteriorly on the cast for approximately 5 mm. This is the outline for the right-angle "foot," which will be imbedded in the casting just lingual to the crest of the residual ridge. Since it should be assumed that only a mechanical attachment with the casting alloy may result, the "foot" is necessary to secure the wrought wire to the casting. However, a gold alloy cast to a PGP (platinum, gold-palladium) type of wire may result in some metallic bonding. Gold or cobalt-chromium alloys cast to a Ticonium wire results in predominantly mechanical fixation.

Illustrated in Figure 17-33 is an alternate conformation of the wrought-wire attachment, which may be utilized for short abutment teeth where two right-angle bends of the wire cannot be accomplished.

b. Determine the length of the wire needed by adapting a piece of 18-gauge round wax to the penciled outline of the wrought-wire retainer. Straighten this wax form and cut a piece of 18-gauge wire about 2 mm. longer than the wax form (Fig. 17-13).

c. Round one end of the wire with an abrasive rubber wheel. Measure the length of the penciled outline of the wrought-wire direct retainer arm on the cast from its proposed terminal tip to its junction with the envisioned minor connector on the distal of the second premolar. With an abrasive rubber wheel, taper the rounded end portion of the wire uniformly the measured length of the retainer arm. The wire should be so tapered that the terminal end of the wire is approximately one half the diameter of the 18-gauge wire.

d. With No. 115 contouring pliers, bend the tapered portion of the wire to contact the buccal surface of the premolar starting the bend near the tapered terminal end of the wire. The wire must accurately follow the ledge index on the cast. Continue bending the wire to contact the tooth slightly lingual to one half the width of the distal surface of the tooth.

e. With the contoured portion of the wire held in position against the abutment tooth, mark the wire with a pencil at the exact spot where the wire must turn inferiorly toward the residual ridge. Also, carefully estimate the length of this upright portion of the wire according to the outline on the cast. With No. 47 pliers, make an acute (right-angle) bend of the wire at the previously marked spot so that the vertical portion of the wire will contact the guiding plane area of the abutment tooth. The wire cannot be placed back on the cast at this time. Having estimated the length of the vertical portion of the wire, make a right-angle bend so that the remaining portion of the wire contacts the residual ridge region of the cast and is directed posteriorly. Two mm. from the untapered end of the wire, make a right-angle bend so that the end of the wire projects vertically upward.

f. The formed wire should accurately and passively conform to the outline on the stone cast (Figs. 17-14 and 17-15). Wrought wire can be accurately and rather quickly adapted, without nicks or having become strain-hardened. Practice first with paper clips. Place the formed wire and cast aside until the wax pattern has been developed on the other stone cast.

3. Adapt one thickness of 24-gauge casting sheet wax (green or pink) or adhesive

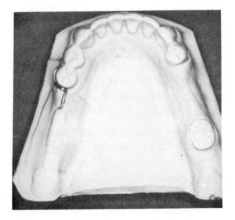

Fig. 17-14. Wrought-wire arm is closely and passively adapted to the abutment tooth. Note the taper of the arm from the distobuccal aspect of the abutment to the retentive end. "Foot" is just lingual to the crest of the residual ridge to provide space for the cervical end of the artificial molar.

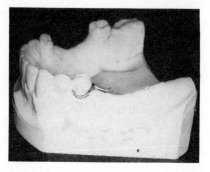

Fig. 17-15. Portion of wrought wire contacting distal of the abutment is placed as far inferiorly as possible since the master cast was blocked out in this area. Such a position will have less of a tendency to "top-load" the tooth in resisting horizontal rotation of the denture. Small angled piece of wire at distal of conformed arm facilitates handling of warm clasp arm with cotton forceps in later waxing procedures.

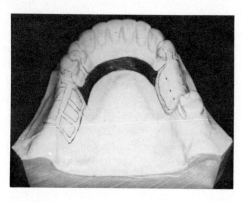

Fig. 17-16. Lingual bar pattern is made of half-pear-shaped, 6-gauge wax form, reinforced on the tissue surface with 24-gauge sheet wax for rigidity. Bar is trimmed to conform to the outline of the denture base on one side and the minor connector outline on the distal extension side.

wax on the lingual aspect of the alveolar ridge to cover the outline of the lingual bar major connector. Be careful not to stretch the wax, thereby altering its thickness.

4. Adapt a piece of 6-gauge half-pear-shaped wax over the sheet wax to conform to the pencil lines denoting the lingual bar and showing through the sheet wax. The greater bulk of the half-pear shape must be at the lower border, with the tapered edge near or along the top pencil line. The thickness of the wax shape and the sheet wax previously adapted plus a small amount of wax added to maintain a half-pear shape will be the thickness of the major connector before polishing.

5. Cut away the sheet wax extending above the outline of the lingual bar and also below the half-pear-shaped wax, which has now become the lingual bar, and cut off both the bar and sheet wax even with the distal aspects of the premolar abutments or according to the outline in these areas (Fig. 17-16). Use a fairly dull instrument (Roach carver) for this purpose to avoid scoring the cast.

6. Seal the inferior and superior borders of the bar to the cast. It is important that

the wax be sealed to the cast throughout its course, yet that the original half-pear shape be preserved. Should any part of the wax pattern not be sealed to the cast, the pattern may become dislodged during the application of the outer investment, resulting in the investment seeping under the pattern. This would result in a false undersurface on the casting.

7. Adapt a piece of 8-gauge half-round wax to the full extent of the guiding plane on the distal surface of the left premolar (flat side to the guiding plane surface). Cut the wax off slightly inferior to the marginal ridge and seal the wax to the cast. Taper the wax superiorly to a feather edge (Fig. 17-17).

8. Adapt a piece of 10-gauge round wax strip from the superior border of the lingual bar up the embrasure between the first and second premolars, then over the marginal ridges, and into the rest seats prepared in the premolars. This minor connector should pass perpendicularly from the lingual bar up the interdental embrasure. A rule previously stated is that any crossing of gingival tissues by components of the framework should be abrupt and definite. A second rule to be followed is that

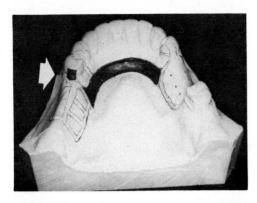

Fig. 17-17. This minor connector (arrow) forms part of the direct retainer assembly for the abutment tooth. Its contact with the guiding plane, in conjunction with guiding plane surfaces on the opposite side of the arch will insure only one path of placement and removal of the completed restoration.

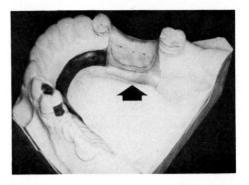

Fig. 17-19. Twenty-four-gauge sheet wax is adapted over the outline of the lingual portion of the cast denture base area. The outline will show through pink sheet wax thus permitting accurate trimming of the wax. Use of 24-gauge sheet wax permits some adjustment of the denture base to alleviate sore spots if such occur after the patient uses the restoration.

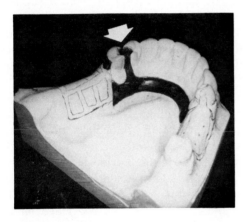

Fig. 17-18. Gingival margins were relieved and interproximal undercuts were blocked out on the master cast parallel to the path of placement. Therefore, this minor connector does not engage an undercut. In fact, the only components of the framework engaging undercuts are the terminal ends of retentive direct retainer arms. See Fig. 4-27 for the interproximal conformation of this component on a finished framework.

minor connectors should conform to interdental embrasures whenever possible and should be so shaped to present as little bulk to the tongue as possible. Seal the wax shape to the cast, converting it to an embrasure form, and wax the occlusal rests to conform to the outline of the rest seat preparations (Fig. 17-18). Strengthen the wax at the marginal ridges if necessary.

The final form of the pattern for the occlusal rests should be representative of the occlusal anatomy before the rest seats were prepared.

9. Cut two pieces of 24-gauge casting sheet wax (green or pink), which, when joined at the crest of the tooth-bounded edentulous ridge, will cover the penciled outline of the cast base (Fig. 17-19). Adapt the lingual portion first, being careful not to stretch the wax. Trim this wax just ½ mm. inferior to the penciled outline of the lingual portion of the cast base area. Seal the wax along its edges and to the adjacent end of the major connector.

10. In a like manner adapt and seal the other piece of 24-gauge sheet wax over the buccal portion of the cast base, joining both pieces over the crest of the ridge in a smooth junction (Fig. 17-20).

11. Adapt a length of 8-gauge half-round wax on the guiding plane, proximal surfaces of the right side abutments (flat side against the guiding plane), attaching one end to the cast base pattern gingivally and carrying the other end over the marginal ridge and into the rest seat preparations (Fig. 17-21). Seal the wax along its edges and to the cast base pattern after the wax has been trimmed to conform to

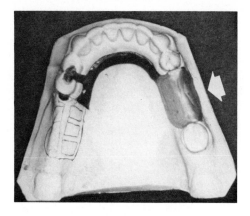

Fig. 17-20. Buccal portion of cast base pattern is added and the wax is trimmed to conform to the outline of the framework. Forming this portion of the cast base pattern is best done in two steps as described to avoid thinning the 24-gauge sheet wax. The two halves are then carefully joined and sealed at the crest of the residual ridge.

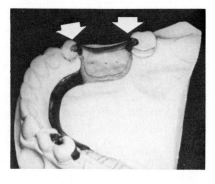

Fig. 17-21. Occlusal rests may be carved to form before other components of the direct retainer assemblies are formed in wax. Rests should conform to the occlusal morphology present before the rest seats were prepared.

the outline of the rests and guiding plane areas.

12. Being guided by the index ledge, adapt a piece of 12-gauge half-round wax on the lingual surface of the right premolar abutment, and connect the distal end of the strip of wax to the previously formed minor connector on the same tooth. On this particular abutment and also on the molar abutment, the retentive clasp arms will be on the buccal surfaces and the reciprocal arms on the lingual surfaces. Reciprocal

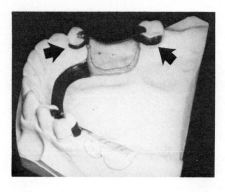

Fig. 17-22. Reciprocal components must be rigid and since they do not engage undercuts need not be tapered for the sake of flexibility. Reciprocal arm on molar restores the lingual anatomy of the abutment crown.

arms are nonretentive and therefore should not be tapered except to avoid abruptness and irritation to the tongue by the terminal end of the clasp arm. Reinforce the junction of the reciprocal arm pattern with the minor connector to which it is attached (Fig. 17-22).

13. Adapt a piece of 8-gauge half-round wax to the lingual surface of the molar abutment, being guided by the lingual ledge of the abutment crown. Connect the strip of wax to the previously formed minor connector. Add sufficient wax to have the lower portion of this reciprocal arm as thick as the lingual extent of the ledge on the crown. Superiorly, wax must be added to restore the normal contour of the lingual surface of the crown and feathered to the lingual height of the crown (Fig. 17-22). The terminal end of the reciprocal arm should have a taper corresponding to the taper of the lingual ledge in this area as viewed from above.

14. Beginning at the inferior border of the reciprocal arm of the right premolar at its junction with the minor connector, adapt a piece of 14-gauge round wax over the outline of the lingual portion of the border of the cast base. Carry the wax form up to the inferior border of the reciprocal arm on the molar abutment. Seal this piece of wax on the outside border without appreciably altering its form. This piece of

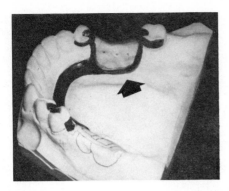

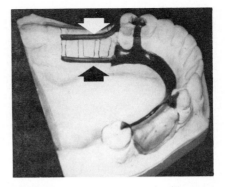

Fig. 17-23. Fourteen-gauge round wax added as described forms a trough to support and retain the acrylic resin supporting the artificial teeth. Therefore, a smooth junction between the framework and the acrylic resin is made without danger of cracks in the resin appearing after the denture has been in use. Since the border of the cast base pattern is thickened by the addition of 14-gauge round wax, the resultant casting can be gently rounded at the borders making it more comfortable for the patient than having the borders finished as sharp edges.

Fig. 17-24. Twelve-gauge half-round wax form is attached to the minor connector on the guiding plane and runs posteriorly just lingual to the crest of the residual ridge. Placed in this position, interference to arranging artificial posterior teeth will be minimized. The lower portion of the ladderlike structure should be superior to the inferior portion of the major connector. Otherwise, a butt-type junction of the major and minor connector would be difficult to construct.

wax will provide an adequate thickness for the border of the cast base and at the same time will form an undercut finishing line on the cast base (Fig. 17-23).

15. Up to this point the forming of the wax pattern has been done primarily on the lingual surfaces of the cast. The rationale of this procedure is to avoid distortion of any buccal components of the pattern by handling of the cast while accomplishing the heavier lingual waxing.

16. Perfect the waxing done thus far by smoothing and adding to the weak points. Smoothing does not mean polishing or flaming the wax pattern, either of which affects only the highest part of the convex surfaces and serves only to flatten and alter the shape of the wax. Rather smoothing should be done by gentle carving, which preserves the original form of the wax pattern. Therefore, as weak areas become evident, reinforce them by flowing on additional wax and blending it into the original waxing with a hot spatula and by carving. In the process of smoothing, gently trim away all excess wax around the borders of the pattern with a Roach carver. Exercise

caution to avoid any alteration of the surface of the cast.

17. Retention for the attachment of resin base on the distal extension side is added next. This consists of two parallel pieces of 12-gauge half-round wax connected with cross rungs to form a ladderlike framework. Beginning at the base of the vertical minor connector on the left second premolar, adapt a piece of 12-gauge half-round wax along the lingual surface of the residual ridge at the ridge crest (convex side up). Extend this piece of wax approximately two-thirds the length of the edentulous area. Seal and blend the proximal end of the wax into the minor connector at its point of origin and just tack the distal end to the cast. The retentive frame need not be sealed to the cast throughout its course (Fig. 17-24).

About 5 to 7 mm. inferior to the longitudinal piece of wax, adapt another piece of 12-gauge half-round wax parallel to the first piece and of the same length. The anterior end of the lower wax strip will be attached to the distal end of the major connector. At its point of origin, add wax to

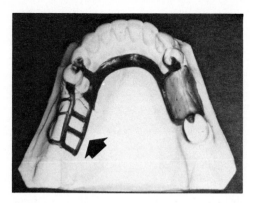

Fig. 17-25. Longitudinal pieces forming a portion of the minor connector are joined with 12-gauge half-round wax forms. Two buccal loops of 18-gauge round wax form are attached to the longitudinal piece of wax near the crest of the residual ridge. A minor connector extending on both the buccal and lingual slopes of the residual ridge will, in all probability, strengthen the acrylic resin denture base.

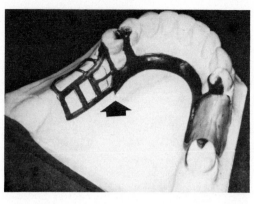

Fig. 17-26. Round 14-gauge wax is used to form a direct connection of the major connector to the minor connector contacting the guiding plane surface. The round form is modified to present a flat surface facing posteriorly and an angled surface anteriorly, thus forming a desired butt joint between the major and minor connector.

reinforce and blend it into the major connector (Fig. 17-24).

At equally spaced intervals of about 4 to 5 mm. join the two longitudinal pieces with connecting bars of 12-gauge half-round wax strips. This forms the rungs of the ladderlike construction (Fig. 17-25). Each end of the rung must be attached securely to the longitudinal pieces with additional wax, so that reinforcement rather than weakness will exist at each junction point. None of these crossbars need be sealed to the cast except at their ends.

From one rung of the ladder, usually the third from the end, curve a piece of 18-gauge round wax over the buccal side of the ridge to join the most distal rung at the end of the framework. This will provide additional support to the buccal flange of the resin denture base. To facilitate casting from lingually placed sprues, this buccal loop should be continuous with any two cross rungs. Attach the buccal loop securely with additional wax but do not seal it to the cast in its entire length. In a long span, such as a distal extension situation from a canine or first premolar abutment, two such buccal loops should be used; otherwise one will usually suffice (Fig. 17-25).

A butt-type joint finishing line of the major connector and the resin base retention ladder (minor connector) is made. The purpose of this type joint and finishing line is twofold. First, a smooth, flat, continuous surface between the major connector and the acrylic resin denture base will result, which is less noticeable to the tongue than is a "hump" surface. Secondly, a butt-type joint is stronger and more resistant to "working" the resin and producing strain fissures than other type joints. Place a strip of 14-gauge round wax about halfway up the lingual surface of the guiding plane minor connector and continue the wax strip inferiorly and on top of the previously formed joint between the ladder and the major connector. Seal this wax to the cast and to the superior border of the major connector. In the process of sealing the 14-gauge round wax, a half-round shape should result. Then additional wax may be added to provide the greatest bulk toward the lingual surface. The minor connector contacting the guiding plane surface is thickest at its gingival portion and tapers

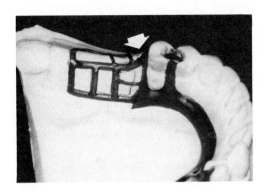

Fig. 17-27. Eighteen-gauge round wax form is used to strengthen connection between the major and minor connector. This could be accomplished with half-round 12-gauge wax form also. It is absolutely necessary that a strong, rigid union exist between the major connector and the minor connector to which the acrylic resin denture base will be attached.

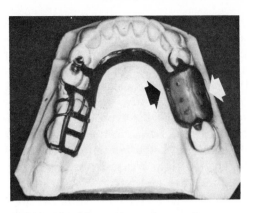

Fig. 17-28. Small mushroom "nailhead" configurations are attached to the cast base portion of the wax pattern. These nailheads serve as additional retentive elements for the acrylic resin supporting the artificial teeth. They should be so positioned that no interference to arranging the artificial teeth will be encountered. Six to eight nailheads are quite sufficient on short-span bases (not more than two missing posterior teeth).

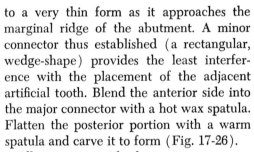

to a very thin form as it approaches the marginal ridge of the abutment. A minor connector thus established (a rectangular, wedge-shape) provides the least interference with the placement of the adjacent artificial tooth. Blend the anterior side into the major connector with a hot wax spatula. Flatten the posterior portion with a warm spatula and carve it to form (Fig. 17-26).

All junctions with the major connector should be reinforced and blended smoothly into its contour (Fig. 17-27). After the butt-type joint is formed, in most instances and especially in those instances where the longitudinal sections of the ladder are separated by more than 4 to 5 mm., an 18-gauge round wax reinforcing element should be provided between the butt joint and the most anterior rung of the ladder (Fig. 17-27).

18. Accomplish the procedure described in 14 on the buccal portion of the cast base pattern.

19. Small "nailheads," as additional acrylic resin retentive elements, are now placed on both the cast base and the minor connector (ladder) for attachment of the resin base on the distal extension side (Fig.

17-28). For the latter, the nailheads serve to attach a resin tray for making a secondary impression and are removed before the denture base is processed.

A nailhead is quickly and easily made by holding one end of a 2 to 3 inch piece of 18-gauge round wax to the area the nailhead is to occupy, sealing the end to the pattern with a hot waxing instrument, holding the strip until the junction has hardened, and then cutting the 18-gauge wax strip about 2 mm. above the junction. With a warm wax spatula, the protruding end of the wax can be "mushroomed" by simply applying a little pressure.

Nailheads on the cast denture base are confined within the undercut finishing lines and must be placed so that they will neither interfere with the arrangement of the artificial teeth nor will protrude through the resin supporting the artificial teeth. Two rows of three or four nailheads are ample. One row should be placed lingually and about halfway between the border of the cast base pattern and the crest of the residual ridge. The other row is similarly located but placed on the buccal side of the cast base pattern.

20. Form the cast retentive direct retainer arms. The creation of the wax pattern has now progressed up to the point of adding the planned retentive clasp arms. These have been classified in Chapter 6. When a cast retentive clasp of any type (other than an I bar type) is to be used, it must be waxed in relation to the height of contour with the terminal one third of the tapered clasp arm progressively engaging a retentive undercut.

The location and extent of the undercut to be utilized as well as the bracing portion of the retentive arm are established first on the master cast and the clasp arm outlined from its origin to its terminus. A wax ledge is carved to establish the location of the inferior border of the clasp arm. In fact, this ledge should be carved the width of a pencil line cervically to the planned inferior border and terminus of the arm to allow for smoothing and polishing the completed casting. Otherwise, the inferior border of the cast arm would occupy a position occlusal to its planned position. This ledge is duplicated on the refractory cast, and the clasp arm is waxed or the plastic pattern is placed with its inferior border along the ledge.

Cast retentive clasp arms are most satisfactorily made utilizing pre-formed plastic patterns that are uniform in dimensions and taper (Fig. 17-7). Students and technicians alike, however, should have had experience in free-hand waxing and in the use of wax shapes. Twelve-gauge half-round wax is used to form the outline of the clasp, which is then sealed to the cast. Some reinforcement at the point of origin and addition of wax along the length of the arm is necessary to create a tapered arm by carving. Of course, some trimming along the sealed edges will also be necessary. The finished pattern should have a uniform taper throughout its course, terminating in a predetermined infrabulge area. With a circumferential clasp, the height of contour is crossed at about two thirds the length of the retentive arm (never less) as the diameter of the clasp arm decreases and the terminal third progressively engages the tooth undercut.

With a bar-type clasp arm, the height of contour is not always crossed by the clasp arm, but the clasp must have a uniform taper from its point of origin to its termination in the undercut area. The point of origin of a bar clasp arm is at the cast denture base or where it emerges from an acrylic resin denture base. Its taper, therefore, should begin at this point rather than at its attachment to minor connectors of the denture framework. Any portion thereof that will be embedded in a resin base must be considered a rigid connector and not part of the retentive clasp; therefore, only the exposed part is tapered to form the bar-type clasp arm.

A cast clasp arm should not be indiscriminately polished and then "pliered" to place. Rather, waxing should be done in such a matter that a minimum of finishing is necessary and its intended relationship to the abutment tooth is maintained.

With the preceding information and suggestions, the patterns for the cast retentive arms may be accomplished. Being guided by the index ledge on the buccal surface of the molar abutment tooth adapt a piece of 12-gauge half-round wax (flat side to abutment) and attach it to the minor connector (body of the direct retainer). Add a small amount of wax to the clasp arm so that it can be carved to a taper that conforms to the relative dimensions of a cast retentive arm as illustrated in Fig. 6-3. Reinforce the junction of the clasp arm with the body of the clasp by adding sufficient wax to provide a uniform taper from the body to the terminal end of the arm (Fig. 17-29). The student is reminded that in forming *all* wax pattern junctions, that the end result must be a solid, homogeneous pattern without pits, voids, cracks, or fissures.

The bar-type retainer is formed next by first adapting a piece of 12-gauge half-round wax (flat side to abutment) on the buccal aspect of the right premolar abutment, being guided by the ledge index on

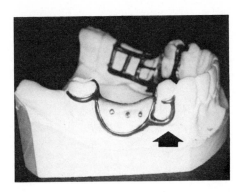

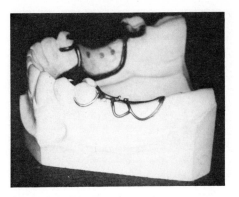

Fig. 17-29. Wax pattern for the cast circumferential retainer arm on the buccal surface of the molar abutment. Since this is a retentive arm, it is tapered from its attachment area to its terminus. Bar-type direct retainer arm (arrow) joins the cast base pattern. From its retentive tip to its junction with the cast base pattern, the clasp is carved to a tapering, half-round form. Note that the inferior portion of the assembly is 6 to 7 mm. inferior to the gingival sulcus to avoid impingement of the tissue and possible strangulation. The only portion of the bar-type retainer arm occupying an undercut is the terminal one-third to one-fourth of the horizontal portion in contact with the tooth.

Fig. 17-30. Previously formed wrought-wire retainer arm is attached to the wax pattern and is in a passive relation to both the abutment tooth and the pattern.

the simulated refractory cast. Carefully cut (vertically) this piece of wax at the designated anterior portion of the retainer. Join another piece of 12-gauge half-round wax (flat side to cast) to the anterior end of the crosspiece on its underneath side. Adapt the wax to follow the inferior border of the outline of the retainer assembly and seal the end to the cast base pattern. Add sufficient wax with a hot spatula to provide a continuous taper from the retentive tip of the bar-type arm to its junction with the pattern for the denture base. The bar retainer is sealed to the cast in its entire length. Carve the wax to the outline form on the cast (Fig. 17-29). The thickest and broadest portion of the bar retainer will be at its junction with the denture base.

21. Perfect the waxing done thus far by carving, smoothing, and adding to weak points. The use of binocular loops (or any magnifying systems) to carefully inspect the pattern at this stage will probably disclose discrepancies heretofore unobserved.

22. Attach the wrought-wire retentive arm. Hold the previously formed wrought-wire retainer in a pair of cotton forceps by the small upright portion of the "foot" and warm it *over* a flame. Place the wire on the cast in its intended position in the wax pattern. It is usually necessary to hold a hot instrument against the retentive arm to dissipate enough heat so that the "foot" and upright portions of the retainer will be passively and completely embedded in the wax pattern (Fig. 17-30). However, the wrought wire need not be hot enough to excessively pool the wax pattern and change its desired form. Carefully inspect the area where the retentive arm emerges from its embedded position in the minor connector to ascertain that the wire arm is positively surrounded by wax without evidence of wax fissures or cracks.

The wax pattern is now completed and ready for spruing and investing (Figs. 17-31 and 17-32). An alternate method for forming the wrought-wire retentive clasp arm is illustrated in Fig. 17-33. The method illustrated is particularly applicable to short abutment teeth and will avoid two acute right-angle bends in the wrought wire.

Waxing metal bases. A technique for forming the retentive framework for the attachment of resin bases has been given. Two basic types of metal bases may be used instead of the resin base. The ad-

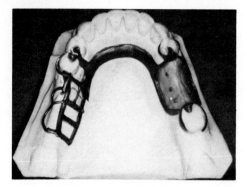

Fig. 17-31. Completed wax pattern for a lower Class II partial denture framework.

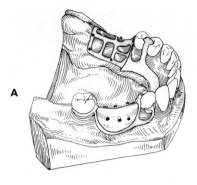

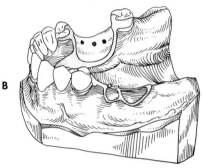

vantages of using cast metal bases in preference to resin bases have been discussed in Chapter 8.

The type of base to be used must be determined prior to blockout and duplication so that the relief over each edentulous ridge may be provided or eliminated as required. For a resin base full relief for the retentive frame must be provided. For a full metal base no relief over the ridge is used. For a partial metal base the junction between metal and resin must be clearly defined by trimming the relief along a definite, previously determined line.

One type of metal base is the full base with a metal border to which tube teeth, cast copings, or a resin superstructure may be attached. If porcelain or plastic tube or grooved teeth are used they must be positioned first and the pattern waxed around them to form a coping (Fig. 17-34). The teeth are then attached to the metal base by cementation or, with the use of resin teeth, attached with additional acrylic resin under pressure, a so-called "pressed-on" method of attaching resin teeth to a metal base. Another method of attaching teeth is to wax the base to form a coping for each tooth, either by carving recesses in the wax or by waxing around dummy teeth. Rather than attaching a ready-made tooth, the full tooth may be waxed into occlusion, the base invested, and the wax patterns replaced with a processed acrylic resin tooth. This method permits some vari-

Fig. 17-32. Meticulous attention to detail and neatness in forming wax patterns not only ensures the quality of the framework but also saves time in finishing the resultant casting. **A,** Right side view. Note the retentive "nailheads" on both the cast base pattern and the minor connector for the denture base. The three nailheads on the minor connector serve to retain the "impression tray" for making a secondary impression and are of no further use after this procedure has been accomplished. **B,** Left side view. The buccal loops have been so placed that they will not interfere with arranging the artificial posterior teeth. In some instances, because of the lack of interresidual ridge space, acrylic resin teeth must be used but most always having their occlusal surfaces duplicated in gold.

ation in the dimension and form of the supplied teeth not possible with ready-made teeth. It is particularly applicable to abnormally long or short spaces or when a stock tooth of desired width is not available. With modern cross-linked acrylic resins, such processed teeth are fairly durable; however, the addition of gold occlusal surfaces is indicated.

Wax patterns of the teeth to be supplied may be waxed directly onto a metal base

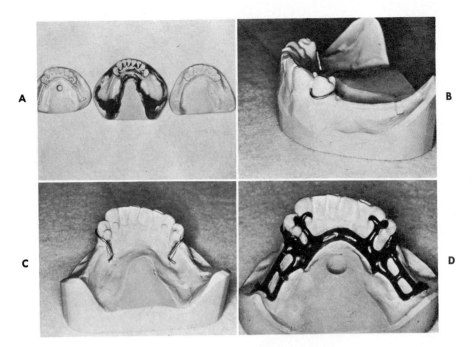

Fig. 17-33. A, Blocked-out master cast is duplicated in refractory investment and also in dental stone. **B,** An 18-gauge, round wrought-wire clasp is carefully adapted to the duplicate stone cast being guided by the ledge index created in wax on the master cast for its placement. The required length of wire for making the clasp is easily determined by laying an 18-gauge, round wax strip to the planned outline and then measuring the wax strip. **C,** Lingually, the wrought wire is bent to conform to the thickest portion of the finishing line at the junction of the lingual bar and the minor connector used to retain the denture base. **D,** The contoured clasp is transferred to the duplicate refractory cast and will occupy the exact position that it occupied on the duplicate stone cast. Waxing the pattern for the framework is completed in the usual manner.

and then cast in gold and attached to the base by soldering. In this method, the denture teeth are carved as for resin veneer fixed partial denture pontics. After attachment to the metal base, resin veneers are then processed to match any adjacent veneered abutment crowns. Teeth visible are generally abutted to the ridge, and cast flanges are used only in the posterior part of the mouth. This method is generally used only in conjunction with full mouth reconstruction. Both the denture framework and the cast pontics are usually made of gold to facilitate assembly by soldering.

When artificial teeth are to be arranged to occlude with an opposing cast or an opposing template, the metal base must be formed with a boxing for the attachment of

the tissue-colored denture resin supporting the teeth. This is the most common method of attaching teeth to a metal base. The wax pattern for the base is formed from one thickness of 24-gauge casting wax, which is then reinforced at the border, and a boxing is formed for the retention of the resin superstructure. Since metal borders are more difficult to adjust than resin, they are usually made somewhat short of the area normally covered with a resin base. Also, since border thickness adds objectionable weight to the denture, it is made with only a slight border roll. This is one disadvantage of the full metal base, in that the border accuracy of the impression registration cannot be used to fullest advantage, and the contouring of facial and lingual sur-

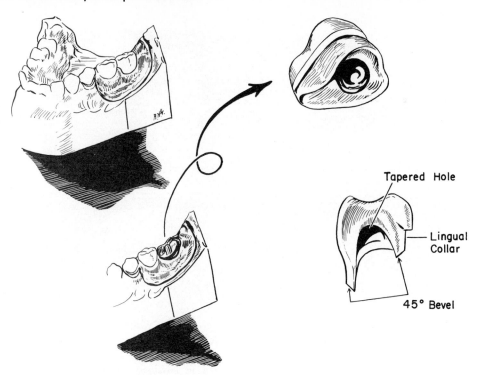

Fig. 17-34. Ready-made porcelain or resin tube tooth, or a denture tooth used as a tube tooth, should be ground to accommodate a cast coping as illustrated. A hole is drilled from the underside of the tooth, or if one is already present it is made larger. When the tooth is ground to fit the ridge with enough clearance for a minimum thickness of metal. A 45-degree bevel is then formed around the base of the tooth, and finally a collar is created on the lingual side, extending to the interproximal area. The tooth is then lubricated and the wax pattern for the denture base formed around it.

faces cannot be as effective as with a resin base in which added bulk can sometimes be used to advantage.

The border is first penciled lightly on the investment cast, and then the 24-gauge sheet casting wax is smoothly adapted. Considerable care must be taken not to stretch and thin the sheet wax in adapting it to the cast. To avoid wrinkling, the wax should be adapted in at least two longitudinal pieces and joined and sealed together at the ridge crest. The wax is then trimmed along the penciled outline with a dull instrument to avoid scoring the investment cast.

A single piece of *14-gauge round* wax is now adapted around the border *over* the sheet wax. With a hot spatula this must be sealed to the cast along its outer border.

The inner half of the round wax form remains untouched. Then, sufficient wax is flowed onto the round wax to blend it smoothly into the sheet wax, thus completing a border roll. Wax is added when needed to facilitate carving without trimming the original 24-gauge thickness. The result should be a rounded border blending smoothly into the sheet wax.

The boxing for the resin, which will in turn support the artificial teeth, is now added, again using *14-gauge round* wax. The proposed outline for the boxing is identified by lightly scoring the sheet wax. Upon this scored line, the 14-gauge round wax is adapted, thus forming the outline of the boxing.

With additional wax, the ditch between the sheet wax and the outer border of the round wax is filled in and blended smoothly onto the sheet wax. This is done in the same manner as the border, adding sufficient wax to allow for smoothing and carving. As mentioned previously, the pattern should not be flamed or polished with a cloth. Instead, the pattern must be smoothed by carving.

The result thus far should be a pattern reinforced at the border and at the boxing and slightly concave in between, with some of the original sheet wax exposed. The inside of the boxing is not sealed to the sheet wax, thus leaving a slight undercut for the attachment of the resin. With a sharp blade, the margins of the boxing are then carved to a knife-edge finishing line. Using the back side of the large end of the No. 7 wax spatula, this margin may be lifted slightly, further deepening the undercut beneath the finishing line.

In addition to the undercut finishing line, retention spurs, loops, or nailheads are added for retention of the resin to be added later. Spurs are usually made of 18-gauge or smaller round wax attached at one end only at random acute angles to the sheet wax. Loops are small-gauge round (wax, resin, or metal) circles attached either vertically or horizontally with space beneath for the resin attachment. Nailheads are made of short pieces of 18-gauge round wax attached vertically to the sheet wax, with the head flattened with a slightly warmed spatula. Any method of providing retention is acceptable if it permits positive attachment of the resin and will not interfere with the placement of artificial teeth.

A metal base waxed as described will provide optimal contours with a minimum of bulk and weight and with adequate provision for the attachment of artificial teeth to the metal base. Properly designed, the more visible portions of the metal base will be covered with the denture resin supporting the supplied teeth.

The second type of metal base is the partial metal base, either without any metal border or without a metal border in visible areas. The most common of these resembles

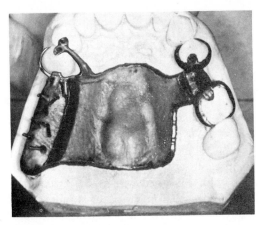

Fig. 17-35. Anatomic replica pattern for an upper Class II, modification 1, partial denture. Note the uniformity of the pattern over the palatal torus. This is waxed for a partial metal base, with diagonal spurs and lingual finishing line for retention of the resin base. The right-angle "foot" of the wrought wire may be seen just above the finishing line distolingual to the abutment. (Modified from McCracken's partial denture construction, ed. 3, St. Louis, 1969, The C. V. Mosby Co.)

a full metal base in all respects except that the buccal border is made short and ends abruptly without a finishing line (Fig. 17-35), or it may be made without any finishing line, with both buccal and lingual borders to be completed with resin. Esthetically and physiologically, a metal base with resin borders offers some advantages over the full metal base in that the thickness and contour may be made similar to a full resin base, yet with many of the advantages of a cast metal base.

Ordinarily no relief on the master cast is necessary when a metal base is to be used. In some instances, however, only the lingual portion of the base is made of metal. This is more often done in the maxillary arch when some changes in buccal ridge contours are anticipated. In such case, relief is used on the buccal half of the ridge only and a retentive frame to support the resin flange is necessary. This permits later relining of the buccal flange to compensate for ridge changes. Any time such a combination is used, relief should be trimmed sharply along a definite line to provide a definite finishing line between the metal and the resin base. This eliminates any unsupported flash of resin, which would later become loosened to permit seepage, resulting in an unclean denture. Since definite undercut finishing lines are not present on partial metal bases, other means of providing mechanical retention must be used. These are usually in the form of numerous spurs at random angles, although numerous small nailheads or loops may be used if preferred. Marginal seepage between the resin and partial metal bases is much more likely to occur over a period of time than in a full metal base with undercut finishing lines. Therefore, every precaution must be taken to provide the best possible mechanical retention.

When a partial metal base or a full metal base without metal borders is used, teeth are arranged in wax, and subsequent steps are completed as for a full resin base. The metal base is visible from the tissue side of the denture only, thus combining the advantages of a metal base with those of a resin base.

ANATOMIC REPLICA PATTERNS

A technique for obtaining a duplication of the palatal portion of a maxillary cast was developed originally by William Thompson as an aid to phonetics. This was called the *Thompson Tru-Rugae technique.* It was soon discovered that many other advantages as well resulted from anatomic replica patterns. It was found that patients became accustomed to an anatomic replica palate much more readily than to a smooth highly polished surface or to the concentrated bulk of palatal bars. It has been claimed that an irregular palatal surface seems to improve mastication by giving the tongue a "washboard" surface against which to press out the softer food particles and thereby separate them for mastication by the teeth.

The appearance of the denture is improved by its anatomic form and by the fact that the surface is never highly polished. This fact is readily recognized and makes the patient aware of the fact that it is a personalized reproduction of his own palate rather than a foreign body to be tolerated.

The irregular contour of the anatomic replica palate adds rigidity to the casting by its corrugated shape, thus permitting the use of thinner castings than would be permissible with a smooth, uncorrugated surface. This adds to patient acceptance and comfort by decreasing both weight and bulk.

To the laboratory, the anatomic replica palate means a saving in polishing time and in finishing and polishing materials.

The original Thompson technique was cumbersome but worthy of note because it led to later developments in anatomic replica techniques. Walker and Orsinger are credited with originating the present technique for palate reproduction, a description of which appeared in 1954. It is now almost a universally accepted technique for making full and partial palate reproductions.

The material is available as a Tru-Rugae kit and contains all the materials needed to make anatomic replica palates for complete and partial dentures. Whether used as a pattern to be burned out and cast or, in slightly thicker form, as an anatomic pattern of the palate to be discarded when boiling out a flasked denture, the technique is essentially the same. Walker and Orsinger listed the equipment and materials required as follows:

Cardboard box approximately 6 by 6 by 2 inches deep [to permit reuse of the polymer]
Camel's-hair brush, large water coloring size, or larger
Small nasal atomizer (DeVilbiss Economy Atomizer No. 182 is satisfactory)*
Wax spatula
Iris or cuticle scissors

---

*Instead of using the hand-operated atomizer, experience has shown that compressed air-operated spray guns give a much finer and more uniform spray and are not subject to clogging. Two of these are the Thayer-Chandler air brush and the Dupli-Color touch-up spray gun, model A, both of which require compressed air for operation.

Powder: Ethyl methacrylate powder, Dupont Lucite HG-24 or equal

Liquid: Methyl methacrylate monomer, or any denture base liquid acrylic resin

Coloring material for liquid: Prussian blue, artist's color ground in oil

Pattern cement: Pre-formed plastic pattern scraps dissolved in acetone

Plasticizers: Methyl salicylate, camphor, rosin, or suitable commercial plasticizers such as Dow Resin 276. . . [The plasticizer is added to the liquid in the atomizer or spray gun only, about six drops to the small atomizer, correspondingly more to the larger spray gun.]*

The following formula for a liquid is used at Lackland Air Force Base and contains a plasticizer:

Camphor	75 ml.
Oil of wintergreen	75 ml.
Acrylic resin monomer	350 ml.
Sudan red	pinch

Procedure for making an anatomic replica pattern. The procedure for making the anatomic replica pattern (or wafer) is as follows:

1. Either save the hydrocolloid mold after removing the investment cast or make an alginate impression of the master cast. The sides of the mold should be cut down to provide better access to the impression. Rinse the mold to remove any loose particles, and remove any excess moisture with compressed air. Leave the surface damp but free of surface moisture.

2. Fill the mold with powder from the cardboard box. (It is suggested that only enough powder be kept in the box to completely fill a hydrocolloid mold rather than to reuse larger quantities. Since this material becomes contaminated, it can be screened to remove foreign particles and replenished with fresh powder from the original container.)

3. Invert the mold over the cardboard box and dump out the surplus powder. Give the back of the hand holding the mold three or four slaps to remove more excess powder. This leaves powder layer

*From Walker, T. J., and Orsinger, W. O.: Palate reproduction by the hydrocolloid-resin method, J. Prosthet. Dent. 4:54-66, 1954.

No. 1 in the mold, which now has a fine sugar-coated appearance.

4. Using the atomizer, or preferably an air gun giving a fine misty spray, spray the face of the mold, as it is held in the other hand, with monomer. In this manner, the liquid is prevented from building up in deeper areas of the mold. The monomer should contain several drops of plasticizer, depending upon the size of the container.

5. Immediately fill the mold again, and dump and tap out the excess powder. This is powder layer No. 2, which is then sprayed with monomer as before. Use sufficient liquid to saturate the powder particles.

Ordinarily, three layers of powder are sufficient to make a pattern thick enough for casting. (For palate reproductions on complete dentures, five or six layers may be necessary.) The thickness will be determined by how hard the operator knocks out the excess powder from the mold and also by the length of time the second and third applications of powder are left on the mold before they are knocked off. The longer they remain on the mold, the thicker the wafer will be, because the powder picks up more liquid as it stands.

6. Set the mold under an inverted container or in a bell jar to prevent evaporation of the monomer and to allow the liquid to penetrate more thoroughly the grains of powder. This results in a finer surface and a more uniform thickness after cementation on the refractory cast. (This precaution applies equally well to any procedure in which denture bases are made by a sprinkling method.) An inverted bowl or glass refrigerator jar prevents evaporation and allows more thorough penetration of the monomer during polymerization.

7. When the plastic wafer has reached a flexible polymerized state (in about thirty minutes), strip it out of the mold completely. With fine iris scissors, trim the wafer to correspond to the outline of the palatal coverage previously penciled lightly on the refractory cast. Discard the cuttings, leaving only the wafer to be cemented to

the refractory cast. If a definite ledge for a finishing line was established on the master cast with relief wax, the plastic wafer should extend about 2 mm. beyond the platform that has been reproduced on the investment cast. This establishes the finishing line on the tissue side of the casting. (The undercut finishing line on the exposed side will be waxed on the plastic wafer about 2 mm. in from its trimmed edge.)

8. With a fine camel's-hair brush, paint a uniform layer of pattern cement on the investment cast inside the penciled outline. If preferred, this cement can be made up by dissolving plastic pattern forms in acetone. If it becomes too thick, it may be thinned with monomer. Excess cement should be avoided because it will cause irregular borders to be reproduced in the casting. Press the plastic wafer to place on the cast, making sure it conforms to the penciled outline. Make sure that the mold is free of debris, and invert the investment cast into it. Add some weight to the base of the cast to assure close contact with the mold while the cement is hardening. In about one hour, the cast with the plastic wafer cemented to it may be removed. The remainder of the denture pattern then may be completed in the usual manner. If it is necessary to store the wafer overnight before completing the pattern, it should be covered with an inverted glass container or placed under a bell jar to maintain its plasticity. Refrigeration will also maintain the plasticity of anatomic replica patterns for extended periods.

In making cast palate reproductions for a complete upper denture the method is essentially the same as that used for a partial denture. For resin palate reproductions, an alginate hydrocolloid impression of the master cast is used rather than a duplication mold, since no refractory cast is involved. The wafer is sprayed into the mold somewhat thicker than for a metal casting, then it is removed after polymerizing and trimmed as above. The wafer is not cemented to the master cast but merely waxed to place to form the palate of the denture. This is done after the denture try-in has been completed. The palate of the original base is then cut out and replaced with the anatomic palate wafer. This is discarded during boilout, leaving a mold that results in an anatomic replica palate on the completed denture.

SPRUING, INVESTING, CASTING, AND FINISHING THE PARTIAL DENTURE FRAMEWORK

Brumfield has listed some of the factors that influence the excellence of a dental casting:

1. Care and accuracy with which the model [cast] is reproduced.
2. Intelligence with which the case [framework] is designed and proportioned.
3. Care and cleanliness in waxing up the model [cast].
4. Consideration of the expansion of the wax due to temperature.
5. The size of the sprues.
6. The length of the sprues.
7. The configuration of the sprues.
8. Points of attachment and manner of attachment of the sprues to the cast.
9. Choice of investment.
10. The location of the pattern in the mold.
11. The mixing water: amount, temperature, and impurities.
12. The spatulation of the investment during mixing.
13. The restraint offered to the expansion of the investment, due to the investment ring.
14. Setting time.
15. Burn-out temperature.
16. Burn-out time.
17. Method of casting.
18. Gases: adhered, entrapped, and absorbed.
19. Force used in throwing the metal into the mold.
20. Shrinkage on cooling.
21. Removal from the investment after casting.
22. Scrubbing, pickling, etc.
23. Polishing and finishing.
24. Heat handling.°

Spruing. Brumfield describes the function of the sprues as follows:

°From Brumfield, R. C.: Dental gold structures, analysis and practicalities, New York, 1949, J. F. Jelenko & Co., Inc.

The sprue channel is the opening leading from the crucible to the cavity in which the appliance [framework] is to be cast. Sprues have the purpose of leading the molten gold from the crucible into the mold cavity. For this purpose, they should be large enough to accommodate the entering stream, and of the proper shape to lead it into the mold cavity as quickly as possible, but with the least amount of turbulence. The sprues have the further purpose of providing a reservoir of molten metal from which the casting may draw during solidification, thus avoiding porosity due to shrinkage. The spruing of the cast may be roughly summarized in three general rules.

1. The sprues should be large enough that the molten metal in them will not solidify until after the metal in the casting proper has frozen. (8 to 12-gauge round wax is usually used for multiple spruing of partial denture castings.)

2. The sprues should lead into the mold cavity as directly as possible and still permit a configuration which will induce a minimum amount of turbulence in the stream of molten metal.

3. Sprues should leave the crucible from a common point and be attached to the case [pattern] at its bulkier sections. That is, no thin sections of casting should intervene between two bulky, unsprued portions.

The configuration of the sprues, from their point of attachment at the crucible, until they reach the mold cavity may be influential in reducing turbulence. One of the more important sources of difficulty in casting is the entrapment of gases in the mold cavity, before they have a chance to escape. If the sprue channels contain sharp right angle turns, great turbulence is induced which is calculated to entrap such gases and so lead to faulty castings. Sprue channels should make long radius, easy turns and also enter the mold cavity from a direction designed to avoid splashing at this point.

As pointed out, the sprues should be attached to the bulky points of the mold [pattern]. If two bulky points exist with a thin section between them, each of the bulky spots should be sprued. The points of attachment should be flared out and local constrictions avoided. If this practice is followed, the sprue, being bulky enough to freeze after the case [framework] has frozen, will continue to feed molten metal to the case [framework] until it has entirely solidified, thus providing sound metal in the casting proper with all shrinkage porosity forced into the sprue rod, which is later discarded.*

There are two basic types of sprues: multiple and single (Figs. 17-36 and 17-37). The majority of partial denture castings require multiple spruing, using 8- to 12-gauge round wax shapes for the main sprues and 12- to 18-gauge round wax shapes for auxiliary sprues. Occasionally, however, a single sprue is preferred for full cast palates and cast metal bases for the mandibular arch when these are used as complete denture bases. With partial dentures, the use of a single sprue is limited to those maxillary frameworks in which, because of the presence of a palatal plate, it is impossible to locate multiple sprues centrally. In such situations, the single sprue may be used advantageously. A single sprue must be attached to the wax pattern so that the direction of flow of the molten metal will be parallel to the long axis of the single sprue. In some instances, the investment cast may have to be cut away anteriorly to make room for the at-

---

*From Brumfield, R. C.: Dental gold structures, analysis and practicalities, New York, 1949, J. F. Jelenko & Co., Inc.

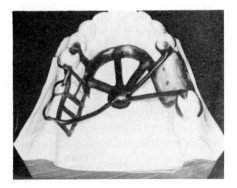

Fig. 17-36. View of a sprued wax pattern. Three 8-gauge sprues attached to the lingual bar and three 12-gauge sprues attached to the retention form and direct retainer assemblies are joined at the central sprue hole in the investment cast.

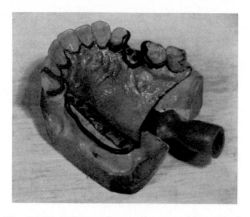

Fig. 17-37. Full cast denture bases and broad palatal coverage patterns are best sprued with a single sprue located posteriorly. Where a cast denture base for a completely edentulous arch is being sprued, the single sprue may be located anteriorly. (Courtesy Ticonium Division, CMP Industries, Inc., Albany, N. Y.)

tachment of the sprue; in others, the sprue may be attached posteriorly. One disadvantage of using a single sprue for large castings is that an extra long investment ring must be used.

Some important points to remember in multiple spruing are as follows:

1. Use a few sprues of larger diameter rather than several smaller sprues.
2. Keep all sprues as short and direct as possible.
3. Avoid abrupt changes in direction; avoid T-shaped junctions as much as possible.
4. Reinforce in all junctions with additional wax to avoid constrictions in the sprue channel and to avoid V-shaped sections of investment that might break away and be carried into the casting.

Step-by-step procedure. The laboratory procedure for multiple spruing is essentially the same for all mandibular castings and maxillary castings except those with a palatal plate. The following technique is given for a typical mandibular Class II partial denture casting:

1. Reduce the base of the cast to about ½-inch thickness. Trim all edges of the cast until it is slightly larger than the wax pat-

tern and tapers from the occlusal aspect toward the base.

2. Cut a ⅜-inch hole through the cast centered on a line joining the distal ends of the major connector on each side. The hole must be large enough to accommodate the main sprue from which other sprues will lead to the framework. (Stainless steel sprue cones may be purchased for forming the main sprue hole. These are available in several sizes and shapes and are used to form the hole in the investment cast at the time the cast is poured into the duplication mold.)

3. Roll one-half sheet of softened pink baseplate wax into a rod of such diameter that it will just pass through the hole cut in the base of the cast when it is inserted from the bottom. Allow the wax rod to protrude slightly on the wax pattern side of the cast. Seal this portion to the cast all around its border. The long portion protruding from the underside of the cast will serve as a handle during investment. The slight projection on the wax pattern side serves as an overjet, with the sprue leads attached approximately 3⁄16 inch below the tip of the main sprue. By using this overjet principle of spruing, the initial thrust of molten metal is directed against the tip of the main sprue reservoir and the turbulence that is created is confined to this area rather than at the entrance to the pattern mold cavity.

4. From this main sprue, attach three pieces of 8-gauge round wax extending radially to the lower border of the lingual bar major connector. Direct one piece to the central portion of the connector and the other two to just anterior to the finishing lines where the major connector joins the base retention on one side and the cast base on the other side. Thus the molten metal is fed to portions of the clasp assembly as well as to the bar itself. Attach these sprues to the bulkiest part of the major connector, being careful not to involve any critical margins. In spruing a tooth-borne partial denture framework consisting of four clasp assemblies, four such sprues

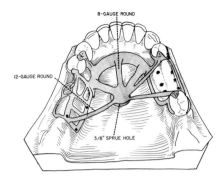

Fig. 17-38. Wax pattern is sprued as illustrated.

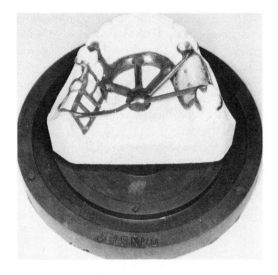

Fig. 17-39. Trimmed investment cast and sprued pattern are secured to the sprue former.

should be used, each attached to the major connector just below the clasp assembly.

5. In a similar manner, using pieces of 12-gauge round wax, connect the main sprue to the retentive framework or to any metal bases. In attaching to a retentive framework, make sure this is at the junction of a crossbar, thus assuring a free flow of metal with a minimum of changes in direction. A 12-gauge, round wax sprue is attached to the body of each direct retainer assembly on the cast denture base side. These sprues so placed will ensure the casting of the bar-type retainer, the circumferential retainer, and the buccal portion of the cast base pattern.

6. Reinforce all points of junction between the sprues and the denture framework with additional wax. The spruing is now completed (Fig. 17-38).

Investing the sprued pattern (Fig. 17-39). The investment for a partial denture casting consists of two parts: the investment cast upon which the pattern is formed and the outer investment surrounding the cast and pattern. The latter is confined within a metal ring, which may or may not be removed after the outer investment has set. If the metal ring is not removed, it must be lined with a layer of asbestos to allow for both setting and thermal expansion of the mold in all directions.

The investment must conform accurately to the shape of the pattern and must preserve the configuration of the pattern as a cavity after the pattern itself has been eliminated through vaporization and oxidation. Brumfield has listed the purposes of the investment as follows:

1. Investment provides the strength necessary to hold the forces exerted by [the] entering stream of molten metal until this metal has solidified into the form of the pattern.
2. It provides a smooth surface for the mold cavity so that the final casting will require as little finishing as possible and in some cases a de-oxidizing agent to keep surfaces bright.
3. It provides an avenue of escape for most of the gases entrapped in the mold cavity by the entering stream of molten metal.
4. It, together with other factors, provides necessary compensation for the dimensional changes of the gold [alloy]* from the molten to the solid, cold state.†

---

*Note the substitution of the word *alloy*, as the same principles apply whether the metal be a precious metal alloy or a chromium-cobalt alloy. In some of the latter alloys, the cobalt is partially replaced by nickel; such alloys are sometimes described as "stellite" alloys.
†From Brumfield, R. C.: Dental gold structures, analysis and practicalities, New York, 1949, J. F. Jelenko & Co., Inc.

The investment for casting gold alloys is a plaster-bound silica material, so compounded that the total mold expansion will offset the casting shrinkage of the gold, which varies from 1% to 1.74% (the highest figure being the shrinkage of pure gold). Generally, the higher the percentage of gold in the alloy, the greater the contraction of the casting upon solidifying.

Only one chromium-cobalt alloy has a sufficiently low melting temperature to be cast into a plaster-silica investment mold. According to Peyton, for the others having a higher melting temperature, an investment containing quartz powder held together by an ethyl silicate or sodium silicate binder is generally used. Expansion to offset casting shrinkage for the chromium-cobalt alloys is accomplished primarily through thermal expansion of the mold and must be sufficient to offset their greater casting shrinkage, which is in the order of 2.3%. For this reason, the metal ring is usually removed after the mold has hardened, to allow for the greater mold expansion necessary with these alloys. Since the investments for chromium-cobalt alloys are generally less porous, there is greater danger of entrapping gases in the mold cavity by the molten metal. Spruing must be done with greater care and, in some instances, provision for venting the mold is necessary to avoid defective castings.

Step-by-step procedure. The technique for applying the outer investment is usually referred to as "investing the pattern." Actually, the cast upon which the pattern is formed is part of the investment also. The following technique is given as being representative of, and applicable to, all partial denture castings:

1. Just before mixing the investment, line the ring with one layer of sheet asbestos. The asbestos should be ¼ inch shorter than the ring at the crucible end. The asbestos permits hot gases to escape at the back through the asbestos; yet some investment in contact with the ring at the crucible end prevents the investment from falling out when handling the ring after heating. Wet the asbestos after it is in place, but do not pack it tightly against the walls of the ring. (Step 1 is omitted if a split-type forming flask is used that will be opened and removed as soon as the investment has set.)

2. Unless the investment cast has been dipped in beeswax, which prevents it from absorbing water from the painting investment, it must be soaked in room-temperature water before painting. In such case, immerse the cast with the sprued pattern in a pan of water at about 85° F. no longer than four minutes. Water saturation of an untreated investment cast assures a good bond between the old investment and the new, but cold water must not be used for fear the pattern will shrink and be loosened from the cast.

3. Mix 100 gm. of investment, using 2 ml. more water than was used to make the investment cast. (If the investment for the cast required 28 ml. of water per 100 gm. of powder, the painting mix should be 30 ml. of water per 100 gm.) Spatulation must be thorough and should continue for about sixty seconds to distribute water throughout the mix when mixed by hand. Remember that a well-spatulated mix gives greater expansion and that mechanical spatulation, under vacuum conditions, usually results in the best mix possible.

Paint the pattern with a wetting agent (debubblizer) to reduce the surface tension of the wax so that the outer investment readily covers and adheres to the pattern, just prior to applying the investment. With a brush carrying the mixed investment, start at one end of the cast and work the investment under the sprues. Use only indirect vibration, the hand supporting the cast being between it and the vibrator. Keep working the investment under the wax sprues, working from one side of the cast around to the other. Proceed to invest the remainder of the pattern in the same manner. Wrought-wire retentive clasp arms also must be covered with investment. The entire pattern should be covered with about ¼ inch of investment. An even layer of investment is necessary to assure uniform expansion of the mold. Set the invested pattern aside until the outer investment has set (unless the vibrator will remain off, do not place the pattern on the same bench or vibration transferred through the bench will cause the investment to pull away from the pattern).

4. After the painting investment has reached its initial set (in about ten minutes), it may be invested in the casting ring or flask former. Just before investing in the casting ring, dip the assembly in water to again wet the outer investment, shaking off any excess water. Four hundred gm. of powder will be ample, mixed with the same proportion of water as before. *Only hand spatulation for about sixty seconds should be used, as some air in the outer investment is necessary to aid in venting the mold.*

One type of casting ring (Ney partial denture casting ring) has no crucible former and consists of a large heavy metal ring with an opening at one end about the diameter of an inlay casting ring. The other end is open to accommodate the invested pattern. To use this ring, the invested pattern is inserted with its main sprue protruding through the center of the smaller opening. The invested cast in this position should have sufficient space above for an adequate bulk of investment to cover it. In this position, connect the main wax sprue with the sides of the ring at its mouth, thus closing the opening. The main sprue protruding through the wax seal may be held between two fingers while the ring is held inverted in the palm of the hand. The invested cast is now completely covered with investment, filling the ring to the top. A glass slab may be slid over the top of the filled ring, to permit inverting the ring on the bench while the investment sets. The crucible is then cut into the hardened investment at the main sprue.

A second type of ring has a crucible former. Representative of this type are the Kerr and Jelenko partial denture casting rings. This type is perhaps the most fre-

quently used. The invested cast is attached to the crucible former by placing the main sprue into the hole and sealing it to the crucible former. Care must be taken that the invested cast is centered in the ring, with sufficient space all around and at the top for adequate thickness of outer investment. The casting ring is seated onto the crucible former and filled with investment, thus embedding the cast in investment as previously outlined.

Dr. Noble G. Wills has developed an innovation to the spruing and investing of a partial denture, which is a valuable aid in securing the investment cast to the sprue former and in regulating the height of the cast in the ring.

For a long time, a tapered sprue cone of metal has been used to form the sprue hole in the investment cast, thus eliminating the need for cutting a ⅜-inch sprue hole in the base of the cast later. The sprue is then reinserted into the cast just prior to investment, where it is retained by friction.

The Wills sprue pin is a machined brass untapered screw ⅜ inch in diameter and threaded with a No. 16 thread. This fits

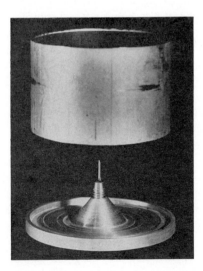

Fig. 17-40. Wills threaded sprue former and matching casting ring. The base and ring may be either the Kerr or the Jelenko size, but both must match. The projection on the ⅜-inch rod threaded with a No. 16 thread is for positioning the lubricated sprue into the duplication mold prior to pouring the investment cast.

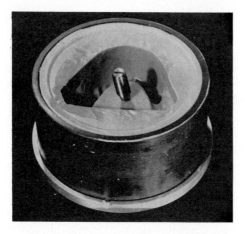

Fig. 17-41. Threaded sprue being held in the duplication mold by the pointed projection. The sprue is first lubricated with petrolatum or silicone jelly. Note the slotted end to facilitate withdrawal from the cast and, later, to adjust with a small screwdriver the height of the wax pattern in the casting ring.

into a threaded hole in a metal sprue former made to accommodate the Kerr or the Jelenko partial denture casting ring (Fig. 17-40). Projecting from the screw is a pin that is used to retain the threaded sprue in the hydrocolloid mold as the investment cast is being poured into it (Fig. 17-41). The threaded sprue must be lubricated with petrolatum or silicone jelly so that it may be removed from the cast with ease. A screwdriver is then used to remove the sprue from the cast, leaving a threaded sprue hole comparable to that in the sprue former.

After the wax pattern is completed and ready to invest, the brass sprue pin is screwed halfway into the base of the cast and the other half is screwed into the sprue former. Thus, the investment cast is held securely to the sprue former, and by inserting a screwdriver through the hole in the sprue former and engaging the slot in the threaded sprue its height in relation to the ring can be adjusted.

Since there is some probability that the sharp edges of investment making up the threaded sprue channel may become broken off by the force of the molten metal and thus be carried into the mold proper,

the threaded sprue hole should be reamed slightly and the particles eliminated just prior to placing the investment in the furnace.

A third type of casting ring is the split-type forming flask, which is opened and removed as soon as the investment has set. This flask is available in various diameters and heights, but the medium size will accommodate about 90% of all wax patterns. This type of casting ring does not use a crucible former. Instead, the flask is placed on a glass slab and nearly filled. Then the invested cast (sprue up) is embedded into it, using the sprue as a handle until the investment reaches a consistency sufficient to support the weight of the cast. Sometimes a copper screen is used inside the split-type flask to support the investment during heating and casting. This is not necessary if care is taken to avoid too rapid burnout or careless handling of the heated mold.

5. Allow the investment to set for at least an hour. At the end of this time, if the first type of ring was used, cut away the wax and protruding main sprue in such a manner as to form a concavity in the investment with the deepest part at the sprue. If the second type was used, merely remove the crucible former, which will leave the investment concaved or funnel shaped. The concavity may be deepened if desired by trimming the walls uniformly smooth, maintaining the funnel shape. If a split-type flask is used, a crucible may be formed by carving a funnel in the mold at the main sprue. Finally, trim the two faces of the mold to be parallel, using the edges of the ring as a guide. This is done by rubbing the mold over a piece of wire mesh screening (Fig. 17-42). If the split-type ring was used, it is now removed by sliding off the retaining clip, which allows the ring to be opened.

Burnout. The burnout operation serves three purposes: it drives off moisture in the mold, it vaporizes and thus eliminates the pattern, leaving a cavity in the mold, and it expands the mold to compensate for contraction of the metal on cooling.

Brumfield has this to say about burnout:

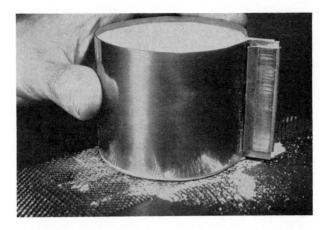

Fig. 17-42. Excess investment may be trimmed flush with the rim of the casting ring or flask by rubbing it over a piece of wire mesh or screening material. (Courtesy Ticonium Division, CMP Industries, Inc., Albany, N. Y.)

The time required to drive off the water is mainly a function of the amount of heat available and of the closeness of the heating element to the investment when placed in the furnace. If the furnace is large and a number of molds are burned out at the same time, the burn-out will require more time than would be the case with a single mold in the same furnace. . . .

The temperature of the mold is held down during early stages of burn-out by the vaporization of the water. Water will not rise appreciably above its boiling point until it is all vaporized. At the end of 60 minutes, the water is practically all driven off and the temperature at the inside of the mold will rise fairly rapidly to near the temperature of the furnace. Complete equalization, however, requires another 70 minutes, giving a total burn-out time of about two and one-quarter hours for eliminating the water and raising the temperature of the mold to approximately 1300° F. The so-called soaking period often recommended to be given the mold, after furnace pyrometer shows the full burn-out temperature, is designed to allow time for the water to be eliminated from the mold and the mold temperature to rise to that of the furnace.

During the time the water is being eliminated, the wax is being eliminated through vaporization and oxidation of carbon. Vaporization of wax ordinarily does not require as much time as that for vaporization of the water and will often have been completed when the temperature on the inside of the furnace has risen to about 1000° F. The carbon residue may

require more time for elimination. The more oxidizing the atmosphere of the eliminating furnace the better from the standpoint of eliminating wax. . . .

It is essential that the time of burn-out be sufficient to entirely eliminate the moisture. If the moisture is not eliminated, its presence has two bad effects on the casting. The casting made from an incompletely eliminated ring is apt to be porous due to the continued emission of steam by the investment. Second, the venting of the mold cavity is largely accomplished through the interstices of the investment itself. Although the investment is finely ground and these interstices are invisible to the eye, they nevertheless exist in very considerable amounts. Most investments contain voids (that is, spaces not occupied by investment particles), which amount to as much as 50 per cent of the total volume occupied. It is through these void spaces that the gases entrapped in the mold cavity by the entering stream of molten metal are able to depart with sufficient rapidity to avoid porosity in the casting. If these spaces are already occupied by steam from the incompletely eliminated mold or by finely divided particles of carbon residue from the wax, the entrapped gases cannot escape and porosity results from their inclusion in the casting. It is better to err on the side of too long a burn-out than in the opposite direction.*

*From Brumfield, R. C.: Dental gold structures, analysis and practicalities, New York, 1949, J. F. Jelenko & Co., Inc.

For the investment to heat uniformly, it should be moist at the start of the burnout cycle. Steam will then carry the heat into the investment during the early stages of the burnout. Therefore, if the investment is not burned out on the same day it is poured, it should be soaked in water for a few minutes before being placed in the burnout furnace.

Just prior to being placed in the furnace, the mold should be placed in the casting machine to balance the weight against the weight of the mold. At this time, the mold should be properly oriented to the machine and its crucible and a scratch line made at the top for later repositioning of the hot mold.

The mold should be placed in the oven with the sprue hole down and the orientation mark forward. Burnout should be started with a cold oven, or nearly so. Then the temperature of the oven should be increased slowly to a temperature of 1200° to 1300° F. over a period of two and one-half to three hours. This temperature then should be maintained for at least a one-half hour "heat-soaking" period to ensure uniform heat penetration. More time must be allowed for plastic patterns, particularly palatal anatomic replica patterns.

It is important that this temperature not be exceeded during the burnout period. (When a high heat investment is used, the manufacturer's instructions as to burnout temperature should be followed.) For all plaster-bound investments, contraction of the mold occurs beyond 1350° F., and breakdown of the binder begins at about 1450° F. To avoid loss of expansion and possible cracking, the soaking temperature should not exceed 1300° F.

Casting. The method of casting will vary widely with the alloy and equipment being used. All methods use force to inject quickly the molten metal into the mold cavity. This force may be either centrifugal or air pressure; the former is more commonly used. In any case, either too much or too little force is undesirable. If too little force is used, the mold is not completely filled before the metal begins to freeze. If too much force is used, excessive turbulence may result in the entrapment of gases in the casting. With centrifugal casting machines this is regulated by the number of turns put on the actuating spring. For the Thermotrol casting machine, for example, this is two to three turns.

The metal may be melted with a gas-oxygen blowtorch or by an electric muffle surrounding the metal. In some commercial casting procedures and in some dental laboratories, the induction method may be used, which provides a rapid and accurate method of melting the metal. The cost of induction equipment prohibits its widespread use.

The blowtorch method may produce consistently excellent results, but the lack of temperature control leaves much responsibility on the skill and judgment of the dentist or technician. Since the temperature at which the metal is thrown into the mold has an important bearing upon the excellence of the casting, the use of controlled melting with an electric muffle, such as the Thermotrol, eliminates many of the variables common to the blow torch method. Properly adjusted, this machine indicates the temperature of the molten metal at the instant it is thrown into the mold.

Removing the casting from the investment. Chromium-cobalt alloys are usually allowed to cool in the mold and are not cleaned by pickling. Finishing and polishing, which are done with special high-speed equipment, require a technical skill in the use of bench lathes not ordinarily acquired by the dental student. The average dentist is more adept in the use of the dental handpiece, whereas the average technician is, by reason of his training, more proficient in the use of bench lathes for finishing and polishing larger castings. The following, therefore, applies specifically to gold alloy castings being completed by the dental student or dentist.

After the casting is completed, allow the mold to cool until the sprue button has changed in color from red to black when viewed in shaded light. This will be about eight to twelve minutes after completion of a large casting. At this time, quench the hot ring in water. With most gold castings, this will produce a fairly soft and ductile condition in the metal. However, the larger the flask and the greater the amount of investment surrounding the casting, the longer the period required for bench cooling prior to quenching. In a recent publication it has been pointed out that when the Ney partial denture flask is used, a cooling period of eight to twelve minutes is sufficient, but that, if a flask with straight sides is used, it will hold approximately 60% more investment and therefore requires considerably more time for cooling. For the latter type of flask (such as the Kerr or Jelenko flask) it is suggested that twenty minutes be allowed for bench cooling to avoid the possibility that the casting will be too soft.

The practice of allowing the casting to completely cool in the investment is not recommended for gold alloys. Although it is true that all gold alloys capable of being hardened because of slow cooling will harden if allowed to cool slowly in the investment, the difference between the outside and the center at any given instant may vary 200° F. or more. Heat hardening by this method is not only uneven but shrinkage also is nonuniform, resulting in an inaccurate casting.

After removal of the investment from the casting by brushing under water with a stiff bristle brush, the casting should be further cleaned by *pickling*. Prior to pickling, detergent powder may be used to aid in removing investment particles.

When the casting is clean, it should be pickled in an acid pickling solution. Prevox, Jel-Pac, dilute sulfuric acid, or 30% to 50% hydrochloric acid may be used for pickling. The latter is objectionable because of the fumes and the fact that these fumes corrode laboratory instruments. It is essential that the pickling acid be clean and relatively colorless rather than have the typical greenish blue color of contaminated acid. Contamination results not only from repeated reuse of the solution but also from handling the casting with metal tongs during pickling. A contaminated acid contains excessive copper and other salts that will contaminate the surface of the casting, leading to tarnish and discoloration in the mouth.

When surface pits and irregularities on the casting become contaminated with foreign salts, later finishing and polishing may fail to remove them completely. When such a restoration comes in contact with sulfur-bearing foods, metallic sulfides are formed that exude from the pits and irregularities. Dark rings of stain and discoloration subsequently spread over a larger area, giving a tarnished appearance to the polished metal. This is the result of using an unclean pickling bath.

Under no conditions should the casting be heated and plunged into the pickling solution. Pickling is properly done by placing the casting in a clean dish and pouring the clean pickling solution over it to a depth sufficient to cover it. The dish then should be heated over a flame until the surface of the casting brightens. The pickling solution is poured off (flushing generously with water or base solution) and the casting washed with an abundance of water. If the acid solution is fresh and clean, no base metal deposits will occur to cause later discoloration of the polished casting in the mouth.

Finishing and polishing. Some authorities hold that the sprues should not be removed from the casting until the majority of the polishing is completed. Although it is true that this policy may prevent accidental distortion, it is difficult to adhere to and is therefore somewhat impractical. Instead, reasonable care should be exercised to avoid any distortion resulting from careless handling.

Actual polishing procedures may vary widely according to personal preference for certain abrasive shapes and sizes. However, several rules in finishing the casting are important. These are as follows:

1. High speeds are preferable to low

speeds. Not only are they effective but in experienced hands there also is less danger of the casting being caught and thrown out of the hands by the rotating instrument.

2. The wheels or points and the speed of their rotation should do the cutting. Excessive pressure heats the work, crushes the abrasive particles, causes the wheels to clog and glaze, and slows up the cutting.

3. A definite sequence for finishing should be adopted and followed in every case. Such a sequence for finishing a gold casting is given by Berger:

(a) Remove sprues with a jeweler's saw rather than separating discs. This saves gold and prevents accidentally cutting into essential parts of the case [framework].

(b) Grind off sprue stubs with ¾" or ⅞" heatless stones, ¹⁄₁₆" thick. Rough grind entire case [framework] and shape bars, clasps, and saddles [metal denture bases]. Always grind bars and clasps lengthwise. Cross-grinding can weaken a bar or clasp by grinding it too thin in spots. [If the location of clasps has been properly surveyed, it should not be necessary to grind the insides of the clasps. Smoothing the inner surface and polishing should be all that is needed.]

(c) Finish grinding with barrel-shaped mounted stones of medium grit. Use above precaution in grinding bars and clasps.

(d) Sandpaper the entire appliance [framework] using fine arbor bands, following the above precautions as to bars and clasps.

(e) . . . . rubber wheel the entire case [framework] carefully to remove all scratches. The better the case [framework] is rubber-wheeled, the easier the subsequent polishing steps become.

(f) The insides of the clasps and other inaccessible points may be polished readily and rapidly with a pointed rubber cylinder. Retentive clasps should be shaped with a uniform taper in both width and thickness throughout their entire length.

(g) The case [framework] is now ready for final polish. Use a B-20, 2-row brush wheel, with pumice or tripoli, or both,

to remove all traces of rubber wheel marks.

(h) Finish this step with a tripoli-charged cloth buff or felt wheel and cones to get a velvety smooth finish.

(i) High gloss is imparted with a rouge-charged cloth or chamois buff.

(j) Boil case [framework] in a solution of [detergent] for several minutes and then with a hard brush remove all traces of polishing media. [This may also be accomplished by brushing with a solution of soap and household ammonia, or with commercial cleaning solutions.]*

4. Clean polishing wheels should be used. If contaminated wheels are used, foreign particles may become embedded in the surface, which will lead to later discoloration.

5. Be sure each finishing operation completely removes all scratches left by the preceding one. Remember that each successive finishing step uses a finer abrasive and therefore cuts more slowly and requires more time to accomplish.

Heat hardening. If the gold casting has been quenched in the investment, it is removed from the investment in its softest and most ductile condition. All grinding and finishing operations are performed while it is in this condition. *After finishing, and just before final polishing, precious metal alloys should be heat hardened.* Although chrome-cobalt alloys cannot be heat hardened, they have satisfactory physical properties in their original state as cast, plus whatever work-hardening occurs from manipulation and use.

Hardening gold castings by heat soaking.† Dental gold castings, which are subject to heat hardening, may be effectively hardened as follows:

1. Quench the casting in the investment by shaking vigorously in an ample volume

---

*From Berger, H. R.: Finishing and polishing requires a careful technic, Jelenko Thermotrol Technician **1:**7, Oct., 1947.

†From information taken from the physical properties chart of J. F. Jelenko & Co., Inc., New York, N. Y.

of water as soon as the sprue button has lost its heat color.

2. Remove the casting from the investment, thoroughly clean, and do all the finishing necessary.

3. When the casting is finished and ready for the final high polish, heat harden it as follows:

a. Stabilize the furnace at the desired temperature by proper adjustment of the dial. See manufacturer's instructions for correct temperature for each alloy. (Yellow casting golds heat harden at temperatures between 600° and 700° F. White gold alloys heat harden more effectively at temperatures as high as 800° F., except Jelenko Palloro and alloys of its type, which require somewhat different treatment. These should be quenched in the investment as soon as the casting machine stops, while the button is still red, and heat hardened by soaking for five minutes in a furnace stabilized at 600° F.)

b. Place the casting on a metal tray in the furnace, close the door, and allow to heat soak for fifteen minutes.

c. Remove the tray at the end of this period with the casting on it (do not touch the casting with cold tongs) and allow to bench cool.

This treatment will produce from 85% to 100% of the strength given by the variable cooling–heat hardening process and avoids any possibility of warpage because of heat treatment.

MAKING OF IMPRESSION TRAYS AND DENTURE BASES

An individual impression tray may be made of self-curing acrylic resin, modeling plastic, or double-thickness baseplate material. Impression trays made from self-curing acrylic resin are preferred in most instances because of their accuracy and lack of dimensional change after being fabricated. Such trays may be made by either the "sprinkle-on" or the "adapting" technique on properly relieved casts. The adapting technique has been illustrated in Fig. 14-8. A sprinkle-on procedure for individual impression trays will be described in this section. However, adapting acrylic resin dough to a properly relieved cast is sufficiently accurate to make individual impression trays. Record or trial denture bases should be made by the sprinkle-on technique because of the requirement for close tissue adaption of these bases.

The resin tray materials are packaged as a powder and liquid with activating chemicals added to induce polymerization when the two are mixed. They are mixed together in a jar in measured proportions and then adapted while in a doughy state to a moistened or lubricated cast. Polymerization is usually rapid with considerable exothermic reaction. They may be trimmed with scissors while soft and further trimmed after polymerizing. Although considered "dead" materials (that is, without elastic memory), they are not accurate enough to use as denture bases for jaw relation records or as trial bases when accuracy is essential.

Trial bases and bases for jaw relation records should either be made of materials possessing accuracy or be relined to provide such accuracy. Relining may be accomplished by seating the previously adapted base onto the tin-foiled or lubricated cast with an intervening mix of some zinc oxide–eugenol paste or with self-curing resin. Some use has been made of the mercaptan and silicone impression materials for this purpose, but the wisdom of using an elastic lining for jaw relation record bases is questionable. However, when rigid setting materials are used for this purpose, any undercuts on the cast must be blocked out with wax or clay to facilitate their removal without damage to the cast.

The ideal jaw relation record base and trial base is one that is processed (or cast) to the form of the master cast, becoming the permanent base of the completed prosthesis. Cast metal bases for either complete or partial dentures offer this advantage over resin-based dentures. Resin bases (either methyl methacrylate, vinyl combinations, or styrene) likewise may be processed directly to the master cast, thus becoming the permanent denture base. In either case, when undercuts are present, the master cast must be destroyed during removal of the base. Then existing undercuts must be blocked out inside the denture base before a cast is poured into it to make an articulator mounting. A second cast, which includes the undercuts, must be poured against the entire base to support it during the processing of the resin superstructure. When both the base and the superstructure are of resin, some care must be taken to avoid visible junction lines between the original resin base and the resin that supports the teeth and establishes facial contours.

Some self-curing acrylic resin materials are sufficiently accurate for use as trial and jaw relation bases. These are used with a sprinkling technique, which, when properly done, permits a base to be made that compares favorably with a processed base. A material must be selected that will polymerize in a reasonable time (usually a twelve-minute monomer) and will retain its form during the sprinkling process. Since polymerization with typical shrinkage toward the cast begins immediately, alternate addition of monomer and polymer in small increments results in reduced overall shrinkage and greater accuracy.

Technique for making a sprinkled acrylic resin denture base or impression tray. The technique for sprinkling a denture base will be given here. Some blockout of the cast is necessary in most instances, depending upon the purpose for which the base is to be used. An individual impression tray requiring space for the impression material may be further relieved with sheet wax or wet asbestos. Sheet asbestos, such as is used to line inlay rings, may be dipped in water and adapted to the cast for this purpose. More than one thickness may be used, or wet asbestos may be added, using the wet asbestos as one would modeling clay. By painting the asbestos relief with a tin-

foil substitute, it may be easily stripped out of the impression tray, leaving no trace of the relief material on either the cast or the tray.

Relief of undercut areas on the cast is best accomplished with a water-soluble modeling clay or baseplate wax. Modeling clay is easily formed and shaped on the cast and is easily removed from either the cast or the base with a natural bristle toothbrush under warm running water. Wax, on the other hand, must be flushed off the cast with hot water. It must be removed from the inside of the base by scraping and with a wax solvent, followed by flushing with water only hot enough to eliminate any residual wax.

Impression trays to be used with an alginate hydrocolloid impression material must be perforated to assure retention of the impression material within the tray. Areas over displaceable soft tissue also require perforation to avoid displacement of those tissues by hydraulic pressure. Perforation is best accomplished by using a bibeveled surgical drill, which fits the dental handpiece but will not become clogged when drilling holes in resin materials.

The amount of relief used for an impression tray will depend upon the type of impression material being used and the quality of the tissues being recorded. Trial bases and bases for jaw relation records, on the other hand, must have maximum contact with the supporting tissues. The accuracy of the base will be in proportion to the total area of intimate tissue contact provided. Those areas most frequently undercut and requiring blockout are the distolingual and retromylohyoid areas of the mandibular cast, the distobuccal and labial aspects of the maxillary cast, and, frequently, small multiple undercuts in the palatal rugae. These areas and any others are blocked out with a minimum of clay, to obliterate as little of the surface of the cast as possible. A close-fitting base may then be made that will have the necessary accuracy and stability and yet may be lifted from and returned to the master cast without abrading it.

Except for the presence of relief, the technique for sprinkling an impression tray is the same as that for a trial or jaw relation record base. The purpose for which it is to be used will influence the relief as follows: (1) an individual impression tray will have overall relief sufficient to accommodate the impression material; (2) an impression tray for making a fluid-wax functional impression prior to the making of the cast framework will have relief over the ridge areas to be recorded, with three or more tooth-bearing areas exposed and a clay matrix over the remainder of the cast; (3) an impression tray attached to the partial denture framework for making a functional impression will have sufficient relief to accommodate the impression material and permit its flow in the mouth; (4) a trial or jaw relation record base will have undercuts blocked out but no relief over the supporting areas of the ridge.

If the impression tray or base is to be attached to a partial denture framework, the framework is first seated on the cast in its terminal position. This is done after the necessary blockout and/or relief has been placed. The cast and the blockout and/or relief is then painted with a tin-foil substitute of a type that may be painted onto a cold surface without leaving a heavy or uneven film, such as Al-Cote. This is essential to the accuracy of a denture base, but not all tin-foil substitutes are suitable for this purpose.

As soon as the tin-foil substitute has dried, the cast is wet with the monomer from a dropper bottle. The ordinary medicine dropper is not suitable for this purpose because the lumen is too large, resulting in an uncontrollable excess of monomer. The glass may be drawn to a fine tip over a flame but is easily broken. Instead, the simple addition of a hypodermic needle of about 23 gauge to the glass lumen by flaming the glass tip around the needle pro-

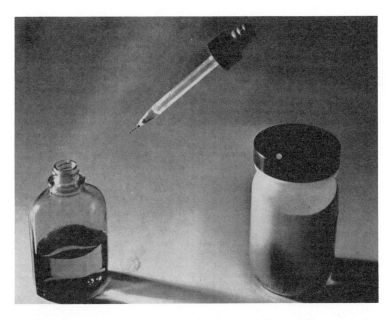

Fig. 17-43. Rapid self-curing acrylic resin in bottles used for sprinkling resin bases, etc. A 23-gauge hypodermic needle has been sealed into the tip of the dropper barrel to limit the size of the drop and facilitate wetting the monomer without flooding. The large-mouthed bottle is of a size that can easily be held in the hand, and it has in the rim a hole the size of a No. 8 or No. 10 round bur to allow the powder to be applied selectively to the area involved.

vides a suitable syringe tip for the application of monomer in small quantities as needed (Fig. 17-43).

After wetting the surface with the monomer, the polymer is sprinkled or dusted onto the wet surface until all of the monomer has been absorbed. Sprinkling is best accomplished using a large-mouthed bottle with a single hole in the lid near the rim. The hole should be about the size of a No. 8 round bur. This facilitates the placement of the polymer without excess in any one area. A flexible bottle with suitable applicator tip also may be used. However, it seems that better control over the application of the polymer is possible when a bottle with a hole in the cap is used. The objective should be the uniform application of polymer over the entire ridge rather than the allowing of excess to accumulate at the border to be trimmed later. A self-curing acrylic resin material must be used that will retain its form during the sprinkling procedure without objectionable flow into low areas.

Once the polymer has been sprinkled in slight excess, the monomer is again added. Flooding must be avoided; therefore, the monomer must be directed over the entire surface gradually until the polymer has just absorbed the monomer. *A few seconds' delay prior to the addition of excess monomer will allow the mass to reach a tacky consistency and prevent it from flowing when more monomer is added.* Then the monomer may be added in excess, which is immediately absorbed by the application of more polymer as before. This process is repeated selectively until a uniform layer has been built up, just thick enough so that none of the underlying cast or relief may be seen. Some areas will require further addition, particularly ridge crests and other prominent areas.

The final step in sprinkling is the addition of monomer sufficient to leave a wet surface. *Immediately,* the cast should be placed in a covered glass dish or covered with an inverted bowl. This permits final polymerization in a saturated atmosphere of monomer and prevents evaporation of surface monomer. The cast should not be placed in water or any attempt made to accelerate polymerization. Slow polymerization is necessary so that shrinkage *toward* the cast will occur, earlier layers polymerizing first. Only thus will overall shrinkage be negligible and accuracy of fit be assured. Whereas this is of little consequence in the making of an impression tray, it is most essential in the making of a sprinkled resin base.

Although polymerization will be about 90% complete within an hour, and an impression tray may even be lifted within a half hour, a sprinkled denture base should be left *overnight* before being separated from the cast. It should then be lifted either dry or under lukewarm tap water. It should not be immersed in hot water or some warpage may occur.

A sprinkled acrylc resin base made with the precautions outlined above will retain its accuracy for days, or even for an indefinite period, comparable to that of a heat-cured resin base (Figs. 17-44 and 17-45). Failure to do so can be attributed to faulty technique rather than to any inherent inaccuracy in the material itself, provided the proper material has been used. As with any resin base, storing in air results in some distortion because of dehydration. However, since the stone cast itself may not be stored in water, possible distortion of the resin from being immersed off of the cast must be weighed against that occurring due to dehydration. Generally, the latter is not sufficient to warrant keeping the resin base in water.

Technique for making an impression tray attached to a framework. Individual impression trays can be conveniently made by adapting a quick-curing acrylic resin dough to the relieved master cast and framework. Less time is required to make the trays by this method than with the sprinkle-on technique, and the required accuracy is not compromised when care is used in fabricating the trays (Fig. 17-46).

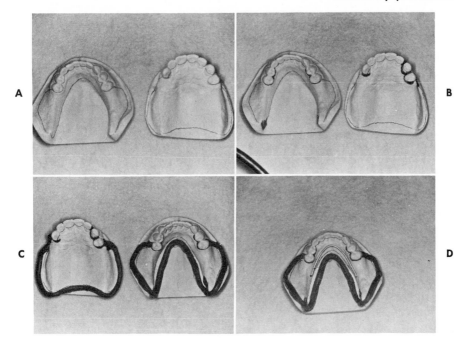

Continued.

Fig. 17-44. Stable record bases are required to correctly orient diagnostic casts representative of distal extension removable partial denture situations. Such bases are made using an auto-polymerizing acrylic resin. **A,** The extent of the record bases are outlined in pencil. Note that the outline includes the cingula of the anterior teeth and the distal surface of prospective terminal abutments. **B,** Interproximal undercuts are blocked out with wax. Other undercut areas involved in the denture base design are also eliminated by blockout. Prominent or undercut rugae must be blocked out or covered with a soft quick-curing acrylic resin, which then becomes a part of the record base. **C,** Utility wax is adapted to the outline of the cast in the edentulous regions to confine the acrylic resin when it is being applied. The wax should be adapted approximately 2 mm. from the penciled outline to provide adequate thickness of the record base borders. **D,** A stiff 16-gauge wire is bent to conform to the lingual alveolar ridge of the lower cast and becomes a part of the record base. This wire will strengthen the final record base and will eliminate some flexibility of the base.

OCCLUSION RIMS

It has been explained that jaw relation records for partial dentures always should be made upon accurate bases that are either part of the denture casting itself or attached to it in exactly the same relation as the final denture base will be. Further, it has been stated that, although the use of the final denture base is best for jaw relation records, a sprinkled or corrected acrylic resin base may be used satisfactorily. In any case, accuracy of the base supporting the occlusion record must be a foregone conclusion before considering the function of occlusion rims.

Occlusion rims may be made of several materials. The material that is most commonly used to establish static occlusal relationships is the baseplate wax rim. However, use of a wax occlusion rim is likely to be inaccurate when the occlusal portion of the rim is pooled with a hot instrument or flamed, because of the fact that uniform softening cannot be assured. Also, some errors in repositioning apposing casts against wax occlusion rims for mounting on the articulator are likely to occur. When some soft material that sets to a rigid state, such as impression plaster or impression paste, is used in conjunction with wax rims to record static occlusal relations, many of the errors common to wax rims are elimina-

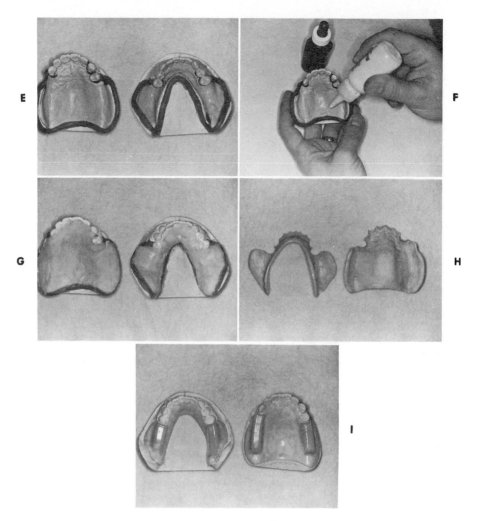

Fig. 17-44, cont'd. **E,** A tin-foil substitute (Al-Cote) is painted on the cast to act as a separator. Two thin coats are applied, allowing the first coat to dry before application of the second coat. **F,** Acrylic resin is sprinkled on the cast, alternating the application of monomer and polymer. **G,** A uniform thickness (2 mm.) of acrylic resin is sprinkled within the record base outline. **H,** The record bases have been removed (after curing) and trimmed to the established outlines. Note the tissue detail and border thickness. **I,** Occlusion rims have been added to the polished record bases.

ted provided some space exists between the occlusion rims and/or opposing teeth at the desired vertical dimension to be recorded.

Modeling plastic may be used rather than wax for occlusion rims, with several advantages over the latter. It may be softened uniformly by flaming, yet becomes rigid and sufficiently accurate when chilled. It may be trimmed with a sharp knife to expose the tips of the opposing cusps to re-

check or position an opposing cast into the record rim. Opposing occlusion rims of modeling plastic may be keyed with greater accuracy than opposing wax rims. Preferably, however, even those should be trimmed short of contact at the vertical dimension of occlusion, and plaster or impression paste should be interposed for the final record. As with wax rims, an adjustable frame to support the final record also may be used.

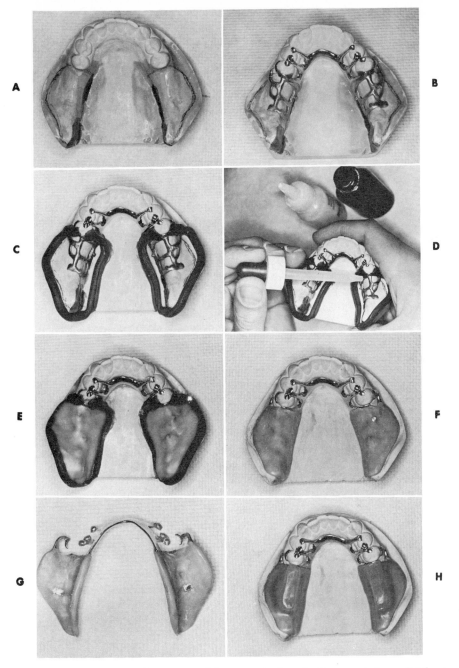

Fig. 17-45. Technique for making a record base attached to the framework for a distal extension removable partial denture. **A,** Tissue undercuts are blocked out only enough to eliminate the undercuts, and the edentulous ridges are painted with a tin-foil substitute (Al-Cote). **B,** The framework is positioned on the cast after the tin-foil substitute has dried. A small amount of wax is added on either side of the minor connector extension touching the distal surface of the premolars to avoid having acrylic resin "run under" the connector at the gingival of the abutment tooth. **C,** Utility wax strips are used to confine the "sprinkled-on" acrylic resin, and they outline the extent of the record base. The wax strips do not cover the finishing lines of the direct retainers and lingual bar. **D,** The cast is wet with monomer in a small area and just enough polymer is added to take up the monomer. This procedure is repeated until an overall thickness of 2 mm. is obtained. **E,** All areas within the wax boxing have been covered by the acrylic resin. **F,** The record base has been removed from the cast and trimmed. Only borders of the record base are polished. **G,** A view of the tissue surfaces. **H,** Occlusion rims are added to the record base.

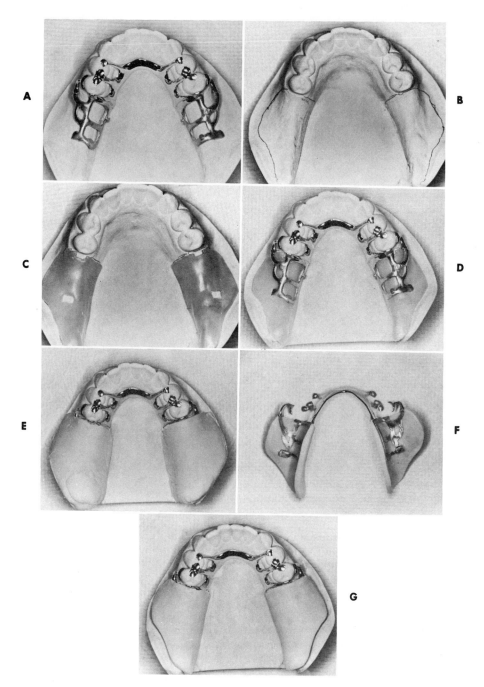

Fig. 17-46. For legend see opposite page.

Occlusion rims of either baseplate wax or modeling plastic may be used to support intraoral central bearing devices and/or intraoral tracing devices. However, because of its greater stability, modeling plastic is preferable for this purpose also, when the edentulous situation permits the use of flat plane tracings. An example of such a situation is when an opposing denture is being made concurrently with the partial denture. In such case, modeling plastic occlusion rims provide greater stability than wax rims, with corresponding improvement in the predictable accuracy of such a jaw relation record. Although the sealing of opposing occlusion rims or the use of clips for complete denture jaw relation records, particularly for an initial articulator mounting, may be acceptable, the existence of a partial denture framework makes this practice hazardous. Since it is necessary that the dentist be able to see that the partial denture framework is in its original relation to the supporting teeth before the casts are articulated, the framework and attached base should be seated accurately on its cast before the opposing cast is repositioned in occlusion to it.

Occlusion rims for recording functional, or dynamic, occlusion must be made of a hard wax that can be carved by the opposing dentition. This method, outlined in Chapter 16, presumes that the opposing arch is intact or has been restored. Functional occlusion records by this method cannot be made when both arches are being restored simultaneously.

Rather, an opposing arch must be as intact as the treatment plan calls for or must be restored by whatever prosthetic means the situation dictates. Opposing partial dentures or an opposing complete denture may be carried concurrently up to the final occlusal record. One denture is then completed and placed and the functional record made in opposition to it. Frequently, this requires that all opposing teeth be articulated first in wax to establish optimal ridge relations and the correct occlusal plane. One denture is then carried to completion, and the teeth remaining in wax on the opposing denture are removed while the functional occlusal record is being made.

No single wax has been manufactured specifically for establishing functional occlusal records. Some inlay waxes are used for this purpose because they can be carved by the opposing dentition and because most of them are hard enough to support occlusion over a period of hours or days. A wax for recording functional crown and bridge occlusion, since it is established entirely in the dental office, is selected on the

Fig. 17-46. Secondary impressions for distal extension mandibular removable partial dentures are made in an individual tray attached to the denture framework. **A,** The framework has been tried in the mouth and fits the mouth and master cast as planned. **B,** An outline of the resin tray is penciled on the cast. **C,** One thickness of baseplate wax is adapted to the outline to act as a spacer so that room for the impression material exists in the finished tray. Windows are cut in the wax spacer corresponding to the regions on the cast contacted by the minor connectors for the denture bases. **D,** The framework is warmed and pressed to position on the relieved master cast. All regions of the cast that will be contacted by the autopolymerizing acrylic resin dough are painted with a tin-foil substitute (Al-Cote). **E,** Quick-curing acrylic resin is mixed, and wafers of the material are made as described in Chapter 14. The resin material is adapted to the cast and over the framework with finger pressure. Excess material over the borders of the cast is removed with a sharp knife while the material is still soft. **F,** The cured resin trays and framework are removed from the cast, and the trays are trimmed to the outline of the wax spacer. **G,** Borders of the trays will be adjusted to extend within 2 mm. of the tissue reflections. Holes then will be placed in the trays corresponding to the crest of the residual ridge and retromolar pads to allow the escape of excess impression material when the impression is made.

basis of how well it may be carved by the opposing dentition in a relatively short period of time. Therefore, a softer wax may be used than is required for the recording of occlusal paths over a period of twenty-four hours or more. For this latter purpose, Peck's purple hard inlay wax seems to satisfy best the requirements for a wax that is durable yet capable of recording a functional occlusal pattern. This wax is packaged in the form of sticks. A layer of sticky wax is first flowed onto the surface of the denture base. Two sticks of the inlay wax are then laid parallel along the longitudinal center of the denture base and secured to it with a hot spatula. This is the only preparation prior to the dental appointment. Since neither the height nor the width of the occlusion rim can be known in advance, and since deep warming of a chilled wax rim is difficult, the rim is not completed prior to the appointment.

With the patient in the chair, a hot spatula is inserted into the crevice between the two sticks of wax, making the center portion fluid between two supporting walls. Some transfer of heat to the supporting walls occurs, resulting in the occlusion rim becoming uniformly softened. The patient is asked to close into this wax rim until the natural teeth are in contact, which establishes both the height and the width of the occlusion rim. Wax is then added or carved away as indicated and the patient asked to go into lateral excursions. Any excess wax is then removed, and any unsupported wax is supported by addition. Finally, wax is added to increase the vertical dimension sufficient to allow (1) for denture settling, (2) for changes in jaw relation brought about by the reestablishment of posterior support, and (3) for carving in all mandibular excursions. When sufficient height has been established, as well as sufficient width to accommodate all excursive movements, the patient is instructed and dismissed.

Although this discussion has been included in this chapter on laboratory procedures, the entire procedure of establishing occlusion rims for recording functional occlusion should be considered a chairside procedure rather than a laboratory procedure. It is necessary, however, that the purpose of a functional occlusal record be clearly understood so that subsequent laboratory steps may be accomplished in a manner that the effect of such an occlusal record may be reproduced on the finished denture.

MAKING A STONE OCCLUSAL TEMPLATE FROM A FUNCTIONAL OCCLUSAL RECORD

After final acceptance of the occlusal record as registered by the patient, the effectiveness of this method for establishing functional occlusion on the partial denture will depend upon how accurately the following procedures are carried out. For this reason it will be given as a step-by-step procedure.

Step-by-step procedure. 1. If the base of the master cast (or processing cast) has not been keyed previously, do this before proceeding. First reduce the thickness of the base if it is so thick that difficulty will be encountered in flasking. The base may not be reduced on this account after removal from the articulator, since the mounting record would be lost.

Keying may be done in several ways, but a method whereby the keyed portions are visible on the articulator mounting eliminates some possibility of remounting error. According to the preferred method, form a 45-degree bevel on the base of the cast by hand or with the model trimmer and then add three V-shaped grooves on the anterior and the posterior aspects of the base of the cast at the bevel (Fig. 17-47). The bevel serves to facilitate reseating the cast on the articulator mounting, and the mounting surfaces are made still more definite by the triangular grooves. Being placed at the beveled margin, the triangular grooves are visible at all times and any discrepancy may be clearly seen.

2. Inspect the underside of the cast framework and denture bases, removing

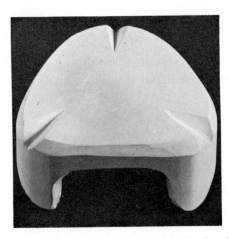

Fig. 17-47. Base of any cast should be beveled and keyed as shown before mounting on the articulator. Petroleum jelly is used as a separating medium to facilitate removal and remounting subsequent to processing. Keying should always be done prior to boxing and pouring an occlusal registration because the cast and template must be mounted on the articulator before they are separated.

any particles of wax or other debris. Similarly, inspect and clean the master cast of any particles of stone, wax, blockout material, or any other debris that might prevent the casting from being seated accurately upon it.

Now seat the denture framework on the cast in its original terminal position. This is the position that was maintained by securing with sticky wax while the trial denture base was being made, with all of the occlusal rests seated. It is also the position that the casting assumed in the mouth while the occlusal record was being made and must be duplicated upon returning the denture framework to the master cast. Holding the framework in this terminal position, secure it again with stick wax. (If a processing cast is being used in place of the master cast, the denture base will have been made upon that cast and the same precautions in returning the framework to its original position apply.)

3. With the denture framework and the occlusal record in position, form a matrix of clay around the occlusal record to confine the hard stone, which will form the stone occlusal template. (If electroforming has been done as mentioned in Chapter 16, the electroforming precedes Step 1. The clay matrix is the same for a metallized surface as for the wax record.)

The clay matrix should rise at a 45-degree angle from the buccal and lingual limits of the occlusal registration. Then arch either clay or a sheet of wax across from one side to the other, forming a vault that will permit lingual access when articulating the teeth.

Leave the occlusal surfaces of the adjacent abutment teeth or the corresponding surfaces of a processing cast exposed so that they may act as vertical stops. This will serve to maintain the vertical relation on the articulator. Unless such stone-to-stone stops are used, the vertical relation on the articulator may be altered by the technician, either accidentally or otherwise. Any change in vertical relations is incompatible with a concept of dynamic occlusion, since the occlusal pattern is directly related to the degree of jaw separation. Although it may be true that vertical dimension may be changed when casts are mounted in relation to the opening axis of the mandible, *as long as natural cusps remain to influence mandibular movement, the vertical relation established with a functional occlusal record must not be changed on the articulator.*

Treat the surfaces of the adjacent abutment teeth left exposed with sodium silicate, Microfilm, or some other separating medium to ensure separation of the stone vertical stops.

4. If the wax record has not been metallized, use a hard dental stone to form the opposing template. This may be an improved stone such as Duroc, but the use of a stone die material such as Vel-Mix is preferred. Only the occluding surface need be poured in the harder stone, a less costly laboratory stone being used to back it up. If this is done, add the second layer to the first before the former takes its initial set, to avoid any possibility of accidental separation between the two materials.

Vibrate the stone only into the wax registration and against the stone stops. Pile on the rest of the stone and leave uneven to facilitate firm attachment to the mounting stone. Attach the occlusal template to the articulator without provision for remounting, since only the working cast need be keyed for remounting.

5. After the stone template has set, attach the occluded casts to both arms of the articulator before separating. The type of atriculating instrument used is of little importance, since all eccentric positions are recorded on the template, and whatever instrument is used acts purely as a simple hinge or a tripod. Therefore, any laboratory articulator or tripod may be used. Because of the easy access afforded in setting teeth and adjusting occlusion, the Hagman Junior Balancer is preferred over most other instruments for this purpose.

Since both casts are not usually attached to the articulator with the same mix of material, the first mounting may be done with plaster without fear of error being introduced by the expansion of the plaster. Mounting to the opposing arm of the articulator, however, should be accomplished with stone to avoid such expansion. (When mounting complete denture casts, the upper cast, being mounted with the aid of a face-bow, should be attached to the upper arm of the articulator with mounting stone. The lower cast is then attached to the lower arm also with mounting stone to avoid error in jaw relations caused by the expansion of plaster.)

It must be remembered which arch is represented by the working cast, and the articulator mounting should be made accordingly. For example, for a mandibular denture the template is attached to the upper arm of the articulator, whereas for a maxillary denture the template is mounted upside down on the lower arm. The keyed base of the working cast attached to the opposing arm must be coated with mineral oil or petroleum jelly to facilitate its separation from the mounting plaster.

6. After the mounting has been completed, separate the casts and remove the clay. The template with its mounting may be removed from the articulator if a mounting ring or mounting stud permits, otherwise trimming must be done on the articulator. With pencil, outline the limits of the occlusal registration and carefully knife-trim any excess stone around its borders. Trim the vertical stops to a sharp edge on the buccal surface where they contact the working cast. Also remove any overhanging stone, leaving the occluding template and vertical stops clearly visible and accessible.

Remove the wax registration preparatory to arranging artificial teeth to the occluding template.

ARRANGING POSTERIOR TEETH TO AN OPPOSING CAST OR TEMPLATE

Whether posterior teeth are to be arranged to occlude with an opposing cast or an occlusal template, unless metal bases are part of the denture framework, the denture base upon which the jaw relation record has been made must first be removed and discarded. Since record bases that are entirely tissue supported have no place in recording occlusal relations for partial dentures, the bases must be attached to the denture framework. Metal bases being part of the prosthesis, present no problem. The teeth may be arranged in wax or replaced on the metal base, depending on the type of posterior tooth being used, and these occluded directly to the opposing cast or template.

Unless occlusal relations are recorded on final resin bases, self-curing acrylic resin bases by the sprinkling method are the most accurate and stable of bases that may be used for this purpose. (An alternate method is the relining of the original impression bases, thus accomplishing the same purpose.) While static relations may be recorded successfully on corrected bases, functional registrations are best accomplished on new resin bases made for that purpose. In either case, the denture cannot be completed on these bases, nor can the bases be removed conveniently from the retentive framework during the boilout after flasking. Therefore, the metal framework must be lifted from the cast and the original record base removed by flaming its underside: *Care must be taken not to allow the resin to catch on fire or the cast framework will become discolored with carbon.* The framework is then returned to its original position on the master cast and secured there with sticky wax before proceeding with the arrangement of artificial teeth.

Posterior tooth forms. Posterior tooth forms for partial dentures should not be selected arbitrarily. One should bear in mind at all times that the objective in partial denture occlusion is harmony between natural and artificial dentition. Whether the teeth are arranged to occlude with an opposing cast or to an occlusal template, they should be modified to harmonize with the existing dentition. In this respect, both partial denture occlusion and occlusion on a single complete denture differ from complete denture occlusion. In the latter, posterior teeth may be selected and articulated according to the dentist's own concept of what constitutes the most favorable complete denture occlusion, whereas partial denture occlusion must be made to harmonize with an existing occlusal pattern. Thus, the occlusal surfaces on the finished partial denture may bear little resemblance to the original occlusal surfaces of the teeth as manufactured.

Posterior teeth for partial dentures should be considered *material from which a suitable occlusal surface may be formed rather than teeth to be articulated as well as possible with opposing surfaces.* The original occlusal form, therefore, is of little importance in forming the posterior occlusion for the partial denture.

Whereas the posterior teeth may be made of porcelain or resin, resin teeth are more easily modified and subsequently reshaped for masticating efficiency by adding grooves and spillways. Resin teeth are also more easily narrowed buccolingually to reduce the size of the occlusal table without sacrificing strength or esthetics. They also may be more easily ground to fit minor connectors and irregular spaces and to avoid retentive elements of the denture-framework. It is again stated that when acrylic resin teeth are used without gold occlusal surfaces, the occlusion must be evaluated quite frequently to make sure that the occlusal surfaces of the resin teeth have not worn out of contact in centric occlusion. Aside from economics, the occlusal surfaces of acrylic resin teeth should be duplicated in gold to prevent excessive wear of the occlusal surfaces (Fig. 17-48).

Arranging teeth to an occluding surface. The procedure for arranging teeth to a static relationship with an opposing cast is essentially the same as for arranging teeth to an occluding template. On the other hand, articulation of artificial teeth on an adjustable instrument, which reproduces to some extent mandibular movement, will follow more closely the customary pattern for complete denture occlusion.

Step-by-step procedure. The procedure for arranging posterior teeth to an occluding template is as follows:

1. First raise the vertical adjustment of the articulator approximately 1 mm. If vertical stops are used, this will separate the stone stops by that amount.

2. With the aid of marking tape or articulating ribbon, mark the mesial and the ridge lap surfaces of the tooth to be placed against the most anterior minor connector on either side. Continue to mark and relieve this tooth until it conforms to and fits around the minor connector, occluding with the opposing surface at the existing vertical dimension. Modify the cusps of this tooth as required to occlude with the opposing surface.

3. Arrange the remaining teeth on that side in order, progressing posteriorly. Relieve the ridge lap and modify the occlusal surfaces as required to occlude optimally with the opposing surfaces. One or more teeth may have to be narrowed mesiodistally to establish a satisfactory mesiodistal relation with the opposing teeth. In other

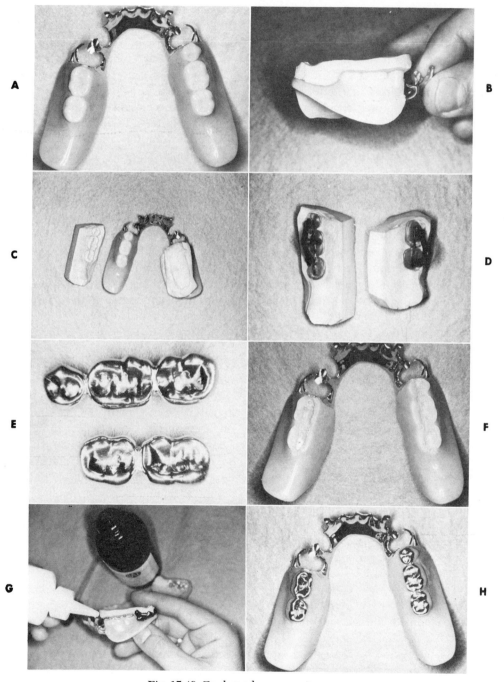

Fig. 17-48. For legend see opposite page.

instances, it may be necessary to leave a space between the first two teeth to accomplish this effect. Although intercuspation is desirable in most instances, it is not absolutely necessary when arranging to an occlusal template, since modified occlusal surfaces will function satisfactorily in any mesiodistal relation.

4. If a posterior abutment is present, the last tooth may have to be narrowed mesiodistally to fit the remaining space. This tooth also should be ground to conform to the contour of the minor connector, thereby effecting a more natural marginal contact relation with the abutment tooth.

5. Proceed to the opposite side of the arch and arrange the tooth or teeth in the same sequence, with each tooth lying adjacent to a minor connector being ground to fit that minor connector.

6. When all teeth have been arranged to the opposing surfaces, having been modified to occlude optimally at the existing vertical dimension, release the vertical element (pin or screw), leaving the occlusion uniformly high. When vertical stops of stone are used, the vertical element on the articulator may be removed entirely, since the absolute vertical dimension will be ultimately maintained by the stone stops. Otherwise, the pin or screw should be returned to its original position. (This is, of course, difficult to reestablish without a calibrated pin, hence the value of having definite stone stops.)

Using marking tape or articulating ribbon as an indicator, the occlusal surfaces are now further modified until an optimal occlusal relationship at the selected vertical dimension of occlusion has been established. At least three factors must be considered:

a. The template surface may be easily abraded or otherwise damaged by repeated closure against the teeth being arranged. This does not apply when opposing artificial teeth are being arranged and modified concurrently. When arranging teeth on a single denture, however, an opposing surface made of hard metal is the only way of

---

Fig. 17-48. Gold occlusal surfaces, duplicating the occlusal morphology of adjusted acrylic resin posterior teeth, are readily fabricated. **A,** Denture has been used by the patient and all necessary occlusal adjustments have been accomplished on the resin teeth in the first two weeks of use. **B,** Stone matrix is poured over the occlusal surfaces and extended over the top one-fourth of the buccal surfaces. **C,** Stone matrix is extended to cover the depth of the lingual flange so that it can be positively relocated in the same position after the artificial teeth have been prepared for the reception of the gold occlusal surfaces. Buccal portion of the matrix is trimmed so that the wax patterns for the gold surfaces will be about 1½ mm. thick. **D,** Stone matrices are painted with a separating medium and wax patterns of the occlusal surfaces are formed by flowing inlay wax into the occlusal portions of the matrix. Small retention loops are placed—one in each individual occlusal pattern. The patterns are sprued and cast in Type III gold. **E,** Wax patterns have been cast and polished. **F,** Acrylic resin artificial teeth are prepared for the reception of the gold occlusal surfaces by reducing their occlusal portion about 2 mm. and making an undercut groove through the central fossa of the resin teeth. The groove should only be deep enough to accommodate the retention loops on the gold occlusal surfaces. **G,** Gold occlusals, stone matrix and denture are assembled. The matrix is held in position with sticky wax. Tooth shade acrylic resin (autopolymerizing) is used to attach the gold occlusal surfaces to the denture by using the "sprinkle in" method of application. **H,** The procedure is completed by finishing and polishing the tooth shade resin. Although the original occlusal surfaces have been duplicated in gold and now occupy the same position as the original resin surfaces. a remounting cast should be made so that any possible resulting occlusal discrepancies can be corrected on an articulator using new interocclusal records to mount the lower cast and denture. (From Morris, A. L., and Bohannon, H. M., editors: Dental specialties in general practice, Philadelphia, 1969, W. B. Saunders Co.)

eliminating this possibility; otherwise, violent tapping must be avoided.

b. Unreliable markings usually result when articulating paper is used. Areas of heavy contact become perforated, leaving only a small mark, whereas areas of lesser contact may make a heavier mark. This may be avoided by using a marking tape or an inked ribbon, which better conforms to irregular occluding surfaces, does not tear or become perforated, and remains constant with repeated use. Markings are thus more reliably interpreted. A ribbon holder has been described in Chapter 16 under the discussion on arranging teeth to an occluding template.

c. Wax from articulating paper eventually is deposited on opposing surfaces, having the effect of increasing the vertical dimension of occlusion and leading to false interpretation of occlusal interference. This too is avoided by using a marking tape or an inked ribbon, since the ink or dye does not create a false surface.

Regardless of the type of indicator used, stone stops are best left unmarked for better interpretation of absolute contact. Wax from articulating paper may create a false surface here also, changing the vertical relation. Although marking ink does not do this, it does make visualization of the vertical relation at the stops more difficult to interpret.

7. Except for the addition of spillways, perfect the occlusion while the teeth are still in wax. Only those errors occurring as a result of processing will then need to be corrected by remounting. Final waxing may be done off of the articulator, but the cast should be returned to it to correct for any tooth displacement resulting from waxing and carving.

TYPES OF ANTERIOR TEETH

Anterior teeth on partial dentures are concerned primarily with esthetics and the function of incising. These are best arranged in the mouth, since an added appointment for try-in would be necessary anyway. They may be arranged arbitrarily on the cast and then tried in, but a stone index of their labial surfaces should be made on the master cast after the final arrangement has been established.

From a purely mechanical standpoint, all missing anterior teeth are best replaced with fixed restorations rather than with the partial denture. However, for economic or cosmetic reasons or in situations in which several missing anterior teeth are involved, such as in a Class IV partially edentulous arch, their replacement with the partial denture may be unavoidable.

Some types of anterior teeth used on partial dentures are as follows:

1. Porcelain or resin teeth, attached to the framework with acrylic resin.

2. Ready-made resin teeth processed directly to retentive elements on the metal framework with a matching resin. This is called a *pressed-on* method and has the advantage of permitting prior selection and try-in of the anterior teeth, plus the advantage of using ready-made resin teeth for labial surfaces. These are then hollowed out on the lingual surface to facilitate their permanent attachment to the denture framework with resin of the same shade.

3. Resin teeth processed to a metal framework in the laboratory. Tooth forms of wax may be carved on the denture framework and tried in the mouth, adjusted for esthetics and occlusion, and then processed in a resin of a suitable shade. There is some question as to whether or not the shade and durability of such teeth are comparable to manufactured plastic teeth, but improvements in materials have led to improved quality and appearance of laboratory-made teeth. Moreover, such teeth may frequently be shaped and characterized to better blend with the adjacent natural teeth.

4. Porcelain or resin facings cemented to the denture framework. These may be tried in the mouth on a baseplate wax base and adjusted for esthetics. Ready-made plastic backings may be used, which become part of the pattern for the partial denture framework, and the teeth are then ultimately cemented to the denture frame-

work. Esthetically, these are less satisfactory than other types of anterior teeth, but they have the advantage of greater strength and are easily replaced. A record of the mold and shade of each tooth should be kept, and only the ridge lap of the replacement teeth need to be ground to fit. When replaceability is the main reason for its use, the stock facing should not be beveled or difficulty will be encountered in replacing it. Replacement also may be accomplished by waxing and processing a resin facing directly to the metal backing. Stock tube or side-groove teeth are not ordinarily used for anterior teeth on partial dentures because of the horizontal forces that tend to dislodge them.

5. The denture pattern may include anterior teeth hollowed out to receive resin veneers, the same as for veneer crowns and veneer pontics on fixed partial dentures. This is most applicable when the denture framework is to be cast in gold. Then labial surfaces may be waxed and the final carving for esthetics done in the mouth. A modification of this method is the waxing of the veneer coping on a previously cast gold base. These are then cast separately and attached to the framework by soldering. Esthetically, the result is comparable to that obtained with resin veneer crowns. This method is particularly applicable when there is a desire to make the replaced teeth match adjacent veneered abutment crowns.

WAXING AND INVESTING THE PARTIAL DENTURE PRIOR TO PROCESSING RESIN BASES OR ATTACHMENTS

Waxing the partial denture base. Waxing the partial denture base prior to investing differs little from the waxing of a complete denture; the only difference is the waxing to and around exposed parts of the metal framework. Here, undercut finishing lines should be provided whenever possible. Then the waxing is merely butted to the finishing line with a little excess to allow for finishing. Otherwise, small voids in the

wax may become filled with investing plaster, or fine edges of the investment may break off during boilout and packing. In either case, small pieces of investment may become embedded in the resin at the finishing lines. This is avoided by slightly overwaxing and then finishing the resin back to the metal finishing line with finishing burs. Abrasive wheels and discs should not be used for this purpose, as they will cut into the metal and may burn the resin. Pumice and a rag wheel should be used sparingly for polishing because it will cut the resin more rapidly than the metal and leave the finishing line elevated above the adjacent resin.

When waxing to polished metal parts not possessing a finishing line, it must be remembered that no attachment will exist and that over a period of time there inevitably will be some seepage, separation, and disco'oration of the resin in this area. This may be avoided to some extent by roughening the metal whenever possible to effect some mechanical attachment. The wax should be left thick enough so that the resin will have some bulk at its junction with the polished metal. Thin films of resin over metal should be avoided, and, in finishing, these should be cut back to an area of bulk with finishing burs. Otherwise, any thin film of resin will eventually separate and become discolored and unclean due to marginal seepage.

Gingival form should be waxed in accordance with modern concepts of cosmetics and should be made as self-cleansing as possible. The dental student should familiarize himself with normal gingival architecture as found on diagnostic casts of natural dentition, beginning with the casts of each other's mouths usually made in basic technique exercises. In this manner he may have a better concept of gingival contours to be reproduced on prosthetic restorations.

In general, students and technicians alike seem to lack a clear concept of natural gingival architecture and are prone to leave too much tooth embedded in wax. Artificial teeth ordinarily should be uncovered fully to expose all the anatomic crown and even beyond when gingival recession is to be simulated. Relatively few prosthodontic patients are in an age bracket in which some gingival recession and exposed cementum would not normally be present, and this should be simulated on prosthodontic restorations in proportion to the patient's age. With partial dentures, gingival contours around the remaining natural teeth should be used as a guide to the gingival contours to be reproduced on the prosthesis. However, interproximal spaces are most always filled particularly between posterior artificial teeth.

The denture should be waxed and carved as for a cast restoration, which it actually is, regardless of the material to be used or the method of processing. The fact that a split-mold technique is used for processing does not alter the fact that the form of the denture base is to be reproduced by a casting procedure. Therefore, the denture pattern should be waxed with care in the same form as that desired for the finished restoration rather than attempt to shape facial contours on the prosthesis during the polishing phase. Polishing should consist primarily of trimming away the flash, stippling polished surfaces when desired, and polishing lightly with brush wheels and pumice followed by final polishing with a soft brush wheel and a nonabrasive shining agent such as "whiting." Gross trimming and polishing with pumice should not be necessary if the denture has been properly waxed prior to investing.

Since the polished surfaces of any denture play an important part in both retention and the control of the food bolus buccal and lingual contours generally should be made concave. Border thickness of the denture should be left as recorded in the impression. The only exceptions are the distolingual aspect of the lower denture base to avoid interference with the tongue, and the distobuccal aspect of the upper denture base to avoid interference with the coronoid process of the mandible.

These are the only areas that cannot ordinarily be waxed to final contour before investing and may need to be thinned *by the dentist* at the time of final polishing.

Investing the partial denture. In investing a partial denture for processing a resin base, it must be remembered that the denture cast must be recovered from the flask intact for remounting. The practice of cutting the teeth off the cast to expose the connectors and retainers, which are then embedded in the upper half of the flask, is permissible only when an existing denture base is being relined and no provision has been made for remounting. (In such case, it seems that this practice has no advantage over investing the denture being so relined upside-down in the lower half of the flask.) Since some increase in vertical dimension has, in the past, been inevitable in any split-mold processing technique, this method results in the denture framework being raised from the supporting teeth by the amount of increase. Whereas occlusal adjustment in the mouth may temporarily reestablish a harmonious occlusal relation with the opposing teeth, the denture framework must then settle into supporting contact with the abutment teeth at the expense of the underlying ridge.

Changes in vertical dimension may be held to a minimum by using denture resins that can be placed in the mold in a fluid rather than a doughy state or those that may be injected in a fluid state into a closed mold. Dimensional changes occurring during relining may also be held to a minimum by using cold-curing resins for this purpose, thus avoiding the thermal expansion of a mold subjected to elevated temperatures.

When two opposing partial dentures are being made concurrently, one is sometimes processed and placed first and then the final occlusion established on the second denture to a fully restored arch. In such case, when there are no natural teeth in opposition, it is not necessary that the first denture be remounted after processing. In all other cases, remounting to correct for errors in occlusion is absolutely necessary. Flasking must be accomplished so that the cast may be recovered from the flask undamaged.

Since the partial denture impression (fluid-wax) may not be boxed prior to pouring the cast, metal mounting plates cannot be used as with complete denture impressions. Adding a mounting plate later with additional stone is not dependable, because if the cast separates between the two layers of stone, the mounting record is lost. The base of the stone cast must therefore be keyed by beveling and notching on at least three sides.

Minute voids in the base of the cast will have been reproduced in the stone-mounting, and although the obvious larger blebs may be trimmed away, smaller blebs will remain. If the voids in the cast become filled with investing material, the effect is two particles trying to occupy the same space. This may be prevented by covering the base with tin foil prior to investing. By coating the base and sides of the cast with petroleum jelly, tin foil may be easily adapted by burnishing it on with a towel. Not only does this keep the base of the cast isolated from investing material but the cast also may be more easily recovered from the surrounding investment.

After tin-foiling, the remainder of the cast should be coated with some reliable separator, such as mineral oil, petroleum jelly, sodium silicate, or tin-foil substitute. The entire cast, except for the wax and teeth, may then be invested in the lower half of the flask (Fig. 17-49). As with a complete denture, only the supplied teeth and wax are left exposed to be invested in the upper half. Also, as with a complete denture, the investment in the lower half must be smooth and free of undercuts, and must be coated with a separator to facilitate separation of the two halves of the flask.

An alternate and preferred procedure is to invest the cast only to the top of the tin-foiled base, smoothing the investment and

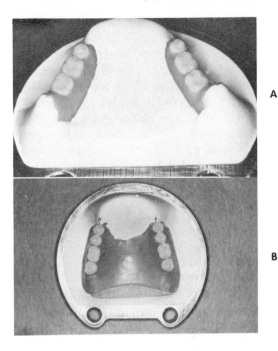

Fig. 17-49. A, Class II mandibular denture invested in the lower half of the flask. Master cast upon which the denture will be processed is completely covered with investing stone exposing only the artificial teeth and waxed denture bases. There are *no* undercuts in the lower half of the flask, thus assuring separation of the flask halves after the investment procedure is completed. B, Maxillary Class II denture invested in the lower half of an investing flask.

applying a reliable separator. Then, a second layer of investment is placed around the anatomic portion of the cast, covering the natural teeth and the exposed parts of the denture framework. This is likewise smoothed and made free of undercuts and coated with a separator prior to pouring the top half of the flask. Recovery of the cast is thus made easier by having a shell of investment over the anatomic portion of the cast, which may be removed separately.

When the denture base is to be characterized by applying tinted resins to the mold, care should be taken not to embed the wax border in the lower half of the flask. Bennett has pointed out the need for investing only to the border of the wax, leaving the entire surface to be tinted reproduced in the upper half of the flask. With this precaution, tinting may be carried all the way to the border and later removal of the flask will not mar the tinted surface. If tinting is not to be done or is to be done only at the cervical margins of the teeth and the interdental papillae, the wax border should be embedded in the lower half where it may be faithfully reproduced and preserved during polishing.

The use of resin materials that require trial packing is complicated by the presence of the retentive framework of the partial denture. With their use, trial packing must be done with a sheet of cellophane between two layers of the resin dough; otherwise, the flask could not be opened without pulling the resin away from either the teeth in one half of the flask or the metal framework in the other. Resin dough is placed in each half of the flask, the sheet of cellophane placed between them, and the flask closed for trial packing. The flask is then opened, the cellophane removed, and the excess flash trimmed away. Final closure is then effected without the intervening sheet of cellophane.

More recently, resin materials that require no trial packing have been developed. These are mixed as usual but are either poured into the mold or placed in the mold in a soft state. They offer little or no resistance to closure of the flask, yet the finished product is comparable to resin materials packed in a doughy state. They must be used in some excess, with the excess escaping between the halves of the flask. Although they are soft enough to allow the escape of gross excess, the use of a land space is advisable to avoid a thin film on the land area. Any film existing on the land area after deflasking may be interpreted as an opening of the flask by that amount, hence the need for some provision for an intervening space to accommodate the excess and to facilitate its escape as the flask is closed.

To provide such a land space, the land area on the lower half of the flask may be painted with melted baseplate wax prior to pouring the top half. After wax elimination, a space then remains to accommodate any excess resin remaining after the flask is completely closed. It is necessary that no plaster or wax be allowed to remain on the rim of the flask and that the flask make metal-to-metal contact before pouring the second half. Only in this way is it possible to see that the flask is completely closed prior to placing it in the curing unit.

The pouring of the top half of the flask follows the same procedure as with a complete denture. Whereas it is not absolutely necessary that the entire top half be poured in stone, it is necessary that a stone cap of some type be used to prevent tooth movement in an occlusal direction. This is due to the inability of plaster to withstand closing pressures. All plaster remaining on the occlusal surfaces of the teeth should be removed and a separator added prior to pouring the stone cap to facilitate its removal during deflasking. If the use of stone investment is preferred, a shell of improved stone or die stone may be painted or applied with the fingers onto the wax and teeth and this allowed to harden before filling the remainder of the flask with plaster. If a full stone investment is preferred, some provision should be made for easy separation during deflasking. Not only should a separate stone cap be used but metal separators or knife cuts radiating out to the walls of the flask should also be placed in the partially set stone. Deflasking is then easily accomplished by removing the stone cap and inserting a knife blade between the sections of stone.

Boilout should be deferred until the investing material has set for several hours or, preferably, overnight. Boilout must effectively eliminate all wax residue; therefore an adequate source of clean hot water must be available. After wax elimination with boiling water, it should be flushed with a solution of grease-dissolving detergent and again with clean boiling water.

Immediately after boilout, the warm mold should be painted with a thin film of tin-foil substitute, being careful not to allow it to collect around the cervical portions of the teeth. A second coat should be applied after the first coat has reasonably dried, and packing of the mold should proceed immediately after this film has dried to the touch. Once the tin-foil substitute becomes completely dry it may wrinkle and lift away from the plaster, defeating the purpose for which it is used.

When the master cast for a distal extension partial denture has been repoured from a secondary impression, the supporting "foot" on the retention frame may not necessarily be in contact with the cast. Closing pressure within the flask may distort the unsupported extension of the metal framework, with subsequent rebound upon deflasking. The finished denture base will then lack contact with the supporting tissues, resulting in denture rotation about the fulcrum line similar to that occurring after tissue resorption. *To provide support for the distal extension of the metal framework during flask closure, a self-curing resin should be sprinkled or painted around the distal end of the framework and allowed to harden before proceeding with packing the denture resin.*

PROCESSING THE DENTURE

Processing follows the same procedure as that for a complete denture. Denture base characterization may be added just prior to packing. This is most desirable when denture base material will be visible. Posterior resin bases alone ordinarily do not require characterization, but the dentist should select a denture base material that closely resembles the color of the surrounding tissues. The ideal resin base material for partial dentures is therefore one that (1) may be used without trial packing, (2) possesses a shade that is compatible with surrounding tissues, and (3) is dimensionally stable and accurate.

Layered silicone rubber flasking. There has never been any question concerning the merits of tin-foiling the denture before investing, which results in a tin-foil-lined matrix and eliminates the need for a separating film. The fact remains, however, that the use of a tin-foil substitute has become almost universal.

At best, any tin-foil substitute creates an undesirable film at the gingival margins of the teeth, resulting in microscopic separation between the teeth and the surrounding resin. This may be shown by sectioning a finished denture and by observing the marginal discoloration around the cervical portions of the teeth after several months in the mouth. To some extent, injection molding obviates this objection to the use of a tin-foil substitute—which is one of the principal advantages of injection molding over compression molding.

Since the use of compression molding is widespread and is likely to continue, some method that eliminates the use of a tin-foil substitute is needed. The layered silicone rubber method results in more complete adaptation of the resin around the cervical portions of porcelain teeth and more complete bonding to resin teeth. In addition, denture base tints may be applied directly to the mold without first applying a separating film.

A room-temperature-curing silicone rubber, which has sufficient body and toughness for the purpose, is applied to the wax surface of the denture and over the teeth just prior to pouring the upper half of the flask. The manufacturer's instructions must be followed as to mixing and time elapsed before adding the outer stone investment to ensure curing and bonding to the overlying investment. Boilout is then completed in the usual way.

A further advantage of the layered silicone rubber method is the ease with which deflasking is accomplished. If the wax carving of the denture has been completed with care prior to flasking, denture tints remain unaltered by unnecessary trimming and polishing of the processed denture.

All resin base materials available up to the present time exhibit some dimensional change, both during processing and in the mouth. The fit of the denture is therefore dependent, to a large extent, upon the accuracy, or lack of accuracy, of the denture base material, since impression and cast materials in use today are themselves reasonably accurate. In an attempt to minimize dimensional changes in the denture base, materials and techniques are constantly being improved. Some of these use injection molding to provide a continuous source of material to the mold as curing shrinkage occurs. One technique utilizes hydraulic pressure within the top half of the flask to limit the shrinkage toward the cast only. It is claimed, by the originator of this technique, that processing by any other means results in both a distorted mold and a distorted cast, because of collapse of the stone or plaster around the myriad of small air voids inevitably present. Evidence of this distortion can be seen when the cast is returned to the remounting surface on the articulator and seems to lend support to the claim that compression molding does result in a slightly distorted cast.

Compression molding resins in a doughy state are giving way to the use of materials that may be poured into the mold or placed into the mold in a soft state, thus eliminating trial packing and excessive pressures, which leads to open flasks and altered vertical dimension. Activated, or cold-curing, resins are sometimes used to avoid mold expansion occurring at higher temperatures. Materials other than acrylic resins are used with various techniques, some of these being styrene, vinyl, and, experimentally, epoxy resins. The main objective behind the development of newer techniques and materials is greater dimensional accuracy and stability, combined with strength and better appearance.

The study of the history of denture base materials is a most interesting one that has been covered elsewhere in dental literature. The future of denture base materials promises to be just as fascinating a study, but such a discussion cannot be included within the scope of this book. With newer materials, the future of methyl methacrylate as a denture base material is uncertain despite its acceptance as the best material available for this purpose since its introduction in 1937. Although it has made possible the simulation of natural tissue color and contours combined with ease of manipulation, the fact remains that it leaves much to be desired as far as accuracy and dimensional stability are concerned. Whether or not other and newer materials will eventually supplant methyl methacrylate as a denture base material remains to be seen. The fact is that the denture base of the future (1) must be capable of accurately reproducing natural tissue tones faithfully through the use of characterizing stains and customizing procedures and (2) must not require elaborate processing procedures and equipment, which would make the cost prohibitive for general usage.

REMOUNTING AND OCCLUSAL CORRECTION

As long as dimensional changes continue to occur during the processing of resin denture bases or the resin attachment of teeth to metal bases, the processed denture will need to be remounted on the articulating instrument for correction of the altered occlusion. Even with improved denture base materials and processing techniques, some movement of artificial teeth will still occur due to the dimensional instability of the wax in which the artificial teeth were arranged. So until both sources of error can be eliminated, remounting will continue to be necessary.

The only alternate to remounting is the correction of the occlusion in the mouth. As has been discussed previously, the limitations to doing so successfully depends upon the number of teeth involved, the stability of the denture bases, the accessibility of the occlusion, and the ability of the dentist to interpret and correct occlusal discrepancies.

How well the occlusion may be perfected by remounting will depend upon the manner in which jaw relations were transferred to an instrument and how closely the instrument is capable of reproducing functional occlusion. But even though the articulator is capable of reproducing only a static centric relation, that relation at least should be reestablished prior to placement of the denture.

Whereas it is admitted that there are limitations to the perfection of eccentric occlusion in the mouth, some believe that it can be done with more accuracy than on an instrument that is incapable of reproducing eccentric positions. Correction for errors in centric occlusion, however, should not be included in this philosophy, for such is based upon a premise that centric occlusion may be established satisfactorily by intraoral adjustment, followed then by a perfecting of eccentric occlusion. Because of denture instability and the inaccessibility of the occlusion for analysis, this is presuming more than anyone can justify. Even occlusal adjustment of natural dentition, in which each tooth has its own support, can best be done when preceded by an analysis of articulated diagnostic casts.

One cardinal premise must be accepted if prosthetic dentistry is to be anything more than a haphazard procedure. This is *that it is possible to transfer centric jaw relations to an instrument with accuracy and to maintain this relation throughout the fabrication of the prosthesis.* If this is true, then centric occlusion, coinciding either with centric jaw relation or with centric occlusion of the remaining natural teeth, or both, must have been established prior to initial placement of the prosthesis. This means that occlusal correction by remounting after final processing is an absolute necessity to the success of the restoration.

The term *remounting* is also applied to the mounting of a completed prosthetic restoration back onto an instrument using some kind of interocclusal records. Errors in occlusion resulting from processing of tooth-borne dentures may be corrected by reattaching the indexed processing cast and denture to the same instrument on which the occlusion was formulated. However, because of some instability inherent in distal extension removable partial dentures,

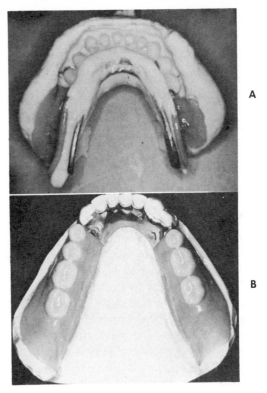

Fig. 17-50. **A**, Stock, perforated tray is used to make an irreversible hydrocolloid (alginate) impression of the denture and the dental arch. Blockout of undercuts in the denture base and of the tips of direct retainers is necessary so that the denture can be readily removed and replaced on a resultant remounting cast, as illustrated in **B**. **B**, Remounting cast poured in stone. The denture can be readily removed and replaced on the cast for occlusal correction procedures using an articulator.

such dentures should be recovered from processing investment, finished, and polished for performing occlusal corrections by the use of new intraoral records. A remounting cast must be made by the dentist before occlusal corrections can be accomplished. This is simply done by first placing the denture in the mouth and making an irreversible hydrocolloid (alginate) impression of the denture and remaining teeth in the arch (Fig. 17-50). When the impression is removed, the denture usually will remain in the impression or can be accurately replaced. Undercuts in the denture bases are blocked out, the retentive elements of the framework are covered with a thin layer of molten wax, and a remounting cast is poured in the impression. The remounting casts are then oriented to the articulator by the same type interocclusal records that were used to orient the casts to formulate the occlusion.

Occlusal harmony must exist before the patient is given possession of the dentures. Delaying the correction of occlusal discrepancies until the dentures have had a chance to settle is not justifiable.

Remounting after processing is accomplished by returning the cast to a keyed relationship with the articulator mounting. Whereas the use of metal mounting plates attached to both surfaces may be desirable, it is not practical to do so with a partial denture cast. Stone to stone, properly keyed and free of debris, provides a sufficiently accurate surface for remounting.

A simple procedure, which greatly enhances the accuracy of the remounting surfaces, is the making of a stone split cast. After beveling and keying the base of the master cast, a separating film is applied and the inverted cast is encircled with a strip of lead boxing material. A thin layer of hard stone of a different color is then vibrated onto the base of the cast, and the exposed surface is left purposely uneven. Paper clips or washers may be partially embedded for added retention. After this thin layer of stone has hardened, it is attached to the articulator with mounting plaster. Separation of the cast from the articulator and any subsequent remounting are then accomplished with opposing stone surfaces, resulting in greater accuracy than is possible with a stone cast against mounting plaster alone.

It is most important that the mounting surfaces be free of particles that would prevent reestablishment of their original relationship. Therefore, tin foil of about 0.002 inch thickness should be applied to the base of the cast prior to investing. This is easily accomplished by coating the surface of the cast with petrolatum and then applying the tin foil smoothly with the aid of a cloth towel. The original mounting surface of the cast is thus protected from contamination, and, on stripping away the tin foil after deflasking, the original surface may be returned to its original position. The opposing mounting surface on the articulator should be brushed and blown free of particles and then the base of the cast secured to it with sticky wax or modeling plastic. Plaster may then be used for additional security, but only after the cast has first been secured with some reliable thermoplastic material. *A layer of cement, such as Duco cement, should never be used as it introduces an intervening film that interferes with the accuracy of the remounting.*

Precautions to be taken in remounting. The following precautions should be taken to assure the accuracy of remounting to make final occlusal adjustment prior to the polishing and initial placement of the denture. These apply to all types of occlusal relationship records but are directed particularly to remounting to an occlusal template, when stone vertical stops are used.

1. Make sure that the base of the cast has been reduced before keying and mounting, so that it will not have to be altered later to get it into the flask.

2. Bevel the margins of the base of the cast so that it will seat in a definite boxlike manner in the articulator mounting.

3. Notch the posterior and the anterior aspects of the base to assure further its return to its original position. Notches at the margins are preferable to depressions within the base, as the former permits a visual check of the accuracy of the remounting.

4. Lubricate lightly the base and sides of the cast before mounting to facilitate easy removal from the mounting plaster.

5. Tin-foil the base and sides of the cast prior to flasking so that traces of investment will not be present to interfere with remounting.

6. When remounting, secure the cast to the articulator with sticky wax or modeling plastic, followed by plaster over both the mounting and the sides of the cast.

7. Before adjusting the occlusion, make certain that no traces of investment remain on the vertical stops.

8. Take care not to abrade the opposing occlusal surface during occlusal adjustment. The use of marking tape or inked ribbon is preferable to articulating paper. The artificial tooth is less likely to cut through and mar the opposing surface, and ink or dye will not build up a false opposing surface as will the wax from articulating paper.

9. Occlusal readjustment to an occlusal template is complete when the stone verticle stops are again in contact. With other types of articulator mountings, readjustment is complete when the vertical pin is again in contact and any valid horizontal excursions are freed of interference.

Occlusal readjustment, as was the original articulation, is at the expense of the original tooth anatomy. Occlusal surfaces should be reshaped by adding grooves and spillways and by reducing the area of the occlusal table, thus improving the masticating efficiency of the artificial tooth. Although this may be done immediately after occlusal readjustment and prior to initial placement of the denture, it may be deferred until final adjustment has been completed. In any event, it is a necessary step in the completion of any removable prosthesis.

Porcelain teeth may be reshaped with abrasive or diamond mounted points. Plastic teeth lend themselves better to reshaping with small burs to restore functional anatomy. Either type should be repolished judiciously to avoid reduction of cuspal contacts. Although cusps may be narrowed, spillways added, and the total area of contact reduced to improve masticating efficiency, critical areas of contact, both vertical and horizontal, must always be preserved.

POLISHING THE DENTURE

The areas to be considered in the polishing of a partial denture are (1) the borders of the denture bases, (2) the facial surfaces, and (3) the teeth and adjacent areas.

The borders on full metal bases will have been established previously. On partial metal bases and full resin bases, the accuracy with which the border may be finished will depend upon the accuracy of the impression record and how well this was preserved on the stone cast. Edentulous areas recorded from impressions in stock trays generally lack the accuracy at the borders that is found on casts made from impressions in individualized trays and by secondary impression methods. Border accuracy is determined also by whether or not the impression recorded a functional or a static relationship of the bordering tissue attachments.

Denture borders. The principal objectives to be considered in making an impression of edentulous areas of a partially edentulous arch are (1) maximum support for the partial denture base and (2) extension of the borders to obtain maximum coverage compatible with moving tissues. Although this second objective may be obtained with an adequate individualized impression tray, it is best accomplished with a secondary impression method. Not only should the *extent* of the border be recorded accurately but also its *width*. Both extent and width as recorded should be preserved on the stone cast. With the exception of certain areas that are arbitrarily thinned in polishing (mentioned previously in this chapter), finishing and polishing the denture borders should consist only of removing any flash and artifactual blebs. Otherwise borders should be left as recorded in the impression.

When the impression is made in a stock tray, both the extent and the width of the border will have been influenced by the tray itself. Some areas will be left short of the total area available for denture support, while others will be extended beyond functional limits by the overextension of the tray. In such areas the technician must interpret the anatomy of the mouth as best he can and arbitrarily trim the denture borders just short of obvious overextension. This presumes an intimate knowledge of the anatomy of the mouth of the patient for whom the restoration is being made, which the technician does not possess. Any overextension remaining after arbitrarily trimming the border has to be corrected in the mouth. We prefer to finish the borders of dentures ourselves, having painstakingly developed them during impression procedures.

Facial surfaces. The facial surfaces of the denture base are those polished surfaces lying between the borders and the supplied teeth. Methods have been proposed for making sectional impression records of buccal contours, thereby permitting the denture base to be made to conform to facial musculature. These have never received wide acceptance and may be considered impractical in removable partial prosthodontics.

Facial surfaces may be established in wax or may be carved into the denture base after processing. Generally, it is desirable that it be done in wax as part of the wax pattern, both because it is easier to do so and because contours can best be established at a time when additions can be made if desired. Buccal surfaces should be made concave to aid in the retention of the denture by border molding, to preserve the border roll and thereby prevent food impacting, and to facilitate return of the food bolus back onto the masticating table. Lingual surfaces should be made concave to provide tongue room and to aid in the retention of the denture. If such contours are established previously in wax, finishing is not only more easily accomplished but border and gingival areas are also less likely to be inadvertently altered. Polishing of concave surfaces is always more difficult than flat and convex surfaces, and this can largely be avoided by taking care to contour and polish the wax pattern prior to investing.

Finishing gingival and interproximal areas. The contouring of gingival and interproximal areas in the cured resin is difficult and generally unsatisfactory. The practice of doing so dates back to the days when vulcanite rubber was trimmed and shaped with Pearson-type chisels and a trimming block was a necessary piece of equipment in any dental laboratory. Finishing was done with vulcanite burs and with brush wheels and pumice, creating the vertical interproximal grooves that for many years were typical of the "denture look." Not only is this contrary to modern concepts of denture esthetics but also gingival and interproximal carving of the denture resin around plastic teeth may not be done without some damage to the teeth themselves.

Modern cosmetic considerations demand that gingival carving be done around each tooth individually, with variations in the height of the gingival curve and in the length of the interdental papillae. Interproximally, the papillae should be convex rather than concave. The gingival attachment should be free of grooves and ditches that would accumulate debris and stain and should be as free-cleansing as possible. All this precludes gross shaping and trimming of gingival areas *after* processing. Gingival carving should be done in wax, and investing should be done with care to avoid blebs and artifacts. Finishing should consist only of trimming around the teeth and the interdental papillae with small round burs to create a more natural simulation of living tissue, plus light stippling with an off-center round bur for the same reason. Polishing should consist only of light buffing with brush wheels and pumice and finally with a soft brush wheel and a nonabrasive polishing agent such as tin oxide.

Pumicing of gingival areas can only serve to polish the high spots, and although it may be done lightly, its use should be limited to light buffing of areas already made as smooth as possible by other means. Not only does heavy pumicing of the denture resin create a typical "denture look" but it also alters the surface of any plastic teeth present. If pumicing must be done, plastic teeth should be protected with adhesive tape during the process.

Any polishing operation on a partial denture done on a lathe is made hazardous by the presence of clasp retainers, which can easily become caught in the polishing wheel. Although the least damage that might occur is the distortion of a clasp arm, there is a greater possibility that the denture may be thrown forceably into the lathe pan with serious damage to the framework or other parts of the denture. The technician must be ever conscious of this possibility and always cover any projecting clasp with the finger while it is near the polishing wheel. In addition, it is wise to keep a pumice pan well filled with wet pumice to cushion the shock should an accident occur. Any other lathe pan used in polishing should be lined with a towel or with a resilient material such as automotive undercoating material for the same reason.

Frush has listed the following rules for varying the height of the gingival tissue at the cervical portion of the teeth:

(a) Slightly below the high lip line at the central incisors.
(b) Lower than the central incisor gum line [gingival margin] at the lateral incisors.
(c) Higher than the central or lateral incisor gum line [gingival margin] at the canine.

(d) Slightly lower than the canine at the premolar and variable for both premolars and molars.*

The correctly formed interdental papilla should be formed so that it will be self-cleansing. It should be carved so that it is in harmony with the interpretation of age and will be the deciding factor in the visible outline form of the tooth. As Frush has pointed out, even a drop of wax properly placed can change the appearance of a square tooth to one of tapering or ovoid appearance. A properly formed interdental papilla further enhances the natural appearance by increasing the color in this area.

The rules for forming the interdental papilla are given by Frush as follows:

(a) The papilla must extend to the point of tooth contact for cleanliness.
(b) The papillae must be of various lengths.
(c) The interdental papilla must be convex in all directions.
(d) The papillae must be shaped according to the age of the patient.
(e) The papilla must end near the labial face of the tooth and never slope in-

*From Frush, J. P.: Dentogenic restorations and dynesthetics, Los Angeles, 1957, Swissdent Foundation.

Table 17-1. Instruments for finishing the denture*

CC trimmers	2B and 5A	Periphery [border] and palate
Fissure bur	No. 562	Frenum
No. 2 bur	Straight	For cleaning the necks [cervical portions] of the teeth and interdental spaces
No. 8 bur	Eccentric	Rough carving of the labial face of the denture
S. S. White	Points No. 12, B2, and B28	Lingual cutaway on the palate of the denture behind the anterior teeth
Torit wet or dry fine water-proof discs ⅞″		Outline the necks [cervical portions] and the papillae
No. 5 bur	Eccentric	Carve the papillae, the labial face of the denture, the necks [cervical portions] of the teeth and finer stippling
Nos. 1 and ½ burs	Eccentric	Refine the carving and facial shape of the papillae

*From Frush, J. P.: Dentogenic restorations and dynesthetics, Los Angeles, 1957, Swissdent Foundation.

ward to terminate towards the lingual portion of the interproximal surface.*

Frush's instructions for finishing a denture that has been carefully waxed prior to investing are as follows:

(1) Trim excess flash from the periphery [border] and, if any, from around the necks [cervical portions] of the teeth.
(2) Trim the lingual of the teeth and established lingual "cutaways" or valleys behind any interior interdental spaces.

(3) Stipple the labial-buccal surfaces with a No. 5 round bur (eccentric).
(4) Refine the papillae with first a No. 1 round and finally with a No. ½ round (eccentric) bur.
(5) Polish the periphery [border] and the palatal or lingual surfaces. Then lightly polish the stippled surface (labial-buccal) with a No. B-12 brush wheel and pumice.
(6) High shine the periphery [border] and palate (and lingual), but not the labial-buccal surface.*

---

*From Frush, J. P.: Dentogenic restorations and dynesthetics, Los Angeles, 1957, Swissdent Foundation.

*From Frush, J. P.: Dentogenic restorations and dynesthetics, Los Angeles, 1957, Swissdent Foundation.

CHAPTER 18

Work authorizations for removable partial dentures

A work authorization is a written direction for laboratory procedures to be performed in the fabrication of dental restorations. The responsibility of a dentist to the public and his profession in safeguarding the quality of prosthodontic services is discharged, in part, through meaningful work authorizations. Properly executed, they provide the means for increased professional satisfaction in a removable partial denture service.

A work authorization by a dentist is the same as granting "power of attorney"; it grants authority for others to act in his behalf. It bears the same relationship to a dental laboratory technician as the sextant does to a navigator—it plots his course.

Work authorizations are effective channels of communication when properly executed. They enhance the quality of the completed restorations by eliminating stereotyped production, and in its place provide for individually, scientifically considered prostheses.

Work authorization

Content. The information contained in a work authorization should include (1) name and address of the dental laboratory, (2) name and address of the dentist originating the work authorization, (3) date of the work authorization, (4) identification of the patient, (5) desired completion date of the request, (6) specific instruc-

tions, (7) signature of the dentist, and (8) registered license number of the dentist. All these requirements can be accommodated in a simple designed form (Fig. 18-1).

Function. The following four important functions are performed by a work authorization: (1) It furnishes definite instructions for the laboratory procedures to be accomplished and establishes the acceptable minimum of quality for the services rendered. (2) It provides a means of protecting the public from the illegal practice of dentistry. (3) It is a protective document for both the dentist and dental laboratory technician if they become participants in a lawsuit to resolve matters between them. (4) It completely delineates the responsibilities of the dentist and the dental laboratory technician.

Characteristics. A work authorization must be legible, clear, concise, and readily understood. It is unreasonable to assume that laboratory technicians are decoding experts. Sufficient information must be included in a work authorization to enable the technician to study and execute the request. Many dentists are overly presumptive in assuming that a request can be acceptably fulfilled without proper directions.

It is sound practice to provide the dental laboratory technician with adequate written instructions for each required laboratory service in the construction of a resto-

WORK AUTHORIZATION — REMOVABLE PARTIAL DENTURES

TO: CENTRAL DENTAL LABORATORY   Date _____

FROM _____

PATIENT IDENTIFICATION: _____

PATIENT SOURCE: ( ) CLINIC ( ) HOSPITAL ( ) PERSONAL CARE ( ) RESEARCH

GENERAL REQUEST: _____

_____

DATE & TIME REQUIRED _____

METAL FOR FRAMEWORK: _____

DENTURE BASE: ( ) ACRYLIC RESIN ( ) METAL ( ) COMBINATION

TOOTH SELECTION: ( ) PORCELAIN ( ) ACRYLIC RESIN ( ) OTHER

MAKE _____ MOLD _____ SHADE _____

SPECIFIC INSTRUCTIONS: _____

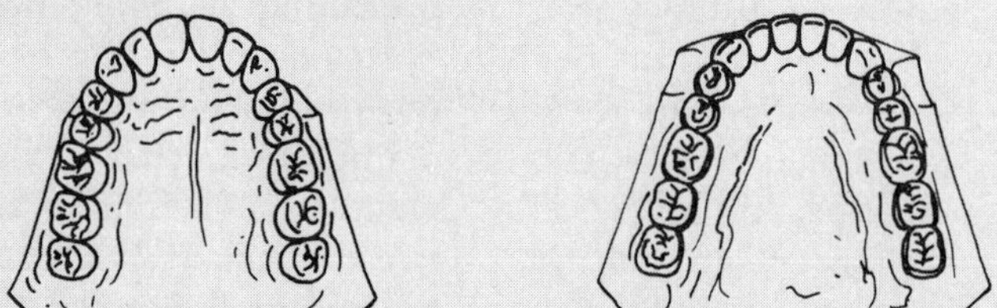

_____

_____

_____

_____

_____

_____

_____

SIGNATURE

COLOR CODE ON CAST: Denture Design (Green), Survey Lines (Black), Finishing Lines (Red)

WAXING SPECIFICATIONS FOR TYPE "D" GOLD; CHROME-COBALT IN PARENTHESIS

1. Lingual Bar—6 GA. ½ Pear + 24(26) GA. Sheet
2. Anterior Palatal Bar—Two 26(28) GA. Sheets
3. Posterior and Single Palatal Bars—Two 26(28) GA. Sheets Reinforced by 12 GA. ½ RD. Strip in Center
4. Lingual Plate Extensions } 24 GA. Sheet
   Guiding Plane Plates
   Cast Bases
   Full Palatal Castings
5. Indirect Retainer—10 GA ½ RD. Strip
6. Finishing Lines—12 GA ½ RD. Strip Inverted
7. Direct Retainer Arms—Molars, Large (Medium) Plastic Preformed Patterns. Premolars and Canines, Medium (Small) Preformed Plastic Patterns
8. Acrylic Resin Retention Mesh—12(14) GA ½ RD. Strip or Preformed Patterns
9. Master Cast Relief for Retention Mesh—Two 26 GA Sheets.

Fig. 18-1. Work authorization form used in undergraduate clinic designed specifically for removable partial dentures to furnish detailed information to the laboratory technician. It is available in tablet form so that a carbon copy of the work authorization can be conveniently made. The original copy is white and goes to the laboratory technician. The carbon copy is yellow and is retained in the files of the dentist.

WORK AUTHORIZATION — REMOVABLE PARTIAL DENTURES

TO: CENTRAL DENTAL LABORATORY   Date *11/27/67*

FROM *Dr. John Doe, Medical Arts Bldg*

PATIENT IDENTIFICATION: *Patient # 3041*

PATIENT SOURCE: ( ) CLINIC   ( ) HOSPITAL   ( ) PERSONAL CARE   ( ) RESEARCH

GENERAL REQUEST: *Please fabricate a maxillary removable partial denture framework.*

DATE & TIME REQUIRED *12/4/67, 10 a.m.*

METAL FOR FRAMEWORK: *Type "D" gold*

DENTURE BASE: ( ) ACRYLIC RESIN   ( ) METAL   ( ) COMBINATION

TOOTH SELECTION: ( ) PORCELAIN   ( ) ACRYLIC RESIN   ( ) OTHER

MAKE _____ MOLD _____ SHADE _____

SPECIFIC INSTRUCTIONS: *See below color code and waxing specs. Orient master cast to surveyor arm by tripod marks. All undercuts in framework design (except retentive tips of clasps) to be blocked out parallel to path of placement. Provide indices to transfer design to refractory cast. Cast and finish framework. Anatomic replica pattern. Please return with blocked out master cast. Thank you.*

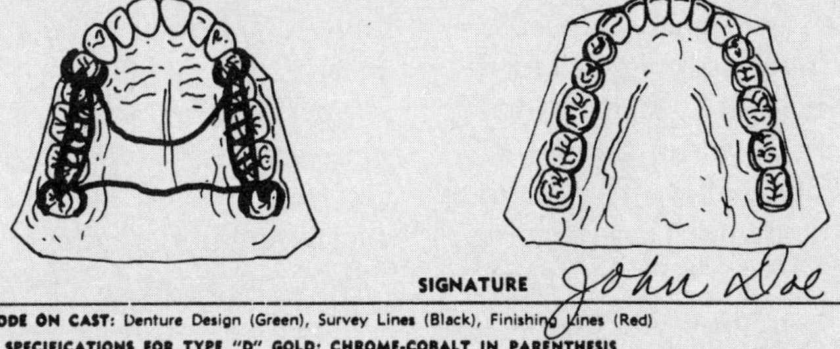

SIGNATURE *John Doe 30112*

COLOR CODE ON CAST: Denture Design (Green), Survey Lines (Black), Finishing Lines (Red)

WAXING SPECIFICATIONS FOR TYPE "D" GOLD; CHROME-COBALT IN PARENTHESIS

1. Lingual Bar—6 GA. ½ Pear + 24(26) GA. Sheet
2. Anterior Palatal Bar—Two 26(28) GA. Sheets
3. Posterior and Single Palatal Bars—Two 26(28) GA. Sheets Reinforced by 12 GA. ½ RD. Strip in Center
4. Lingual Plate Extensions
   Guiding Plane Plates } 24 GA. Sheet
   Cast Bases
   Full Palatal Castings
5. Indirect Retainer—10 GA ½ RD. Strip
6. Finishing Lines—12 GA ½ RD. Strip Inverted
7. Direct Retainer Arms—Molars, Large (Medium) Plastic Preformed Patterns. Premolars and Canines, Medium (Small) Preformed Plastic Patterns
8. Acrylic Resin Retention Mesh—12(14) GA ½ RD. Strip or Preformed Patterns
9. Master Cast Relief for Retention Mesh—Two 26 GA Sheets.

Fig. 18-2. This work authorization accompanies the master cast upon which *the dentist* has designed and drawn the outline for the removable partial denture framework. It is simple and nontime-consuming to execute, yet furnishes detailed information so that the request can be properly fulfilled.

ration. Therefore, a new work authorization should accompany the material returned to the laboratory for continuing progress in completing the restoration. In a modern dental practice it is highly improbable that a "one trip" laboratory service is adequate to provide a truly professional removable restoration.

No single work authorization form is adequate to furnish detailed instructions for accomplishing the laboratory phases in the construction of removable partial dentures, crowns and fixed partial dentures, and complete dentures or for accomplishing orthodontic laboratory procedures. Inherent differences in the many types of restorations themselves and differences in the laboratory phases necessary for their construction establish a requirement for individual work authorization forms.

Definitive instructions by work authorizations

Work authorizations forms may be designed so that only a minimum of writing is necessary to relay thorough instructions (Fig. 18-2). The form can contain printed listings of materials and specifications that require either a *check mark* or a *fill in* for authorizing their use.

A reminder space to designate the choice of metal for the framework is included. Frameworks for removable partial dentures are usually cast in either a type "D" gold or a chrome-cobalt alloy. The nature of the material of the denture base may be indicated by check mark. It is difficult to elicit this information from the markings on master casts.

Space is reserved on the work authorization form to furnish the technician with information on the dentist's selection of teeth. The responsibility for tooth selection must remain with the dentist. Success of the removable partial denture partly depends on the consideration given to the size, number, and placement of the denture teeth as well as the material from which they are made.

A display of courtesy deserved by, and a demonstration of respect for, the laboratory

technician are indicated. The general request is prefaced by *please* and the specific instructions are ended with *thank you*. Do any other three words promote better relations?

A good work authorization form not only assures clarity, but it also simplifies correct execution. Figures can be provided on which diagrams may be drawn to enhance written descriptions when necessary. These diagrams may show the occlusal and lingual surfaces of the posterior teeth and the lingual surfaces of the anterior teeth. The palatal region of the upper dental arch and the lingual slopes of the mandibular alveolar ridge also can be included. These features allow a clear, diagrammatic representation of the location of major connectors, which will compliment the outline of the framework on the master cast.

A color code index can be used to explain the markings on the master cast when it is submitted to the laboratory for the fabrication of a framework. A green pencil is used to outline the framework; red designates the desired location of finishing lines on the framework; and black lines denote the height of contour on teeth and soft tissues created during the survey of the cast. The color code eliminates confusion in interpreting the markings on the master cast.

Specifications for waxing the framework components for gold or chrome-cobalt alloy castings must be furnished for the technician and are an integral part of the work authorization form. Specifications that are adequate for most removable partial denture frameworks may be listed. This feature alone saves time and effort in preparing the work authorization and *is also a handy reference for the laboratory technician.* The listing of average specifications does not preclude altering a specification when the situation requires other characteristics in a given component.

The specific instructions in a work authorization must be so constructed that they will be a constant source of direction and supervision for the laboratory phases of a removable partial denture service. Instructions should leave no doubt of the dentist's requirements in a request for laboratory services. It is foolish to use undercut dimensions of 0.01 to 0.02 inch when surveying a master cast unless directions for incorporating these dimensions in the finished framework are included.

Work authorization blanks should be available in tablet form so that a carbon duplicate can be conveniently made, supplying a copy for both the dentist and the dental laboratory technician. The original may be of a different color than is the carbon copy for ready identification.

Legal aspects of work authorizations

No national statutory restrictions exist on dental laboratory operations. Regulation of dental laboratories and dental laboratory technicians is invested in the states. Fortunately, all states exercise this control.

Interpretations of acts constituting the practice of dentistry are moderately uniform. However, statutory restrictions on dental laboratory operations vary widely from state to state in stringency and requirements for legal operations.

Prosecution and conviction of persons engaged in the illegal practice of dentistry is a time-consuming and difficult proceeding. This situation could be alleviated if duly executed work authorizations were required to be presented by all dental laboratories or dental technicians on demand of a duly authorized agency.

Many states require that work authorizations be made in duplicate and that both the dentist and dental laboratory technician retain a copy for a period of two years or more from the date of the work authorization. Thus documents are available to substantiate or refute claims and counterclaims concerning the illegal practice of dentistry or to aid in the settlement of misunderstandings between a dentist and a dental laboratory technician.

Delineation of responsibilities by work authorizations

The dentist is responsible for all phases of a removable partial denture service in the strict sense of the word. He may request the dental laboratory technician to perform certain mechanical phases of the service; *however, the laboratory technician is responsible to the dentist and never to the patient.* A dentist who relegates the design of a removable partial denture to a less qualified individual immediately eliminates the opportunity for a preventive removable partial denture service.

A dentist who imposes on auxiliary personnel responsibilities that are legally and morally his own does a great injustice to his patients, his technicians, and the dental profession. There is little doubt but that the "denturist" movement and the presently existing impasse between dentist and dental laboratory organizations are due, in part, to many individual dentists imposing unrealistic responsibility on their laboratory technicians. Furthermore, this unwelcomed relationship is partly due to the submission of poor impressions, casts, records, and instructions to the laboratory technician with the demand of impossible quality in the returned restoration under threat of economic boycott.

Most dental laboratory technicians are ethical and earnestly desire to contribute their talents to the dental profession. The dental profession is vitally interested in increasing the numbers of serious-minded dental auxiliary personnel to share in providing oral health. However, until such time as the dental profession elevates itself in the eyes of laboratory technicians, and also elevates the stature of dental laboratory technology, greater availability of responsible auxiliary personnel is more fancied than real.

The dental laboratory technician is a member of a team whose objectives are the prevention of oral disease and the maintenance of oral health as adjuncts to the physical and mental well-being of the public. A good dental laboratory technician is a valuable asset to the dentist and contributes much to the team effort in providing oral health for patients. To paraphase statements by Dr. G. P. Smith, the degree and quality of the team effort is the responsibility of the dentist and depends upon his knowledge, experience, technical skill, administrative ability, integrity, and ability to communicate effectively.

Much of the technical phase of a removable partial denture service may be delegated by a dentist. Work authorizations help to fulfill the moral obligation to supervise and direct those technical phases that can be accomplished by dental laboratory technicians.

There are substantial indications that many members of the dental profession either are not cognizant of the rewards of writing good work authorizations or are not proficient in their execution. It is not a secret that some dentists submit no instructions when availing themselves of commercial dental laboratory services.

If the practice of prosthodontics is to remain in the control of dentists, each member of the dental profession must avoid delegating responsibility to those who are less qualified to accept the responsibility.

CHAPTER 19

Initial placement, adjustment, and servicing of the removable partial denture

Initial placement of the completed partial denture should never be sandwiched in between other scheduled appointments. Too often this is done in the appointment for initial placement of both complete and removable partial denture restorations. Both, being removable restorations not requiring the elaborate preparations common to the cementation of fixed restorations, can be quickly placed and the patient dismissed with instructions to return when soreness or discomfort develops. Perhaps this is where the word *patient* originated, because of the patience and fortitude required in accommodating to a new denture.

Although it is true that this is a necessary part of adjusting to new dentures, many other factors are also pertinent. Among these are how well the patient has been informed as to the mechanical and biologic problems involved in the fabrication and wearing of a removable prosthetic restoration and how much confidence he has acquired in the excellence of the finished product through his own observation of the various steps in its construction. Knowing in advance that every step has been carefully planned and executed with skill, and having acquired confidence both in the dentist and in the excellence of the restoration, the patient is better able to accept the adjustment period as a necessary, but transient, step in learning to wear the prosthesis. Much of this confidence can be dissipated when the dentist places the prosthesis with an air of finality as though to imply that "my part in the fabrication of this restoration is now completed. The rest is up to you, including payment of the fee on your way out of the office."

The term *adjustment* has two connotations, each of which must be considered separately. First is the adjustments to the bearing surfaces of the denture and the occlusion made by the dentist at the time of initial placement and thereafter. Second is the adjustment or accommodation by the patient, psychologically and biologically, to the presence of a foreign body, which is to serve as a prosthetic restoration of some missing part or parts of the body, in this particular instance, an oral prosthesis.

It must be presumed that the partial denture has been fabricated with care and that the prosthesis is representative of the best that the dentist is capable of producing. Certainly it is not within the scope of this book to suggest ways and means of adjusting a faulty designed or poorly fabricated prothesis to fit the patient's mouth. But, as in industry, a casting is rarely, if ever, considered a precision product. Certain machining operations are necessary before the casting is considered finished and acceptable. So it is with a partial denture restoration. First, the rough metal alloy casting must be finished and polished to fit an accurate stone cast of the patient's mouth. After the processing of resin bases, the occluding teeth must be altered to perfect the occlusal relationship between opposing artificial dentition or between artificial dentition and an opposing cast or template. Denture bases then must be finished to eliminate excess and to perfect the contours of polished surfaces for the best functional and esthetic result. All these are machining operations made necessary by the inadequacies of casting procedures, for actually both the metal and resin parts of a prosthetic restoration are produced by casting methods. Unfortunately, such machining operations in the laboratory rarely eliminate the need for final adjustment in the mouth, which is also, in effect, a machining process to perfect the fit of the restoration to the oral tissues.

Included in this final step in a long sequence of machining procedures necessary to produce a biologically acceptable prosthetic restoration are the adjustment of the occlusion to accommodate the occlusal rests and other metal parts of the denture, the adjustment of the bearing surfaces of the denture bases in harmony with the supporting soft tissues, and the final adjustment of occlusion on the artificial dentition to harmonize with natural occlusion in all mandibular positions.

Occlusal interference from the denture framework. Any occlusal interference from occlusal rests and other parts of the denture framework should have been eliminated prior to or during the establishment of occlusal relations. Assuming that the denture framework will have been tried in the mouth before establishing a final jaw relation, any such interference should have been detected and eliminated. *Much of this need not exist at all if mouth preparations and the design of the denture framework are carried out with a specific treatment plan in mind.* In any event, occlusal interference from the framework itself should not ordinarily require further adjustment at the time the finished denture is initially placed. *For the dentist to have sent an impression or casts of the patient's mouth to the laboratory and to receive a finished partial denture prosthesis without having once tried the cast framework in the mouth is not only a dereliction of his responsibility to the patient but is also, in effect, handing the practice of prosthetic dentistry over to the dental laboratory technician.* However, when such is done, it is obvious that occlusal interference from the casting itself must be first detected and eliminated before proceeding with other adjustments to the denture.

Adjustments to the bearing surfaces of the denture bases. The machining of bearing surfaces to perfect the fit of the denture to the supporting tissues should be accomplished by the use of some indicator paste. The paste must be one that will be readily displaced by positive tissue contact and will not adhere to the tissues of the mouth. An area of the denture base showing through the film of indicator paste may be erroneously interpreted as a pressure spot, when actually the paste had adhered to the tissues in that area. Therefore, only those areas showing through an intact film of indicator paste should be interpreted as pressure areas and be relieved accordingly.

Rather than dismiss the patient with instructions to return when soreness develops and then over-relieve the denture over a traumatized area to restore patient comfort, the use of pressure indicator paste should be routine with any tissue-bearing prosthetic restoration. The paste should be applied in a thin layer over the bearing surfaces and then both occlusal and digital pressure applied to the denture. The patient cannot be expected to apply a heavy enough force to the new denture to register all of the pressure areas present. Therefore, the dentist should apply both vertical and horizontal forces with his fingers in excess of that which might be expected of the patient. The denture is then removed and inspected. Any areas heavy enough to displace a thin film of indicator paste should be relieved and the procedure repeated with a new film of indicator until pressure areas have been eliminated.

Pressure areas most frequently encountered are as follows: in the mandibular arch—the lingual slope of the mandibular ridge in the premolar area, the mylohyoid ridge, the border extension into the retromylohyoid space, and the distobuccal border in the vicinity of the ascending ramus and the external oblique ridge; in the maxillary arch—the inside of the buccal flange of the denture over the tuberosities, the border of the denture lying at the molar prominence, and at the hamular notch where the denture may impinge on the pterygomandibular raphe or the pterygoid hamulus itself. In addition, in either arch there may be bony spicules or spicules of the denture base itself that will require specific relief.

The amount of relief by machining that will be necessary will depend upon the accuracy of the impression registration, the master cast, and the denture base. Despite the accuracy of modern impression and cast materials many denture base materials leave much to be desired in this regard, and the element of technical errors is also always present. It is therefore essential that discrepancies in the denture base be detected and corrected before the tissues of the mouth are subjected to the stress of supporting a prosthetic restoration. This is one of our major responsibilities to the patient, that trauma be always held to a minimum. *Therefore, the appointment time for the initial placement of the denture must be adequate to permit such adjustment.*

Adjustment of occlusion in harmony with natural and artificial dentition. The final step in the adjustment of the partial denture at the time of initial placement is the adjustment of the occlusion to harmonize with the natural occlusion in all mandibular excursions. When opposing partial dentures are placed concurrently, the adjustment of the occlusion will parallel, to some extent, the adjustment of occlusion on complete dentures. This is particularly true

when the few remaining natural teeth are out of occlusion. But where *one or more* natural teeth may occlude in any mandibular position, those teeth will influence mandibular movement to some extent. It is necessary, therefore, that artificial dentition on the partial denture be made to harmonize with whatever natural occlusion remains.

Occlusal adjustment of tooth-borne removable partial dentures may be performed accurately by any of several intraoral methods. *It has been our experience, however, that occlusal adjustment of distal extension removable partial dentures is accomplished more conveniently and accurately by using an articulator than by any intraoral method.* Since distal extension denture bases will exhibit some movement under a closing force, intraoral indications of occlusal discrepancies, whether by inked ribbon or disclosing waxes, are difficult to interpret. Distal extension dentures, positioned on remounting casts, can conveniently be related to the articulator with new, nonpressure interocclusal records, and the occlusion can be adjusted accurately as a laboratory procedure at the appointment for initial placement of the dentures.

The methods by which occlusal relations may be established and recorded have been discussed in Chapter 16. In this chapter the advantages of establishing a functional occlusal relationship with an intact opposing arch have been discussed and also the limitations that exist to the perfecting of harmonious occlusion on the finished prosthesis by intraoral adjustment alone. Even when the occlusion on two opposing partial dentures is being adjusted entirely in the mouth, it is best that one arch be considered an intact arch and the other one adjusted to it. This is accomplished by first eliminating any occlusal interference to mandibular movement imposed by one denture and adjusting any opposing natural dentition to accommodate to the denture teeth. Then the opposing partial denture is placed, and occlusal adjustments are made to harmonize with both the natural dentition and the opposing denture, which is now considered part of an intact dental arch. Which denture is adjusted first and which one is made to occlude with it is somewhat arbitrary, with the following exceptions: If one partial denture is entirely tooth supported and the other has a tissue-supported base, the tooth-supported denture is adjusted to final occlusion with any opposing natural teeth and then that arch is treated as an intact arch and the opposing denture adjusted to occlude with it. If both partial dentures are entirely tooth borne, the one occluding with the most natural teeth is adjusted first and the second denture then adjusted to occlude with an intact arch. Tooth-borne segments of a composite (tooth- and tissue-supported) partial denture are likewise adjusted first to harmonize with any opposing natural dentition. The final adjustment of occlusion on opposing tissue-supported bases is usually done on the mandibular denture since this is the moving member, and the occlusion is made to harmonize with the maxillary denture, which is treated as part of an intact arch.

Intraoral occlusal adjustment is accomplished by using some kind of indicator and suitable mounted points and burs. Diamond or other abrasive points must be used to reduce enamel and metal contacts. These also may be used to reduce plastic tooth surfaces, but burs may be used for plastic with greater effectiveness. Articulation paper may be used as an indicator if one recognizes that heavy interocclusal contacts may become perforated, leaving only a light mark, while secondary contacts, being lighter and frequently sliding, may make a heavier mark. Although articulation ribbon does not become perforated, it is not easy to use in the mouth, and the differentiation between primary and secondary contacts is difficult to ascertain.

In general, occlusal adjustment of multiple contacts between natural and/or artificial dentition when tooth-borne partial dentures are involved follows the same principles as those for natural dentition alone.

This is because the partial dentures are retained by devices attached to the abutment teeth, whereas with complete dentures no mechanical retainers are present. The use of more than one color of articulation paper or ribbon to record and differentiate between centric and eccentric contacts is just as helpful in adjusting partial denture occlusion as natural occlusion, and for the initial adjustment this method may be used.

For final adjustment, however, since one denture will be adjusted to occlude with an intact arch, the use of an occlusal wax may be necessary to establish points of excessive contact and interference. This cannot be done by articulation paper alone. An occlusal wax, such as Kerr occlusal indicator, which is adhesive on one side, or strips of 28-gauge Kerr green casting wax or other similar soft wax, may be used. It should always be used bilaterally, with two strips folded together at the midline. Thus the patient is not as likely to deviate to one side as he is when wax is introduced unilaterally. (See Fig. 19-1.)

For centric contacts, the patient is guided to tap into the wax and then the wax is removed and inspected under transillumination for perforations. All perforated areas are either premature contacts or excessive contacts and must be adjusted. One of two methods may be used to locate specific areas to be relieved. Articulation ribbon may be used to mark the occlusion, and then those marks representing areas of excessive contact are identified by referring to the wax record and are relieved accordingly. A second method is to introduce the wax strips a second time, this time adapting them to the buccal and lingual surfaces for retention. After having the patient tap into the wax, perforated areas are marked with waterproof pencil. The wax is then stripped off and the penciled areas are relieved. This procedure has been outlined in some detail by Jankelson.

Whichever method is used, it must be repeated until occlusal balance in centric occlusion has been established and more uniform contacts without perforations are

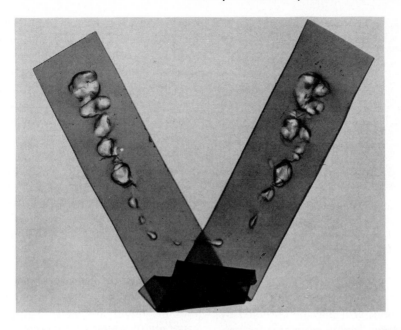

Fig. 19-1. Two strips of 28-gauge soft green (casting) wax are placed in the mouth between opposing dentition. These are first folded over anteriorly to unite the two halves, and then the patient is guided to tap in centric occlusion two or three times. Viewed out of the mouth, against a source of light, uniform contacts free of perforations may be considered to be simultaneous contacts. Perforations in the wax represent occlusal prematurities that should be relieved. The accuracy of this method or any other intraoral method is dependent not only upon the dentist's interpretation of marks (perforations) but also on the stability of denture bases.

evident from a final interocclusal wax record. After adjustment in centric occlusion has been completed, Jankelson suggests that the patient should be asked to "open and eat the wax lightly" several times. Any remaining areas of interference are then reduced, thus assuring that there is no interference during the chewing stroke. Adjustments to relieve interference during the chewing stroke should be confined to buccal surfaces of mandibular teeth and lingual surfaces of maxillary teeth. This serves to narrow the cusps so that they will go all the way into the opposing sulci without wedging as they travel into centric contact. Skinner proposed that the patient be given a small bite of soft banana to chew rather than to expect him to chew without food actually being present. The small bolus of banana promotes normal functional activity of the chewing mechanism, yet by its soft consistency does not itself cause indenta-

tions in the soft wax. Any interfering contacts encountered during the chewing stroke are thus detected as perforations in the wax, which are marked with pencil and relieved accordingly.

Kyes has described some of the advantages to be had with an alginate interocclusal record, supplementing or replacing the use of soft wax strips for this purpose (Fig. 19-2). An alginate hydrocolloid impression material is applied to the occlusal surfaces of the mandibular teeth, and the patient is asked to bring the teeth together, as previously rehearsed, until the first point of contact is made. This occlusion is then held until the material has set. The gelled hydrocolloid is carefully removed from the open mouth and the excess carefully trimmed away with scissors; it is then dropped into a plaster bowl of water until it has become firmer and easier to handle without tearing. This record of occlusion

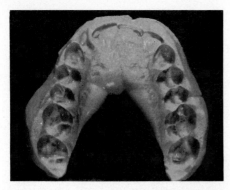

Fig. 19-2. Alginate hydrocolloid interocclusal record. Perforations in the alginate are interpreted as areas of hyperocclusion. These are then located on the teeth with articulating ribbon and relieved accordingly.

may be observed in water with a dark bowl as a background, or it may be observed by transillumination. In any case, areas of prematurity may be seen as perforations in the alginate and the overall areas of occlusal contact interpreted for evidence of hyperocclusion. Occlusal adjustment may then proceed, using either articulating ribbon or perforations in suitable wax strips as a specific indication of areas to be relieved.

This method is primarily diagnostic and is usually supplemented by the use of articulating ribbon or occlusal wax. However, it has definite advantages over the latter two as a diagnostic aid because the impression materials offer no resistance to closure. Further, because of its soft consistency and because it is applied over all occluding surfaces simultaneously, a natural stimulus to closure is effected. This method may be used effectively between a natural, artificial, or mixed dentition.

Adjustments to occlusion should be repeated at a reasonable interval after the dentures have reached a point of equilibrium and the musculature has become adjusted to the changes brought about by restoration of occlusal contacts. This second occlusal adjustment usually may be considered sufficient until such time as tissue-supported denture bases no longer support the occlusion and corrective measures, either by reoccluding the teeth or relining

the denture, must be employed. However, a periodic recheck of occlusion at intervals of six months is advisable to avoid traumatic interference resulting from changes in denture support or tooth migration.

After the adjustment of occlusion, the anatomy of the artificial teeth should be restored to maximum efficiency by restoring grooves and spillways (food escapeways) and by narrowing the teeth buccolingually to increase the sharpness of the cusps and reduce the width of the food table. Mandibular buccal and maxillary lingual surfaces in particular should be narrowed to assure that these areas will not interfere with closure into the opposing sulci. Since artificial teeth used on partial dentures opposing natural or restored dentition should always be considered *material* out of which a harmonious occlusal surface is created, final adjustment of the occlusion always should be followed by the meticulous restoration of the most functional occlusal anatomy possible. Although this may be done after a subsequent occlusal adjustment at a later date, the possibility that the patient may fail to return on schedule is always present and, in the meantime, broad and inefficient occlusal surfaces may cause an overloading of the supporting structures, which would be traumatogenic. Therefore, the restoration of an efficient occlusal anatomy is an essential part of the denture adjustment at the time of placement. Again, this requires that sufficient time be allotted for the initial placement of the partial denture to permit all necessary occlusal corrections to be accomplished.

Instructions to the patient. Finally, before dismissing the patient, the difficulties that may be encountered and the care that must be given the prosthesis and the abutment teeth must be reviewed with the patient.

The patient should be advised that he will probably experience some discomfort or minor annoyance initially. Whereas this is to some extent due to the presence of bulk, which the tongue in particular must become accustomed to, any strange object, however comfortable, must be accepted biologically and psychologically before it can become an integral part of the oral mechanism.

The patient must be advised also of the possibility of soreness developing despite every attempt on the part of the dentist to prevent its occurrence. Since patients vary widely in their ability to tolerate discomfort, it is perhaps best to advise every patient as though soreness is inevitable, with every assurance that any needed adjustments will be made. On the other hand, the dentist himself should be aware of the fact that some patients are unable to accommodate ever to the presence of a removable prosthesis. Fortunately, these are few in any practice. However the dentist must avoid any positive statements that might be interpreted or construed by the patient to be positive assurance tantamount to a guarantee that he will be able to use the prosthesis with comfort and acceptance. Too much depends upon the patient's ability to accept a foreign object and to tolerate reasonable pressures to make such assurance possible.

Discussing phonetics with the patient in regard to his new dentures may indicate that this is a unique problem to be overcome because of the influence of the prosthesis on speech. With few exceptions, which are usually due to excessive and avoidable bulk in the denture design or to improper placement of teeth and the contour of denture bases, the average patient will experience little difficulty in wearing the partial denture. Most of the hindrances to normal speech will disappear in a few days.

Similarly, perhaps little or nothing should be said to the patient about the possibility of gagging or the tongue's reaction to a foreign object. Most patients will experience little or no difficulty in this regard, and the tongue will normally accept smooth, nonbulky contours without objection. Contours that are too thick, too bulky, or improperly placed should be avoided in the construction of the denture, but, if present, these should be detected and eliminated at the time of placement of the denture. The dentist should palpate the prosthesis in the mouth and reduce excessive bulk accordingly before the patient has an opportunity to object to it. The area most frequently needing thinning is the distolingual flange of the mandibular denture. Here the denture flange should almost always be thinned during the finishing and polishing of the denture base. Sublingually, the denture flange should be reproduced as recorded in the impression, but distal to the second molar the flange should be trimmed somewhat thinner. Then, upon placing the denture, the dentist should palpate this area to ascertain that a minimum of bulk exists that might be encountered by the side and base of the tongue. If this needs further reduction, it should be done and the denture repolished before dismissing the patient.

The patient should be advised of the need for keeping the dentures and the abutment teeth meticulously clean. If cariogenic processes are to be prevented, the accumulation of debris should be avoided as much as possible, particularly around abutment teeth and beneath minor connectors. Furthermore, inflammation of gingival tissues is prevented by removing accumulated debris and by substituting toothbrush massage for the normal stimulation of tongue and food contact with areas that will be covered by the denture framework.

The mouth and partial denture should be cleaned after eating and before retiring. Brushing before breakfast also may be effective in reducing the bacterial count, which may help to lessen acid formation in the caries-susceptible individual after eating. A partial denture may be effectively cleaned by the use of a small, stiff-bristle brush. Debris may be effectively removed through the use of dentifrices, since they contain the essential elements for cleaning. Household cleaners should not be used because they are too abrasive for use on resin surfaces. The patient, and the elderly or handicapped patient in particular, should be advised to clean the denture over a basin partially filled with water so that the fall will be broken if the denture is dropped accidentally during cleaning.

In addition to brushing with a dentifrice, additional cleaning may be accomplished by the use of a solvent cleaning solution such as D.O.C. (denture oxygen cleanser) or a solution made of one part Clorox to two parts Calgon. The patient should be advised to soak the dentures in the solution for fifteen minutes once daily, followed by a thorough brushing with a dentifrice.

In some mouths, the precipitation of salivary calculus on the partial denture necessitates the taking of extra measures for its removal. Such patients may need to be provided with a small bottle of Taxi liquid stain detergent, with instructions to apply the solution to the denture at weekly intervals to dissolve the accumulated calculus. The Taxi should be used on the denture only when it is out of the mouth and then the denture should be rinsed thoroughly before returning it to the mouth.

Since many patients will dine away from home, the informed patient should provide some means of carrying out midday oral hygiene. Simply rinsing the partial denture and the mouth with water after eating is beneficial if brushing is not possible.

Opinion is divided on the question of whether or not a partial denture should be worn during sleep. Conditions should determine the advice given the patient, *although generally the tissues should be allowed to rest by removing the denture at night.* In such a case, the denture should be placed in a container and covered with water to prevent its dehydration, with subsequent dimensional change. About the only situation that possibly justifies the wearing of partial dentures at night is when stresses generated by bruxism would be more destructive since they then would be concentrated on fewer teeth. Broader distribution of the stress load, plus the splinting effect of the partial denture, may

make the wearing of the denture at night advisable. However, an individual, latex rubber mouth protector should be worn at night until the cause of the bruxism is eliminated.

There occurs frequently the question of whether an opposing complete denture should be worn when a partial denture in the other arch is out of the mouth. The answer is that if the partial denture is to be removed at night, the opposing complete denture should not be left in the mouth. There is no more certain way of destroying the alveolar ridge, which supports a maxillary complete denture, than to have it occlude with a few remaining anterior mandibular teeth.

After all necessary adjustments to the partial denture have been made and the patient has been advised as to the proper care of the denture, he must also be advised as to the future care of the mouth to ensure health and longevity of the remaining structures. How often the mouth and denture should be examined by the dentist depends upon the oral and physical condition of the patient. If the patient is caries-susceptible or has tendencies toward periodontal disease or alveolar atrophy, his mouth should be examined more frequently. Every six months should be the rule if conditions are normal. At least once a year a roentgenographic examination should supplement clinical examination and oral prophylaxis.

The need for increasing retention on clasp arms to make the denture more secure will depend upon the type of clasp that has been used. Increasing retention should be accomplished by adjusting the clasp arm to engage a deeper part of the retention undercut rather than by bending the clasp in toward the tooth. The latter creates only frictional retention, which violates the principle of clasp retention. Being an active force, such retention contributes to tooth and/or restoration movement in a horizontal direction, disappearing only when either the tooth has been moved or the clasp arm returns to a *passive* relationship with the abutment tooth. Unfortunately, this is almost the only adjustment that can be made to a half-round cast clasp arm. On the other hand, the round wrought-wire clasp arm may be adjusted cervically and brought into a deeper part of the retentive undercut. Thus the passivity of the clasp arm in its terminal position is maintained, but retention is increased by its being forced to flex more to withdraw from the deeper undercut. The patient should be advised that the abutment tooth and the clasp will serve longer if the retention is held to a minimum, which is only that amount necessary to resist reasonable dislodging forces.

Denture rocking or looseness developing in the future may be due to a change in the form of the supporting ridges rather than to a lack of retention. This should be detected as early as possible after it occurs and corrected by relining or rebasing. The loss of tissue support is usually so gradual that the patient may be unable to detect the need for relining. This usually must be determined by the dentist at subsequent examinations as evidenced by rotation of the distal extension denture about the fulcrum line. If the partial denture is opposed by natural dentition, the loss of base support causes a loss of occlusal contact, which may be detected by having the patient close upon wax strips placed bilaterally. If, however, a complete denture or distal extension partial denture opposes the partial denture, the interocclusal wax test is not dependable since occlusal contact may have been maintained by posterior closure, changes in the temporomandibular joint, and/or migration of the opposing denture. In such case, evidence of loss of ridge support is determined solely by the indirect retainer leaving its seat as the distal extension denture rotates about the fulcrum line.

No assurance can be given to the patient that uncrowned abutment teeth will not decay at some future time. Even with full cast crowns, there can be no positive assurance that the tooth will not ever decay gingival to the crown, as a result of gingival recession and caries attack of exposed cementum. The patient can be assured, however, that prophylactic measures in the form of meticulous oral hygiene and the avoidance of carbohydrates, coupled with routine care by the dentist, will be rewarded by greater health and longevity of the remaining teeth.

The patient should be advised that maximum service may be expected from the partial denture if he observes the following rules:

1. Avoid careless handling of the denture, which may lead to distortion or breakage. Damage to the partial denture occurs while it is out of the mouth, as a result of dropping it during cleaning or an accident occurring when the denture is not being worn. Fractured teeth and denture bases can be repaired, as can broken clasp arms, but a distorted framework can rarely, if ever, be satisfactorily readapted or repaired.

2. Teeth should be protected from caries by proper oral hygiene, proper diet, and frequent dental care. The teeth will be no less susceptible to caries when a partial denture is being worn but may be more so because of the retention of debris. At the same time, the remaining teeth have become all the more important as a result of oral rehabilitation, and abutment teeth have become even more valuable because of their importance to the success of the partial denture. Therefore, the need for a rigid regime of *oral hygiene, diet control, and periodic clinical observation and treatment* is essential to the future health of the entire mouth. *Also the patient must be more conscientious about responding to being recalled at stated intervals by the dentist for examination and necessary treatment.*

3. Periodontal damage to the abutment teeth can be avoided by maintaining tissue support of any distal extension bases. As a result of periodic examination this can be detected and corrected by relining or whatever procedure is indicated.

4. Partial denture treatment must be accepted as something that cannot be considered permanent but must receive regular and continuous care by both the patient and the dentist. The obligations for maintaining caries control and for returning at stated intervals for treatment must be clearly understood, as well as the fact that regular charges will be made by the dentist for whatever treatment is rendered.

The partial denture patient should not be dismissed as completed without at least one subsequent appointment for observation and minor adjustment if needed. This should be made at an interval of twenty-four hours after initial placement of the denture. It need not be a lengthy appointment but should be made as a definite rather than a drop-in appointment. Not only does this give the patient assurance that any necessary adjustments will be made and provide the dentist with an opportunity to check on the patient's acceptance of the prosthesis but it also avoids giving the patient any idea that he may break into the dentist's schedule at will and serves to give notice that an appointment is necessary for future adjustments.

CHAPTER 20

Relining and rebasing the removable partial denture

Differentiation between relining and rebasing has been discussed previously in Chapter 1. Briefly, *relining* is the resurfacing of a denture base with new material to make it fit the underlying tissues more accurately, whereas *rebasing* is the replacement of a denture base with new material without changing the occlusal relations of the teeth.

In either case, a new impression registration is necessary, using the existing denture base as an impression tray for either a close-mouth or an open-mouth impression procedure. One of several types of impression materials may be used. The impression may be made with a metallic oxide impression paste, with one of the rubber-base or silicone impression materials, with an activated resin used as an impression material, or with a mouth-temperature wax.

In making the decision between a closed-mouth and an open-mouth impression method for relining, one must first consider the reasons for doing so and the objectives to be obtained. Again, it is necessary to differentiate between the two basic types of partial dentures, one being the all-tooth-borne restoration and the other being the tooth-and-tissue-supported restoration.

RELINING TOOTH-BORNE DENTURE AREAS

When total abutment support is available, but for one reason or another a re-movable partial denture has been the restoration of choice, support for that restoration is derived entirely from the abutment teeth at each end of each edentulous span. This support is effective through the use of occlusal rests, boxlike internal rests, internal attachments, and/or supporting ledges on abutment restorations. Except for intrusion of abutment teeth under functional stress, settling of the restoration toward the tissues of the residual ridge is prevented by the supporting abutments. Tissue changes occurring beneath tooth-borne denture bases does not affect the support of the denture and therefore relining or rebasing is usually done for other reasons. These are (1) unhygienic conditions and the trapping of debris between the denture and the residual ridge, (2) an unsightly condition due to the space that has developed, and/or (3) patient discomfort associated with lack of tissue contact arising from open spaces between the denture base and the tissues. Anteriorly, some loss of support beneath a denture base may lead to some denture movement, despite occlusal support and direct retainers located posteriorly. Rebasing might be the treatment of choice if the artificial teeth are to be replaced or rearranged, or if the denture base needs to be replaced for esthetic reasons or because it has become defective.

For either relining or rebasing to be accomplished, the original denture base must have been made of a resin material that can be relined or replaced. Frequently, tooth-borne partial denture bases are made of metal as part of the cast framework. These cannot be satisfactorily relined, although they may sometimes be altered by drastic grinding to provide mechanical retention for the attachment of an entirely new resin base. Ordinarily, a metal base, with its several advantages, is not used in a tooth-borne area in which early tissue changes are anticipated. A metal base should not be used after recent extractions or other surgery, nor for a long span when relining to provide secondary tissue support may become necessary. (A distal extension metal base is ordinarily used only when a partial denture is being made over tissues that have become conditioned to supporting a previous denture base.)

Since the tooth-borne denture base cannot be depressed beyond its terminal position with the occlusal rests seated and the teeth in occlusion, and since it cannot rotate about a fulcrum, a closed-mouth impression method is used. Virtually any impression material may be used, provided sufficient space is allowed beneath the denture base to permit the excess material to flow to the borders, at which it is either turned by the bordering tissues or, as in the palate, allowed to escape through holes without unduly displacing the underlying tissues. The qualities of each type of impression material must be kept in mind when selecting the material to be used for this purpose. Ordinarily, an impression material is used that will record the anatomic form of the oral tissues.

A word should be said in favor of relining a tooth-borne resin base with one of the immediate reline materials, such as Durbase or Self-Set. When one or more relatively short spans are to be relined the making of an impression for that purpose requires that the denture be flasked and processed. The possibilities of an increased vertical dimension of occlusion resulting and the denture becoming distorted during laboratory procedures must be weighed

against the disadvantages of using a direct reline material. Fortunately these materials are constantly being improved with greater predictability and color stability. The possibility that the original denture base will become crazed or distorted by the action of the activated monomer is relatively nonexistent when the base is made of modern cross-linked resin. However, for this reason earlier resin bases should not be subjected to relining with direct reline resins.

When relining in the mouth with a resin reline material is done with a definite technique, the results can be quite satisfactory, with complete bonding to the existing denture base, good color stability, and with permanence and accuracy. The procedure for applying a direct reline of an existing resin base is as follows:

1. Relieve generously the tissue side of the denture base and just over the borders. This not only provides space for an adequate thickness of new material but also eliminates the possibility of tissue impingement because of confinement of the material.

2. Apply masking or adhesive tape over the polished surfaces from the relieved border to the occlusal surfaces of the teeth.

3. Mix the powder and liquid in a glass jar according to the proportions recommended by the manufacturer. First stir red fibers into the monomer, if not already incorporated into the powder, according to the color characteristics of the base being relined.

4. While the material is reaching the desired consistency, have the patient rinse the mouth with cold water. At the same time, wipe the fresh surfaces of the dried denture base with a cotton pellet saturated with some of the monomer. This facilitates bonding and makes sure that the surface is free of any contamination.

5. When the material has first begun to take on some body, but while still quite fluid, apply it to the tissue side of the denture base and over the borders. Immediately place the denture in the mouth in its terminal position and have the patient close

into occlusion. Then, with the mouth open, manipulate the cheeks to turn the excess at the border and establish harmony with bordering attachments. If a mandibular denture is being relined, have the patient move the tongue into each cheek and then against the anterior teeth to establish a functional lingual border. It is necessary that the direct retainers be effective to prevent displacement of the denture while molding of the borders is accomplished. Otherwise the denture must be held in its terminal position with finger pressure on the occlusal surfaces.

6. Immediately remove the denture from the mouth and with fine curved iris scissors trim away gross excess material and any material that has flowed onto proximal tooth surfaces and other components of the denture framework. While this is being done, have the patient again rinse the mouth with cold water. Then replace the denture in its terminal position, bringing the teeth into occlusion. Then repeat the border movements with the mouth open. By this time or soon thereafter the material will have become firm enough to maintain its form out of the mouth.

7. Remove the denture, rinse quickly in water, and dry the relined surface with compressed air. Apply a generous coating of glycerine or Tect-ol with a brush or cotton pellet to prevent frosting of the surface because of evaporation of monomer. The material is then allowed to bench cure, thus eliminating patient discomfort and tissue damage from exothermic heat or prolonged contact with raw monomer. Although it is preferable that twenty to thirty minutes elapse before trimming and polishing, it may be done as soon as the material hardens. The masking tape must be removed before trimming but should be replaced over the teeth and polished surfaces below the junction of the new and old materials to protect those surfaces during final polishing.

Properly done, a direct reline is entirely acceptable for most tooth-borne partial denture bases made of a resin material except when some tissue support is desired for long spans between abutment teeth. In the latter case, a reline impression in wax may be accomplished, the denture then flasked, and a processed reline added for optimal tissue contact and support.

RELINING DISTAL EXTENSION PARTIAL DENTURE BASES

A distal extension partial denture, deriving its major support from the tissues of the residual ridge, requires relining much more frequently than tooth-supported denture areas. Because of this, distal extension bases are usually made of a resin material that can be relined to compensate for loss of support because of tissue changes. Whereas tooth-supported areas are relined for other reasons, the sole reason for relining a distal extension base is to reestablish tissue support for that base.

The need for relining a distal extension base is determined by evaluating the stability and occlusion at reasonable intervals after initial placement of the denture. Prior to the time of initial placement, the patient must be advised that periodic examination and also relining when it becomes necessary are imperative and that the success of the partial denture and the health of the remaining tissues and abutment teeth depends upon periodic examination and servicing of both the denture and the abutment teeth. The patient also should be told that a charge will be made in proportion to the treatment required.

There are two indications of the need for relining a distal extension partial denture base. First, a loss of occlusal contact between opposing dentures or between the denture and opposing natural dentition may be evident. This is determined by having the patient close on two strips of 28-gauge soft green or blue (casting) wax. If occlusal contact between artificial dentition is weak or lacking while the remaining natural teeth in opposition are making firm contact, the distal extension denture needs to have occlusion reestablished on the present base either by altering the occlusion or by reestablishing the original position of the denture framework and base and sometimes both. In most instances, reestablishing the original relationship of the denture is necessary and the occlusion will automatically be reestablished.

Second, a loss of tissue support causing rotation and settling of the distal extension base or bases is obvious when alternate finger pressure is applied on either side of the fulcrum line. Although checking for occlusal contact alone may be misleading, such rotation is positive proof that relining is necessary. If occlusal inadequacy is detected without any evidence of denture rotation toward the residual ridge, all that needs be done is to reestablish occlusal contact by rearranging the teeth or by adding to the occlusal surfaces with resin or cast gold onlays. On the other hand, if occlusal contact is adequate but denture rotation can be demonstrated, it is usually due to migration or extrusion of opposing teeth or to a shift in position of an opposing maxillary denture, thus maintaining occlusal contact at the expense of the stability and tissue support of that denture. This is frequently the situation when a partial denture is opposed by a maxillary complete denture. It is not unusual for a patient to complain of looseness of the maxillary complete denture and request relining of that denture when actually it is the partial denture that needs relining. Relining and thus repositioning the partial denture results in repositioning of the maxillary complete denture with a return of stability and retention in that denture. Therefore, evidence of rotation of a distal extension partial denture about the fulcrum line must be the deciding factor as to whether or not relining needs to be done.

Rotation tissueward about the fulcrum line always results in a lifting of the indirect retainer(s). The framework of any distal extension partial denture must be in its original terminal position with indirect retainers fully seated during and at the end of any relining procedure. Any possibility of rotation about the ful-

crum line because of occlusal influence must be prevented, and therefore the framework must be held in its original terminal position during the time the impression is being made. This all but eliminates the practicability of using a closed-mouth impression procedure effectively when relining unilateral or bilateral distal extension bases. Steffel has outlined in detail one procedure for making a functional reline impression (see Chapter 15). The use of posterior stops of modeling plastic does not entirely eliminate the possibility of tissue displacement and denture rotation occurring when the mouth is closed and the teeth are in occlusion. Although adjusting the occlusion helps to prevent such rotation when the final impression is being made, one cannot always be sure that some rotation and lifting of the indirect retainers does not occur.

The only sure method, therefore, of making a reline impression for a distal extension partial denture is with an open-mouth procedure done in exactly the same manner as the original secondary impression. The denture to be relined is first relieved generously on the tissue side and then is treated the same as the original impression base for a functional impression. The step-by-step procedure is the same, with the dentist's three fingers placed on the two principal occlusal rests and at a third point between, preferably at an indirect retainer farthest from the axis of rotation. The framework is thus returned to its original terminal position, with all tooth-supported components fully seated. The tissues beneath the distal extension base are then registered in a relationship to the original position of the denture that will assure (1) the denture framework being returned to its intended relationship with the supporting teeth, (2) the reestablishment of optimal tissue support for the distal extension base, and (3) the restoration of the original occlusal relationship with the opposing teeth.

Although it is true that the teeth are not allowed to come into occlusion during an open-mouth impression procedure, the original position of the denture is positively determined by its relationship with the supporting abutment teeth. Since this is the relationship upon which the original occlusion was established, returning the denture to that position should bring about a return to the original occlusal relationship if two conditions are satisfied. First of these is that the laboratory procedures during relining must be done accurately without any increase in vertical dimension. This is essential with any reline procedure, but particularly with a partial denture because any change in vertical dimension will prevent occlusal rests from seating and will result in overloading and trauma to the underlying tissues. The second condition is that the opposing teeth have not extruded or migrated or that the position of an opposing denture has not become irreversibly altered. In the latter situation some adjustment of the occlusion will be necessary, but this should be deferred until the opposing teeth or denture and the structures associated with the temporomandibular joint have had a chance to return to their original position before denture settling occurred. One of the greatest satisfactions of a job well done is to be found in the execution of an open-mouth reline procedure as described above, which results in the restoration not only of the original denture relationship and tissue support but the original occlusal relationship as well.

In rare instances, after the relining of a distal extension partial denture by this method, the occlusion is found to be negative rather than positive or the same as it was before relining. This may be due to wear of occlusal surfaces over a period of time, to the original occlusion being high with resulting depression of opposing teeth, or to other reasons. In such case, occlusion on the denture must be restored to reestablish an even distribution of occlusal loading over both natural and artificial dentition. Otherwise, the natural dentition must carry the burden of mastication unaided, and the

denture becomes only a space-filling or cosmetic device.

METHODS OF REESTABLISHING OCCLUSION ON A RELINED PARTIAL DENTURE

Occlusion on a relined partial denture may be reestablished by one of several methods.

One method involves making a remounting cast, as previously described, and correctly relating the opposing casts to an articulator. The articulator then may be adjusted by interocclusal records. If the artificial teeth to be corrected are acrylic resin, the occlusion can be reestablished either by adding autopolymerizing acrylic resin to occlusal surfaces or by fabricating gold occlusal surfaces, which can be attached to the original replaced teeth. The original teeth also may be removed from the denture base and replaced by new teeth arranged to harmonize with the opposing occlusal surfaces. Baseplate wax may be used to support the teeth as they are being arranged. The wax should be carved to restore the lingual anatomy of the teeth and the portion of the denture base that was eliminated when the original teeth were removed. A stone matrix is made covering the occlusal and lingual surfaces of the teeth and denture flange. Then wax may be removed from the denture base and teeth. Those areas on the stone matrix, intimate to the new acrylic resin to be added, should be painted with a tin-foil substitute. The new teeth are placed in the stone matrix, and the matrix is accurately attached to the denture base with sticky wax. Autopolymerizing acrylic resin is then used to attach the teeth and is conveniently sprinkled on by a buccal approach. The buccal surface of the denture base adjacent to the teeth should be overfilled slightly so that the correct shape may be restored to this portion of the base during finishing and polishing procedures. Occlusal discrepancies as a result of this procedure should be corrected on the articulator by new jaw relation records if the denture involved has a distal extension base.

Another method is to remove the original teeth and replace them with a hard inlay wax occlusion rim upon which a functional registration of occlusal pathways is then established (Chapter 16). Either the original teeth or new teeth may then be arranged to occlude with the template thus obtained and subsequently attached to the denture base with processed or self-curing resin. If the latter is used, the need for flasking may be eliminated by securing the teeth to a stone matrix while the resin attachment is applied with a brush technique. Regardless of the method used for reattaching the teeth, the occlusion thus established should require little adjustment in the mouth and should be typical of the occlusal harmony that is possible by this method.

The third method is a functional method obtained by establishing occlusal pathways in wax, but it results in cast gold onlays being cemented to the original replacement teeth. Recesses must be ground into the occlusal surfaces that are to be restored, and some lubricant must be used to ensure removal of the wax patterns. A hard inlay wax is used to record functional occlusion in all excursions, preferably over a period of twenty-four hours or more. The wax record is then carved as for full coverage inlay patterns, except that they are left in one piece for all adjacent teeth. Some occlusal anatomy should be carved into the patterns to provide escapeways and promote greater efficiency and less occlusal loading than do the broad occlusal contacts registered in wax. The inlays are then cast in a B-type gold and cemented to the denture teeth.

Tissue conditioning prior to relining a partial denture base. Distal extension partial denture bases frequently need relining within a few months because of initial tissue changes after the placement of a first partial denture. This is not usually observed when the patient has been wearing a previous partial denture. Applegate has shown the beneficial effects of a treatment base prior to completion of the final base. Whether as a result of wearing a treatment base or a previous partial denture, gross tissue changes are not as likely to occur once the tissues have become conditioned to supporting a denture base.

There has been much interest in the use of fluid resins for tissue-conditioning purposes prior to relining a complete denture. This is due to the stabilizing effect of a soft resin reline rather than to any medicinal action of the treatment material. It has been clearly shown that tissues that are unhealthy and edematous because of an ill-fitting denture base may be returned to a normal, healthy state by repeated applications of a soft relining material in conjunction with sound prosthodontic principles.

Tissues under a partial denture base generally remain healthy because of the supporting and stabilizing effect of the denture framework. Therefore, treatment with tissue-conditioning material is not usually indicated if the denture can be conveniently removed from the mouth for varying periods prior to relining. On the other hand, utilizing one of the tissue treatment materials for stabilizing the denture is indicated —but only for treatment purposes. These are not meant to be impression materials, nor can they provide the support necessary to restore the proper relationship of the denture framework to the supporting teeth. An open-mouth relining procedure as outlined previously in the chapter should follow any tissue treatment procedures. However, all restorations to be relined should remain out of the mouth twenty-four hours prior to the relining procedure to permit the tissues to return to as near a normal state as possible.

CHAPTER 21

Repairs and additions to removable partial dentures

Inevitably, the need for repairing or adding to a partial denture will occasionally arise. However, the frequency of this occurring should be held to a minimum by careful diagnosis, intelligent treatment planning, adequate mouth preparations, and carrying out an effective partial denture design with all component parts properly constructed. Any need for repairs or additions will then be due to unforeseen complications arising in abutment or other teeth in the arch or to breakage or distortion of the denture through accident or careless handling by the patient rather than to faulty design or construction.

It is important that the patient be instructed in the proper placement and removal of the restoration so that undue strain is not placed upon clasp arms or other parts of the denture nor upon the abutment teeth contacted. The patient also should be advised that care must be given the restoration when it is out of the mouth and that distortion occurring due to careless handling may be irreparable. It should be made clear that there can be no guarantee against breakage or distortion occurring from causes other than obvious structural defects.

CLASSIFICATION OF REPAIRS AND ADDITIONS

Repairs and additions to partial dentures may be classified according to the cause of occurrence—broken clasp arms, broken occlusal rests, distortion or breakage of other components, loss of an additional tooth, and miscellaneous causes.

Broken clasp arms. There are several reasons for breakage.

1. Breakage may result from repeated flexure into and out of too severe an undercut. If the periodontal support is greater than the fatigue limit of the clasp arm, failure of the metal occurs first; otherwise, the abutment tooth is loosened and eventually lost due to the persistent strain placed upon it. This type of breakage can be avoided by locating clasp arms only where an acceptable minimum of retention exists, as determined by an accurate survey of the master cast. The amount of retention is predictable only by the proper utilization of guiding planes during placement and removal.

2. Breakage may occur due to structural failure of the clasp arm itself. A cast clasp arm that is not uniformly tapered because the pattern was not properly formed or because of careless finishing and polishing will eventually break at its weakest point because of repeated flexure at that point. This can be avoided by providing a uniform taper to flexible retentive clasp arms and uniform bulk to all rigid nonretentive clasp arms.

Wrought-wire clasp arms may eventually fail because of repeated flexure at the point at which a nick or constriction occurred due to careless use of the contouring pliers. They also may break at the point of origin from the casting because of excessive manipulation during initial adaptation to the tooth or subsequent readaptation. The latter can best be avoided by cautioning the patient against repeatedly lifting the clasp arm away from the tooth by application of the fingernail during removal of the denture. A wrought-wire clasp arm can normally be adjusted several times over a period of years without failure. It is only when the number of adjustments are excessive that breakage is likely to occur.

Wrought-wire clasp arms also may break at the point of origin because of crystallization of the metal. This usually occurs during initial adaptation or soon after completion of the restoration. It can be prevented by proper selection of the wrought wire used and by avoiding too high burnout and casting temperatures when a cast-to method is used. When the wrought wire is attached to the framework by soldering, as must be done with all but one of the chromium-cobalt alloys, the soldering technique must avoid crystallization of the wire. For this reason, it is best that soldering be done electrically to prevent overheating the wrought wire.

3. Breakage may occur due to careless handling by the patient. Any clasp arm will become distorted or will break if subjected to excessive abuse by the patient. The most common cause of failure of a cast clasp arm is distortion caused by accidentally dropping the denture into the lavatory basin or onto other hard surfaces. The most common cause of failure of a wrought-wire clasp is due to repeated readjustment made necessary by the patient lifting improperly against the wrought wire during removal of the denture. This is avoided by instructing the patient before a mirror in how to remove the denture without distorting the wrought-wire clasp arms. Removal should be accomplished by lifting against some other part of the framework or at the point of origin of the wrought-wire clasp arm

rather than along its course. It is also avoided by placing wrought-wire clasp arms on the lingual surface of abutment teeth whenever possible, where they are inaccessible to the fingernail during removal.

Broken occlusal rests. Breakage of an occlusal rest almost always occurs at the point at which it crosses the marginal ridge, because of weakness at this point. Improperly prepared occlusal rest seats are usually the cause of such weakness, because an occlusal rest crossing a marginal ridge that was not lowered sufficiently during mouth preparations is either made too thin or is thinned by adjustment in the mouth to avoid occlusal interference. Failure of an occlusal rest is rarely due to a structural defect in the metal and rarely if ever due to accidental distortion. Therefore, the blame for such failure must frequently be assumed by the dentist for not having provided sufficient space during mouth preparations for the placement of an occlusal rest of adequate bulk.

Distortion or breakage of other components, such as major and minor connectors. Assuming that these components were made with adequate bulk originally, distortion can occur only from abuse by the patient. All such components should be designed and fabricated with sufficient bulk to assure their rigidity and permanace of form under normal circumstaces. In such case, any distortion or breakage occurring when the restoration is out of the mouth is then the fault and obligation of the patient, the dentist's responsibility being limited to its repair or replacement at a reasonable fee.

Major and minor connectors occasionally become weakened by adjustment to avoid or eliminate tissue impingement. Such adjustment at the time of initial placement is due to inadequate survey of the master cast or to faulty design or fabrication of the casting. This is inexcusable and reflects upon the dentist, and such a restoration should be remade rather than weaken the restoration by attempting to compensate for its inadequacies by relieving the metal. Similarly, tissue impingement arising from inadequately relieved components is due to faulty construction, and the casting should be remade with enough relief to avoid impingement. Failure of any component that was weakened by adjustment at the time of initial placement is the responsibility of the dentist. However, adjustment made necessary by settling of the restoration because of abutment teeth becoming intruded under functional loading may be unavoidable, and subsequent failure due to the weakening effect of such adjustment may necessitate the making of a new restoration as a consequence of tissue changes. Frequently, repeated adjustment to a major or minor connector to relieve tissue impingement may not result in actual breakage but results in a loss of rigidity to the point that the connector can no longer function effectively. In such case, either a new restoration must be made or that part replaced by casting a new section and then reassembling the denture by soldering. This occasionally requires disassemby of denture base areas and replaced teeth, and the cost and probable success must then be weighed against the cost of an entirely new restoration. Frequently, the latter course is advisable.

Loss of an additional tooth or teeth not involved in the support or retention of the restoration. Such additions to a partial denture are usually simply made when the bases are made of resin. The addition of teeth to metal bases is more complex and necessitates either casting a new component, and attaching it by soldering, or creating retentive elements for the attachment of a resin extension. In most instances, when a distal extension denture base is extended, the need for subsequent relining the entire base should be considered. After the extension of the denture base, a relining procedure of both the new and old base then should be carried out to provide optimal tissue support for the restoration.

Loss of an abutment tooth necessitating not only its replacement but also the substi-

tution of a new clasp assembly on another abutment. This is usually the next adjacent tooth, which may or may not have to undergo restorative treatment. In the latter case, any new restoration should be done to conform to the original path of placement, with proximal guiding plane, occlusal rest seat, and suitable retentive areas. Otherwise, modifications to the existing tooth should be done the same as would be done during any other mouth preparations, with proximal disking, preparation of an adequate occlusal rest seat, and any reduction in tooth contours necessary to accommodate retentive and stabilizing components. A new clasp assembly then may be cast for this tooth and the denture reassembled with the new replacement tooth added.

The most frequent cause of the loss of an abutment tooth is periodontal involvement. If an abutment tooth becomes carious or fractures, it can frequently be restored with a crown made to fit the existing denture clasp. Early pulpal involvement is usually amenable to endodontic treatment, by gaining access through the existing restoration. However, an abutment tooth that becomes periodontally involved is too often lost. In many instances this could have been avoided initially by more careful evaluation of the periodontal support of a tooth that is to serve as an abutment and by the use of multiple abutments by splinting whenever advisable. When an adjacent tooth must be substituted as the new abutment, it must be considered as potentially a periodontally weakened tooth and treated accordingly. Occasionally, splinting of two teeth with double restorations is necessary before the denture is extended to include the new abutment. This is often made more necessary by the fact that the edentulous area is increased by one tooth and, in a distal extension situation, the leverage on the abutment is increased correspondingly.

Other types of repairs and replacements. Included in this category is the replacement of a broken or lost denture tooth, the repair of a broken resin base, or the reattachment of a loosened resin base to the metal framework. Breakage is sometimes due to poor design, faulty construction, or the use of the wrong material for a given situation. Other times it is due to an accident that will not necessarily repeat itself. If the latter occurs, repair or replacement usually suffices. On the other hand, if fracture has occurred due to structural causes or if it occurs a second time after having been repaired once before, then some change in the design, either by modification of the original denture or with a new denture, may be necessary. Usually the share of responsibility by dentist and patient will depend upon the length of service given by the denture before breakage occurred and upon other contributing factors, such as the existence of an abnormal occlusion. Such matters are best approached by a frank and honest appraisal of all the factors involved, based on the patient's understanding that the permanence or longevity of any prosthetic restoration, since it is dependent upon the changing characteristics of living tissues, can never be assured.

PROCEDURES FOR MAKING REPAIRS AND ADDITIONS

Although most repairs or additions to partial dentures may be done by the laboratory technician through work authorizations, impressions and other chairside procedures must be done in accordance with the laboratory procedures to follow.

If a new clasp assembly is to be made, an impression is made for a new master cast. This is poured and surveyed, and the design of the new clasp outlined. The same applies to the making of any new component part to be cast and subsequently attached to the original framework. Frequently the patient can continue to wear the denture while the new part is being made and must be without it only for the brief period of time it takes to reassemble the parts. Jaw relations are usually made with the original denture in the mouth, and at the same time an impression is made for an occluding cast.

For more simple repairs and additions, it is usually preferable that the impression be made with the denture in place, the denture being removed in the impression. An alginate hydrocolloid impression material should be used that has sufficient toughness upon setting to permit withdrawal of the denture in the impression.

The impression should be poured immediately, either in stone or in a mixture of stone and plaster to facilitate later removal without difficulty. If a resin repair or addition is to be done, the stone and plaster mixture will be sufficiently strong. But if a new clasp arm is to be adapted, the cast should be made of the harder stone for obvious reasons. If an occlusal rest or some soldered clasp assembly is to be made, the soldering will be done on a refractory duplicate of the stone cast and the original stone cast will be used for the final fitting and finishing.

REPLACING A BROKEN CLASP ARM WITH A WROUGHT-WIRE RETENTIVE ARM

A broken retentive clasp arm, regardless of its type, may be replaced with a wrought-wire retentive arm embedded in a resin base or attached to a metal base by electric soldering. Frequently this avoids the necessity of constructing an entirely new clasp assembly. Eighteen-gauge wrought wire is used to replace the original clasp arm.

When a resin base is present, the wire may be embedded into it with repair resin, thus eliminating the need for soldering (Fig. 21-1). The method for replacing a clasp in this manner is as follows:

The remains of the original clasp arm is first cut off flush with its point of origin. A hole is then drilled just below the adjacent artificial tooth as close as possible to the minor connector from which it originated. This hole must be angled downward toward the opposite side, emerging approximately midway on the opposite side of the resin base. From this hole a groove is cut in the resin base long enough to accommodate a sufficient length of the wrought wire

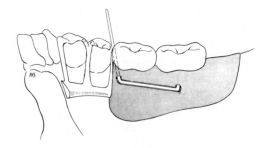

Fig. 21-1. Lingual view of the technique for replacing a broken retentive clasp arm with an 18-gauge wrought wire. The wrought wire is embedded securely with self-curing repair resin in a groove cut in the resin base.

for adequate retention. At the opposite end of this groove, a hole is made that will accommodate a right-angle turn in the wire. A piece of 18-gauge wrought wire to be used as a clasp arm is shaped with a right-angle bend at one end, adapted to fit the lingual groove, and then bent to fit the hole passing through to the opposite side. A straight portion sufficient to be adapted later as a clasp arm is left emerging from the resin base at the point of origin of the new clasp arm.

After securing the projecting wrought wire with sticky wax, self-curing repair resin is painted into the resin base until the defect is overfilled. After polymerizing, this is trimmed and polished. The projecting wrought wire is then cut off to the required length and adapted to serve as a new retentive clasp arm. The abutment tooth must be surveyed to determine the location of the desired undercut. The terminal portion of the adapted clasp arm is then rounded and tapered slightly.

This method is suitable any time a retentive clasp arm must be replaced and avoids any disassembly of the original denture. Because of the flexibility of wrought wire, it cannot be used to replace a stabilizing arm when rigidity is needed. In such case, when a rigid clasp arm has been lost, it is best that an entirely new clasp assembly be cast and attached to the framework by soldering.

REPAIRING BY SOLDERING

It has been said that 80% of all soldering in dentistry can be done electrically. Electric soldering units are available for this purpose, and most dental laboratories are so equipped. Electric soldering permits soldering close to a resin base without removing that base, because of the rapid localization of heat at the electrode. The resin base needs only to be protected with wet asbestos during soldering.

Gold solder is used for soldering both gold and chromium-cobalt alloys. For electric soldering, triple-thick solder should be used so that the additional bulk of the solder will retard melting momentarily while the carbon electrode conducts heat to the area being soldered. For chromium-cobalt alloys a color-matching white 19K gold solder, which melts at about 1675° F., is used. An application of flux is essential to the success of any soldering operation.

Following is a procedure* for electric soldering:

1. Roughen both sections to be joined.

2. Adapt platinum foil to the master cast to serve as a backing upon which the solder will flow. Lift the edges of the foil to form a trough to confine the flow of the solder.

3. Seat the pieces to be soldered onto the master cast and secure them temporarily with sticky wax. Over each piece add enough soldering investment or plaster to secure them after the sticky wax is eliminated, but leave as much metal exposed as possible.

4. After flushing off the sticky wax with hot water, secure the cast to the soldering stand. Cut sufficient solder and place conveniently nearby. Insert tweezers into the grounding terminal and the size carbon into the electrode holder that is best suited to the size and bulk of the sections to be joined (the smaller the piece of carbon used, the less power output needed).

---

*Adapted from Ticonium Technique Manual, Ticonium Division, Consolidated Metal Products Corp., Albany, N. Y.

5. Place the points of the tweezers so that both sections are grounded. Flux both sections. Put sufficient triple-thick solder on or in the joint to complete the soldering in one operation, always starting with enough solder to complete the job.

6. Wet the carbon tip with water to aid conduction of the current and then touch the carbon to the solder. Press the foot pedal, allowing time for the solder to flow freely, and then let up on the foot pedal. Do not push the solder with the carbon tip, but let the heat alone make the solder flow. Do not remove the carbon from the solder while the soldering operation is in progress, as this will cause surface pitting because of arcing as the carbon is removed. After the solder has flowed and the foot pedal is released, remove the carbon and grounding tweezers and proceed to remove the work from the cast for finishing.

Torch soldering requires an entirely different approach. It is used when the solder joint is long or unusually bulky, and when a larger quantity of solder has to be used. The procedure* for torch soldering is as follows:

1. Roughen both sections to be joined.

2. Adapt platinum foil to the master cast so that it extends under both sections.

3. Seat the sections on the master cast in the correct relationship and secure them temporarily with sticky wax. Flow sticky wax also into the joint to be soldered.

4. Attach a dental bur or nail over the two sections with a liberal amount of sticky wax. Attach a second and even a third nail or bur across other areas to lend additional support. Never use pieces of wood for this purpose, because the wood will swell if it gets wet, thus distorting the relationship of the two sections.

---

*Adapted from Ticonium Technique Manual, Ticonium Division, Consolidated Metal Products Corp., Albany, N. Y.

5. Remove the assembled casting from the master cast carefully. Adapt a stock of utility wax directly under each section, on either side of the platinum foil. After boil-out, investment will remain in the center to support the platinum foil.

6. Invest the casting in sufficient soldering investment to secure it, leaving as much of the area to be soldered exposed as possible. When the investment has set, boil out the sticky and utility waxes. Then place the investment in a drying oven at a temperature not exceeding 200° F. until the contained moisture has been eliminated. Do not preheat the investment with a torch or oxides will be formed that will interfere with the flow of the solder.

7. Use the reducing part of the flame, which is that feathery part just outside the blue inner cone. Flux the joint thoroughly and dry out the flux with the outer part of the flame until it has a powdery appearance. Heat the casting until it is dull red and then, holding a strip of solder in the soldering tweezers, dip it into the flux and feed it into the joint while the casting is being held at a dull red heat with the torch. Once the soldering operation has begun do not remove the flame, as any cooling will cause oxides to be formed. The heat from the casting should be sufficient to melt the solder; so do not put the flame directly on the solder or it will become overheated, resulting in pitting.

8. After the soldering has been completed, allow the investment to cool slowly before quenching and proceeding with finishing. Remember that any soldering operation that heats the entire casting is in effect a heat-treating operation, and heat-hardening of a repaired gold alloy casting is desirable to restore its optimal physical properties.

CHAPTER 22

Interim, transitional, and treatment removable partial dentures

Removable partial dentures designed to span short intervals of time, often must be fabricated as a part of a total prosthodontic treatment. Such restorations serve many useful purposes and may be classified according to the purpose for which they are used. It is not our intent to introduce new terminology; however, for the sake of clarity, it seems justifiable to discuss these restorations under several headings.

Interim partial dentures. Interim partial dentures are made for economic or other reasons when the use of such a restoration is justified. For example, a patient may be preparing to make a trip and time does not permit the making of adequate mouth preparations and the rendering of a more complete partial denture service. Another example is that the patient may be in poor health or be facing some medical or surgical emergency. Also, a young person may have lost teeth prematurely through an accident or for other reasons. Either for the sake of appearance or for the purpose of maintaining a space, or both, an interim partial denture must be made until such time as fixed restorations can be fabricated or more definitive partial denture service is possible.

When recent extractions must be replaced temporarily while tissues heal or, in younger patients, until the adjacent teeth have reached sufficient maturity to be used as abutments for fixed restorations, the use of an interim patial denture maintains mesiodistal and occlusal relations until other restorative treatment can be done. An acceptable esthetic result usually can be obtained. It is important, however, that the patient or the parents of the younger patient be made aware that any such removable restoration is *temporary* and may jeopardize the integrity of the adjacent teeth and the health of the supporting soft tissues if worn for extended periods without supportive care. The need for strict oral hygiene and diet control also must be clearly understood, and provisions made therefore while an interim partial denture is being worn. Generally, the younger patient is even more susceptible to caries when wearing a removable restoration, and adequate prophylactic measures must be taken to prevent decalcification and carries in the teeth contacted.

An interim partial denture may replace only one or more missing anterior teeth, or it may replace several teeth, both anterior and posterior, in a partially edentulous dental arch. Such a restoration is usually made of acrylic resin, either by a sprinkling method or by waxing, flasking, and processing with either self-curing or thermal-curing resin. It may be retained by wraparound wrought-wire clasps, Crozat-type clasps, interproximal spurs, or wire loops.

In rare instances, separate cast circumferential type clasps may be used, attached to the resin base by a retaining lug.

Whatever the materials and methods of retention used, such partial dentures are *temporary* and a distinction must be made between this type of restoration and a partial denture prosthesis with prepared abutments and rigid all-cast framework construction. *Too frequently a partial denture is constructed by dental laboratories on order from the dentist, who then represents it to the patient as a "partial denture," with a fee that is a multiple of the laboratory cost. However it should be considered nothing more than a temporary restoration.* The patient is being misled (perhaps the word "fleeced" is more appropriate) when such a temporary restoration is purported to be representative of modern restorative dentistry.

Interim partial dentures are made for one or more of the following reasons: (1) to maintain a space, (2) to reestablish occlusion, (3) to replace visible missing teeth while definitive restorative procedures are being accomplished, (4) to serve while the patient is undergoing periodontal or other treatment, and (5) to condition the patient to wearing a removable prosthesis. In the latter instance, the patient's response to wearing a more costly restoration may be evaluated, and, on some rare occasions, further treatment may be interrupted while the patient becomes conditioned to the wearing of a removable restoration.

In some instances an existing partial denture can be used with modifications as an interim partial denture. Such modifications may include relining and the adding of teeth and clasps to an existing denture. In other instances an existing partial denture may be converted to a transitional complete denture for immediate placement while tissues heal and an opposing arch is prepared to receive a partial denture. Sometimes an interim partial denture must be made to replace missing anterior teeth in a partially edentulous arch, which are ultimately to be replaced with fixed restora-

tions. On occasion the anterior portion of the restoration is cut away when the fixed restorations are placed, leaving the remainder of the denture to be worn while posterior abutment teeth are being prepared.

Still another type of interim denture is one on which missing posterior teeth are replaced temporarily with a resin occlusion rim rather than with occluding teeth. In dental school clinics it is sometimes impossible to complete treatment in a school year and the continuing student may desire to resume treatment after the summer recess. In such instances occlusion may be maintained, and, as in the case of treatment dentures, the tissues may be conditioned by having the patient wear a temporary restoration with posterior occlusion rims that have been adjusted to occlusal harmony.

Transitional partial dentures. A transitional partial denture is made to aid the patient in making the transition to complete dentures when total loss of teeth is inevitable. Such a partial denture also may be considered a treatment restoration, since the patient is at the same time being conditioned to the wearing of a removable prosthesis. It should be considered strictly a temporary measure that provides the patient with a restoration for the remaining life of the natural teeth when further restorative treatment of those teeth is impractical or economically or technically impossible.

Such a partial denture may be worn for prolonged periods, in the meantime undergoing revision, modification to include additional teeth lost, and/or relining when such becomes necessary or advisable. The dentist should agree to provide such a partial denture only under the following conditions: (1) that a definite fee for the treatment is impossible to predict and that the cost will depend upon the servicing necessary and (2) that when, in his opinion, further wearing of the transitional denture is unwise and jeopardizes the health of the remaining tissues, the transition to complete dentures will proceed.

Treatment partial dentures. Treatment

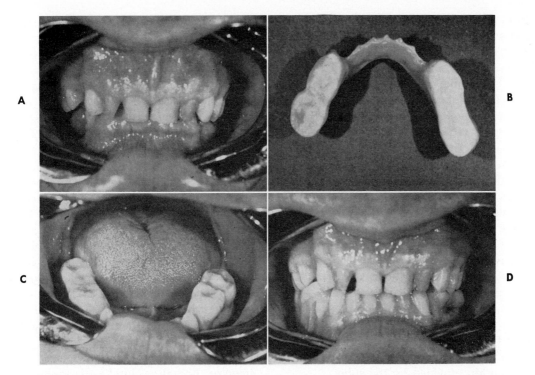

Fig. 22-1. Four views showing the use of a removable occlusal splint. **A,** Evidence of over-closure to be corrected by occlusal reconstruction. **B,** A removable occlusal splint for the lower arch using tooth-colored acrylic resin for occlusal surfaces. **C,** The removable splint in the mouth. The occlusal anatomy is the result of an occlusal registration done in wax on the resin base, which is then invested, and to which tooth-colored resin is added to reproduce the functional occlusal surfaces that were recorded in wax. **D,** The resulting occlusion with removable splint. This may be adjusted until satisfactory, and then it signifies the vertical dimension, to be maintained by oral rehabilitation.

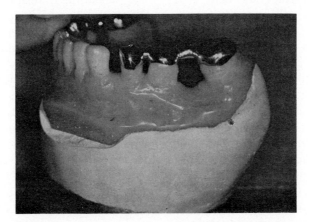

Fig. 22-2. Cast gold occlusal splints. Following occlusal adjustment, the splints are cemented to the teeth. Since these are made to fit the unprepared natural teeth, they cannot extend beyond the height of contour of each tooth. Surveying is therefore necessary prior to their construction. The splints may be eliminated tooth by tooth as subsequent restorations are being done, thus maintaining the established vertical relationship.

partial dentures are used for the following reasons: (1) to establish a new occlusal relationship or vertical dimension and (2) to condition teeth and ridge tissues to support better the partial denture to follow.

Treatment partial dentures may be used as occlusal splints in much the same manner as cast or resin occlusal splints are used on natural teeth (Figs. 22-1 and 22-2). When total tooth support is available, there is little difference between a fixed and a removable occlusal splint except that a removable splint is too likely to be left out of the mouth unless the patient is actually made more comfortable by its presence. This is usually true when temporomandibular joint pathology is alleviated by the wearing of an occlusal splint. In other situations, it may be advisable to cement the removable restoration to the teeth until such time as the patient has become accustomed to, and dependent upon, the jaw relationship provided by the splint.

Both fixed and removable tooth-supported occlusal splints have much in common. Either of them may be eliminated sectionally as restorative treatment is being done, thus maintaining the established jaw relation until all restorative treatment has been completed. The dentist usually decides whether these are to be fixed or removable and whether they are made of a cast (silver or gold) alloy or of a resin material.

When one or more distal extension bases exist on an occlusal splint, a different situation exists. The establishment of a new occlusal or vertical relation depends too much upon the quality of support the splint receives to ignore the need for the best possible support for any existing distal extension base. Both broad coverage and functional basing of tissue-supported bases are desirable, as well as some type of occlusal rest on the nearest abutments. Any tissue-supported occlusal splint should at least be relined in the mouth with a self-curing reline resin to afford optimal coverage and support for the distal extension base.

O. C. Applegate, in an article on the choice of partial or complete denture treatment, has emphasized the advantages of conditioning edentulous areas to provide stable support for distal extension partial dentures. This is accomplished by having the patient wear a treatment partial denture for a period of time prior to construction of the final base. In the absence of opposing occlusion, stimulation of the underlying tissues by applying intermittent finger pressure to the denture base is advised. Whether the stimulation is from occlusal or finger pressure, there seems to be little doubt that the tissues of the residual ridge become more capable of supporting a distal extension partial denture when they have been conditioned by the wearing of a previous restoration.

Abutment teeth also benefit from the wearing of a treatment restoration when such a restoration applies an occlusal load to those teeth, either through occlusal coverage or through occlusal rests. Frequently a tooth that is to be used as an abutment for a partial denture has been out of occlusion for some time. Immediately upon applying an occlusal load to that tooth sufficient to support any type of removable prosthesis, some intrusion of the tooth will occur. If such intrusion is allowed to occur after initial placement of the final prosthesis, the occlusal relationship of the prosthesis and its relation to the adjacent gingival tissues will be altered. Perhaps this is one reason for gingival impingement, which occurs after the denture has been worn for some time, even though seemingly adequate relief had been provided initially. When a treatment partial denture is worn, such abutment teeth have an opportunity to become stabilized under the loading of the treatment restoration, and intrusion will have occurred prior to making the impression for the master cast. There is sufficient reason to believe that both abutment teeth and supporting ridge tissues are better capable of providing continuing support for the partial denture when they have been previously conditioned by the wearing of a treatment restoration.

Another example of the use of a treatment partial denture is to facilitate the eruption of posterior teeth through the use of an acrylic resin bite plane. Particularly in the younger patient, early loss of some posterior teeth results in either depression or incomplete eruption of the remaining teeth. The most frequently seen example of this is when the molar teeth in one arch are missing and the premolar teeth remain in occlusion. These are then either depressed or were never able to erupt fully because of excessive occlusal loading. Overclosure results, with anterior teeth likewise in excessive contact, leading to orthodontic movement of these teeth and/or excessive vertical overlap. Prosthetic replacement of missing teeth with a partial denture can thus only perpetuate an overclosed relationship unless one of two objectives is accomplished first. One is to increase the occlusal height of the remaining teeth arbitrarily with restorations. The other is to permit the remaining posterior teeth to attain full eruption by increasing the vertical dimension of occlusion. Usually the latter method is preferable.

For such treatment an acrylic resin restoration is made that causes the lower anterior teeth to close against an acrylic resin plane while the posterior teeth remain out of occlusion. Some depression of the lower anterior teeth may occur but without ill effect. More important, posterior teeth that have become depressed or were not fully erupted may migrate into a new vertical occlusion as dictated by the amount of opening anteriorly. Once this has occurred, prosthetic replacement of the missing teeth may proceed and the established vertical dimension be maintained with fixed or removable restorations or a combination of both.

. . .

These are the various types of prosthetic restorations for the partially edentulous mouth that are, and must be, considered temporary restorations. It is imperative that a distinction be made between these and a true partial denture service and that the patient be advised of the purposes and limitations of such restorations. In no instance should the patient be misled into believing that an inadequate, interim partial denture is representative of modern prosthetic dentistry.

CHAPTER 23

Miscellaneous partial prosthodontics

John J. Sharry, B.S., D.M.D.*

The prosthetic replacement of tissue defects, which were either surgically or developmentally acquired, often depends upon removable restorations that are retained by clasps on the teeth.

Certain considerations will be discussed that do not supplant but rather supplement those general principles of design that apply to the usual removable partial denture. Such components as the pharyngeal portion of a cleft palate restoration and the obturator that closes the defect resulting from a hemisection of the maxilla impose further burdens on the usual designs. Resultant dislodging forces must be considered and included in the design that will be used for any particular patient.

Several types of prostheses depend on a partial denture framework for their retention. An attempt to describe only a representative few is made, since the variations are myriad and do not lend themselves to classification.

CLEFT PALATE PROSTHESES

The cleft palate obturator is one of the most common obturators and is the one about which most has been written. (Various other restorations, often referred to as maxillofacial prostheses, will be discussed in general rather than specific terms later.)

---

*Dean, College of Dental Medicine, Medical University of South Carolina, Charleston, S. C.

Classification. Cleft palates lend themselves to morphologic classifications. The simplest and perhaps the most easily remembered is that of Veau. He proposed four classes: Class I, in which the cleft involves only the soft palate; Class II, which involves the soft and hard palates but not the alveolus; Class III, which involves the soft and hard palates, continuing through the alveolus on one side of the premaxillary area; and Class IV, which involves the soft and hard palates, the cleft continuing through the alveolus on both sides, leaving a free premaxilla (Fig. 23-1). The latter two classes are usually, though not always, associated with a cleft lip.

Etiology. The etiology of cleft palate is not clear but seems at the present time to have some basis in heredity, although many other factors have been mentioned, such as infectious diseases of the mouth, mechanical interferences in the fetus, nutritional inadequacies, and various changes in the intrauterine environment.

Personality evaluation. The personality range of individuals with a cleft palate is not much different from that of the general population. Perhaps more of them fall into the quiet, unresponsive, withdrawn category and a few exhibit a brashness or bravado (which generally disappears with continued association). However, a large share are well-adjusted, pleasant people. Sometimes one wonders how so many can

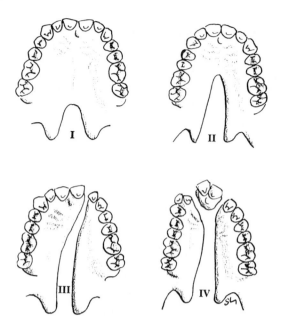

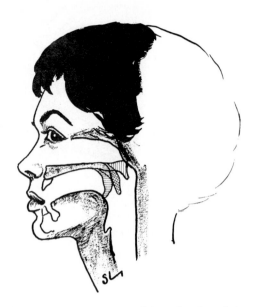

Fig. 23-1. Veau's classification of cleft palates.

Fig. 23-2. Three positions of the soft palate during normal activity.

be happy when the attitude of the parents and the public is often such that a considerable degree of overprotection or rejection is the fate of these cleft palate individuals when they are children.

It should be noted here that so many factors influence diagnosis and treatment of these patients that a "team approach" (dentist, surgeon, pediatrician, speech therapist, and so forth) to management of these patients is essential.

There are a few areas in which certain differences of approach are necessary in treating such persons. For example, it is often found that their speaking habits are so poor that they cannot be understood. This difficulty will usually disappear with continued association, but initially a relative can interpret for them. If they are alone, then a paper and pencil will solve the problem.

Anatomy. During the examination of clefts that have not been operated upon, the dentist should examine the nasal and pharyngeal cavities and their component structures and, by using a blunt instrument or finger, ascertain the tissue consistency of various areas. It should be noted

here that the gag reflex of the person with a cleft palate is markedly diminished and does not usually hinder palpatory examination.

The knowledge of the anatomic structure of these cavities serves not merely to satisfy intellectual curiosity but, more important, it places the dentist on familiar ground when and if it becomes necessary to remove impression materials that may inadvertently be forced through the cleft or perforation while obtaining impressions of the dental arches.

The normal soft palate either closes the nasal cavity from the pharynx or the oral cavity from the pharynx, or it just relaxes as the occasion demands (Fig. 23-2). If this "valve" is not whole, then, of course, it cannot effectively perform these closing functions but rather allows food to enter the nasopharynx during deglutition and air to enter the nasal cavity during the production of those speech sounds wherein the air should be directed into the oral cavity. Further, it makes the production of such sounds as "puh" and "kuk" practically impossible.

A group of muscles is attached to the

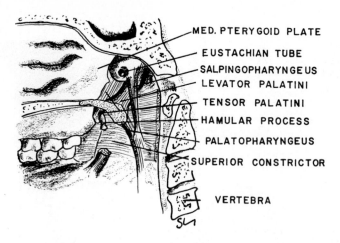

Fig. 23-3. Dissection of the velopharyngeal area as seen from the side.

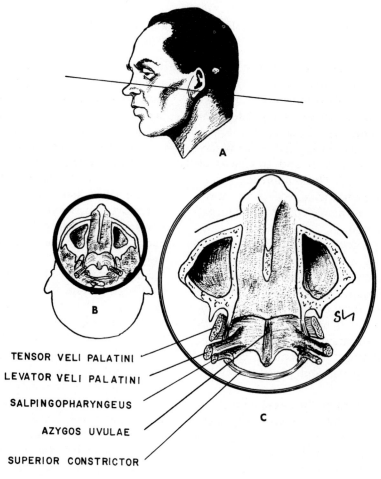

Fig. 23-4. Musculature of the soft palate as seen from above. **A,** The area of section. **B,** The portion of section used. **C,** Detail of section.

soft palate and is responsible for the closure of the nasal cavity. This total action (closing off the nasal cavity) is called the *velopharyngeal closure.* To accomplish this the following, more or less simultaneous, muscular contractions take place.

The levator veli palatini muscle, which originates on the petrous portion of the temporal bone and the cartilage of the eustachian tube and runs downward and forward to insert into the palatine aponeurosis, contracts, pulling the soft palate upward and backward (Fig. 23-3). This is a paired muscle, and upon entering the soft palate it merges with its fellow of the opposite side, forming a sling. At the same time, the tensor veli palatini, which arises from the scaphoid fossa, the sphenoid spine, and eustachian cartilage, travels downward and forward to the lateral aspect of the hamulus (which is used as a pulley), swings medially to enter the soft palate, contracts, and effects tension on the soft palate. Now the soft palate has been pulled backward and upward.

However, the pull is not sufficient to close the gap between the distal limits of the soft palate and the pharynx, so the pharynx accommodates by moving forward and medially. This is accomplished by the joint action of three muscles. The pterygopharyngeal portion of the superior constrictor, which originates usually on the medial pterygoid plate, travels backward fanwise to terminate in a median raphe in the posterior pharynx. It contracts and pulls the posterior pharyngeal wall forward to meet the soft palate. (See Fig. 23-4.) Meanwhile, since this action may not be quite enough in certain instances, the palatopharyngeus muscle, which we can see in the throat as the posterior pillars of the tonsil and which has two parts, the thyropalatal and pharyngopalatal portions, comes into play. The latter part, which arises in the palatal aponeurosis and travels backward and downward to insert in a fanwise fashion in the posterior pharynx anterior to, but interlaced with, the superior constrictor fibers, contracts strongly. It is

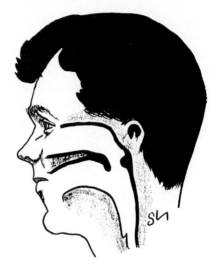

Fig. 23-5. Passavant's cushion in the posterior pharyngeal wall.

more or less circular, and it further attempts to approximate the soft palate and pharynx and, in doing so, produces a ridge or "bunching up" of the posterior pharyngeal musculature, called Passavant's cushion (Fig. 23-5). This is usually, though not always, visible in the patient with a cleft palate. It is located at levels varying from as high as the region of the atlas to as low as the level of the distally projected mandibular occlusal plane. Now the soft palate is touching the posterior pharyngeal wall, but there is a leak when the lateral aspect of the soft palate does not meet the lateral aspect of the pharynx. This will be closed by the salpingopharyngeus muscle. This muscle arises from the cartilage of the eustachian tube and travels downward and laterally to fan out and insert in the lateral pharyngeal wall. When it contracts it pulls the lateral wall medially, thus closing the last gap in velopharyngeal closure. All these muscle contractions take place almost simultaneously. The velopharyngeal mechanism has now closed the nasal cavity from the oral cavity and pharynx. This movement is used in deglutition to prevent food from entering the nose and in speech when pronouncing the so-called polsive sounds, puh, buh, tuh, duh, kuh, guh. These sounds are produced by closing off the nose and building up pressure in the mouth and suddenly releasing it. Thus the name "plosive."

The second position, the closure of the oral cavity, is a result of the contraction of the following. The thyropalatal portion of the palatopharyngeus muscle arises from the posterolateral rim of the thyroid cartilage and courses upward through the posterior pillar to insert into the palatine aponeurosis, where it merges with its fellow of the opposite side, forming an inverted **U**. When it contracts it pulls the soft palate down toward the tongue. Meanwhile, the tensor is flattening the dome of the soft palate to bring down the portion of the structure that may not come down with the action of the thyropalatal muscle. Concurrently, the tongue is forced upward and backward. To finally eliminate the possibility of a leak, the palatoglossus muscle, which is attached superiorly to the palate and inferiorly to the tongue, forming more or less a sphincteric structure in this motion, contracts and completes the approximation. Therefore, it can now be seen that velopharyngeal closure *is not* a simple sphincteric action of the superior constrictor and palatopharyngeus muscles (which run in a nearly horizontal direction) but is instead the resultant contraction of these and others running in a vertical direction, such as the levator, tensor, and the salpingopharyngeus muscles. This second position is used in sucking and in the pronunciation of sounds such as "ng" in the word sing. The third position finds the palate relaxed as in normal breathing.

Pathology. The patient with a cleft palate, because of his inability to close off the nose, is constantly the victim of nasal infections and middle ear infections sometimes resulting in deafness. He cannot pronounce correctly the plosive sounds and tries to overcompensate with his tongue. He tries to make the latter obturate the cleft and articulate at the same time. These habits are an obstacle to the speech correctionist who must attempt to train the patient to forget these habits and learn a new set of movements.

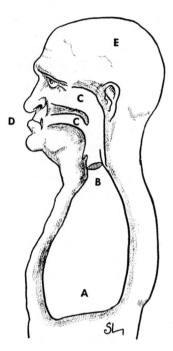

Fig. 23-6. Mechanisms of speech. **A,** Respiratory organ (lungs). **B,** Phonating organ (vocal cords). **C,** Resonating chambers (oral and nasal cavities). **D,** Articulating organs (lips, tongue, and teeth). **E,** Integrating center (brain).

Despite some of these difficulties, the patient can be nourished adequately, and aside from the possibility of constant nasal and pharyngeal infections, he may be generally quite healthy although many cleft palate patients have other defects also, such as heart and skeletal congenital abnormalities. The inability to speak properly constitutes his greatest problem.

Physiology of speech. Speech is a function of respiration, phonation, resonation, articulation, and integration. Respiration is, of course, concerned with the exchange of air by the lungs; phonation is accomplished by the abduction and adduction of the vocal cords, which change the pitch of the voice; resonation is realized in the nasal, oral, and pharyngeal cavities, which are the prime resonation chambers. The teeth, tongue, lips, and palate serve as articulatory mechanisms, and all, of course, would be nothing without the integrating facilities of the human brain. (See Fig. 23-6.)

The soft palate performs any one of the following basic functions in speech. It closes off the nasal cavity, as in producing "k" and hard "g"; it closes off the oral cavity for production of the sounds "m," "n," and "ng" (as in "ring"), or it may close neither cavity completely but allow varying portions of the air stream to enter the appropriate resonating chambers.

Although the soft palate is but one part of the velopharyngeal mechanism (the other part being the pharyngeal muscles), it is of such importance that when cleft, the individual cannot effect velopharyngeal closure.

Surgical treatment. Two general types of physical treatment can restore partially or completely the function of the soft palate. The first concerns surgical procedures to close the soft palate (and the hard palate when involved). The other utilizes an artificial restoration, called an *obturator,* which serves not to close the soft palate but rather to fill the space between the two halves of the palate. (Both the surgical and prosthetic approaches are usually of little avail without speech therapy, given previously, conjointly, or subsequently.) The surgical approach is generally concerned with the closure and, in many instances, the lengthening of the palate. Closure is achieved by denuding the opposing edges of the two halves of the cleft palate and suturing them together. This may necessitate lateral relaxing incisions paralled to the long axis of the cleft, which will allow it to be apposed and sutured together (Fig. 23-7, *A* and *B*). Lengthening of the palate may be accomplished by an anterior incision of the palatine mucosa, which may run from the area of the molars on one side around back of the anterior teeth (avoiding the anterior palatine foramen) to the molars on the opposite side (Fig. 23-7, *C* and *D*). The palatine mucosa posteriorly and medially to this incision is dissected from the palatine bone and displaced backward, thus lengthening the soft palate. The denuded palatine bone anteriorly becomes epithelized via granulation tissue.

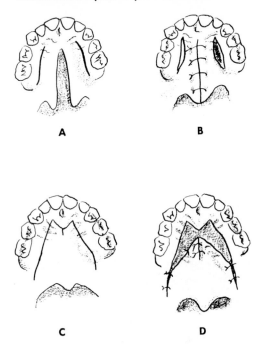

Fig. 23-7. Surgical procedures in cleft palate therapy. **A,** Relaxing incisions in the palatal mucosa. **B,** Mucosa elevated and displaced medially where freshened edges of the cleft are sutured together. **C,** Incision for push-back operation. **D,** Push-back completed and sutured.

When the general types of operation are not feasible, the surgeon may perform a pharyngeal flap operation, wherein a longitudinal flap is dissected from the posterior pharyngeal wall (its attachment being located either below or above) and is brought forward and sutured to the denuded posterior edge of the soft palate (Fig. 23-8). This then forms a continuous tissue bridge between the soft palate and the pharynx, which functions well as part of the velopharyngeal mechanism. The flap, as dissected, tends to curl medially, leaving lateral space for air transmission through the nasal cavity. Since much of the pharyngeal closing movement is in a medial direction, one can see that this action can aid in velopharyngeal closure because the lateral walls converge medially toward the flap. There are more definitive surgical approaches to the cleft palate, but they are generally concerned with either of these two aims.

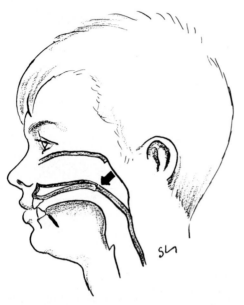

Fig. 23-8. Pharyngeal flap operation viewed from the side. The flap is based below.

Prosthodontic treatment. The prosthetic approach utilizes a metal framework that is similar to a partial denture framework in which is included a posterior latticework extension into the area of the cleft (Fig. 23-9). This extension supports an acrylic resin bulb, which is the obturator.

The *preservation* of the patient's teeth is of *prime importance* because although obturators have been made for edentulous patients, they can never be as efficient as those that utilize the teeth for stabilization. Therefore, all necessary restorative dentistry must be accomplished immediately. In a large percentage of patients the dentist is faced with the problem of restoring occlusal harmony, and therefore the patient may first require orthodontic treatment. However, an obturator often can be combined with the orthodontic appliance. When a patient has good occlusion, no active caries, and no periodontal disease or other oral lesions, construction of the permanent prosthetic restoration may be undertaken.

Fig. 23-9

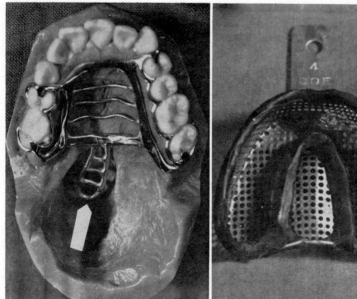

Fig. 23-10

Fig. 23-9. Ladderlike extension of the framework into the area of the cleft.
Fig. 23-10. Use of utility wax to confine impression material to the tissues.

Impressions with alginate hydrocolloid impression materials. The examination will reveal the nature of the unrepaired cleft or, if repaired, those perforations that sometimes result from tissue breakdown. One should look particularly in the anterior mucobuccal fold for minute oronasal perforations after the repair of Classes III and IV clefts.

A resilient impression material must be used because of the many tissue undercuts. The alginate hydrocolloid impression materials serve this purpose adequately.

The problems incident to impressions are divided into two groups; the unrepaired cleft presenting one situation and the repaired cleft another. The unrepaired cleft palate, Classes II, III, and IV, will be considered first. (The method of obtaining impressions of the teeth are not modified by Class I clefts.) When using a hydrocolloid impression material, the posterior portion of the tray should be modified with boxing or utility wax to prevent material from flowing down the patient's throat. In addition, the use of this wax adjacent to the cleft or perforation will record more accurately the mucosal detail by confining the impression material to those areas. (See Fig. 23-10.)

The material should be prevented from entering the nasal cavity in such a large quantity that it may fracture from the main body of material. Such an accident requires a tedious process of fragmentation and removal. To prevent this, simply underload the tray in the area of cleft. The tooth-bearing section of the tray is completely filled with the alginate, but the area corresponding to the cleft is loaded to a height of only 2 to 3 mm. Thus, when the tray is seated, the material is not likely to be forced upward into the cleft in sufficient quantity to "lock."

Cleft palates previously repaired present slightly different problems. The palatal repair itself may look adequate, and yet an oronasal perforation may exist in the labial mucobuccal fold as previously mentioned. If it is present, either pack this perforation with wet gauze (in many instances the perforations are too small for this approach) or else the tray must be "underloaded" in this area so that a large amount of the impression material will not be forced into the nasal cavity.

Amounts small enough to be dislodged by blowing the nose should not be of concern. Larger amounts, however, require a considerable degree of skill in their fragmentation and removal as *they cannot be pushed into the mouth as in unrepaired defects and must be manipulated within the nasal cavity.*

Those perforations that may exist on the palate itself should be approached in a similar manner. If the area is large enough to pack off with wet gauze, then this is the method of choice. If the diameter is a half inch or more, then perhaps it is better to handle it like an open cleft, using utility wax damming and underloading the tray in that area.

Framework. The design of the framework is of primary importance, as it must be balanced to eliminate, as much as possible, harmful torque effects on the teeth. The essential requirements for the casting consist of the following: (1) the metal to be used should be as thin as possible commensurate with strength so that metal bulk does not cause an added obstacle to speech. (2) The tip of the clasp should engage a distal undercut on the posterior abutments to support the obturator. On abutments further anterior, the clasp should engage mesial undercuts when anterior replacements are necessary (Fig. 23-11). If proper undercuts are not present or if the teeth must be restored with full crowns because of caries or for other reasons such as fixed splinting, adequate embrasure crossing space must be planned in the restorations. It is wise to utilize continuous lingual bracing, even on teeth not used for retentive clasps, in order to distribute widely the torquing forces often developed by these restorations.

The pharyngeal portion is usually attached to the framework by a distal loop or

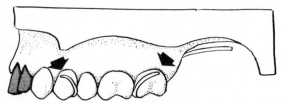

Fig. 23-11. When anterior replacements are necessary (shaded teeth), the clasp on anterior abutments should engage a mesial undercut. The clasp on the distal abutments should engage a distal undercut.

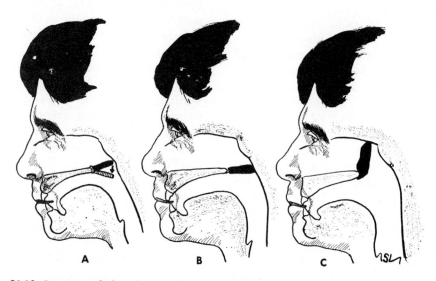

Fig. 23-12. Location of the pharyngeal portion of the several obturators. **A,** Hinge type. **B,** Fixed type. **C,** Meatus type.

"ladder" from the casting. The superoinferior position of the loop will vary according to the type of prosthesis.

Obturator design. Following are the three main types of obturators: the so-called hinge or movable type, the fixed type, and the meatus type (Fig. 23-12). The hinged type is connected to the main framework by means of a hinge. Its bulk is located above the cleft edges and supposedly serves an anatomic purpose in that it moves up and back, supported by the soft palate edges, as does the normal soft palate to effect velopharyngeal closure. Theoretically, this is workable, but in practice it is not quite true because many cleft palates have limited motion and many authors believe that this type of obturator is limited in use other than for a few patients. The fixed

type is stationary and is directed toward Passavant's pad. It depends on the forward movement of the pad and lateral movement of the pharynx to effect closure. This is the obturator in most general use today and, if made well, is relatively efficient. The meatus obturator will be discussed later because of the difference in construction.

PHARYNGEAL IMPRESSIONS. The method of obtaining impressions for the hinge type or the fixed type is essentially the same. It involves the following steps: A mound of modeling plastic approximating the pharyngeal defect in shape and size is placed on the distal extension and warmed. This bulk is directed as high above the area of Passavant's pad as feasible and is placed into the patient's mouth while still warm. When the

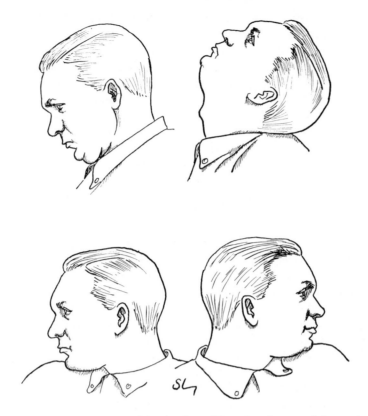

Fig. 23-13. Positions of the head for border-molding the pharyngeal impression.

framework is seated properly on the teeth, the patient is instructed to swallow, tilt the head back, and then place the chin on the chest. Keeping it there, he should turn the head from left shoulder to right shoulder. (See Fig. 23-13.) This total routine should be accomplished quickly to mold the modeling plastic while it is still warm. The resultant impression is then removed from the mouth and compared with the defect. Gross inadequacies are noted and, if necessary, more material is added. The modeling plastic impression is then removed and all excess trimmed. It should have a superoinferior thickness of not more than 5 to 6 mm. to keep it as lightweight as possible.

Experience in making impressions for a fixed type of restoration (and occasionally the hinge type) has demonstrated that attempts to obtain accurate detail in impressions by means of the "wash" materials may be abandoned. There is a certain amount of leakage that will occur around any obturator, and this leakage does not materially affect the efficiency of the restoration. When the patient swallows, there is a vigorous excursion of the pharyngeal musculature; when he talks, there is less movement of it. Because the restoration must be made comfortable enough to enable the patient to swallow, an air leak will occur during ordinary speech. Furthermore, the musculature changes its shape, and the detail obtained from a wash impression will not be maintained on tissue topography for any length of time.

The procedures used for making impressions for cleft palate prostheses may well be due for reevaluation. Recently, several children for whom orthodontic appliances were to be constructed were examined jointly by an orthodontist and a prosthodontist. It was decided that removable appliances that combined orthodontic and prosthodontic treatment should be constructed. However, it was believed that it would be wise to provide the prosthodontic treatment in several progressing steps to avoid any antagonism on the part of the child toward the obturating section.

Accordingly, impressions of the pharyngeal area were avoided, and some firm wax was attached to the palatal portion of the acrylic resin appliance, which had been finished. The wax extension was constructed initially to such a dimension that it would not contact the pharyngeal tissues at any time. Acrylic resin was then substituted for the wax, and the patient wore this "bulb" for one week. The next week the "bulb" was enlarged to contact one or two small areas during swallowing. It was planned to accustom the child gradually to a mass of material in the nasopharynx and then to obtain an impression of the tissues in that region. However, it was noted that when the "bulb" was enlarged (by means of hand molding), there was a marked improvement in the nasal quality of the voice.

Further empirical enlargement of the "bulb" was made at the next appointment. There was some further improvement of the voice, but it was not as dramatic as that of the second appointment. Finally, the pharyngeal impression was made, and the finished restoration was placed. The voice quality was not improved over that of the previous week. The results in several succeeding patients treated in this same manner suggested that it may not be necessary to obtain detailed impressions for pharyngeal obturators.

It has been interesting to note again and again the secondary role that surgical and prosthetic procedures play in the correction of cleft palate speech. We may work hard and provide our patients with an excellent technical result, but even with our understandable enthusiasm, we are not entirely satisfied with the vocal results. Conversely, we often see patients for whom relatively little has been done, and yet with all their lack of physical equipment, they speak reasonably well. We are convinced that the procedures per se do not always make the correction. They merely provide the equipment, and personality, either the patient's or the therapist's, or both, heals. Nevertheless, we need to provide the best equipment possible.

MEATUS OBTURATOR. The pharyngeal impression for a meatus obturator is considered as a separate section here. The meatus obturator is formulated on the presumption that complete occlusion of the oropharynx from the nasopharynx is not necessary for good cleft palate speech. It is believed, rather, that the partial occlusion of the nasal cavity will result in a marked diminution and, in many instances, complete elimination of the nasal sound that is so apparent and so objectionable in the patient with a cleft palate. If the restoration fulfills this objective, the logopedist, who, when using other appliances, has to train certain muscles to reduce the hypernasality and others to conquer the articulative defects, need direct his efforts only toward correcting the latter. He need not concern himself with the muscle-training incident to reducing nasality. This in turn should reduce the number of training sessions necessary to improve speech for any particular patient.

This type of obturator ignores Passavant's pad and the posterior pharyngeal wall. Instead it makes contact with the superior aspect of the nasal cavity at the junction of nasal and pharyngeal cavities.

In other words, whereas the usual fixed type of obturator is directed in a line more or less parallel to, and continuous with, the palate, this type is inclined perpendicularly to the palate (Fig. 23-14).

The construction is not complicated. The upper casting is finished with the usual loop projecting into the cleft and is checked in the mouth for accuracy. Using this framework as a vehicle, softened modeling plastic is molded around the distal loop with its greatest bulk directly above the loop. When the modeling plastic is hard, it is removed. More softened material is added and the denture framework is repo-

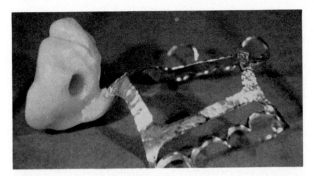

Fig. 23-14. Side view of a meatus obturator showing its relation to the framework.

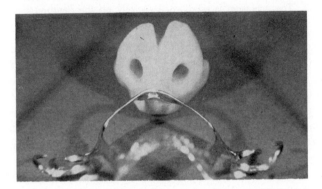

Fig. 23-15. Frontal view of the meatus obturator showing the vents.

sitioned in the mouth. Then an attempt by the patient is made to blow air through the nose. If air escapes, then small amounts of modeling plastic are added in likely areas until no air escapes through the nose and the patient talks as though he had a bad cold (the so-called rhinolalia clausa). The impression is removed from the mouth, and at this time any projection of material into the eustachian tubes should be cut from the impression to allow free interchange of air.

The completed impression is invested, boiled out, and processed in acrylic resin. After polishing, it is placed in the patient's mouth to check for gross errors in processing. When it is satisfactory, a vent about 3 mm. in diameter is cut in an anteroposterior direction, approximately in the center and free of turbinates and vomer. If the later is very large, it may be necessary to make two smaller holes on either side. (See Fig. 23-15.)

This opening serves as a means of breathing through the nose. The restoration is put back into the mouth and the patient is instructed to speak. If the voice sounds "closed," the aperture is enlarged until a balance between the closed and open "nose" is reached. Immediately upon placing the prosthesis and balancing the size of the hole, the resultant nasality should improve. Only the articulative defects remain and these are not as unpleasant because of the normal nasal quality. There is usually no gagging tendency and no irritation of the mucous membrane. When the physical situation permits the use of any type of obturator, the decision as to which should be used must be determined by individual preference rather than by intrinsic value.

It was apparent early that a classic meatus type could be constructed in too few instances. Therefore a compromise between the fixed type and the meatus type

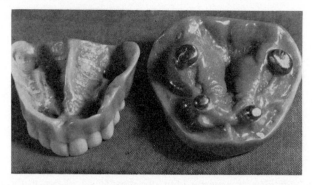

Fig. 23-16. Model of repaired cleft palate with its restoration. Four remaining maxillary teeth, which do not occlude with mandibular teeth, are crowned and act as retentive mechanism for a façade prosthesis. The occlusion is established entirely on the denture.

is now attempted, rarely getting the impression as high as the latter and never as low as the former. It is my opinion that the obturator should be as high in the pharynx as is feasible. This compromise obturator does not usually require vents.

Psychologic aspects. The psychologic aspects of cleft palate prostheses cannot be overemphasized. Underdeveloped maxillary dental arches are often seen in those patients who have had early surgical closure. If the orthodontist is unable for any reason to correct these malocclusions, the patient is left with an underdeveloped middle third of the face. This pseudo-Class III appearance can be somewhat diminished by a facade prosthesis. In these instances, all teeth have to be crowned and the prosthesis is fashioned anterior to these teeth for proper appearance. Fig. 23-16 shows an extreme situation in which only four teeth remained and these were not occluding with any of the mandibular teeth. The facade prosthesis was fashioned to improve the appearance and also to provide a masticating unit.

MAXILLOFACIAL PROSTHESIS

Many oral defects are the results of corrective surgery or of accidental trauma. The prosthetic replacement of lost oral structure has to be approached with some caution since the remaining tissues are often scarred and more reactive to pressures. The presence of teeth is a great boon to the prosthodontist who may treat such persons. It is well known that attempts to replace the tissue lost in a hemisection of the palate is extremely difficult *in the edentulous patient.* If worn at all, such prostheses are maintained largely by the active will of the patient and to a lesser degree by the usual biophysical factors.

When teeth are present in the mouth, the construction of the prosthesis is divided into three phases: (1) the complete and perfect restoration of all the remaining teeth and periodontal tissues; (2) the design and construction of the metal framework; and (3) the construction of the tissue replacement section. The first phase should include full crown coverage whenever necessary for restoration of carious areas, for protection from carious processes, and whenever necessary to provide retentive areas for clasp arms.

As in cleft palate therapy, the loss of any of the teeth places a burden on remaining teeth, and the loss of all teeth is catastrophic. The dentist should resort to any measures that will preserve the integrity of the remaining teeth, including the splinting together of several teeth.

Although the detailed design of the metal framework will vary for each patient, two general principles must be considered. First, the bracing aspects of the design must be emphasized. For example, every molar and premolar tooth remaining after a hemisection of the maxilla should have

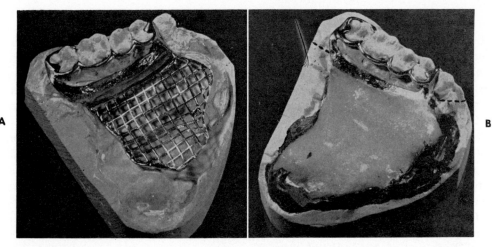

Fig. 23-17. Prosthetic treatment of maxillary hemisection. **A,** All posterior teeth remaining after a hemisection of the maxilla should have reciprocal arms to distribute widely the downward dislodging force of the unsupported side. **B,** When the corrected impression is obtained, all the original cast except the teeth and adjacent gingival tissues is cut away, and a new cast is poured into the corrected impression. The dotted line separates the new section from the original section of the cast.

a bracing arm, to distribute torque forces adequately (Fig. 23-17). Second, retentive clasp arms should be designed so that they resist the displacement forces of the finished restoration. It must be remembered that weight alone is often an important displacing force for these restorations.

The tissue replacement section of the prosthesis is important because, of course, it serves the primary function of this type of restoration. When the framework has been checked in the mouth for accurate fit, an acrylic resin impression tray is fashioned as part of the framework. This impression tray is underextended at least 1 mm. in all directions. The border is now accurately recorded in a low-fusing stick modeling plastic. When this is done, all modeling plastic areas that contact tissue are scraped 0.5 mm. and the final impression is obtained in a rubber-base impression material.

The original cast is now altered by removing all the tissue-borne section, retaining only the teeth and the adjacent gingival portion. The impression and framework are replaced accurately on the remainder of the cast, and a new tissue section is poured into the final impression. Thus a corrected cast is available for processing.

The utmost care must be exercised to avoid even the slightest displacement of remaining soft tissue. This is extremely important in patients whose defects are due to cancer surgery because any tissue irritation in these areas is potentially dangerous. This is especially true if irradiation therapy followed surgery. Mechanical attempts to lock restorations into tissue undercuts by ingenious sectional devices are hazardous.

Many of the patients who have a defect that is the result of cancer therapy have received radiation therapy in combination with the surgical procedures. This therapy greatly diminishes the normal blood supply and makes the tissues particularly susceptible to infections and traumatic injury. Because the original blood supply to the maxilla is greater than to the mandible the effects of radiation are more serious on the mandible. Patient responses to a therapeutic dose of 7,000 roentgens vary considerably so an individual assessment of the patient should guide the placement of a prosthesis. The degree and duration of the acute reaction to the therapy along with the appearance of the tissues (particularly color) as it relates to blood supply dictate the prosthetic treatment. The surgery usually diminishes the sensory nerve supply to the area so that these patients may develop an ulcer without the usual symptom of pain. Therefore all patients who have been irradiated should be closely followed for possible trauma caused by the prosthesis.

It follows naturally that there is a correlation between the tissue resistance and the amount of trauma required to produce a breakdown in the tissues. The amount of time the denture is worn and the way it is used (speech, deglutition, mastication) will influence the total amount of trauma produced. Each patient should therefore gradually increase the time and activities performed with the prosthesis until it is determined how much trauma he can safely tolerate.

As was mentioned previously, weight is a considerable displacing factor, and when prostheses demand thickness and bulk, they should be constructed in such a way that they are hollow. This is an easy process today with the autopolymerizing resins. These resins enable us to process hollow restorations, which may be capped and sealed with additional autopolymerizing resin.

When constructing prostheses after radical surgery of the face and neck, one must be prepared to alter them to accommodate for changes in tissue topography. The latter result from altered physiology in connection with lymph drainage in general. Sometimes these patients will have a marked difference in the tissue-fluid content of their facial tissues from morning to night. This may prove difficult to the prosthodontist because if the prosthesis fits in the morning, it will be loose in the afternoon, and if it fits in the afternoon, it may cause sore spots in the morning. In general, the former situation is to be preferred. Accordingly, it may be better to make all impressions in the morning.

Furthermore, the process of scar contraction may continue for several weeks or months, which will demand continual revision of the prosthesis.

One final word should be added about scarring. Restoration of facial contour should never be attempted when considerable pressure against scar tissue is required to do so. This again may cause ulceration, displacement of the restoration, movement of the teeth, or all three.

When arranging teeth for a restoration, replacing a hemisection of the maxilla, it should be remembered that the remaining tissue bearing the force of occlusion is of poor quality. Therefore, the occlusion should be arranged to contact just lightly on the affected side. In some instances, it may be preferable to eliminate occlusal contact entirely, to avoid any pressure. The patient should be instructed to avoid chewing on the affected side. He now has a difficult situation, but it is better for him to eat only on one side without soreness than to eat on both and develop constantly irritated tissue areas.

It must be realized that these particular patients have been through a difficult period. The thoughts of losing large tissue blocks are matters of concern to even the most callous. The realization that the resultant defects in speech or appearance may be permanent does not encourage the patient. Therefore he should be informed that the prostheses are available, and a clear assessment of their role should be offered to him.

The dentist should neither dispel this hope with talk of failure or build false hopes with talk of great success. Indeed, he should consider his own chances of creating a successful prosthesis. Then the patient should be encouraged to cooperate in the construction of the restoration and be encouraged to wear it. Negative approaches are poor. If one dwells unduly on the chance of failure, he is making a bad mistake. Instead, tell the truthful story of the many people who wear these restorations successfully.

It occurs to me that there is a great deal of difference between the following statements:

1. There are 40% of people who wear

these restorations happily and successfully.

2. There are 60% of people who cannot wear these restorations.

The former is encouraging, the latter deadening. Use a positive bright approach, being careful not to build up false hopes. Building a bleak picture can seriously affect the patient's attitude toward the prosthesis.

Years of constructing these cleft palate and surgical prostheses have convinced me that it is perhaps the most rewarding branch of prosthetic dentistry. These patients are not petty, arrogant people; they are indeed appreciative, cooperative, and a pleasure to know.

The patient can often tell the dentist much about how the restoration should serve and can offer constructive suggestions concerning its design. Always listen to, and weigh carefully, these suggestions. It has been my experience that near failures have been converted to successful restorations by following the patient's directions in certain aspects of construction. This is true primarily in the design of the metal framework.

In addition, I find that denture adhesives are less objectionable to me now than they were previously. They can be healthy aids to retention, partially relieving the teeth of burden, thus extending tooth longevity. Of course, scrupulous cleansing of oral tissues and restorations must be maintained.

I am grateful to Dr. Stephen Bartlett, Professor of Prosthetic Dentistry at the College of Dental Medicine, Medical University of South Carolina, for his helpful suggestions for revision of this chapter.

Selected references

TEXTBOOKS

Applegate, O. C.: Essentials of removable partial denture prosthesis, Philadelphia, 1965, W. B. Saunders Co.

Austin, K. P., and Lidge, E. F., Jr.: Partial dentures, St. Louis, 1957, The C. V. Mosby Co.

Boucher, C. O., editor: Swenson's complete dentures, ed. 6, St. Louis, 1970, The C. V. Mosby Co.

Brecker, S. C.: Clinical procedures in occlusal rehabilitation, Philadelphia, 1966, W. B. Saunders Co.

Brecker, S. C.: Crowns, Philadelphia, 1961, W. B. Saunders Co.

Brumfield, R. C.: Dental gold structures, New York, 1949, J. F. Jelenko & Co., Inc.

Craddock, F. W.: Prosthetic dentistry, St. Louis, 1951, The C. V. Mosby Co.

Denton, G. B.: The vocabulary of dentistry and oral science, Chicago, 1958, American Dental Association.

Dykema, R. W., Cunningham, D. M., and Johnston, J. F.: Modern practice in removable partial prosthodontics, Philadelphia, 1969, W. B. Saunders Co.

Ewing, J. E.: Fixed partial prosthesis, Philadelphia, 1959, Lea & Febiger.

Farrell, J.: Partial denture designing, London, 1970, Henry Kimpton Publishers.

Fenn, H. R. B., Liddelow, K. P., and Gimson, A. P.: Clinical dental prosthetics, London, 1953, Staples Press, Ltd.

Fish, E. W.: Principles of full denture prosthesis, London, 1964, Staples Press, Ltd.

Gehl, D. H., and Dresen, O. M.: Complete denture prosthesis, Philadelphia, 1958, W. B. Saunders Co.

Goldman, H. M., and Cohen, D. W.: Periodontal therapy, ed. 4, St. Louis, 1968, The C. V. Mosby Co.

Granger, E. R.: Practical procedures in oral rehabilitation, Philadelphia, 1962, J. B. Lippincott Co.

Harkins, C. S.: Principles of cleft palate prosthesis, New York, 1960, Columbia University Publications.

Heartwell, C. M., Jr.: Syllabus of complete dentures, Philadelphia, 1968, Lea & Febiger.

Johnston, J. F., Phillips, R. W., and Dykema, R. W.: Modern practice in crown and bridge prosthodontics, Philadelphia, 1971, W. B. Saunders Co.

Kazis, H., and Kazis, A. J.: Complete mouth rehabilitation through crown and bridge prosthodontics, Philadelphia, 1956, Lea & Febiger.

Kennedy, E.: Partial denture construction, Brooklyn, 1942, Dental Items of Interest Publishing Co.

Langley, L. L., and Cheraskin, E.: The physiological foundation of dental practice, ed. 2, St. Louis, 1956, The C. V. Mosby Co.

Lee, J. H.: Dental aesthetics, Bristol, 1962, Stonebridge Press.

Lucia, V. O.: Modern gnathological concepts, St. Louis, 1961, The C. V. Mosby Co.

McNeil, C. K.: Oral and facial deformity, New York, 1954, Pitman Publishing Corp.

Miller, E. R.: Removable partial prosthodontics, Baltimore, 1972, The Williams & Wilkins Co.

Morley, M. E.: Cleft palate and speech, Edinburgh, 1954, E. & S. Livingstone, Ltd.

Morris, A. L., and Bohannon, H. M., editors: Dental specialties in general practice, Philadelphia, 1969, W. B. Saunders Co.

Nagle, R. J., Sears, V. H., and Silverman, S. I.: Denture prosthetics, ed. 2, St. Louis, 1962, The C. V. Mosby Co.

Osborne, J., and Lammie, G. A.: Partial dentures, Oxford, 1952, Blackwell Scientific Publications.

Peyton, F. A., and Craig, R. G.: Restorative dental materials, St. Louis, 1971, The C. V. Mosby Co.

Phillips, R. W.: Elements of dental materials, Philadelphia, 1971, W. B. Saunders Co.

Preiskel, H. W.: Precision attachments in dentistry, St. Louis, 1968, The C. V. Mosby Co.

Rahn, A. O., and Boucher, L. J.: Maxillofacial prosthetics, Philadelphia, 1970, W. B. Saunders Co.

Ramfjord, S. P., and Ash, M. M., Jr.: Occlusion, ed. 2, Philadelphia, 1971, W. B. Saunders Co.

Rebassio, A. D.: Protesis parcial removable, Buenos Aires, 1960, Editorial Mundi Republica Argentina.

Sarnat, B. F., editor: The temporomandibular joint, Springfield, Ill., 1951, Charles C Thomas, Publisher.

Scheu, R.: Wrought-wire technique for partial dentures, Bristol, 1960, Stonebridge Press.

Schwartz, L.: Disorders of the temporomandibular joint, Philadelphia, 1959, W. B. Saunders Co.

Schweitzer, J. M.: Oral rehabilitation problem cases, St. Louis, 1964, The C. V. Mosby Co.

Sharry, J. J., editor: Complete denture prosthodontics, ed. 2, New York, 1968, McGraw-Hill Book Co.

Shillington, G. B.: Fundamentals of partial denture planning, Ottawa, 1957, Queen's Printer.

Sicher, H., and DuBrul, E. L.: Oral anatomy, ed. 5, St. Louis, 1970, The C. V. Mosby Co.

Silverman, M. M.: Occlusion in prosthodontics and in the natural dentition, Washington, D. C., 1963, Mutual Publishing Co.

Singer, F., and Schon, F.: Partial dentures, Chicago, 1966, Year Book Medical Publishers, Inc.

Skinner, E. W., and Phillips, R. W.: The science of dental materials, Philadelphia, 1967, W. B. Saunders Co.

Steiger, A. A., and Boitel, R. H.: Precision work for partial dentures, Zurich, 1959, Buchdruckerei Berichthaus.

Terkla, L. G., and Laney, W. R.: Partial dentures, ed. 3, St. Louis, 1963, The C. V. Mosby Co.

Tylman, S. D.: Theory and practice of crown and fixed partial prosthodontics (bridge), ed. 6, St. Louis, 1970, The C. V. Mosby Co.

Wilson, W. H., and Lang, R. L.: Practical crown and bridge prosthodontics, New York, 1963, McGraw-Hill Book Co.

ABUTMENT RETAINERS: EXTERNAL AND INTERNAL ATTACHMENTS

Adisman, I. K.: The internal clip attachment in fixed-removable partial denture prosthesis, N. Y. J. Dent. 32:125-129, 1962.

Ainamo, J.: Precision removable partial dentures with pontic abutments, J. Prosthet. Dent. 23: 289-295, 1970.

Augsburger, R. H.: The Gilmore attachment, J. Prosthet. Dent. 16:1090-1102, 1966.

Blatterfein, L.: Study of partial denture clasping, J. Am. Dent. Assoc. 43:169-185, 1951; Design and positional arrangement of clasps for partial dentures, N. Y. J. Dent. 22:305-306, 1952.

Breisach, L.: Esthetic attachments for removable partial dentures, J. Prosthet. Dent. 17:261-265, 1967.

Brodbelt, R. H. W.: A simple paralleling template for precision attachments, J. Prosthet. Dent. 27:285-288, 1972.

Caldarone, C. V.: Attachments for partial dentures without clasps, J. Prosthet. Dent. 7:206-208, 1957.

Cohn, L. A.: The physiologic basis for tooth fixation in precision-attached partial dentures, J. Prosthet. Dent. 6:220-244, 1956.

DeVan, M. M.: Fortn. Rev. Chic. Dent. Soc. 27: 7-12 (portrait), 1954; Preserving natural teeth through the use of clasps, J. Prosthet. Dent. 5:208-214, 1955.

Dietz, W. H.: Modified abutments for removable and fixed prosthodontics, J. Prosthet. Dent. 11: 1112-1116, 1961.

Dolder, E. J.: The bar joint mandibular denture, J. Prosthet. Dent. 11:689-707, 1961.

Farrell, J.: Wrought wire retainers—a method of increasing their flexibility, Br. Dent. J. 131:327, 1971.

Gilson, T. D.: A fixable-removable prosthetic attachment, J. Prosthet. Dent. 9:247-255, 1959.

Gindea, A. E.: A retentive device for removable dentures, J. Prosthet. Dent. 27:501-508, 1972.

Green, J. H.: The hinge-lock abutment attachment, J. Am. Dent. Assoc. 47:175-180, 1953.

Grosser, D.: The dynamics of internal precision attachments, J. Prosthet. Dent. 3:393-401, 1953; Harvard Dent. Alumni. Bull. 14:7-9, 1954.

Handlers, M., Lenchner, N. H., and Weissman, B.: A retaining device for partial dentures, J. Prosthet. Dent. 7:483-488, 1957.

Hekneby, M.: The spring-slide joint for lower free end removable partial dentures, J. Prosthet. Dent. 11:256-263, 1961.

Hollenback, G. M., and Oaks, S.: Role of the precision attachment in partial denture prosthesis, J. Am. Dent. Assoc. 41:173-182, 1950.

Isaacson, G. O.: Telescope crown retainers for removable partial dentures, J. Prosthet. Dent. 22: 436-448, 1969.

James, A. G.: Self-locking posterior attachment for removable tooth-supported partial dentures, J. Prosthet. Dent. 5:200-205, 1955.

Johnson, J. F.: The application and construction of the pinledge retainer, J. Prosthet. Dent. 3: 559-567, 1953.

Knodle, J. M.: Experimental overlay and pin partial denture, J. Prosthet. Dent. 17:472-478, 1967.

Knowles, L. E.: A dowel attachment removable partial denture, J. Prosthet. Dent. 13:679-687, 1963.

Leff, A.: Precision attachment dentures, J. Prosthet. Dent. 2:84-91, 1952.

Mann, A. W.: The lower distal extension partial denture using the Hart-Dunn attachment, J. Prosthet. Dent. 8:282-288, 1958.

Morrison, M. L.: Internal precision attachment retainers for partial dentures, J. Am. Dent. Assoc. 64:209-215, 1962.

Morrow, R. M.: Tooth-supported complete dentures: an approach to preventive prosthodontics, J. Prosthet. Dent. 21:513-522, 1969.

Myers, G. E., Wepfer, G. G., and Peyton, F. A.: The thiokol rubber base impression materials, J. Prosthet. Dent. 8:330-339, 1958.

Nelson, E. A., and Hinds, F. W.: Abutments as applied to fixed as well as removable partial denture prosthesis, J. Am. Dent. Assoc. 29:534-542, 1942.

Oddo, V. J., Jr.: The movable-arm clasp for complete passivity in partial denture construction, J. Am. Dent. Assoc. 74:1009-1015, 1967.

Phillips, R. N.: A problem of retention in a lower partial denture, J. Prosthet. Dent. 6:213-219, 1956.

Plotnick, I. J.: Internal attachment for fixed removable partial dentures, J. Prosthet. Dent. 8:85-93, 1958.

Pound, E.: Cross-arch splinting vs. premature extractions, J. Prosthet. Dent. 16:1058-1068, 1966.

Preiskel, H.: Precision attachments for free-end saddle prostheses, Br. Dent. J. 127:462-468, 1969; Screw retained telescopic prosthesis, Br. Dent. J. 130:107-112, 1971.

Prince, I. B.: Conservation of the supportive mechanism, J. Prosthet. Dent. 15:327-338, 1965.

Rispler, C. J.: Evaluation of precision attachments in partial denture construction, J. Soc. Dent. Res. 1:8-12, 1952; Bull. San Diego Cty. Dent. Soc. 25:8-9, 15, 1955.

Rosen, M. H.: Fixed-movable partial dentures with interlocking onlay attachments: review of a practical case, J. Am. Dent. Assoc. 41:306-307, 1950.

Rubin, J. G.: Precision attachment partial dentures with hydrocolloid impression: an accurate, rapid procedure, Dent. Dig. 60:504-508, 1954.

Schuyler, C. H.: Analysis of the use and relative value of the precision attachment and the clasp in partial denture planning, J. Prosthet. Dent. 3:711-714, 1953.

Singer, F.: Improvements in precision—attached removable partial dentures, J. Prosthet. Dent. 17:69-72, 1967.

Smith, R. A., and Rymarz, F. P.: Cast clasp transitional removable partial dentures, J. Prosthet. Dent. 22:381-385, 1969.

Terrell, W. H.: Specialized frictional attachments and their role in partial denture construction, Aust. J. Dent. 55:119-128, 1951; Dent. J. Aust. 22:471-483, 1950; J. Prosthet. Dent. 1:337-350, 1951.

Vasic, S., et al.: An aesthetic clasp for acrylic partial dentures, J. Can. Dent. Assoc. 37:38-39, 1971.

Vig, R. G.: Splinting bars and maxillary indirect retainers for removable partial dentures, J. Prosthet. Dent. 13:125-129, 1963.

Williams, A. G.: Technique for provisional splint with attachment, J. Prosthet. Dent. 21:555-559, 1969.

ANATOMY

Barker, B. C. W.: Dissection of regions of interest to the dentist from a medical approach, Aust. Dent. J. 16:163-171, 1971.

Bennett, N. G.: A contribution to the study of the movements of the mandible, J. Prosthet. Dent. 8:41-54, 1958.

Boucher, C. O.: Anatomy of the mouth in relation to complete dentures, J. Wis. State Dent. Soc. 19:161-166, 1943; Complete denture impressions based upon the anatomy of the mouth, J. Am. Dent. Assoc. 31:1174-1181, 1944.

Brodie, A. G.: Anatomy and physiology of head and neck musculature, Am. J. Orthod. 36:831-844, 1950.

Craddock, F. W.: Retromolar region of the mandible, J. Am. Dent. Assoc. 47:453-455, 1953.

Haines, R. W., and Barnett, S. G.: The structure of the mouth in the mandibular molar region, J. Prosthet. Dent. 9:962-974, 1959.

Last, R. J.: The muscles of the mandible, Dent. Dig. 61:165-169, 1955.

Martone, A. L., et al.: Anatomy of the mouth and related structures, J. Prosthet. Dent. Part I, 11:1009-1018, 1961; Part II, 12:4-27, 1962; Part III, 12:206-219, 1962; Part IV, 12:409-419, 1962; Part V, 12:629-636, 1962; Part VI, 12:817-834, 1962; Part VII, 13:4-33, 1963; Part VIII, 13:204-228, 1963.

Merkeley, H. J.: The labial and buccal accessory muscles of mastication, J. Prosthet. Dent. 4:327-334, 1954; Mandibular rearmament. Part I. Anatomic considerations, J. Prosthet. Dent. 9:559-566, 1959.

Pendleton, E. C.: Anatomy of the face and mouth from the standpoint of the denture prosthetist, J. Am. Dent. Assoc. 33:219-234, 1946; Changes in the denture supporting tissues, J. Am. Dent. Assoc. 42:1-15, 1951.

Roche, A. F.: Functional anatomy of the muscles of mastication, J. Prosthet. Dent. 13:548-570, 1963.

Silverman, S. I.: Denture prosthesis and the functional anatomy of the maxillofacial structures, J. Prosthet. Dent. 6:305-331, 1956.

BIOMECHANICS

Abel, L. F., and Manly, R. S.: Masticatory function of partial denture patients among navy personnel, J. Prosthet. Dent. 3:382-392, 1953.

Applegate, O. C.: Use of the paralleling surveyor in modern partial denture construction, J. Am. Dent. Assoc. 27:1397-1407, 1940.

Avant, W. E.: Fulcrum and retention lines in

planning removable partial dentures, J. Prosthet. Dent. **25**:162-166, 1971; Factors that influence retention of removable partial dentures, J. Prosthet. Dent. **25**:265-270, 1971.

Brudevold, F.: Basic study of the chewing forces of a denture wearer, J. Am. Dent. Assoc. **43**: 45-51, 1951.

Brumfield, R. C.: Load capacities of posterior dental bridges, J. Prosthet. Dent. **4**:530-547, 1954.

Cecconi, B. T., Asgar, K., and Dootz, E.: The effect of partial denture clasp design on abutment tooth movement, J. Prosthet. Dent. **25**:44-56, 1971; Removable partial denture abutment tooth movement as affected by inclination of residual ridges and types of loading, J. Prosthet. Dent. **25**:375-381, 1971; Clasp assembly modifications and their effect on abutment tooth movement, J. Prosthet. Dent. **27**:160-167, 1972.

Clayton, J. A., and Jaslow, C.: A measurement of clasp forces on teeth, J. Prosthet. Dent. **25**:21-43, 1971.

DeVan, M. M.: The nature of the partial denture foundation: suggestions for its preservation, J. Prosthet. Dent. **2**:210-218, 1952.

Frechette, A. R.: The influence of partial denture design on distribution of force to abutment teeth, J. Prosthet. Dent. **6**:195-212, 1956.

Goodman, J. J., and Goodman, H. W.: Balance of force in precision free-end restorations, J. Prosthet. Dent. **13**:302-308, 1963.

Henderson, D., and Seward, T. E.: Design and force distribution with removable partial dentures; a progress report, J. Prosthet. Dent. **17**:350-364, 1967.

Hindels, G. W.: Stress analysis in distal extension partial dentures, J. Prosthet. Dent. **7**:197-205, 1957.

Howell, A. H., and Manly, R. S.: An electronic strain gauge for measuring oral forces, J. Dent. Res. **27**:705-712, 1948.

Kaires, A. K.: Partial denture design and its relation to force distribution and masticatory performance, J. Prosthet. Dent. **6**:672-683, 1956.

Knowles, L. E.: The biomechanics of removable partial dentures and its relationship to fixed prosthesis, J. Prosthet. Dent. **8**:426-430, 1958.

Kratochvil, F. J.: Influence of occlusal rest position and clasp design on movement of abutment teeth, J. Prosthet. Dent. **13**:114-124, 1963.

Lowe, R. O., et al.: Swallowing and resting forces related to lingual flange thickness in removable partial dentures, J. Prosthet. Dent. **23**:279-288, 1970.

Moses, C. H.: Biomechanics and artificial posterior teeth, J. Prosthet. Dent. **4**:782-802, 1954.

Shohet, H.: Relative magnitudes of stress on abutment teeth with different retainers, J. Prosthet. Dent. **21**:267-282, 1969.

Skinner, E. W., and Chung, P.: The effect of surface contact in the retention of a denture, J. Prosthet. Dent. **1**:229-235, 1951.

Smyd, E. S.: Bio-mechanics of prosthetic dentistry, J. Prosthet. Dent. **4**:368-383, 1954; The role of tongue, torsion, and bending in prosthodontic failures, J. Prosthet. Dent. **11**:95-111, 1961.

Yurkstas, A., and Curby, W. A.: Force analysis of prosthetic appliances during function, J. Prosthet. Dent. **3**:82-87, 1953.

Yurkstas, A., Fridley, H. H., and Manly, R. S.: A functional evaluation of fixed and removable bridgework, J. Prosthet. Dent. **1**:570-577, 1951.

Zoeller, G. N.: Block form stability in removable partial dentures, J. Prosthet. Dent. **22**:633-637, 1969.

Zoeller, G. N., and Kelly, W. J., Jr.: Block form stability in removable partial prosthodontics, J. Prosthet. Dent. **25**:515-519, 1971.

CLASSIFICATION

Applegate, O. C.: The rationale of partial denture choice, J. Prosthet. Dent. **10**:891-907, 1960.

Avant, W. E.: A universal classification for removable partial denture situations, J. Prosthet. Dent. **16**:533-539, 1966.

Miller, E. L.: Systems for classifying partially dentulous arches, J. Prosthet. Dent. **24**:25-40, 1970.

Skinner, C. N.: A classification of removable partial dentures based upon the principles of anatomy and physiology, J. Prosthet. Dent. **9**:240-246, 1959.

CLEFT PALATE

Aram, A., and Subtelny, J. D.: Velopharyngeal function and cleft palate prostheses, J. Prosthet. Dent. **9**:149-158, 1959.

Baden, E.: Fundamental principles of orofacial prosthetic therapy in congenital cleft palate, J. Prosthet. Dent. **4**:420-433, 1954.

Calvan, J.: The error of Gustan Passavant, Plast. Reconstr. Surg. **13**:275-289, 1954.

Cooper, H. K.: Integration of service in the treatment of cleft lip and cleft palate, J. Am. Dent. Assoc. **47**:27-32, 1953.

Fox, A.: Prosthetic correction of a severe acquired cleft palate, J. Prosthet. Dent. **8**:542-546, 1958.

Gibbons, P., and Bloomer, H.: A supportive-type prosthetic speech aid, J. Prosthet. Dent. **8**:362-369, 1958.

Graber, T. M.: Oral and nasal structures in cleft palate speech, J. Am. Dent. Assoc. **53**:693-706, 1956.

Harkins, C. S.: Modern concepts in the prosthetic rehabilitation of cleft palate patients, J. Oral Surg. **10**:298-312, 1952.

Harkins, C. S., and Ivy, R. H.: Surgery and prosthesis in the rehabilitation of cleft palate patients, J. South. Calif. Dent. Assoc. **19**:16-24, 1951.

Landa, J. S.: The prosthodontist views the rehabilitation of the cleft palate patient, J. Prosthet. Dent. **6**:421-427, 1956.

Lloyd, R. S., Pruzansky, S., and Subtelny, J. D.: Prosthetic rehabilitation of a cleft palate patient subsequent to multiple surgical and prosthetic failures, J. Prosthet. Dent. 7:216-230, 1957.

Malson, T. S.: Complete denture for the congenital cleft palate patient, J. Prosthet. Dent. 5:567-578, 1955.

Merkeley, H. J.: Cleft palate prosthesis, J. Prosthet. Dent. 9:506-513, 1959.

Nidiffer, T. J., and Shipmon, T. H.: The hollow bulb obturator for acquired palatal openings, J. Prosthet. Dent. 7:126-134, 1957.

Olinger, N. A.: Cleft palate prosthesis rehabilitation, J. Prosthet. Dent. 2:117-135, 1952.

Rosen, M. S.: Prosthetics for the cleft palate patient, J. Am. Dent. Assoc. 60:715-721, 1960.

Sharry, J. J.: The meatus obturator in cleft palate prosthesis, Oral Surg. 7:852-855, 1954; Meatus obturator in particular and pharyngeal impressions in general, J. Prosthet. Dent. 8:893-896, 1958.

Strain, J. C.: A simplified device to attach the distal extension to the denture of a cleft palate patient, J. Prosthet. Dent. 3:727-730, 1953.

Torn, D. B.: Speech and cleft palate partial denture prosthesis, J. Prosthet. Dent. 2:413-417, 1952.

Vale, W. A.: Fixed bridge for a cleft palate, Br. Dent. J. 96:65-66, 1954.

Webster, R. C.: Cleft palate treatment, Oral Surg. 1:647-669, 943-980, 1948; 2:99-153, 485-542, 1949.

COMPLETE MOUTH AND OCCLUSAL REHABILITATION

Bronstein, B. R.: Rationale and technique of biomechanical occlusal rehabilitation, J. Prosthet. Dent. 4:352-367, 1954.

Chestner, S. B.: Cold cure acrylic resin splints in occlusal rehabilitation, J. Prosthet. Dent. 5:228-231, 1955.

Cohn, L. A.: Occluso-rehabilitation. Principles of diagnosis and treatment planning, Dent. Clin. North Am., pp. 259-281, March, 1962.

Dubin, N. A.: Advances in functional occlusal rehabilitation, J. Prosthet. Dent. 6:252-258, 1956.

Goldman, I.: The art and science of full mouth rehabilitation, Dent. Dig. 59:17-22, 1953.

Kazis, H.: Functional aspects of complete mouth rehabilitation, J. Prosthet. Dent. 4:833-841, 1954.

Kornfeld, M.: The problem of function in restorative dentistry, J. Prosthet. Dent. 5:670-676, 1955.

Landa, J. S.: An analysis of current practices in mouth rehabilitation, J. Prosthet. Dent. 5:527-537, 1955.

Mann, A. W., and Pankey, L. D.: Oral rehabilitation utilizing the Pankey-Mann instrument and a functional bite technique, Dent. Clin. North Am. pp. 215-230, March, 1959; Oral rehabilitation. Part I. Use of the P-M instrument in treatment planning and restoring the lower posterior teeth, J. Prosthet. Dent. 10:135-150, 1960; Part II. Reconstruction of the upper teeth using a functionally generated path technique, 10:151-162, 1960.

Rubinstein, M. N.: Approach to mouth reconstruction, Dent. Dig. 61:24-28, 1955.

Schuyler, C. H.: An evaluation of incisal guidance and its influence on restorative dentistry, J. Prosthet. Dent. 9:374-378, 1959.

Schweitzer, J. M.: Open bite from the prosthetic point of view, Dent. Clin. North Am., pp. 269-283, March, 1957.

Thompson, M. J.: Hydrocolloid: its role in restorative dentistry, Dent. Clin. North Am., pp. 101-112, March, 1959.

CROWNS AND FIXED PARTIAL DENTURES

Alexander, P. C.: Analysis of the cuspid protective occlusion, J. Prosthet. Dent. 13:309-317, 1963.

Baraban, D. J.: Cementation of fixed bridge prosthesis with zinc oxide-rosin-eugenol cements, J. Prosthet. Dent. 8:988-991, 1958.

Bartlett, A. A.: Some principles of modern fixed bridge construction, J. Am. Dent. Assoc. 29:2166-2173, 1942.

Beeson, P. E.: The use of acrylic resins as an aid in the development of patterns for two types of crowns, J. Prosthet. Dent. 13:493-498, 1963.

Boyd, H. R., Jr.: Pontics in fixed partial dentures, J. Prosthet. Dent. 5:55-64, 1955.

Brotman, I. N.: The roentgenogram as an aid in veneer crown preparation, J. Prosthet. Dent. 4:349-351, 1954.

Caplan, J.: Maintenance of full coverage fixed-abutment bridges, J. Prosthet. Dent. 5:852-854, 1955.

Cavanagh, W. D.: Crown and bridge prosthesis, J. Can. Dent. Assoc. 21:222-226, 1955.

Chestner, S. B.: Cold acrylic resin splints in occlusal rehabilitation, J. Prosthet. Dent. 5:228-231, 1955.

Coelho, D. H.: The ultimate goal in fixed bridge procedures, J. Prosthet. Dent. 4:667-672, 1954; Criteria for the use of fixed prosthesis, Dent. Clin. North Am. pp. 299-311, March, 1957.

Collett, H. A.: Cast shell veneer crowns, J. Prosthet. Dent. 25:177-182, 1971.

Cooper, T. M., et al.: Effect of venting on cast gold full crowns, J. Prosthet. Dent. 26:621-626, 1971.

Cowgen, G. T.: Retention, resistance and esthetics of the anterior three-quarter crown, J. Am. Dent. Assoc. 62:167-171, 1961.

Davis, M. C., and Klein, G.: Combination gold and acrylic restorations, J. Prosthet. Dent. 4:510-522, 1954.

Ewing, J. E.: Re-evaluation of the cantilever principle, J. Prosthet. Dent. 7:78-92, 1957.

Freese, A. S.: Impressions for temporary acrylic

resin jacket crowns, J. Prosthet. Dent. **7**:99-101, 1957.

Gerson, I.: Cementation of fixed restorations, J. Prosthet. Dent. **7**:123-125, 1957.

Guyer, S. E.: Nonrigid subocclusal connector for fixed partial dentures, J. Prosthet. Dent. **26**:433-436, 1971.

Hagerman, D. A., and Arnim, S. S.: The relation of new knowledge of the gingiva to crown and bridge procedures, J. Prosthet. Dent. **5**:538-542, 1955; Dent. Abstr. **1**:44, 1956.

Henderson, D., et al.: The cantilever type of posterior fixed partial dentures: A laboratory study, J. Prosthet. Dent. **24**:47-67, 1970.

Herschfus, L.: Procedure for immediate temporary bridge, Dent. Dig. **60**:550-551, 1954.

Johnson, E. A., Jr.: Combination of fixed and removable partial dentures, J. Prosthet. Dent. **14**:1099-1106, 1964.

Johnston, J. F., Dykeman, R. W., Mumford, G., and Phillips, R. W.: Construction and assembly of porcelain veneer gold crowns and pontics, J. Prosthet. Dent. **12**:1125-1137, 1962.

Kahn, A. E.: Reversible hydrocolloids in the construction of the unit-built porcelain bridge, J. Prosthet. Dent. **6**:72-79, 1956.

Leff, A.: New concepts in the preparation of teeth for full coverage, J. Prosthet. Dent. **5**:392-400, 1955; Reproduction of tooth anatomy and positional relationship in full cast or veneer crowns, J. Prosthet. Dent. **6**:550-557, 1956.

Ludwick, R. W., Jr., and Lynn, L. M.: A method to reduce pain during cementation of restorations, J. Am. Dent. Assoc. **53**:563-566, 1956.

Malson, T. S.: Anatomic cast crown reproduction, J. Prosthet. Dent. **9**:106-112, 1959.

Miller, I. F.: Full coverage abutment, N. Y. J. Dent. **22**:339-340, 1952.

Nuttall, E. B.: Clinical and technical aspects of crown and bridge prosthesis, Bull. Phila. Cty. Dent. Soc. **14**:128-133, 1950.

Patur, B.: The role of occlusion and the periodontium in restorative procedures, J. Prosthet. Dent. **21**:371-379, 1969.

Phillips, R. W., and Price, R. R.: Some factors which influence the surface of stone dies poured in alginate impressions, J. Prosthet. Dent. **5**:72-79, 1955.

Phillips, R. W., and Biggs, D. H.: Distortion of wax patterns as influenced by storage time, storage temperature, and temperature of wax manipulation, J. Am. Dent. Assoc. **41**:28-37, 1950.

Phillips, R. W., and Swartz, M. L.: A study of adaptation of veneers to cast gold crowns, J. Prosthet. Dent. **7**:817-822, 1957.

Pound, E.: The problem of the lower anterior bridge, J. Prosthet. Dent. **5**:543-545, 1955.

Pruden, K. C.: A hydrocolloid technique for pin-ledge bridge abutments, J. Prosthet. Dent. **6**:65-71, 1956.

Pruden, W. H.: Full coverage, partial coverage, and the role of pins, J. Prosthet. Dent. **26**:302-306, 1971.

Rheuben, R. P.: Full mouth reconstruction for the general practitioner, Dent. Dig. **60**:294-301, 1954.

Rubin, M. K.: Full coverage: the provisional and final restorations made easier, J. Prosthet. Dent. **8**:664-672, 1958.

Rubinstein, M. N.: Immediate acrylic temporary crown and bridge, Dent. Dig. **60**:12-13, 1954.

Saklad, M. J.: An esthetic provisional cast gold and acrylic splint, J. Prosthet. Dent. **4**:653-655, 1954.

Sheets, C. E.: Dowel and core foundations, J. Prosthet. Dent. **23**:58-65, 1970.

Shooshan, E. D.: The reverse pin-porcelain facing, J. Prosthet. Dent. **9**:284-301, 1959.

Smith, G. P.: The marginal fit of the full cast shoulderless crown, J. Prosthet. Dent. **7**:231-243, 1957; Objectives of a fixed partial denture, J. Prosthet. Dent. **11**:463-473, 1961.

Staffanou, R. S., and Thayer, K. E.: Reverse pin-porcelain veneer and pontic technique, J. Prosthet. Dent. **12**:1138-1145, 1962.

Stibbs, G. D.: Impression and pattern technique for anterior three-quarter crowns, J. Prosthet. Dent. **6**:558-562, 1956.

Talkov, L.: The copper band splint, J. Prosthet. Dent. **6**:245-251, 1956.

Terkla, L. G.: Crown morphology in relation to operative and crown and bridge dentistry, Dent. Abstr. **1**:394-396, 1956.

Troxell, R. R.: The polishing of gold castings, J. Prosthet. Dent. **9**:668-675, 1959.

Wagman, S. S.: Tissue management for full cast veneer crowns, J. Prosthet. Dent. **15**:106-117, 1965.

Wagner, A. W., Burkhart, J. W., and Fayle, H. E., Jr.: Contouring abutment teeth with cast gold inlays for removable partial dentures, J. Prosthet. Dent. **201**:330-334, 1968.

Wallace, F. H.: Resin transfer copings, J. Prosthet. Dent. **8**:289-292, 1958.

Wheeler, R. C.: Complete crown form and the periodontium, J. Prosthet. Dent. **11**:722-734, 1961.

Willey, R. E.: The preparation of abutments for veneer retainers, Dent. Abstr. **2**:28, 1957.

Woolson, A. H.: Restorations made of porcelain baked on gold, J. Prosthet. Dent. **5**:65, 1955.

Wyrick, W.: An anterior fixed bridge replacing a missing tooth where abnormally large interproximal spaces exist, J. Prosthet. Dent. **2**:829-830, 1952.

Yalisone, I. L.: Crown and sleeve-coping retainers for removable partial prostheses, J. Prosthet. Dent. **16**:1069-1085, 1966

Zola, A.: The acrylic resin transfer pattern, J. Prosthet. Dent. **9**:278-283, 1959.

DENTAL LABORATORY PROCEDURES

Asgar, K., and Peyton, F. A.: Casting dental alloys to embedded wires, J. Prosthet. Dent. **15:**312-321, 1965.

Benfield, J. W., and Lyons, G. V.: Precision dies from elastic impressions, J. Prosthet. Dent. **12:**737-752, 1962.

Blanchard, C. H.: Filling undercuts on refractory casts with investment, J. Prosthet. Dent. 3:417-418, 1953.

Collett, H. A.: Casting chrome-cobalt alloys in small laboratories, J. Prosthet. Dent. 21:216-266, 1969.

Dirksen, L. C., and Campagna, S. J.: Mat surface and rugae reproduction for upper partial denture castings, J. Prosthet. Dent. 4:67-72, 1954.

Dootz, E. R., Craig, R. G., and Peyton, F. A.: Influence of investments and duplicating procedures on the accuracy of partial denture castings, J. Prosthet. Dent. 15:679-690, 1965; Simplification of the chrome-cobalt partial denture casting procedure, J. Prosthet. Dent. 17:464-471, 1967; Aqueous acrylamide gel duplicating material, J. Prosthet. Dent. 17:570-577, 1967.

Elbert, C. A., and Ryge, G.: The effect of heat treatment on hardness of a chrome-cobalt aloy, J. Prosthet. Dent. 15:873-879, 1965.

Elliott, R. W.: The effects of heat on gold partial denture castings, J. Prosthet. Dent. 13:688-698, 1963.

Enright, C. M.: Dentist-dental laboratory harmony, J. Prosthet. Dent. 11:393-394, 1961.

Gilson, T. D., Asgar, K., and Peyton, F. A.: The quality of union formed in casting gold to embedded attachment metals, J. Prosthet. Dent. 15:464-473, 1965.

Grunewald, A. H., Paffenbarger, G. C., and Dickson, G.: The effect of molding processes on some properties of denture resins, J. Am. Dent. Assoc. 44:269-284, 1952; Dentist, dental laboratory, and the patient, J. Prosthet. Dent. 8:55-60, 1958; The role of the dental technician in a prosthetic service, Dent. Clin. North Am., pp. 359-370, July, 1960.

Johnson, H. B.: Technique for packing and staining complete or partial denture bases, J. Prosthet. Dent. 6:154-159, 1956.

Jones, D. W.: Thermal analysis and stability of refractory investments, J. Prosthet. Dent. 18:234-241, 1967.

Lanier, B. R., et al.: Making chromium-cobalt removable partial dentures: a modified technique, J. Prosthet. Dent. 25:197-205, 1971.

Mahler, D. B., and Ady, A. B.: The influence of various factors on the effective setting expansion of casting investments, J. Prosthet. Dent. 13:365-373, 1963.

Peyton, F. A.: Cast chromium-cobalt alloys, Dent. Clin. North Am. 759-771, Nov. 1958.

Peyton, F. A., and Anthony, D. H.: Evaluation of dentures processed by different techniques, J. Prosthet. Dent. 13:269-281, 1963.

Ryge, G., Kozak, S. F., and Fairhurst, C. W.: Porosities in dental gold castings, J. Am. Dent. Assoc. 54:746-754, 1957.

Schmidt, A. H.: Repairing chrome-cobalt castings, J. Prosthet. Dent. 5:385-387, 1955.

Smith, G. P.: The responsibility of the dentist toward laboratory procedures in fixed and removable partial denture prosthesis, J. Prosthet. Dent. 13:295-301, 1963.

Suffert, L. W., and Mahler, D. B.: Reproducibility of gold castings made by present day dental casting technics, J. Am. Dent. Assoc. 50:1-6, 1955.

Tuccillo, J. J., and Nielsen, J. P.: Compatibility of alginate impression materials and dental stones, J. Prosthet. Dent. 25:556-566, 1971.

Walker, T. J., and Orsinger, W. O.: Palate reproduction by the hydrocolloid-resin method, J. Prosthet. Dent. 4:54-66, 1954.

DENTURE ESTHETICS: TOOTH SELECTION AND ARRANGEMENT

Culpepper, W. D.: A comparative study of shade-matching procedures, J. Prosthet. Dent. 24:166-173, 1971.

DeVan, M. M.: The appearance phase of denture construction, Dent. Clin. North Am., pp. 255-268, March, 1957.

Eich, F. A.: The construction of a metal mold for acrylic teeth, J. Prosthet. Dent. 1:594-600, 1951.

French, F. A.: The selection and arrangement of the anterior teeth in prosthetic dentures, J. Prosthet. Dent. 1:587-593, 1951.

Frush, J. P., and Fisher, R. D.: Introduction to dentogenic restorations, J. Prosthet. Dent. 5:586-595, 1955; How dentogenic restorations interpret the sex factor, J. Prosthet. Dent. 6:160-172, 1956; How dentogenics interprets the personality factor, J. Prosthet. Dent. 6:441-449, 1956.

Geiger, E. C. K.: Duplication of the esthetics of an existing immediate denture, J. Prosthet. Dent. 5:179-185, 1955.

Hughes, G. A.: Facial types and tooth arrangement, J. Prosthet. Dent. 1:82-95, 1951.

Krajicek, D. D.: Natural appearance for the individual denture patient, J. Prosthet. Dent. 10:205-214, 1960.

Myerson, R. L.: The use of porcelain and plastic teeth in opposing complete dentures. J. Prosthet. Dent. 7:625-633, 1957.

Payne, A. G. L.: Factors influencing the position of artificial upper anterior teeth, J. Prosthet. Dent. 26:26-32, 1971.

Pound, E.: Lost—fine arts in the fallacy of the ridges, J. Prosthet Dent. 4:6-16, 1954; Recapturing esthetic tooth position in the edentulous patient, J. Am. Dent. Assoc. 55:181-191, 1957;

Applying harmony in selecting and arranging teeth, Dent. Clin. North Am., pp. 241-258, March, 1962.

Proctor, H. H.: Characterization of dentures, J. Prosthet. Dent. 3:339-349, 1953.

Roraff, A. R.: Instant photographs for developing esthetics, J. Prosthet. Dent. 26:21-25, 1971.

Tillman, E. J.: Molding and staining acrylic resin anterior teeth, J. Prosthet. Dent. 5:497-507, 1955; Dent. Abstr. 1:111, 1956.

Tustison, H. W.: Gold inlays cast into porcelain teeth, J. Prosthet. Dent. 3:181-183, 1953.

Van Victor, A.: Positive duplication of anterior teeth for immediate dentures, J. Prosthet. Dent. 3:165-177, 1953; The mold guide cast—its significance in denture esthetics, J. Prosthet. Dent. 13:406-415, 1963.

Vig, R. G.: The denture look, J. Prosthet. Dent. 11:9-15, 1961.

Wallace, D. H.: The use of gold occlusal surfaces in complete and partial dentures, J. Prosthet. Dent. 14:326-333, 1964.

Wolfson, E.: Staining and characterization of acrylic teeth, Dent. Abstr. 1:41, 1956.

Young, H. A.: Denture esthetics, J. Prosthet. Dent. 6:748-755, 1956.

DIAGNOSIS AND TREATMENT PLANNING

Applegate, O. C.: Evaluating oral structures for removable partial dentures, J. Prosthet. Dent. 11:882-885, 1961.

Bartels, J. C.: Diagnosis and treatment planning, J. Prosthet. Dent. 7:657-662, 1957.

Bennett, C. G.: Transitional restorations for function and esthetics, J. Prosthet. Dent. 15:867-872, 1965.

Blatterfein, L.: The planning and contouring of acrylic resin veneer crowns for partial denture clasping, J. Prosthet. Dent. 6:386-404, 1956.

Bolender, C. L., Swenson, R. D., and Yamane, G.: Evaluation of treatment of inflammatory papillary hyperplasia of the palate, J. Prosthet. Dent. 15:1013-1022, 1965.

Contino, R. M., and Stallard, H.: Instruments essential for obtaining data needed in making a functional diagnosis of the human mouth, J. Prosthet. Dent. 7:66-77, 1957.

Dreizen, S.: Nutritional changes in the oral cavity, J. Prosthet. Dent. 16:1144-1150, 1966.

Dunn, B. W.: Treatment planning for removable partial dentures, J. Prosthet. Dent. 11:247-255, 1961.

Foster, T. D.: The use of the face-bow in making permanent study casts, J. Prosthet. Dent. 9:717-721, 1959.

Frankel, H. J.: Uses of autopolymerizing acrylic resins in fixed partial prosthesis, J. Prosthet. Dent. 8:1003-1006, 1958.

Frechette, A. R.: Partial denture planning with special reference to stress distribution, J. Prosthet. Dent. 1:700-707 (disc., 208-209), 1951.

Friedman, S.: Effective use of diagnostic data, J. Prosthet. Dent. 9:729-737, 1959.

Gill, J. R.: Treatment planning for mouth rehabilitation, J. Prosthet. Dent. 2:230-245, 1952.

Harvey, W. L.: A transitional prosthetic appliance, J. Prosthet. Dent. 14:60-70, 1964.

Henderson, D., Hickey, J. C., and Wehner, P. J.: Prevention and preservation—the challenge of removable partial denture service, Dent. Clin. North Am. July, 1965.

House, M. M.: The relationship of oral examination to dental diagnosis, J. Prosthet. Dent. 8:208-219, 1958.

Killebrew, R. F.: Crown construction and splinting of mobile partial denture abutments, J. Am. Dent. Assoc. 70:334-338, 1965.

Lambson, G. O.: Papillary hyperplasia of the palate, J. Prosthet. Dent. 16:636-645, 1966.

Landa, J. S.: Diagnosis of the edentulous mouth and the probable prognosis of its rehabilitation, Dent. Clin. North Am., pp. 187-201, March, 1957.

McCracken, W. L.: Differential diagnosis: fixed or removable partial dentures, J. Am. Dent. Assoc. 63:767-775, 1961.

McGill, W. J.: Acquiring space for partial dentures, J. Prosthet. Dent. 17:163-165, 1967.

Moulton, G. H.: The importance of centric occlusion in diagnosis and treatment planning, J. Prosthet. Dent. 10:921-926, 1960.

Payne, S. H.: Diagnostic factors which influence the choice of posterior occlusion, Dent. Clin. North Am., pp. 203-213, March, 1957.

Rudd, K. D., and Dunn, B. W.: Accurate removable partial dentures, J. Prosthet. Dent. 18:559-570, 1967.

Sauser, C. W.: Pretreatment evaluation of partially edentulous arches, J. Prosthet. Dent. 11:886-893, 1961.

Schuyler, C. H.: Elements of diagnosis leading to full or partial dentures, J. Am. Dent. Assoc. 41:302-305, 1950.

Seiden, A.: Occlusal rests and rest seats, J. Prosthet. Dent. 8:431-440, 1958.

Uccellani, E. L.: Evaluating the mucous membranes of the edentulous mouth, J. Prosthet. Dent. 15:295-303, 1965.

Wagner, A. G.: Instructions for the use and care of removable partial dentures, J. Prosthet. Dent. 26:481-490, 1971.

Waldron, C. A.: Oral leukoplakia, carcinoma, and the prosthodontist, J. Prosthet. Dent. 15:367-376, 1965.

Wilson, J. H.: The general principles of diagnosis and prognosis of partial dentures, Dent. J. Aust. 11:69-77, 1939.

Young, A. C.: Indications and the diagnosis for fixed partial denture prosthesis, J. Am. Dent. Assoc. 41:289-295, 1950.

Young, H. A.: Diagnostic survey of edentulous patients, J. Prosthet. Dent. 5:5-14, 1955.

IMPRESSION MATERIALS AND METHODS; THE PARTIAL DENTURE BASE

Applegate, O. C.: The partial denture base, J. Prosthet. Dent. **5**:636-648, 1955; An evaluation of the support for the removable partial denture, J. Prosthet. Dent. **10**:112-123, 1960.

Bailey, L. R.: Acrylic resin tray for rubber base impression materials, J. Prosthet. Dent. **5**:658-662, 1955; Rubber base impression techniques, Dent. Clin. North Am., pp. 156-166, March, 1957.

Beckett, L. S.: Partial denture impressions, Dent. J. Aust. **27**:135-138, 1955.

Boucher, C. O.: A critical analysis of mid-century impression techniques for full dentures, J. Prosthet. Dent. **1**:472-491, 1951.

Chase, W. W.: Adaptation of rubber-base impression materials to removable denture prosthetics, J. Prosthet. Dent. **10**:1043-1050, 1960.

Chong, M. P., et al.: The tear test as a means of evaluating the resistance to rupture of alginate impression materials, Aust. Dent. J. **16**:145-151, 1971.

Clark, R. J., and Phillips, R. W.: Flow studies of certain dental impression materials, J. Prosthet. Dent. **7**:259-266, 1957.

Davis, M. C.: The use of rubber base impression materials in the construction of inlays, J. Prosthet. Dent. **8**:123-134, 1958.

Feinberg, E.: Technique for master impressions in fixed restorations, J. Prosthet. Dent. **5**:663-666, 1955.

Frank, R. P.: Analysis of pressures produced during maxillary edentulous impression procedures, J. Prosthet. Dent. **22**:400-403, 1969.

Fusayama, T., and Nakazato, M.: The design of stock trays and the retention of irreversible hydrocolloid impressions, J. Prosthet. Dent. **21**:136-142, 1969.

Gilmore, W. H., Schnell, R. J., and Phillips, R. W.: Factors influencing the accuracy of silicone impression materials, J. Prosthet. Dent. **9**:304-314, 1959.

Harris, W. T., Jr.: Water temperature and accuracy of alginate impressions, J. Prosthet. Dent. **21**:613-617, 1969.

Heartwell, C. M., et al.: Comparison of impressions made in perforated and nonperforated rimlock trays, J. Prosthet. Dent. **27**:494-500, 1972.

Hindels, G. W.: Load distribution in extension saddle partial dentures, J. Prosthet. Dent. **2**:92-100, 1952.

Holmes, J. B.: Influence of impression procedures and occlusal loading on partial denture movement, J. Prosthet. Dent. **15**:474-481, 1965.

Hudson, W. C.: Clinical uses of rubber impression materials and electroforming of casts and dies in pure silver, J. Prosthet. Dent. **8**:107-114, 1958.

Johnston, J. F., Cunningham, D. M., and Bogan, R. G.: The dentist, the patient, and ridge preservation, J. Prosthet. Dent. **10**:288-295, 1960.

Kramer, H. M.: Impression technique for removable partial dentures, J. Prosthet. Dent. **11**:84-92, 1961.

Leupold, R. J.: A comparative study of impression procedures for distal extension removable partial dentures, J. Prosthet. Dent. **16**:708-720, 1966.

Leupold, R. J., and Kratochvil, F. J.: An altered-cast procedure to improve support for removable partial dentures, J. Prosthet. Dent. **15**:672-678, 1965.

McCracken, W. L.: An evaluation of activated methyl methacrylate denture base materials, J. Prosthet. Dent. **2**:68-83, 1952.

Mitchell, J. V., and Damele, J. J.: Influence of tray design upon elastic impression materials, J. Prosthet. Dent. **23**:51-57, 1970.

Morrow, R. M., et al.: Compatibility of alginate impression materials and dental stones, J. Prosthet. Dent. **25**:556-566, 1971.

Myers, G. E.: Electroformed die technique for rubber base impressions, J. Prosthet. Dent. **8**:531-535, 1958.

Pfeiffer, K. A.: Clinical problems in the use of alginate hydrocolloid, Dent. Abstr. **2**:82, 1957.

Phillips, R. W.: Factors influencing the accuracy of reversible hydrocolloid impressions, J. Am. Dent. Assoc. **43**:1-17, 1951; Factors affecting the surface of stone dies poured in hydrocolloid impressions, J. Prosthet. Dent. **2**:390-400, 1952; Elastic impression materials—a second progress report of a recent conference, J. South. Calif. Dent. Assoc. **26**:150-153, 1958; Physical properties and manipulation of rubber impression materials, J. Am. Dent. Assoc. **59**:454-458, 1959.

Prieskel, H. W.: Impression techniques for attachment-retained distal extension removable partial dentures, J. Prosthet. Dent. **25**:620-628, 1971.

Rapuano, J. A.: Single tray dual-impression technique for distal extension partial dentures, J. Prosthet. Dent. **24**:41-46, 1970.

Rosenstiel, E.: Rubber base elastic impression materials, Dent. Abstr. **1**:55, 1956.

Rudd, K. D., Morrow, R. M., and Bange, A. A.: Accurate casts, J. Prosthet. Dent. **21**:545-554, 1969.

Rudd, K. D., Morrow, R. M., and Strunk, R. R.: Accurate alginate impressions, J. Prosthet. Dent. **22**:294-300, 1969.

Rudd, K. D., et al.: Comparison of effects of tap water and slurry water on gypsum casts, J. Prosthet. Dent. **24**:563-570, 1970.

Silver, M.: Impressions and silver-plated dies from a rubber impression material, J. Prosthet. Dent. **6**:543-549, 1956.

Smith, P. K.: The effect on the accuracy of polysulphide impression material after treating preparations with various agents, Aust. Dent. J. **16:** 337-339, 1971.

Smith, R. A.: Secondary palatal impressions for major connector adaptation, J. Prosthet. Dent. **24:**108-110, 1970.

Stafford, G. D., and MacCulloch, W. T.: Radiopaque denture base materials, Br. Dent. J. **131:**22-24, 1971.

Steffel, V. L.: Relining removable partial dentures for fit and function, J. Prosthet. Dent. **4:**496-509, 1954; J. Tenn. Dent. Assoc. **36:**35-43, 1956.

Tilton, G. E.: The denture periphery, J. Prosthet. Dent. **2:**290-306, 1952.

Wilson, J. H.: Partial dentures—relining the saddle supported by the mucosa and alveolar bone, J. Prosthet. Dent. **3:**807-813, 1953.

MAXILLOFACIAL PROSTHESIS

Ackerman, A. J.: Maxillofacial prosthesis, Oral Surg. **6:**176-200, 1953; The prosthetic management of oral and facial defects following cancer surgery, J. Prosthet. Dent. **5:**413-432, 1955.

Brown, K. E.: Fabrication of a hollow-bulb obturator, J. Prosthet. Dent. **21:**97-103, 1969.

Cantor, R. et al.: Methods for evaluating prosthetic facial materials, J. Prosthet. Dent. **21:**324-332, 1969.

Edgerton, M. T., and Pyott, J. E.: Surgery and prosthesis in jaw reconstruction, J. Prosthet. Dent. **4:**257-262, 1954.

Emory, L.: Partial denture prosthesis for war injuries, J. Am. Dent. Assoc. **35:**643-644, 1947.

Grunewald, A. H.: The prosthodontist's role in cranioplasty, J. Prosthet. Dent. **5:**235-243, 1955.

Kelly, E. K.: Partial denture design applicable to the maxillofacial patient, J. Prosthet. Dent. **15:**168-173, 1965.

Lazzari, J. B.: Intraoral splint for support of the lip in Bell's palsy, J. Prosthet. Dent. **5:**579-581, 1955.

Nethery, W. J., and Delclos, L.: Prosthetic stent for gold-grain implant to the floor of the mouth, J. Prosthet. Dent. **23:**81-87, 1970.

Olin, W. H.: Maxillofacial prosthesis, J. Am. Dent. Assoc. **48:**399-409, 1954.

Nadeau, J.: Maxillofacial prosthesis with magnetic stabilizers, J. Prosthet. Dent. **6:**114-119, 1956.

Smith, E. H., Jr.: Prosthetic treatment of maxillofacial injuries, J. Prosthet. Dent. **5:**112-128, 1955.

Strain, J. C.: A mechanical device for duplicating a mirror image of a cast or moulage in three dimensions, J. Prosthet. Dent. **5:**129-132, 1955.

Young, J. M.: The prosthodontist's role in total treatment of patients, J. Prosthet. Dent. **27:**399-412, 1972.

MISCELLANEOUS

Academy of Denture Prosthetics: Principles, concepts and practices in prosthodontics; Progress Report III, J. Prosthet. Dent. **13:**283-294, 1963.

Adisman, I. K.: What a prosthodontist should know, J. Prosthet. Dent. **21:**409-416, 1969.

Anthony, D. H., and Gibbons, P.: The nature and behavior of denture cleansers, J. Prosthet. Dent. **8:**796-810, 1958.

Applegate, O. C.: Conditions which may influence the choice of partial or complete denture service, J. Prosthet. Dent. **7:**182-196, 1957; The removable partial denture in the general practice of tomorrow, J. Prosthet. Dent. **8:**609-622, 1958; Factors to be considered in choosing an alloy, Dent. Clin. North Am., pp. 583-590, Nov., 1960.

Asgar, K., et al.: A new alloy for partial dentures, J. Prosthet. Dent. **23:**36-43, 1970.

Atwood, D. A.: Practice of prosthodontics: past, present, and future, J. Prosthet. Dent. **21:**393-401, 1970.

Augsburger, R. H.: Evaluating removable partial dentures by mathematical equations, J. Prosthet. Dent. **22:**528-543, 1969.

Baker, C. R.: Difficulties in evaluating removable partial dentures, J. Prosthet. Dent. **17:**60-62, 1967; Occlusal reactive prosthodontics, J. Prosthet. Dent. **17:**566-569, 1967.

Barrett, D. A., and Pilling, L. O.: The restoration of carious clasp-bearing teeth, J. Prosthet. Dent. **15:**309-311, 1965.

Bates, J. F.: Studies related to fracture of partial dentures, Br. Dent. J. **120:**79-83, 1966.

Beck, H. O.: A clinical evaluation of the Arcon concept of articulation, J. Prosthet. Dent. **9:**409-421, 1959; Alloys for removable partial dentures, Dent. Clin. North Am., pp. 591-596, Nov., 1960.

Beck, H. O., and Morrison, W. E.: Investigation of an Arcon articulator, J. Prosthet. Dent. **6:**359-372, 1956.

Beckett, L. S.: Some fundamentals of partial denture construction, Aust. J. Dent. **44:**363-367, 1940; The influence of saddle classification on the design of partial removable restorations, J. Prosthet. Dent. **3:**506-516, 1953.

Blatterfein, L.: Role of the removable partial denture in the restoration of lost vertical dimension, N. Y. Univ. J. Dent. **10:**274-276, 1952.

Blatterfein, L., et al.: Minimum acceptable procedures for satisfactory removable partial denture service, J. Prosthet. Dent. **27:**84-87, 1972.

Boucher, C. O., editor: Current clinical dental terminology, St. Louis, 1963, The C. V. Mosby Co.; Writing as a means for learning, J. Prosthet. Dent. **27:**229-234, 1972.

Boucher, L. J., et al.: Guidelines for advanced prosthodontic education, J. Prosthet. Dent. **23:**104-110, 1970.

Breitbart, A. R.: Converting a tooth-supported denture to a distal extension removable partial denture, J. Prosthet. Dent. **18:**233, 1967.

Brockhurst, P. J.: Comparison of the performance of materials for spring members in dental appliances, using the theory of simple bending, Aust. Dent. J. **15:**119-125, 1970.

Cummer, W. E.: Partial denture service. In Anthony, L. P., editor: American textbook of prosthetic dentistry, Philadelphia, 1942, Lea & Febiger, pp. 670-840.

Dale, J. W.: A full and partial denture survey, Aust. Dent. J. **15**:225-227, 1970.

Derry, A., and Bertram, U.: A clinical survey of removable partial dentures after 2 years usage, Acta Odontol. Scand. **28**:581-598, 1970.

DeVan, M. M.: The additive partial denture: its principles and design (partial dentures) North West Dent. **35**:303-307, 312, 1956; Dent. Abstr. **2**:468, 1957.

Elliott, R. W.: The effects of heat on gold partial denture castings, J. Prosthet. Dent. **13**:688-698, 1963.

Ewing, J. E.: Temporary cementation in fixed partial prosthesis, J. Prosthet. Dent. **5**:388-391, 1955; The construction of accurate full crown restorations for an existing clasp by using a direct metal pattern technique, J. Prosthet. Dent. **15**:889-899, 1965.

Federation of Prosthodontic Organizations: Guidelines for evaluation of completed prosthodontic treatment for removable partial dentures, J. Prosthet. Dent. **27**:326-328, 1972.

Fish, S. F.: Partial dentures, Br. Dent. J. **128**:243-246, 289-293, 339-344, 398-402, 446-453, 495-502, 547-551, 590-592, 1970.

Fish, S. F., et al.: A study of prosthetic dentistry, Br. Dent. J. **127**:59-70, 1969.

Fisher, A. A.: Allergic sensitization of the skin and oral mucosa to acrylic resin denture materials, J. Prosthet. Dent. **6**:593-602, 1956.

Gecker, L. M.: Bruxism—a rationale of therapy, J. Am. Dent. Assoc. **66**:14-18, 1963.

Giglio, J. J., Lace, W. P., and Arden, H.: Factors affecting retention and stability of complete dentures, J. Prosthet. Dent. **12**:848-856, 1962.

Girardot, R. L.: The physiologic aspects of partial denture restorations, J. Prosthet. Dent. **3**:689-698, 1953.

Glossary of Prosthodontic Terms, J. Prosthet. Dent. **20**:447-480, 1968.

Hardcourt, H. J., et al.: The properties of nickel-chromium casting alloys containing boron and silicon, Br. Dent. J. **129**:419-423, 1970.

Harrison, W. M., and Stansbury, B. E.: The effect of joint surface contours on the transverse strength of repaired acrylic resin, J. Prosthet. Dent. **23**:464-472, 1970.

Herlands, R. E.: Removable partial denture terminology, J. Prosthet. Dent. **8**:964-972, 1958.

Hickey, J. C.: Responsibility of the dentist in removable partial dentures, J. Ky. Dent. Assoc. **17**:70-87, 1965.

Hickey, J. C.: Charge to workshop on advanced prosthodontic training, J. Prosthet. Dent. **21**:388-392, 1969.

Hobdell, M. H., et al.: The prevalence of full and partial dentures in British populations, Br. Dent. J. **128**:437-442, 1970.

Jankelson, B. H.: Adjustment of dentures at time of insertion and alterations to compensate for tissue changes, J. Am. Dent. Assoc. **64**:521-531, 1962.

Johnson, W.: Gold alloys for casting dentures: an investigation of some mechanical properties, Br. Dent. J. **102**:41-49, 1957.

Jones, R. R.: The lower partial denture, J. Prosthet. Dent. **2**:219-229, 1952.

Kaires, A. K.: A study of partial denture design and masticatory pressures in a mandibular bilateral distal extension case, J. Prosthet. Dent. **8**:340-350, 1958.

Kelly, E. K.: The physiologic approach to partial denture design, J. Prosthet. Dent. **3**:699-710, 1953.

Kelly, E.: Fatigue failure in denture base polymers, J. Prosthet. Dent. **21**:257-266, 1969; Changes caused by a mandibular removable partial denture opposing a maxillary complete denture, J. Prosthet. Dent. **27**:140-150, 1972.

Kessler, B.: An analysis of the tongue factor and its functioning areas in dental prosthesis, J. Prosthet. Dent. **5**:629-635, 1955.

Klein, I. E., et al.: Minimum clinical procedures for satisfactory complete denture, removable partial denture, and fixed partial denture services, J. Prosthet. Dent. **22**:4-10, 1969.

Kratochvil, F. J.: Maintaining supporting structures with a removable partial prosthesis, J. Prosthet. Dent. **25**:167-174, 1971.

Landa, J. S.: The troublesome transition from a partial lower to a complete lower denture, J. Prosthet. Dent. **4**:42-51, 1954.

Lenchner, N. H., Handlers, M., and Weissman, B.: A modification of a special retaining device for partial dentures, J. Prosthet. Dent. **8**:973-980, 1958.

Lew, I.: Free-end saddle prosthesis, Part 2, Dent. Dig. **63**:456-460, 1957.

Maison, W. G.: Instructions to denture patients, J. Prosthet. Dent. **9**:825-831, 1959.

Martone, A. L.: The fallacy of saving time at the chair, J. Prosthet. Dent. **7**:416-419, 1957; The effects of oral prostheses on the production of speech sounds, 1956, Ohio State Univ. Dent. Abstr. **2**:508, 1957; The challenge of the partially edentulous mouth, J. Prosthet. Dent. **8**:942-954, 1958.

McCracken, W. L.: A comparison of tooth-borne and tooth-tissue–borne removable partial dentures, J. Prosthet. Dent. **3**:375-381, 1953; Auxiliary uses of cold-curing acrylic resins in prosthetic dentistry, J. Am. Dent. Assoc. **47**:298-304, 1953; A philosophy of partial denture treatment, J. Prosthet. Dent. **13**:889-900, 1963.

Means, C. R., and Flenniken, I. E.: Gagging—a problem in prosthetic dentistry, J. Prosthet. Dent. **23**:614-620, 1970.

Mehringer, E. J.: The saliva as it is related to the wearing of dentures, J. Prosthet. Dent. **4:** 312-318, 1954.

Morden, J. F. C., Lammie, G. A., and Osborne, J.: Effect of various denture cleaning solutions on chrome cobalt alloys, Dent. Dig. 1:682, 1956.

Morse, P. K., and Boucher, L. J.: What a prosthodontist does, J. Prosthet. Dent. **21:**402-408, 1969.

Mosteller, J. H.: Use of prednisolone in the elimination of postoperative thermal sensitivity, J. Prosthet. Dent. **12:**1176-1179, 1962.

Neufeld, J. O.: Changes in the trabecular pattern of the mandible following the loss of teeth, J. Prosthet. Dent. **8:**685-697, 1958.

Öatlund, S. G.: Saliva and denture retention, J. Prosthet Dent. **10:**658-663, 1960.

Osborne, J., and Lammie, G. A.: The bilateral free-end saddle lower denture, J. Prosthet. Dent. **4:**640-652, 1954.

Overton, R. G., and Bramblett, R. M.: Prosthodontic services: a study of need and availability in the United States, J. Prosthet. Dent. **27:**329-339, 1972.

Phillips, R. W., and Leonard, L. J.: A study of enamel abrasion as related to partial denture clasps, J. Prosthet. Dent. **6:**657-671, 1956.

Plainfield, S.: Communication distortion. The language of patients and practitioners of dentistry, J. Prosthet. Dent. **22:**11-19, 1969.

Ramsey, W. O.: The relation of emotional factors to prosthodontic service, J. Prosthet. Dent. **23:**4-10, 1970.

Raybin, N. H.: The polished surface of complete dentures, J. Prosthet. Dent. **13:**236-239, 1963.

Reynolds, J. M.: Crown construction for abutments of existing removable partial dentures, J. Am. Dent. Assoc. **69:**423-426, 1964.

Rothman, R.: Phonetic considerations in denture prosthesis, J. Prosthet. Dent. **11:**214-223, 1961.

Rudd, K. D., and Dunn, B. W.: Accurate removable partial dentures, J. Prosthet. Dent. **18:**559-570, 1967.

Savage, R. D., and MacGregor, A. R.: Behavior therapy in prosthodontics, J. Prosthet. Dent. **24:**126-132, 1970.

Schabel, R. W.: Dentist-patient communication— a major factor in treatment prognosis, J. Prosthet. Dent. **21:**3-5, 1969; The psychology of aging, J. Prosthet. Dent. **27:**569-573, 1972.

Schole, M. L.: Management of the gagging patient, J. Prosthet. Dent. **9:**578-583, 1959.

Schopper, A. F.: Removable appliances for the preservation of the teeth, J. Prosthet. Dent. **4:** 634-639, 1954; Loss of vertical dimension: causes and effects: diagnosis and various recommended treatments, J. Prosthet. Dent. **9:**428-431, 1959.

Schuyler, C. H.: Stress distribution as the prime requisite to the success of a partial denture,

J. Am. Dent. Assoc. **20:**2148-2154, 1933; Planning the removable partial denture to restore function and maintain oral health; N. Y. Dent. J. **13:**4-10, 1947.

Sears, V. H.: Comprehensive denture service, J. Am. Dent. Assoc. **64:**531-552, 1962.

Skinner, E. W., and Gordon, C. C.: Some experiments on the surface hardness of dental stones, J. Prosthet. Dent. **6:**94-100, 1956.

Skinner, E. W., and Jones, P. M.: Dimensional stability of self-curing denture base acrylic resin, J. Am. Dent. Assoc. **51:**426-431, 1955.

Smith, F. W., and Applegate, O. C.: Roentgenographic study of bone changes during exercise stimulation of edentulous areas, J. Prosthet. Dent. **11:**1086-1097, 1961.

Stahl, D. G.: A simplified procedure for fabricating a temporary removable acrylic bite plane, Dent. Abstr. **1:**719, 1956.

Steiger, A. A.: Progress in partial denture prosthesis, Int. Dent. J. **2:**542-573, 1952.

Stoner, C.: The use of self-curing acrylic resin in the temporary splinting of teeth, Dent. Dig. **61:**296-301, 1955.

Sweeney, W. T., Myerson, R. L., Rose, E. E., and Semmelman, J. O.: Proposed specification for plastic teeth, J. Prosthet. Dent. **7:**420-424, 1957.

Tallgren, A.: Alveolar bone loss in denture wearers as related to facial morphology, Acta Odontol. Scand. **28:**251-270, 1970.

Tomlin, H. R., and Osborne, J.: Cobalt-chromium partial dentures; a clinical survey, Br. Dent. J. **110:**307-310, 1961.

Trainor, J. E., and Elliott, R. W., Jr.: Removable partial dentures designed by dentists before and after graduate level instruction: a comparative study, J. Prosthet. Dent. **27:**509-514, 1972.

Van Huysen, G., Fly, W., and Leonard, L.: Artificial dentures and the oral mucosa, J. Prosthet. Dent. **4:**446-460, 1954.

Wallace, D. H.: The use of gold occlusal surfaces in complete and partial dentures, J. Prosthet. Dent. **14:**326-333, 1964.

Wilson, J. H.: Some clinical and technical aspects of partial dentures, Dent. J. Aust. **26:**176-183, 1954.

Wright, W. H.: Partial denture prosthesis: a preventive oral health service, J. Am. Dent. Assoc. **43:**163-168, 1951,

Young, H. A.: Factors contributory to success in prosthodontic practice, J. Prosthet. Dent. **5:**354-360, 1955.

Zerosi, C.: A new type of removable splint: its indications and function, Dent. Abstr. **1:**451-452, 1956.

MOUTH PREPARATIONS

Boitel, R. H.: The parallelometer; a precision instrument for the prosthetic laboratory, J. Prosthet. Dent. **12:**732-736, 1962.

Brown, H.: Alignment of abutments for fixed partial dentures, J. Prosthet. Dent. **12**:940-946, 1962.

Gaston, G. W.: Rest area preparations for removable partial dentures, J. Prosthet. Dent. **10**:124-134, 1960.

Glann, G. W., and Appleby, R. C.: Mouth preparations for removable partial dentures, J. Prosthet. Dent. **10**:698-706, 1960.

Johnston, J. F.: Preparation of mouths for fixed and removable partial dentures, J. Prosthet. Dent. **11**:456-462, 1961.

Kahn, A. E.: Partial versus full coverage, J. Prosthet. Dent. **10**:167-178, 1960.

McCracken, W. L.: Mouth preparations for partial dentures, J. Prosthet. Dent. **6**:39-52, 1956.

Mills, M.: Mouth preparation for removable partial denture, J. Am. Dent. Assoc. **60**:154-159, 1960.

Phillips, R. W.: Report of the Committee on Scientific Investigation of the Academy of Restorative Dentistry, J. Prosthet. Dent. **13**:515-535, 1963.

Schorr, L., and Clayman, L. H.: Reshaping abutment teeth for reception of partial denture clasps, J. Prosthet. Dent. **4**:625-633, 1954.

Sollé, W.: The parallelo-facere: a parallel drilling machine for use in the oral cavity, J. Am. Dent. Assoc. **63**:344-352, 1961.

OCCLUSION; JAW RELATION RECORDS; TRANSFER METHODS

Applegate, O. C.: Loss of posterior occlusion, J. Prosthet. Dent. **4**:197-199, 1954.

Baraban, D. J.: Establishing centric relation and vertical dimension in occlusal rehabilitation, J. Prosthet. Dent. **12**:1157-1165, 1962.

Beck, H. O.: A clinical evaluation of the Arcon concept of articulation, J. Prosthet. Dent. **9**:409-421, 1959; Selection of an articulator and jaw registration, J. Prosthet. Dent. **10**:878-886, 1960; Choosing the articulator, J. Am. Dent. Assoc. **64**:468-475, 1962.

Beckett, L. S.: Accurate occlusal relations in partial denture construction, J. Prosthet. Dent. **4**:487-495, 1954.

Berke, J. D. and Moleres, I.: A removable appliance for the correction of maxillomandibular disproportion, J. Prosthet. Dent. **17**:172-177, 1967.

Berman, M. H.: Accurate interocclusal records, J. Prosthet. Dent. **10**:620-630, 1960.

Beyron, H. L.: Occlusal relationship, Int. Dent. J. **2**:467-496, 1952; Characteristics of functionally optimal occlusion and principles of occlusal rehabilitation, J. Am. Dent. Assoc. **48**:648-656, 1954; Occlusal changes in adult dentition, J. Am. Dent. Assoc. **48**:674-686, 1954.

Block, L. S.: Preparing and conditioning the patient for intermaxillary relations, J. Prosthet.

Dent. **2**:599-603, 1952; Tensions and intermaxillary relations, J. Prosthet. Dent. **4**:204-207, 1954.

Boos, R. H.: Occlusion from rest position, J. Prosthet. Dent. **2**:575-588, 1952; Basic anatomic factors of jaw position, J. Prosthet. Dent. **4**:200-203, 1954; Maxillomandibular relations, occlusion, and the temporomandibular joint, Dent. Clin. North Am., pp. 19-35, March, 1962.

Borgh, O., and Posselt, U.: Hinge axis registration: experiments on the articulator, J. Prosthet. Dent. **8**:35-40, 1958.

Boucher, C. O.: Occlusion in prosthodontics, J. Prosthet. Dent. **3**:633-656, 1953.

Braly, B. V.: Occlusal analysis and treatment planning for restorative dentistry, J. Prosthet. Dent. **27**:168-171, 1972.

Brown, S. W.: Disharmony between centric relation and centric occlusion as a factor in producing improper tooth wear and trauma, Dent. Dig. **52**:434-440, 1946.

Cerveris, A. R.: Vibracentric equilibration of centric occlusion, J. Am. Dent. Assoc. **63**:476-483, 1961.

Christensen, P. B.: Accurate casts and positional relation records, J. Prosthet. Dent. **8**:475-482, 1958.

Clayton, J. A., et al.: Pantographic tracings of mandibular movements and occlusion, J. Prosthet. Dent. **25**:389-396, 1971.

Cohn, L. A.: Factors of dental occlusion pertinent to the restorative and prosthetic problem, J. Prosthet. Dent. **9**:256-277, 1959.

Cohn, R.: The relationship of anterior guidance to condylar guidance in mandibular movement, J. Prosthet. Dent. **6**:758-767, 1956.

Collett, H. A.: Balancing the occlusion of partial dentures, J. Am. Dent. Assoc. **42**:162-168, 1951.

Colman, A. J.: Occlusal requirements for removable partial dentures, J. Prosthet. Dent. **17**:155-162, 1967.

Craddock, F. W.: The accuracy and practical value of records of condyle path inclination, J. Am. Dent. Assoc. **38**:697-710, 1949.

Craddock, F. W., and Thompson, J. R.: Functional analysis of occlusion, J. Am. Dent. Assoc. **39**:404-406, 1949.

D'Amico, A.: Functional occlusion of the natural teeth of man, J. Prosthet. Dent. **11**:899-915, 1961.

Draper, D. H.: Forward trends in occlusion, J. Prosthet. Dent. **13**:724-731, 1963.

Emmert, J. H.: A method for registering occlusion in semiedentulous mouths, J. Prosthet. Dent. **8**:94-99, 1958.

Fedi, P. F.: Cardinal differences in occlusion of natural teeth and that of artificial teeth, J. Am. Dent. Assoc. **62**:482-485, 1962.

Fountain, H. W.: Seating the condyles for centric

relation records, J. Prosthet. Dent. **11**:1050-1058, 1961.

Frank, L.: The opening axis of the jaw, Dent. Dig. **62**:16-19, 1956.

Gilson, T. D.: Theory of centric correction in natural teeth, J. Prosthet. Dent. **8**:468-474, 1958.

Goodfriend, D. J.: New facebow for dentist-laboratory cooperation, J. Am. Dent. Assoc. **68**:866-872, 1964.

Granger, E. R.: The articulator and the patient, Dent. Clin. North Amer., pp. 527-539, Nov., 1960.

Hardy, I. R.: The developments in the occlusal patterns of artificial teeth, J. Prosthet. Dent. **1**:14-28, 1951.

Harris, E.: Occlusion, J. Prosthet. Dent. **1**:301-306, 1951.

Hausman, M.: Interceptive and pivotal occlusal contacts, J. Am. Dent. Assoc. **66**:165-171, 1963.

Henderson, D.: Occlusion in removable partial prosthodontics, J. Prosthet. Dent. **27**:151-159, 1971.

Hindels, G. W.: Occlusion in removable partial denture prosthesis, Dent. Clin. North Am., pp. 137-146, March, 1962.

Hughes, G. A., and Regli, C. P.: What is centric relation? J. Prosthet. Dent. **11**:16-22, 1961.

Jaffe, V. N.: The functionally generated path in full denture construction, J. Prosthet. Dent. **4**:214-221, 1954.

Jankelson, B.: Considerations of occlusion on fixed partial dentures, Dent. Clin. North Am., pp. 187-203, March, 1959.

Jeffreys, F. E., and Platner, R. L.: Occlusion in removable partial dentures, J. Prosthet. Dent. **10**:912-920, 1960.

Kapur, K. K.: The comparison of different methods of recording centric relation, 1956, Tufts Univ. Dent. Abstr. **2**:508, 1957.

Kingery, R. H.: A review of some of the problems associated with centric relation, J. Prosthet. Dent. **2**:307-319, 1952.

Kurth, L. E.: Balanced occlusion, J. Prosthet. Dent. **4**:150-167, 1954.

Lauritzen, A. G., and Bodner, G. H.: Variations in location of arbitrary and true hinge axis points, J. Prosthet. Dent. **11**:224-229, 1961.

Lindblom, G.: Balanced occlusion with partial reconstructions, Int. Dent. J. **1**:84-98, 1951; The value of bite analysis, J. Am. Dent. Assoc. **48**:657-664, 1954.

Long, J. H., Jr.: Location of the terminal hinge axis by intraoral means, J. Prosthet. Dent. **23**:11-24, 1970.

Lucia, V. O.: Centric relation—theory and practice, J. Prosthet. Dent. **10**:849-956, 1960.

Lucia, V. O.: The gnathological concept of articulation, Dent. Clin. North Am., pp. 183-197, March, 1962.

Mann, A. W., and Pankey, L. D.: The P. M. philosophy of occlusal rehabilitation, Dent. Clin. North Am., pp. 621-636, Nov., 1963.

McCollum, B. B.: The mandibular hinge axis and a method of locating it, J. Prosthet. Dent. **10**:428-435, 1960.

McCracken, W. L.: Functional occlusion in removable partial denture construction, J. Prosthet. Dent. **8**:955-963, 1958; Impression materials in prosthetic dentistry, Dent. Clin. North Am., pp. 671-684, Nov., 1958; Occlusion in partial denture prosthesis, Dent. Clin. North Am., pp. 109-119, March, 1962.

Mehta, J. D., and Joglekar, A. P.: Vertical jaw relations as a factor in partial dentures, J. Prosthet. Dent. **21**:618-625, 1969.

Meyer, F. S.: The generated path technique in reconstruction dentistry, Parts I and II, J. Prosthet. Dent. **9**:354-366, 432-440, 1959.

Millstein, P. L., et al.: Determination of the accuracy of wax interocclusal registrations, J. Prosthet. Dent. **25**:189-196, 1971.

Moore, A. W.: Ideal versus adequate dental occlusion, J. Am. Dent. Assoc. **55**:51-56, 1957.

Moses, C. H.: The significance of some natural laws in the practice of preventive and restorative dentistry, J. Prosthet. Dent. **3**:304-322, 1953; Human tooth form and arrangement from the anthropologic approach, J. Prosthet. Dent. **9**:197-212, 1959.

Moulton, G. H.: The importance of centric occlusion in diagnosis and treatment planning, J. Prosthet. Dent. **10**:921-926, 1960.

Nuttall, E. B.: Establishing posterior functional occlusion for fixed partial dentures, J. Am. Dent. Assoc. **66**:341-348, 1963.

O'Leary, T. J., et al.: Tooth mobility in cuspid-protected and group-function occlusions, J. Prosthet. Dent. **27**:21-25, 1972.

Olsson, A., and Posselt, U.: Relationship of various skull reference lines, J. Prosthet. Dent. **11**:1045-1049, 1961.

Payne, S. H.: A comparative study of posterior occlusion, J. Prosthet. Dent. **2**:661-666, 1952; Selective occlusion, J. Prosthet. Dent. **5**:301-304, 1955.

Pearson, W. D.: Reducing frictional resistance in the occlusion of dentures, J. Prosthet. Dent. **5**:338-341, 1955.

Pruden, W. H.: Occlusion related to fixed partial denture prosthesis, Dent. Clin. North Am., pp. 121-136, March, 1962.

Rapp, R.: The occlusion and occlusal patterns of artificial posterior teeth, J. Prosthet. Dent. **4**:461-480, 1954.

Reitz, P. V.: Technique for mounting removable partial dentures on an articulator, J. Prosthet. Dent. **22**:490-494, 1969.

Reynolds, J. M.: Occlusal wear facets, J. Prosthet. Dent. **24**:367-372, 1970.

Ricketts, R. M.: Occlusion—the medium of dentistry, J. Prosthet. Dent. **21**:39-60, 1969.

Robinson, M. J.: Centric position, J. Prosthet. Dent. **1**:384-386, 1951.

Robinson, S. C.: Equilibrated functional occlusions, J. Prosthet. Dent. **2**:462-476, 1952; Hydraulic equilibration in complete and partial artificial dentures, Dent. Rec. **74**:114-119, 1954.

Scaife, R. R., Jr., and Holt, J. E.: Natural occurance of cuspid guidance, J. Prosthet. Dent. **22**:225-229, 1969.

Schireson, S.: Grinding teeth for masticatory efficiency and gingival health, J. Prosthet. Dent. **13**:337-345, 1963.

Schuyler, C. H.: Fundamental principles in the correction of occlusal disharmony—natural and artificial (grinding), J. Am. Dent. Assoc. **22**: 1193-1202, 1935; Correction of occlusal disharmony of the natural dentition, N. Y. Dent. J. **13**:445-462, 1947; Factors of occlusion applicable to restorative dentistry, J. Prosthet. Dent. **3**: 772-782, 1953; An evaluation of incisal guidance and its influence in restorative dentistry, J. Prosthet. Dent. **9**:374-378, 1959; Factors contributing to traumatic occlusion, J. Prosthet. Dent. **11**:708-715, 1961.

Sears, V. H.: Occlusion: the common meeting ground in dentistry, J. Prosthet. Dent. **2**:15-21, 1952; Occlusal pivots, J. Prosthet. **6**:332-338, 1956; Centric and eccentric occlusions, J. Prosthet. Dent. **10**:1029-1036, 1960; Mandibular equilibration, J. Am. Dent. Assoc. **65**:45-55, 1962.

Shanahan, T. E. J.: Physiologic and neurologic occlusion, J. Prosthet. Dent. **3**:631-632, 1953.

Shanahan, T. E. J., and Leff, A.: Interocclusal records, J. Prosthet. Dent. **10**:842-848, 1960.

Silverman, M. M.: Determination of vertical dimension by phonetics, J. Prosthet. Dent. **6**:465-471, 1956; Dent. Abstr. **2**:221, 1957.

Skurnik, H.: Accurate interocclusal records, J. Prosthet. Dent. **21**:154-165, 1969.

Stuart, C. E.: Accuracy in measuring functional dimensions and relations in oral prosthesis, J. Prosthet. Dent. **9**:220-236, 1959.

Teteruck, W. R., and Lundeen, H. C.: The accuracy of an ear face-bow, J. Prosthet. Dent. **16**: 1039-1046, 1966.

Trapozzano, V. R.: Occlusal records, J. Prosthet. Dent. **5**:325-332, 1955. An analysis of current concepts of occlusion, J. Prosthet. Dent. **5**:764-782, 1955; Occlusion in relation to prosthodontics, Dent. Clin. North Am., pp. 313-325, March, 1957; Laws of articulation, J. Prosthet. Dent. **13**: 34-44, 1963. Discussion by C. O. Boucher follows.

Weinberg, L. A.: The transverse hinge axis: real or imaginary, J. Prosthet. Dent. **9**:775-787, 1959; An evaluation of the face-bow mounting, J. Prosthet. Dent. **11**:32-42, 1961; Arcon principle in the condylar mechanism of adjustable articulators, J. Prosthet. Dent. **13**:263-268, 1963; An evaluation of basic articulators and their concepts. Parts I and II, J. Prosthet. Dent. **13**:622-663, 1963.

Wilson, J. H.: The use of partial dentures in the restoration of occlusal standards, Aust. Dent. J. **1**:93-101, 1956.

Winslow, M. B.: The preventive role of occlusal balancing of the natural dentition, J. Am. Dent. Assoc. **48**:293-296, 1954.

PARTIAL DENTURE DESIGN

Atkinson, H. F.: Partial denture problems. Designing about a path of withdrawal, Aust. J. Dent. **57**:187-190, 1953.

Avant, E. W.: Indirect retention in partial denture design, J. Prosthet. Dent. **16**:1103-1110, 1966.

Blatterfein, L.: A systematic method of designing upper partial denture bases, J. Am. Dent. Assoc. **46**:510-525, 1953; The use of the semiprecision rest in removable partial dentures, J. Prosthet. Dent. **22**:301-306, 1969.

Chick, A. O.: Correct location of clasps and rests on dentures without stress-breakers, Br. Dent. J. **95**:303-309, 1953.

Collett, H. A.: Biologic approach to clasp partial dentures, Dent. Dig. **61**:309-313, 1955.

Craddock, F. W., and Bottomley, G. A.: Second thoughts on clasp surveying, Br. Dent. J. **96**: 134-137, 1954.

Firtell, D. N.: Effect of clasp design upon retention of removable partial dentures, J. Prosthet. Dent. **20**:43-52, 1968.

Fish, E. W.: A new principle in partial denture design, Br. Dent. J. **92**:135-144, 1952.

Frechette, A. R.: Partial denture planning with special reference to stress distribution, J. Ont. Dent. Assoc. **30**:318-329, 1953.

Giradot, R. L.: History and development of partial denture design, J. Am. Dent. Assoc. **28**: 1399-1408, 1941.

Jordan, L. G.: Designing removable partial dentures with external attachments (clasps), J. Prosthet. Dent. **2**:716-722, 1952.

Kelly, E. K.: The physiologic approach to partial denture design, J. Prosthet. Dent. **3**:699-710, 1953.

Knodle, J. M.: Experimental overlay and pin partial denture, J. Prosthet. Dent. **17**:472-478, 1967.

Krikos, A. A.: Artificial undercuts for teeth which have unfavorable shapes for clasping, J. Prosthet. Dent. **22**:301-306, 1969.

Lammie, G. A., et al.: Use of onlays in partial denture construction, Br. Dent. J. **100**:33-42, 1956.

Lazarus, A. H.: Partial denture design, J. Prosthet. Dent. **1**:438-442, 1951.

Lorencki, S. F.: Planning precision attachment restorations, J. Prosthet. Dent. 21:506-508, 1969.

MacKinnon, K. P.: Indirect retention in partial denture construction, Dent. J. Aust. 27:221-225, 1955.

McCracken, W. L.: Contemporary partial denture designs, J. Prosthet. Dent. 8:71-84, 1958; Survey of partial denture designs by commercial dental laboratories, J. Prosthet. Dent. 12:1089-1110, 1962.

Moore, D. S.: Some fundamentals of partial denture design to conserve the supporting structures, J. Ont. Dent. Assoc. 32:238-240, 1955.

Nairn, R. I.: The problem of free-end denture bases, J. Prosthet. Dent. 16:522-532, 1966.

Neurohr, F. G.: Health conservation of the periodontal tissues by a method of functional partial denture design, J. Am. Dent. Assoc. 31:58-70, 1944.

Osborne, J., and Lammie, G. A.: The bilateral free-end saddle lower denture, J. Prosthet. Dent. 4:640-653, 1954.

Perry, C.: Philosophy of partial denture design, Bull. St. Louis Dent. Soc. 25:48-49, 1954 (digest); J. Prosthet. Dent. 6:775-784, 1956.

Pipko, D. J.: Combinations in fixed-removable prostheses, J. Prosthet. Dent. 26:481-490, 1971.

Potter, R. B., Appleby, R. C., and Adams, C. D.: Removable partial denture design: a review and a challenge, J. Prosthet. Dent. 17:63-68, 1967.

Ryan, J.: Technique of design in partial denture construction, J. Dent. Assoc. S. Afr. 9:123-133, 1954.

Rybeck, S. A., Jr.: Simplicity in a distal extension partial denture, J. Prosthet. Dent. 4:87-92, 1954.

Schmidt, A. H.: Planning and designing removable partial dentures, J. Prosthet. Dent. 3:783-806, 1953.

Schuyler, C. H.: The partial denture as a means of stabilizing abutment teeth, J. Am. Dent. Assoc. 28:1121-1125, 1941.

Scott, D. C.: Suggested designs for metal partial dentures, Dent. Tech. 2:21, 26, 1954.

Shohet, H.: Relative magnitudes of stress on abutment teeth with different retainers, J. Prosthet. Dent. 21:267-282, 1969.

Steffel, V. L.: Simplified clasp partial dentures designed for maximum function, J. Am. Dent. Assoc. 32:1093-1100, 1945; Fundamental principles involved in partial denture designs—with special reference to equalization of tooth and tissue support, Aust. J. Dent. 54:328-333, 1950; Dent. J. Aust. 23:68-77, 1951; Fundamental principles involved in partial denture design, J. Am. Dent. Assoc. 42:534-544, 1951.

Sykora, O., and Calikkocaoglu, S.: Masillary removable partial denture designs by commercial dental laboratories, J. Prosthet. Dent. 22:633-640, 1970.

Tench, R. W.: Fundamentals of partial denture design, J. Am. Dent. Assoc. 23:1087-1092, 1936.

Tsao, D. H.: Designing occlusal rests using mathematical principles, J. Prosthet. Dent. 23:154-163, 1970.

Weinberg, L. A.: Lateral force in relation to the denture base and clasp design, J. Prosthet. Dent. 6:785-800, 1956.

Wills, N. G.: Practical engineering applied to removable partial denture designing, Proc. Dent. Centenary, pp. 319-331, 1940.

PERIODONTAL CONSIDERATIONS

Amsterdam, M., and Fox, L.: Provisional splinting—principles and technics, Dent. Clin. North Am., pp. 73-99, March, 1959.

Applegate, O. C.: The interdependence of periodontics and removable partial denture prosthesis, J. Prosthet. Dent. 8:269-281, 1958.

Fish, E. W.: Periodontal diseases: Occlusal trauma and partial dentures, Brit. Dent. J. 95:199-206 (disc. 206-210), 1953.

Glickman, I. J.: Interrelation of local and systemic factors in periodontal disease: bone factor concept, J. Am. Dent. Assoc. 45:422-429, 1952; The role of systemic therapy in the treatment of periodontal disease, J. Am. Dent. Assoc. 62:414-423, 1961.

Ivancie, G. P.: Interrelationship between restorative dentistry and periodontics, J. Prosthet. Dent. 8:819-830, 1958.

Jordan, L. G.: Treatment of advanced periodontal disease by prosthodontic procedures, J. Prosthet. Dent. 10:908-911, 1960.

Kimball, H. D.: The role of periodontia in prosthetic dentistry, J. Prosthet. Dent. 1:286-294, 1951.

Krogh-Poulsen, W.: Partial denture design in relation to occlusal trauma in periodontal breakdown, Acad. Rev. 3:18-23, 1955; Int. Dent. J. 4:847-867, 1954.

McCall, J. O.: Periodontist looks at the clasp partial denture, J. Am. Dent. Assoc. 43:439-443, 1951; The periodontal element in prosthodontics, J. Prosthet. Dent. 16:585-588, 1966.

McKenzie, J. S.: Mutual problems of the periodontist and prosthodontist, J. Prosthet. Dent. 5:37-42, 1955.

Morris, M. L.: Artificial crown contours and gingival health, J. Prosthet. Dent. 12:1146-1155, 1962.

Nevin, R. B.: Periodontal aspects of partial denture prosthesis, J. Prosthet. Dent. 5:215-219, 1955.

Orban, B. S.: Biologic principles in correction of occlusal disharmonies, J. Prosthet. Dent. 6:637-641, 1956.

Osborne, J.: Free-end saddle and the periodontal patient, Dent. Pract. 4:287-297, 1954.

Overby, G. E.: Esthetic splinting of mobile periodontally involved teeth by vertical pinning, J. Prosthet. Dent. 11:112-118, 1961.

Perel, M. L.: Periodontal consideration of crown

contours, J. Prosthet. Dent. **26**:627-630, 1971.

Rubinstein, M. N.: Splinting: periodontal and prosthetic support, Dent. Dig. **60**:342-348, 1954.

Rudd, K. D., and O'Leary, T. J.: Stabilizing periodontally weakened teeth by using guide plane removable partial dentures: a preliminary report, J. Prosthet. Dent. **16**:721-727, 1966.

Schopper, A. F.: Partial denture and its relation to periodontics, J. Am. Dent. Assoc. **45**:415-421, 1952.

Schuyler, C. H.: The partial denture and a means of stabilizing abutment teeth, J. Am. Dent. Assoc. **28**:1121-1125, 1941.

Souder, W., and Paffenbarger, G. C.: Physical properties of dental materials, Circular of the National Bureau of Standards C433, Washington, 1942, United States Government Printing Office.

Sternlicht, H. C.: Prosthetic treatment planning for the periodontal patient, Dent. Abstr. **2**:81-82, 1957.

Talkov, L.: Survey for complete periodontal prosthesis, J. Prosthet. Dent. **11**:124-131, 1961.

Thomas, B. O. A., and Gallager, J. W.: Practical management of occlusal dysfunctions in periodontal therapy, J. Am. Dent. Assoc. **46**:18-31, 1953.

Trapozzano, V. R., and Winter, G. R.: Periodontal aspects of partial denture design, J. Prosthet. Dent. **2**:101-107, 1952.

Waerhaug, J.: Justification for splinting in periodontal therapy, J. Prosthet. Dent. **22**:201-208, 1969.

Ward, H. L., and Weinberg, L. A.: An evaluation of periodontal splinting, J. Am. Dent. Assoc. **63**: 48-54, 1961.

PHYSIOLOGY; MANDIBULAR MOVEMENT

Brekke, C. A.: Jaw function. Part I. Hinge rotation, J. Prosthet. Dent. **9**:600-606, 1959; Part II. Hinge axis, hinge axes, **9**:936-940, 1959; Part III. Condylar placement and condylar retrusion, **10**:78-85, 1960.

Brotman, D. N.: Contemporary concepts of articulation, J. Prosthet. Dent. **10**:221-230, 1960.

Claspp, G. W.: Accurate tracings of mandibular movements, J. Prosthet. Dent. **4**:179-182, 1954.

Emig, G. E.: The physiology of the muscles of mastication, J. Prosthet. Dent. **1**:700-707, 1951.

Fountain, H. W.: The temporomandibular joints—a fulcrum, J. Prosthet. Dent. **25**:78-84, 1971.

Gibbs, C. H., et al.: Functional movements of the mandible, J. Prosthet. Dent. **26**:604-620, 1971.

Jankelson, B.: Physiology of human dental occlusion, J. Am. Dent. Assoc. **50**:664-680, 1955.

Jankelson, B., Hoffman, G. M., and Hendron, J. A., Jr.: The physiology of the stomatognathic system, J. Am. Dent. Assoc. **46**:375-386, 1953.

Kurth, L. E.: Mandibular movement and articulator occlusion, J. Am. Dent. Assoc. **39**:37-46, 1949; Centric relation and mandibular movement, J. Am. Dent. Assoc. **50**:309-315, 1955.

McMillen, L. B.: Border movements of the human mandible, J. Prosthet. Dent. **27**:524-532, 1972.

Messerman, T.: A concept of jaw function with a related clinical application, J. Prosthet. Dent. **13**:130-140, 1963.

Naylor, J. G.: Role of the external pterygoid muscles in temporomandibular articulation, J. Prosthet. Dent. **10**:1037-1042, 1960.

Posselt, U.: Studies in the mobility of the human mandible, Acta Odontol. Scand. **10**:(supp. 10) 19-160, 1952; movement areas of the mandible, J. Prosthet. Dent. **7**:375-385, 1957; Terminal hinge movement of the mandible, J. Prosthet. Dent. **7**:787-797, 1957.

Saizar, P.: Centric relation and condylar movement, J. Prosthet. Dent. **26**:581-591, 1971.

Schweitzer, J. M.: Masticatory function in man, J. Prosthet. Dent. **11**:625-647, 1961.

Shanahan, T. E. J.: Dental physiology for dentures: the direct application of the masticatory cycle to denture occlusion, J. Prosthet. Dent. **2**:3, 1952.

Shore, N. A.: Educational program for patients with temporomandibular joint dysfunction (ligaments), J. Prosthet. Dent. **23**:691-695, 1970.

Sicher, H.: Positions and movements of the mandible, J. Am. Dent. Assoc. **48**:620-625, 1954.

Skinner, C. N.: Physiology of the occlusal coordination of natural teeth, complete dentures, and partial dentures, J. Prosthet. Dent. **17**:559-565, 1967.

Söstenbö, H. R.: C. E. Luce's recordings of mandibular movement, J. Prosthet. Dent. **11**:1068-1073, 1961.

Thompson, J. R.: The rest position of the mandible and its significance to dental science, J. Am. Dent. Assoc. **33**:151-180, 1946.

Ulrich, J.: The human temporomandibular joint: kinematics and actions of the masticatory muscles, J. Prosthet. Dent. **9**:399-406, 1959.

Vaughan, H. C.: The external pterygoid mechanism, J. Prosthet. Dent. **5**:80-92, 1955.

REBASING AND RELINING

Beckett, L. S.: Partial denture. The rebasing of tissue borne saddles. Theory and practice, Aust. Dent. J. **16**:340-346, 1971.

Blatterfein, L.: Rebasing procedures for removable partial dentures, J. Prosthet. Dent. **8**:441-467, 1958.

Steffel, V. L.: Relining removable partial dentures for fit and function, J. Prosthet. Dent. **4**:496-509, 1954.

Wilson, J. H.: Partial dentures—rebasing the saddle supported by the mucosa and alveolar bone, Dent. J. Aust. **24**:185-188, 1952; Partial dentures—relining the saddle supported by the mucosa and alveolar bone, J. Prosthet. Dent. **3**: 807-813, 1953.

STRESSBREAKER DESIGNS

Bartlett, A. A.: Duplication of precision attachment partial dentures, J. Prosthet. Dent. **16:** 1111-1115, 1966.

Bickley, R. W.: Combined splint-stress breaker removable partial denture, J. Prosthet. Dent. **21:**509, 512, 1969.

Cody, L. G.: Broken stress and splinting in the field of partial dentures, J. Colo. Dent. Assoc. **23:**87-92, 1945.

Hekneby, M.: The "spring slide joint," a new attachment for lower partial dentures, Dent. Abstr. **1:**679-680, 1956.

Hirschtritt, E.: Removable partial dentures with stress-broken extension bases, J. Prosthet. Dent. **7:**318-324, 1957.

James, A. G.: Stress breakers which automatically return the saddle to rest position following displacement. Mandibular distal extension partial dentures, J. Prosthet. Dent. **4:**73-81, 1954.

Kabcenell, J. L.: Stress breaking for partial dentures, J. Am. Dent Assoc. **63:**593-602, 1961.

Kane, B. E.: Buoyant stress equalizer, J. Prosthet. Dent. **14:**698-704, 1964; Improved buoyant stress equalizer, J. Prosthet. Dent. **17:**365-371, 1967.

Lane, R. P.: Practical stress breaking in partial dentures, Dent. J. Aust. **19:**314-322, 1947.

Levitch, H. C.: Physiologic stress-equalizer, J. Prosthet. Dent. **3:**232-238, 1953.

Marris, F. N.: The precision dowel rest attachment, J. Prosthet. Dent. **5:**43-48, 1955.

McGee, G. F.: The use of stressbreakers in tissue borne partial dentures, J. Am. Dent. Assoc. 1949.

Neill, D. J.: The problem of the lower free-end removable partial denture, J. Prosthet. Dent. **8:** 623-634, 1958.

Parker, H. M.: Impact reduction in complete and partial dentures, a pilot study, J. Prosthet. Dent. **16:**227-245, 1966.

Plotnik, I. J.: Stress regulator for complete and partial dentures, J. Prosthet. Dent. **17:**166-171, 1967.

Schopper, A. F.: Value of stressbreakers for unilateral partial denture with free-end saddles, J. Am. Dent. Assoc. **38:**183-187, 1949; Value of stress breaker for universal partial dentures with free end-saddles, J. South. Calif. Dent. Assoc. **23:**34-36, 1955.

Simpson, D. H.: Considerations for abutments, J. Prosthet. Dent. **5:**375-384, 1955.

Terrell, W. H.: Split bar technic applicable to both precision attachment and clasp cases, J. South. Calif. Dent. Assoc. **9:**10-14, 1942.

Turkheim, H. J.: Modified stressbreaker, Dent. Pract. **3:**197-198, 1953.

Van Minden, F.: Ideal stressbreaking for partial dentures, J. Am. Dent. Assoc. **30:**657-669, 1943.

SURVEYING

Applegate, O. C.: Use of paralleling surveyor in modern partial denture construction, J. Am. Dent. Assoc. **27:**1317-1407, 1940.

Atkinson, H. F.: Partial denture problems: surveyors and surveying, Aust. J. Dent. **59:**28-31, 1955.

Chestner, S. G.: A methodical approach to the analysis of study cases, J. Prosthet. Dent. **4:**622-624, 1954.

Katulski, E. M., and Appleyard, W. N.: Biological concepts of the use of the mechanical cast surveyor, J. Prosthet. Dent. **9:**629-634, 1959.

Sollé, W.: An improved dental surveyor, J. Am. Dent. Assoc. **60:**727-731, 1960.

WORK AUTHORIZATIONS

Dutton, D. A.: Standard abbreviations (and definitions) for use in dental laboratory work authorizations, J. Prosthet. Dent. **27:**94-95, 1972.

Brown, E. T.: The dentist, the laboratory technician, and the prescription law, J. Prosthet. Dent. **15:**1132-1138, 1965.

Gehl, D. H.: Investment in the future, J. Prosthet. Dent. **18:**190-201- 1968.

Henderson, D.: Writing work authorizations for removable partial dentures, J. Prosthet. Dent. **16:**696-707, 1966.

Quinn, I.: Status of the dental laboratory work authorization, J. Am. Dent. Assoc. **79:**1189-1190, 1969.

Index

A

Abutment, 4
Abutment teeth, 214-237
  for anterior splint bar, 35-36
  anterior teeth and, 228-229
  cast crowns and, 219-220
  cast inlays and, 216-219
  classification of, 214-215
  crowns and inlays for existing retainers and, 234-237
  fixed restorations and, 186-187
    cementation for, 237
  galvanic shocks to, 194
  isolated teeth as, 227-228
  ledges on abutment crowns and, 220-224
  loss of, 417
  minor connectors and, 36-37
  modification of, 172
  molar
    interference and, 148
    third, 169-170
  in mouth preparations, 210-213
  multiple, 226
  oral hygiene and, 405
  posterior, mediodistal clasping of, 79-80
  preservation of, 189
  rest seat preparations and, 212-213
  roentgenographic evaluation of, 166-170
  root morphology and, 169
  sound enamel or existing restorations and, 215-216
  splinting of, 186-187, 226-227
  temporary crowns and, 232-234
  temporary dentures and, 229-232, 424
  treatment dentures and, 424
  in treatment planning, 9
  unopposed for extended time, 206
  veneer crowns and, 224-226
  working casts and, 249-251
Academy of Denture Prosthetics, Nomenclature Committee of, 1, 6
Acrylic resin, 2
  in copings of abutment teeth, 253
  in crowns
    for clasp arms support, 224-226
    for existing dentures, 236
    temporary, 229-234

Acrylic resin—cont'd
  denture base of
    maxillary major connector and, 32, 33
    minor connectors and, 38
    sprinkling technique for, 366-368
  in impression trays, 365
    floor of mouth and, 23
    for functional impression, 266
    impression techniques and, 11-12
    individual, 253-260
    maxillofacial prostheses and, 439
    rubber-base impression materials and, **242**
    selective tissue placement impressions and, 274-275
    sprinkling technique for, 366-368
  for interim dentures, 421
  jet repair, 231
  occlusal registration for fixed denture and, 319
  record bases and
    for arranging posterior teeth, 376
    occlusion of partial denture opposing complete denture and, 324
  relining procedures and, 413-414
  in splints, 206
  teeth of
    anterior, 380
    posterior, 307-311, 377-380
Additions to removable dentures, 415-420
Adjustable frame
  interocclusal wax records and, 301
  for recording centric relation, 181, 182
Adjustment of denture, initial, 399-408; *see also* Initial placement, adjustment, and servicing
Agar hydrocolloids; *see* Hydrocolloids, agar or reversible
Air-turbine handpiece, 199
Al-Cote tin-foil substitute, 234, 367, 370
Alginate hydrocolloids; *see* Hydrocolloids, alginate or irreversible
Alloys
  chromium-cobalt; *see* Chromium-cobalt alloys
  flexibility of, 194
  gold; *see* Gold, alloys of
  for investment casts, 325-326, 358
  metal, 192-195
    low-fusing, 250-251
    tissue reaction to, 99-100